I0065873

Hepatology: A Comprehensive Guide

Hepatology: A Comprehensive Guide

Edited by Dinah Beck

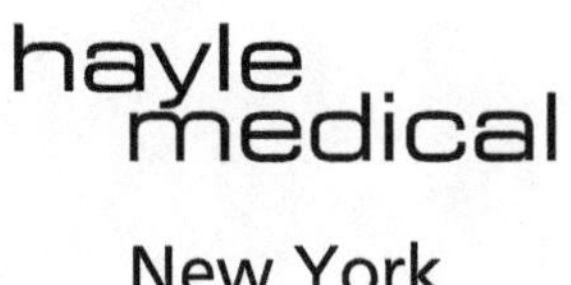

New York

Hayle Medical,
750 Third Avenue, 9th Floor,
New York, NY 10017, USA

Visit us on the World Wide Web at:
www.haylemedical.com

ISBN: 978-1-63241-636-0

Cataloging-in-Publication Data

Hepatology : a comprehensive guide / edited by Dinah Beck.
p. cm.
Includes bibliographical references and index.
ISBN 978-1-63241-636-0
1. Hepatology. 2. Gastroenterology. I. Beck, Dinah.

RC802 .H47 2019
616.33--dc23

Contents

Preface

The main aim of this book is to educate learners and enhance their research focus by presenting diverse topics covering this vast field. This is an advanced book which compiles significant studies by distinguished experts in the area of analysis. This book addresses successive solutions to the challenges arising in the area of application, along with it; the book provides scope for future developments.

The liver is a vital organ of the human body. It supports all other organs. It is prone to a number of diseases and infections passing from the abdominal cavity to the thoracic cavity. Hepatitis is a common medical condition characterized by an inflamed liver. It is caused by hepatitis A, B, C, D and E infections. Herpes simplex virus may also be responsible for such inflammation. Chronic hepatitis B and hepatitis C infections are the main cause of liver cancer. An accumulation of toxins in the bloodstream can cause hepatic encephalopathy, which can be fatal. The excessive consumption of alcohol leads to a host of alcoholic liver conditions, such as alcoholic hepatitis, cirrhosis and fatty liver. The susceptibility of each individual to such diseases varies and may depend on genetics, gender and liver insult. Many liver conditions are typically accompanied by jaundice. All such diseases can be diagnosed by liver function tests and blood tests. This book brings forth some of the most innovative concepts and elucidates the unexplored aspects of hepatology. The objective of this book is to give a general view of the different conditions of the liver and their management strategies. The extensive content herein provides the readers with a thorough understanding of the subject.

It was a great honour to edit this book, though there were challenges, as it involved a lot of communication and networking between me and the editorial team. However, the end result was this all-inclusive book covering diverse themes in the field.

Finally, it is important to acknowledge the efforts of the contributors for their excellent chapters, through which a wide variety of issues have been addressed. I would also like to thank my colleagues for their valuable feedback during the making of this book.

Editor

1

The Association between Female Genital Cutting and Spousal HCV Infection in Egypt

Chris R. Kenyon[1] and Robert Colebunders[2]

[1] *Sexually Transmitted Infections, HIV/STI Unit, Institute of Tropical Medicine, Nationalestraat 155, 2000 Antwerpen, Belgium*
[2] *Infectious Diseases, University of Antwerp (UA), HIV/STD Unit, Institute of Tropical Medicine, Nationalestraat 155, 2000 Antwerpen, Belgium*

Correspondence should be addressed to Chris R. Kenyon; ckenyon@itg.be

Academic Editor: Matthias Bahr

Objective. To identify the risk factors for HCV infection within married couples in Egypt. *Methods.* In 2008 Egypt conducted its first nationally representative survey of HCV prevalence. 11126 of the 12780 individuals aged 15–59 year who were sampled agreed to participate and provided information via a questionnaire about demographic and behavioural characteristics and blood for HCV antibody and RNA analysis. We assessed the risk factors for HCV infection in a subsample of 5182 married individuals via multivariate logistic regression. *Results.* Overall HCV antibody prevalence in the married couples was 18.2% (95% CI, 16.8–19.6). HCV antibody prevalence was higher in the husbands (23.7%) than the wives (12.1%; $P < 0.001$). Having a spouse who was infected with HCV was an independent risk factor for HCV infection with odds ratios of 2.1 (95% CI, 1.6–2.9) and 2.2 (95% CI, 1.6–3.1) for women and men, respectively. Husbands whose wives had experienced female genital cutting (FGC) had a higher prevalence of HCV and this relationship was driven by a strong association in urban areas. Amongst the women there was no association between FGC and HCV overall but in urban areas only women who had experienced FGC were HCV infected. *Conclusions.* This study provides additional evidence of the importance of intrafamilial transmission of HCV in Egypt.

1. Introduction

With 14.7% of 15–59-year-olds testing anti-HCV positive, Egypt has the highest HCV prevalence in the world [1]. Although parenteral antischistosomiasis therapy (PAT) was important in the genesis of Egypt's HCV epidemic this was stopped over 25 years ago and HCV incidence remains high estimated between 150 000 and 500 000 new infections per year [2–4]. Infection from inadequate sterility of dental and medical devices has been shown to play a role in this regard [1, 2, 5–12]. Intrafamilial transmission is an alternative explanation [6]. Support for this theory comes from studies such as a longitudinal study of incidence in two villages in Egypt, which found that the strongest predictor of incident of HCV was having an anti-HCV positive family member [13]. Among those that did and did not have a family member infected with HCV, HCV incidence was 5.8 and 1.0/1000 person years, respectively. Parenteral exposure increased the risk of HCV but was not statistically significant.

This elevated risk of incident of HCV of family members could be due to sharing of implements such as razors or toothbrushes or due to sexual transmission between family members [14, 15]. Alternatively, the elevated risk may be due to shared risk factors (such as the family members all attending a particular health practitioner) rather than being caused by direct transmission between family members [13].

To disentangle these relationships it would be useful to know how HCV is patterned within families. If a husband, is infected is this associated with an increased risk of his wife being infected and vice versa? Is the risk higher for a spouse than nonspousal family members? Are these relationships affected by whether the affected individuals are HCV RNA as opposed to antibody positive?

In 2008 Egypt conducted its first nationally representative survey of HCV prevalence—the 2008 Egyptian Demographic and Health Survey (EDHS). A recently published analysis of this survey found that HCV prevalence increased steadily with age but more so in men than women, reaching, in the

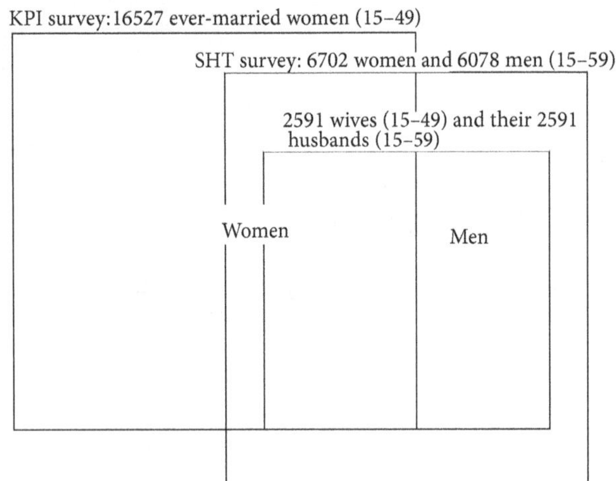

FIGURE 1: The structure of the Egyptian DHS 2008 and the derivation of the married couples subsample. 16527 ever-married women aged 15–49 were sampled in the key population indicators (KPI) survey. In a subsample of households surveyed in the KPI, 6702 women and 6078 men aged 15–49 were sampled in the special health topics (SHT) component. 2591 wives (aged 15–49) and their 2591 husbands (aged 15–59) could be linked to generate the married couples subsample.

50–59-year-age group, 46.3% in men and 30.8% in women [1]. HCV was also more prevalent in rural than urban areas and on multivariate analysis it was found to be associated with male sex, age, poverty, past history of PAT, and blood transfusion. In urban regions, those with a lack of education and females with genital cutting were more likely to be HCV infected.

This analysis did not however examine the extent to which HCV infection covaried within couples and families. The EDHS is the first HCV survey in the world that is both nationally representative and done in a way which enables researchers to link the HCV status of husbands and wives. In this paper we assess the correlates of HCV infection in 2591 married couples from the EDHS.

2. Materials and Methods

The EDHS entailed a three-stage probability sample that provided a nationally representative sample of 16527 ever-married women aged 15–49 who were interviewed about a range of key population indicators (KPI). In addition, in a subsample of 4953 households, 6702 women and 6078 men aged 15–59 were sampled for a special health topics (SHT) component (see Figure 1). The overall response rate for this latter section was 96.2% and 87.6% for the men and women, respectively. 11126 (87.1%) of these agreed to provide blood for HCV testing. This SHT component was selected so as to provide a sample which was representative for Egypt and the six major areas that the EDHS was stratified by: Urban and Frontier governorates and Upper and Lower Egypt (each of the latter two was divided into rural and urban areas). In order to link husbands and wives, we made use of the fact that 3877 women completed both questionnaires. These were the women who had ever been married, were 14–49 years old, and completed the KPI questionnaire. If the respondent was currently married, then the KPI questionnaire specified the husband's line number within their house. This provides a unique identifier for each husband. Via this mechanism, we established that, in the case of 2591 individuals, the husband of a respondent also completed the SHT component of the EDHS. In this paper we study the relationships between HCV and various risk factors in these 2591 husband-wife pairs. Apart from the 5182 individuals in this married subgroup, further 2338 persons aged 15–59 years, living in the same houses as the married couples, were included in the SHT survey. Although the outcome variable used in this study is the presence of anti-HCV antibodies in the 5182 members of the married subgroup, the relationship between the HCV serostatus of the married couples and that of the other household members is also of relevance. We therefore included the HCV antibody and RNA status of these 2338 individuals as exposure variables in our analyses. We also calculated the HCV prevalence for each of Egypt's 26 governorates. These were used as a measure of local or community HCV prevalence.

Unless otherwise stated the terms "HCV prevalence" and "infection" refer to HCV antibody prevalence. The HCV antibody prevalence rates were calculated for a range of potential risk factors available in the special health topics questionnaire. Because of the strong association between age and HCV prevalence all the odds ratios and P values given are age-adjusted. Logistic regression was used to explore the strength of the association of each variable with HCV infection in the 5192 individuals in the married couples cohort.

Tests for interaction between variables were conducted. These tests revealed that the effect of several of the variables varied according to urban/rural location and men/women. As a result, separate models were constructed for men and women as well as urban and rural areas. All the urban women who had not undergone female genital cutting were HCV negative. To avoid the collinearity that this created in the analyses, for the analysis limited to urban women, we randomly selected one urban woman who had not undergone female genital cutting and changed her HCV status as positive. The final models were constructed by including all variables with P values <0.2 on univariate logistic regression. The education variable was not included due to significant collinearity with the income variable. The HCV status of the spouse and that of the other household members (both exposure variables) were represented by HCV RNA instead of HCV antibody positivity in the multivariate models due to exerting a stronger effect on the outcome variable (and considerable collinearity between the RNA and antibody HCV tests). All analyses were weighted to account for the sampling and survey design. Statistical analysis was conducted using STATA version 12.0 (StataCorp, College Station, TX).

The HCV prevalence rates for the husbands and wives were also stratified by the wives' excision status to explore how HCV prevalence in both husbands and wives varies according to the excision status of the woman. The terms excision and female genital cutting (FGC) are used synonymously in the paper. The FGC variable was defined as follows: both the women who had experienced FGC and the men whose wives had undergone FGC were coded as 1 and the women and men whose wives had not undergone FGC were coded as 0. To assess the impact of whether HCV prevalence in women was associated with who conducted the FGC, a second FGC variable, termed FGC-operator, was constructed as follows: women with no history of FGC coded 0, FGC performed by doctor and nondoctor coded as 1 and 2, respectively. The multivariate models for women were run separately with the FGC and FGC-operator variables.

A third generation enzyme-linked immunosorbent assay was used to detect HCV antibodies (Adaltis EIAgen HCV Ab, Casalecchio di Reno, Italy). Positive tests were confirmed by a chemiluminescent microplate immunoassay (CIA). Seropositive specimens were tested for HCV RNA using the RealTime_m2000 system (Abbott Laboratories, Abbott Park, IL, USA). Full details of the survey and sampling strategy have been previously published [1, 16].

3. Results

Overall HCV antibody prevalence in the married couples was 18.2% (95% CI, 16.8–19.6). HCV antibody prevalence was higher in the husbands (23.7%) than the wives (12.1%; $P < 0.001$; see Table 1). Restricting this analysis to the 15–49-year-olds reduced the difference in HCV between the husbands and wives (18.8% and 11.6% resp. $P < 0.001$). HCV prevalence was also higher in rural (20.4%) than urban (12.0%) regions ($P < 0.001$). HCV prevalence increased steadily with age reaching 30.2% (95% CI, 26.8–33.8) in men and 23.9% (95% CI, 20.4–27.7) in women in the 41–49-year-old category. Amongst women, there was a stepwise increase in HCV prevalence with increasing number of children: 6.9% if 0–2 children, 14.1% if 3–5 children, and 24.5% if more than 5 children. There was a lower HCV prevalence in those who had completed secondary level education (14.3%) compared to those with no education (23.5%; $P = 0.001$) and those in the top two income quintiles (12.1 and 12.9%) compared to those in the poorest quintile (22.8%; $P < 0.001$). HCV prevalence in persons who had received PAT (32.1%) was higher than in those who had not (16.5%; $P < 0.001$). Women with excision had a trend to higher HCV prevalence (12.5%) than those without (3.9%; $P = 0.096$; see Tables 1 and 2). Men whose wives had been excised had a higher HCV prevalence than those whose wives had not (23.7% versus 8.3%; $P = 0.003$). Women who had been excised by a doctor had a lower HCV prevalence than those excised by a nondoctor (5.6% versus 13.7%; $P = 0.003$). Respondents who had received a blood transfusion had nonsignificantly higher HCV prevalence rates than those who had not (26.9% versus 17.8%; $P = 0.132$). HCV prevalence increased with length of marriage, increasing from 8.2% to 17.6 and 29.6% in those married for ten years or less, 11–20 years, and over 20 years, respectively. Having received injections and dental treatment were not associated with HCV seropositivity.

Persons with an HCV seropositive partner had a higher HCV prevalence than those who did not (32.6% versus 15.1%; $P < 0.001$). This effect was also evident if one's partner was RNA positive for HCV (34.7% versus 15.9%; $P < 0.001$). The effect was not as marked if it was another member of the household who was HCV antibody (23.3% versus 17.7%; $P = 0.004$) or RNA positive (23% versus 17.9%; $P = 0.015$).

In the multivariate logistic regression analyses, three variables were associated with HCV infection in all models; see Table 3. These were age, local HCV prevalence, and having a spouse who was infected with HCV. Having a nonspousal household member who was HCV infected was not independently associated with HCV. For both men and women HCV was less prevalent in the richer quintiles but in the case of men this effect was evident in the urban but not the rural areas.

HCV was associated with a blood transfusion in women but this association only applied to the rural areas. PAT was associated with HCV in all the models except in the men in the rural and the women in the urban areas. Being married for longer than 20 years was associated with HCV, but only for men. FGC was associated with HCV infection in the men but not the women overall. This relationship in men was driven by a relatively strong association in urban areas. Amongst the women, there was no association between FGC and HCV overall but in urban areas none of the women who were not excised were HCV infected. In the second set of women's models substitution of the FGC variable with the FGC-operator variable had little effect. FGC had no effect in rural areas and a strong effect in urban areas regardless of whether it was conducted by a doctor or nondoctor (data not shown).

The EDHS reveals that, of the women who had undergone FGC, 99.9% had done so by the age of 18. Of the women aged 15–18 surveyed in the EDHS, the HCV prevalence was significantly higher in those who had been excised (39/723; 5.4%) than those who had not (0/164; 0%, $P = 0.028$).

There was no evidence of interaction between the wife's FGC status and HCV status of the partner variables.

4. Discussion

Linking husbands and wives allowed us to test the association of HCV infection between husbands and wives. This represents the first time that this has been done in a nationally representative HCV survey. The sampling strategy used to describe the epidemiology of HCV in the USA, although nationally representative, does not include sexual partners in a linked way that would allow a similar analysis [17]. We found an association between the HCV status of the respondent and their partner. This is true for analyses limited to rural and urban areas and for subanalyses of men and women within these areas. The association remains after controlling for other members of the household being HCV infected. The relationship is slightly stronger when the HCV in the partner is measured with an RNA-based as opposed to an antibody-based test.

If not due to confounding, this association may be due to nonsexual intrafamilial transmission (such as shared utensils, toothbrushes, and razors), sexual transmission, or shared risk exposures (such as attending to the same health care practitioner). If the former was predominant then we should

TABLE 1: HCV seroprevalence and age-adjusted odds ratios for selected characteristics (Egyptian DHS 2008).

Risk factors	Number of exposed (%)[a]	Number of HCV antibody positive (%)[b]	Age-adjusted OR (95% CI)	*P* value (age-adjusted)
Place of residence				
Rural	3234 (37.6)	661 (20.4)	2.4 (1.9–3.0)	<0.001
Urban	1948 (62.4)	233 (12.0)	1	
Region				
Urban governorates	610 (11.8)	76 (12.6)	1	
Lower Egypt—urban	554 (10.7)	69 (12.3)	1.0 (0.7–1.5)	0.994
Lower Egypt—rural	1608 (31.0)	364 (22.9)	2.7 (1.9–3.8)	<0.001
Upper Egypt—urban	600 (11.6)	79 (13.5)	1.1 (0.7–1.7)	0.778
Upper Egypt—rural	1524 (29.4)	294 (20.1)	2.1 (1.5–3.0)	<0.001
Frontier governorates	286 (5.5)	12 (4.5)	0.3 (0.2–0.6)	0.001
Gender				
Women	2591 (50)	300 (12.1)	0.7 (0.6–0.9)	<0.001
Men	2591 (50)	594 (23.7)	1	
Men's age (years)				
15–20	9 (0.4)	0 (0)		
21–30	524 (20.2)	50 (9.5)	1	
31–40	877 (33.9)	117 (13.3)	1.5 (1.0–2.1)	0.034
41–49	827 (31.9)	268 (32.4)	4.5 (3.3–6.3)	0.000
50–59	354 (13.7)	159 (44.9)	7.7 (5.4–11.1)	0.000
Women's age (years)				
15–20	154 (5.9)	5 (3.3)	1	
21–30	1018 (39.3)	60 (5.9)	1.8 (0.7–4.7)	0.188
31–40	860 (33.2)	104 (12.1)	4.1 (1.6–10.2)	0.002
41–49	559 (21.6)	131 (23.4)	9.1 (3.6–22.7)	0.000
Educational attainment				
Secondary completed	2424 (46.8)	282 (14.3)	0.7 (0.6–0.9)	0.001
Incomplete secondary or less	1473 (28.4)	282 (19.9)	0.9 (0.7–1.1)	0.219
No education	1285 (24.8)	330 (23.5)	1	
Wealth index quintile				
Richest	1010 (19.5)	118 (12.1)	0.4 (0.3–0.5)	<0.001
Rich	942 (18.2)	112 (12.9)	0.5 (0.4–0.7)	<0.001
Middle	1128 (21.7)	225 (21.2)	0.9 (0.7–1.2)	0.413
Poor	1056 (20.4)	220 (22.0)	0.9 (0.7–1.2)	0.600
Poorest	1046 (20.2)	219 (22.8)	1	
Parenteral antischistosomiasis therapy				
No	4582 (88.4)	707 (16.5)	1	
Yes	600 (11.6)	187 (32.1)	1.7 (1.4–2.2)	<0.001
Women: reports FGC[c]				
No	132 (5.1)	4 (3.9)	1	
Yes	2459 (94.9)	296 (12.5)	2.9 (0.8–10.1)	0.096
Men: his wife reports FGC[d]				
No	132 (5.1)	11 (8.3)	1	
Yes	2459 (94.9)	583 (23.7)	3.1 (1.5–6.6)	0.003
FGC performed by[g]				
Doctor	386 (15.7)	21 (5.6)	1	

TABLE 1: Continued.

Risk factors	Number of exposed (%)[a]	Number of HCV antibody positive (%)[b]	Age-adjusted OR (95% CI)	P value (age-adjusted)
Nondoctor	2073 (84.3)	275 (13.7)	1.4 (1.1–1.7)	0.003
Blood transfusion				
No	4931 (95.3)	832 (17.8)	1	
Yes	244 (4.7)	60 (26.9)	1.3 (0.9–1.8)	0.132
Multiple injections[e]				
No	4301 (83.0)	751 (18.4)	1	
Yes	881 (17.0)	143 (17.1)	0.9 (0.7–1.1)	0.312
Dental treatment[e]				
No	1829 (35.3)	270 (15.3)	1	
Yes	3353 (64.7)	624 (19.6)	1.1 (0.8–1.2)	0.609
Total number of children[h]				
0–2	1098 (42.4)	73 (6.9)	1	
3–5	1162 (44.9)	154 (14.1)	1.2 (1.0–1.6)	0.427
≥6	331 (12.8)	73 (24.5)	2.1 (1.0–2.5)	0.035
Partner is seropositive for HCV				
No	4288 (82.8)	608 (15.1)	1	
Yes	894 (17.3)	286 (32.6)	2.1 (1.6–2.7)	<0.001
Partner is HCV RNA positive				
No	4569 (88.2)	686 (15.9)	1	
Yes	613 (11.8)	208 (34.7)	2.3 (1.7–2.9)	<0.001
Wife is HCV RNA positive				
No	2291 (88.4)	451 (20.4)	1	
Yes	300 (11.6)	143 (47.4)	2.6 (2.0–3.4)	<0.001
Husband is HCV RNA positive				
No	1997 (77.0)	157 (8.3)	1	
Yes	594 (22.9)	143 (24.3)	2.5 (1.9–3.3)	<0.001
Another household member is seropositive for HCV				
No	4760 (91.9)	798 (17.7)	1	
Yes	422 (8.1)	96 (23.3)	1.6 (1.2–2.1)	0.004
Another household member is HCV RNA positive				
No	4896 (94.5)	834 (17.9)	1	
Yes	286 (5.5)	60 (23.0)	1.5 (1.1–2.1)	0.015
Length of marriage				
0–10 years	2430 (46.9)	258 (8.2)	1	
11–20 years	1574 (30.4)	339 (17.6)	1.2 (1.0–1.5)	0.051
>20 years	1178 (22.7)	461 (29.8)	1.4 (1.1–1.8)	0.016

FGC: female genital cutting.
[a]Unweighted percentage.
[b]Weighted percentage.
[c]Numbers for this row are for women only.
[d]Numbers for this row are for men only.
[e]Defined as 2 or more injections reported in the preceding 6 months.
[f]Ever received dental treatment of any sort.
[g]Of all women who report undergoing FGC
[h]The total number of children that women report giving birth to.

TABLE 2: Prevalence of HCV antibodies in 2591 husband-wife pairs, stratified by female genital cutting (FGC) status of the woman (Egyptian DHS 2008).

	Wife's HCV antibody status (%)		
	Negative	Positive	Total[b] (%)
Wife has undergone FGC			
Husband HCV negative	1721	155	1876 (76.3)
Husband HCV positive	442	141	583 (23.7)
Total[a] (%)	**2163 (88.0)**	**296 (12.0)**	**2459 (100)**
Wife has not undergone FGC			
Husband HCV negative	119	2	121 (91.7)
Husband HCV positive	9	2	11 (8.3)
Total[a] (%)	**128 (97.0)**	**4 (3.0)**	**132 (100)**

[a]Row percentages.
[b]Column percentages.

expect an association between HCV infection in nonspousal family members and in respondents. There was no evidence of such an association in any of the multivariate models. In our models we controlled for a large number of plausible, shared risk exposure types (such as blood transfusions, multiple injections, and PAT), but these did not affect the strength of the relationship between respondent and partner HCV status. The stronger association between the respondent's HCV status and that of their wife/husband as opposed to that of other family members may be mediated by the greater length of time they spent together. The fact that there is a relationship between length of marriage and HCV infection (for men) could be interpreted as supporting evidence for this idea. It does not however explain why this relationship only applies to men. An alternative explanation, and one that is also supported by the relationship between HCV infection and length of marriage, is that sexual transmission between partners is responsible for the relationship of HCV infection in married couples.

We cannot however exclude the possibility that the reason why the association between the wife and the husband's HCV status remains strongly positive after controlling for the HCV status of the other household members is due to the partner's HCV status being a better measure of general (nonsexual) infection pressure than the HCV status of the other household members. In the models we do control for the HCV in the surrounding community, but this is defined at the level of the governorate. This may not be a local enough measure of community HCV prevalence.

The relationship between HCV and FGC is complex. There is a strong relationship between HCV infection and FGC in the urban areas but none in the rural areas. There was little sex-based difference. For the men in the urban areas there is an association between HCV infection and having a wife who was excised (OR 3; 95% CI, 1.1–7.9). In the case of women, none of the nonexcised women had HCV infection.

How do we explain the discrepancy between the rural and urban areas? One possibility is that circumcision in urban areas is more likely to transmit HCV. Though this is possible, it should be noted that it is circumcision by nondoctors that is most strongly correlated with HCV infection [18] and in rural areas the proportion of FGC performed by nondoctors is higher (84.2%) than in urban areas (73.0%; $P < 0.001$) [18]. Another possibility is that FGC is so prevalent in the rural areas (97.2%) that there are too few nonexcised women to be able to demonstrate an effect of FGC on HCV prevalence. For example, in two of the other studies, to consider the impact of FGC on HCV in Egypt, no effect was found, but this may have been due to the extremely low numbers of persons not excised. In the first study there was only one person (out of 1989 individuals in the survey over the age of 20) who was not excised [5]. In the second study, only 4 women out of 1051 (0.4%) over the age of 30 were not excised. This study found a nonsignificant increase in the risk of HCV infection in those women who had been excised by an informal health care provider as opposed to those nonexcised combined with those excised by a formal health care provider (OR 1.6; 95% CI, 0.7–3.8). In a separate analysis of the EDHS a strong ecological association was found between the prevalence of FGC and HCV at the governorate level [18].

FGC has been associated with range of infections [19]. A population-based, cross-sectional study from the Gambia, for example, found a strong association between prevalent FGC and herpes simplex virus-2 infection (OR 4.7, 95% CI, 3.7–6.4) and a weaker association between FGC and bacterial vaginosis [20]. A case-control study of primary infertility in Sudan found more extensive forms of FGC to be more prevalent in the cases [21]. There were too few cases and controls without FGC in Sudan study to allow any analysis of those with versus those without FGC. The evidence from Egypt is mixed. A case control study of the determinants of infertility found that cases were more likely to have been excised by a traditional practitioner and more likely to have had more extensive forms of FGC [22]. A later study found no association between FGC and infertility [23].

What could be the possible mechanisms for FGC to result in increased rates of HCV for both men and women? Inadequate sterilization of implements used to perform FGC could be a factor. The higher HCV prevalence in excised versus nonexcised 15–18-year-olds in the EDHS could be interpreted as evidence supporting this nonsterility hypothesis. In addition, HCV transmission at the time of FGC could have been greater in the past when a considerably greater proportion of FGC procedures were performed by nondoctors [18]. Two

Table 3: Factors associated with 5182 husbands and wives testing seropositive for hepatitis C in the 2008 Egyptian Demographic and Health Survey: multivariate logistic regression model results (odds ratios, 95% confidence intervals, and P values).

	Women			Men			Urban women			Urban men			Rural women			Rural men		
	Odds ratio	95% CI	P value	Odds ratio	95% CI	P value	Odds ratio	95% CI	P value	Odds ratio	95% CI	P value	Odds ratio	95% CI	P value	Odds ratio	95% CI	P value
N	2546			2546			953			953			1593			1593		
Wife had FGC	2.0	0.7–5.1	0.166	2.1	1.1–3.9	0.026	4.0	0.5–31	0.188	3.0	1.1–7.9	0.025	0.9	0.3–2.5	0.85	1.4	0.6–3.3	0.458
Spouse is HCV RNA positive	2.1	1.6–2.9	0.000	2.2	1.6–3.1	0.000	2.4	1.3–4.4	0.005	2.5	1.2–5.1	0.015	2.0	1.4–2.8	0.000	2.2	1.5–3.2	0.000
Wealth index quintile																		
Poorest	Ref																	
Poor	1.2	0.9–1.8	0.260	0.9	0.7–1.3	0.698	1.9	0.5–7.6	0.379	0.2	0.1–0.6	0.002	1.2	0.8–1.8	0.333	1.1	0.8–1.5	0.527
Middle	1.0	0.6–1.5	0.922	1.2	0.9–1.6	0.248	0.9	0.2–3.5	0.855	0.4	0.2–0.9	0.035	1.1	0.7–1.7	0.670	1.4	1.0–1.9	0.063
Rich	0.7	0.4–1.1	0.097	0.7	0.5–0.9	0.017	0.8	0.2–3.1	0.796	0.2	0.1–0.5	0.000	0.8	0.4–1.4	0.378	0.9	0.6–1.5	0.727
Richest	0.5	0.3–0.8	0.003	0.7	0.5–1.0	0.087	0.6	0.2–2.5	0.508	0.3	0.1–0.6	0.001	0.5	0.2–1.1	0.082	1.3	0.7–2.2	0.381
Age[b]	1.1	1.0-1.1	0.000	1.1	1.0-1.1	0.000	1.1	1.1-1.2	0.000	1.1	1.0-1.1	0.000	1.1	1.0-1.1	0.000	1.1	1.0-1.1	0.000
Blood transfusion	1.9	1.1–3.5	0.028	1.1	0.7–1.7	0.604	1.2	0.4–3.3	0.789	1.4	0.8–2.7	0.273	2.3	1.1–4.7	0.025	0.9	0.6–1.6	0.820
Parenteral antischistosomiasis therapy	1.7	1.1–2.8	0.016	1.3	1.0–1.7	0.025	1.9	0.6–5.8	0.254	2.3	1.4–3.8	0.002	1.7	1.1–2.9	0.028	1.1	0.9–1.5	0.412
Another household member is HCV RNA positive	0.8	0.5–1.4	0.455	1.2	0.8–1.9	0.361	1.1	0.3–4.1	0.915	1.5	0.5–4.6	0.518	0.7	0.4–1.4	0.319	1.2	0.7–1.9	0.496
Length of marriage																		
0–10 years	Ref																	
11–20 years	1.0	0.7–1.6	0.887	1.3	1.0–1.8	0.044	0.6	0.2–1.5	0.285	1.4	0.8–2.3	0.243	1.2	0.7–2.1	0.416	1.4	1.0-2.0	0.056
>20 years	1.0	0.5–1.9	0.941	1.6	1.1–2.4	0.019	0.6	0.2–1.9	0.355	1.5	0.7–3.0	0.264	1.2	0.6–2.6	0.601	1.7	1.0-2.8	0.036
Local HCV prevalence[c]	1.1	1.1-1.1	0.000	1.1	1.0-1.1	0.000	1.1	1.0–1.2	0.001	1.0	1.0-1.1	0.033	1.1	1.1-1.1	0.000	1.1	1.0-1.1	0.000
Number of children[d]	1.0	0.9–1.1	0.674	NA			1.0	0.8–1.3	0.695		NA		1.0	0.9-1.0	0.347	NA		

NA: not applicable.

[a]Not entered into model due to collinearity; all nonexcised women were HCV negative (see text).

[b]Age is defined continuously in years.

[c]Local HCV prevalence is defined as the HCV prevalence in the surrounding governorate.

[d]The total number of children that women report giving birth to, here defined continuously.

studies from Egypt have found an association between male circumcision performed by informal health care providers and prevalent HCV infection [5, 24].

The anatomical changes produced by FGC, particularly the more extensive forms of FGC, could also promote subsequent female to male and male to female HCV transmission. It is biologically plausible that FGC could both enhance women's susceptibility to the sexual transmission of HCV and increase the chances that HCV is transmitted to their partner [23]. We cannot however exclude the possibility that the relationship between FGC and HCV is due to an unmeasured confounding variable.

There is considerable controversy in the literature about the extent to which HCV can be transmitted by sexual contact and cohabitation. In general most studies and two systematic reviews have found that HCV can be transmitted sexually but that the risk of infection is low [14, 25]. The most recent systematic review tried to make sense of the conflicting results by dividing the studies into those from high (Japanese) and low (non-Japanese) prevalence regions [14]. They found that pooling the results of studies along these lines provided strong evidence of increased HCV prevalence in offspring of affected persons in endemic areas but no such effect in nonendemic areas. In contrast they found evidence of an increased HCV prevalence amongst the spouses of persons who were HCV seropositive in nonendemic areas but no evidence for this effect in endemic areas. One interpretation of these apparently discordant findings is that HCV prevalence in spouses of HCV seropositive persons was not higher than controls in endemic areas as the prevalence in the controls was so high [14]. In endemic settings, transmission rates may be so high that close to all susceptible persons are infected by the time they are married. This may mask any effect that domestic and sexual transmission may play. An analogous effect was observed with hepatitis B virus. Sexual transmission was shown to occur in low prevalence areas such as USA but not in high prevalence areas such as East Asia [26, 27]. More recent studies have found evidence of spousal transmission of HCV in endemic areas [5, 6, 11, 13, 28–30]. Genotypic studies provide further evidence of the spousal transmission of HCV [8, 15, 30, 31].

In Egypt there is an increasing amount of evidence that intrafamilial transmission is an important source of new infections [5, 13, 29]. Two prospective studies investigating the correlates of incident of HCV in Egypt have found evidence of intrafamilial transmission [13, 32]. One of these was a study that followed up a cohort of 6734 HCV antibody negative persons from 2 rural villages over a median of 1.6 years [13]. In this time there were 33 new HCV infections, 27 of which occurred in families with an anti-HCV positive member. Parenteral factors were not associated with an elevated HCV incidence and in 21 of the cases there was no history of any parenteral exposure. HCV incidence per 1000 person years was higher in spouses of HCV antibody positive as opposed to antibody negative persons (13.1 versus 1.9; $P = 0.08$). Men and women with anti-HCV positive spouses were 7 and 2 times as likely to seroconvert as those with seronegative spouses. HCV incidence in children increased in a stepwise manner if they had one of two parents who is HCV antibody positive. A number of other studies have found marriage to be a risk factor for HCV infection but not all of these are controlled for age, which is likely a significant confounder [5, 6, 29]. One study found that parenteral factors only play a part in explaining prevalent cases in those over the age of 20 in Egypt [6].

One way of tying together the seemingly discordant findings about the extent of intrafamilial HCV transmission from different studies around the world is to apply the insight from hepatitis B virus epidemiology that the predominant mode of transmission may vary considerably between different regions of the world. Hepatitis B transmission in East Asia is predominantly perinatal, in USA it is largely sexual and intravenous drug use [33, 34], and in sub-Saharan Africa an important cause is horizontal transmission between children through poorly defined mechanisms [35–37].

In USA, iatrogenic and intravenous drug usage have been shown to be the dominant modes of HCV transmission [17]. There is mounting evidence that sexual transmission is important in HCV outbreaks of men who have sex with men [38]. The best quality evidence however suggests that sexual transmission has not played a large role in HCV transmission among heterosexuals in the USA [17, 39].

The composite evidence from Egypt reveals a somewhat different epidemiology for HCV. PAT was clearly important in the initial amplification of HCV in Egypt [3]. What perpetuated the spread of HCV thereafter? Perinatal transmission can take place. However, most individuals infected by this route clear the virus spontaneously [6, 40]. Unsterile procedures have clearly played an important role [1, 2, 6–8, 11]. A large proportion of cases are however not explained by these factors [1, 6, 9, 13]. Our study backs up the evidence from elsewhere of the likelihood of horizontal spread between family/household members [5, 9]. Some of this may be sexual but much is likely to be via other, as yet unclearly defined, mechanisms [13]. The findings presented here also build on the evidence from elsewhere [1] that FGC may have played a role in the spread of HCV—both at the time of the procedure and via enhancing the sexual transmission of HCV.

This analysis has a number of serious limitations. The EDHS was a cross-sectional survey and thus the direction of any implied causation cannot be established. Only 5182 individuals (out of 11126 individuals surveyed in the special health topics sample) could be linked together to provide the wife-husband dyad sample used for this analysis. Furthermore the limitations imposed by the linking process meant that the ages of the husbands were from a wider age-band (15–59 years old) than that of the wives (15–49). Because of these limitations, the sample we used cannot be assumed to be representative of whole Egypt.

The uni- and multivariate analyses of the married couple subsample are, however, remarkably similar to those found in analyses of the entire sample of 11126 respondents (presented in Guerra et al. [1]). This suggests that our subsample is not significantly biased.

Given the ongoing high incidence of HCV in Egypt [2], further research is needed to better define the mechanisms for intrafamilial spread so as to guide new prevention strategies.

In particular further research is needed to ascertain if FGC is an effect-modifier in the sexual transmission of HCV.

Acknowledgment

The authors would like to thank Measure DHS (http://www.measuredhs.com) for making these data available.

References

[1] J. Guerra, M. Garenne, M. K. Mohamed, and A. Fontanet, "HCV burden of infection in Egypt: results from a nationwide survey," *Journal of Viral Hepatitis*, vol. 19, no. 8, pp. 560–567, 2012.

[2] F. D. Miller and L. J. Abu-Raddad, "Evidence of intense ongoing endemic transmission of hepatitis C virus in Egypt," *Proceedings of the National Academy of Sciences of the United States of America*, vol. 107, no. 33, pp. 14757–14762, 2010.

[3] C. Frank, M. K. Mohamed, G. T. Strickland et al., "The role of parenteral antischistosomal therapy in the spread of hepatitis C virus in Egypt," *The Lancet*, vol. 355, no. 9207, pp. 887–891, 2000.

[4] R. Breban, W. Doss, G. Esmat et al., "Towards realistic estimates of HCV incidence in Egypt," *Journal of Viral Hepatitis*, vol. 20, pp. 294–296, 2013.

[5] M. Habib, M. K. Mohamed, F. Abdel-Aziz et al., "Hepatitis C virus infection in a community in the Nile Delta: risk factors for seropositivity," *Hepatology*, vol. 33, no. 1, pp. 248–253, 2001.

[6] N. Arafa, M. El Hoseiny, C. Rekacewicz et al., "Changing pattern of hepatitis C virus spread in rural areas of Egypt," *Journal of Hepatology*, vol. 43, no. 3, pp. 418–424, 2005.

[7] M. Talaat, A. Kandeel, O. Rasslan et al., "Evolution of infection control in Egypt: achievements and challenges," *American Journal of Infection Control*, vol. 34, no. 4, pp. 193–200, 2006.

[8] A. Paez Jimenez, N. Sharaf Eldin, F. Rimlinger et al., "HCV iatrogenic and intrafamilial transmission in Greater Cairo, Egypt," *Gut*, vol. 59, no. 11, pp. 1554–1560, 2010.

[9] D. A. Saleh, F. M. Shebl, S. S. El-Kamary et al., "Incidence and risk factors for community-acquired hepatitis C infection from birth to 5 years of age in rural Egyptian children," *Transactions of the Royal Society of Tropical Medicine and Hygiene*, vol. 104, no. 5, pp. 357–363, 2010.

[10] D. A. Saleh, F. Shebl, M. Abdel-Hamid et al., "Incidence and risk factors for hepatitis C infection in a cohort of women in rural Egypt," *Transactions of the Royal Society of Tropical Medicine and Hygiene*, vol. 102, no. 9, pp. 921–928, 2008.

[11] A. P. Jimenez, M. K. Mohamed, N. S. Eldin et al., "Injection drug use is a risk factor for HCV infection in urban Egypt," *PLoS ONE*, vol. 4, no. 9, Article ID e7193, 2009.

[12] G. Esmat, M. Hashem, M. El-Raziky et al., "Risk factors for hepatitis C virus acquisition and predictors of persistence among Egyptian children," *Liver International*, vol. 32, no. 3, pp. 449–456, 2012.

[13] M. K. Mohamed, M. Abdel-Hamid, N. N. Mikhail et al., "Intrafamilial transmission of hepatitis C in Egypt," *Hepatology*, vol. 42, no. 3, pp. 683–687, 2005.

[14] Z. Ackerman, E. Ackerman, and O. Paltiel, "Intrafamilial transmission of hepatitis C virus: a systematic review," *Journal of Viral Hepatitis*, vol. 7, no. 2, pp. 93–103, 2000.

[15] N. P. de Cavalheiro, A. de la Rosa, S. Elagin, F. M. Tengan, and A. A. Barone, "Hepatitis C virus: molecular and epidemiological evidence of male-to-female transmission," *Brazilian Journal of Infectious Diseases*, vol. 14, no. 5, pp. 427–432, 2010.

[16] E. Z. Fatma and A. Way, *Egypt Demographic and Health Survey 2008*, Ministry of Health, Cairo, Egypt, 2009.

[17] G. L. Armstrong, A. Wasley, E. P. Simard, G. M. McQuillan, W. L. Kuhnert, and M. J. Alter, "The prevalence of hepatitis C virus infection in the United States, 1999 through 2002," *Annals of Internal Medicine*, vol. 144, no. 10, pp. 705–714, 2006.

[18] C. Kenyon, J. Buyze, L. Apers, and R. Colebunders, "female genital cutting and hepatitis C spread in Egypt," *ISRN Hepatology*, vol. 2013, Article ID 617480, 3 pages, 2013.

[19] C. Iavazzo, T. A. Sardi, and I. D. Gkegkes, "Female genital mutilation and infections: a systematic review of the clinical evidence," *Archives of Gynecology and Obstetrics*, vol. 287, no. 6, pp. 1137–1149, 2013.

[20] L. Morison, C. Scherf, G. Ekpo et al., "The long-term reproductive health consequences of female genital cutting in rural Gambia: a community-based survey," *Tropical Medicine and International Health*, vol. 6, no. 8, pp. 643–653, 2001.

[21] L. Almroth, S. Elmusharaf, N. El Hadi et al., "Primary infertility after genital mutilation in girlhood in Sudan: a case-control study," *The Lancet*, vol. 366, no. 9483, pp. 385–391, 2005.

[22] M. C. Inhorn and K. A. Buss, "Infertility, infection, and iatrogenesis in Egypt: the anthropological epidemiology of blocked tubes," *Medical anthropology*, vol. 15, no. 3, pp. 217–244, 1993.

[23] K. M. Yount and J. S. Carrera, "Female genital cutting and reproductive experience in Minya, Egypt," *Medical Anthropology Quarterly*, vol. 20, no. 2, pp. 182–211, 2006.

[24] M. K. Mohamed, L. S. Magder, M. Abdel-Hamid et al., "Transmission of hepatitis C virus between parents and children," *American Journal of Tropical Medicine and Hygiene*, vol. 75, no. 1, pp. 16–20, 2006.

[25] G. Rooney and R. J. C. Gilson, "Sexual transmission of hepatitis C virus infection," *Sexually Transmitted Infections*, vol. 74, no. 6, pp. 399–404, 1998.

[26] A. S. Lok, C. L. Lai, P. C. Wu, V. C. Wong, E. K. Yeoh, and H. J. Lin, "Hepatitis B virus infection in Chinese families in Hong Kong," *American Journal of Epidemiology*, vol. 126, pp. 492–499, 1987.

[27] W. Szmuness, M. I. Much, and A. M. Prince, "On the role of sexual behavior in the spread of hepatitis B infection," *Annals of Internal Medicine*, vol. 83, no. 4, pp. 489–495, 1975.

[28] Y. Akahane, M. Kojima, Y. Sugai et al., "Hepatitis C virus infection in spouses of patients with type C chronic liver disease," *Annals of Internal Medicine*, vol. 120, no. 9, pp. 748–752, 1994.

[29] L. S. Magder, A. D. Fix, N. N. H. Mikhail et al., "Estimation of the risk of transmission of hepatitis C between spouses in Egypt based on seroprevalence data," *International Journal of Epidemiology*, vol. 34, no. 1, pp. 160–165, 2005.

[30] J.-H. Kao, P.-J. Chen, P.-M. Yang et al., "Intrafamilial transmission of hepatitis C virus. The important role of infections between spouses," *Journal of Infectious Diseases*, vol. 166, no. 4, pp. 900–903, 1992.

[31] C. J. Healey, D. B. Smith, J. L. Walker et al., "Acute hepatitis C infection after sexual exposure," *Gut*, vol. 36, no. 1, pp. 148–150, 1995.

[32] A. Mostafa, S. M. Taylor, M. El-Daly et al., "Is the hepatitis C virus epidemic over in Egypt? Incidence and risk factors of new hepatitis C virus infections," *Liver International*, vol. 30, no. 4, pp. 560–566, 2010.

[33] M. J. Alter, S. C. Hadler, H. S. Margolis et al., "The changing epidemiology of hepatitis B in the United States. Need for alternative vaccination strategies," *Journal of the American Medical Association*, vol. 263, no. 9, pp. 1218–1222, 1990.

[34] A. Wasley, S. Grytdal, and K. Gallagher, "Surveillance for acute viral hepatitis—United States, 2006," *MMWR Surveillance Summaries: Morbidity and Mortality Weekly Report Surveillance Summaries/CDC*, vol. 57, no. 2, pp. 1–24, 2008.

[35] F. E. A. Martinson, K. A. Weigle, R. A. Royce, D. J. Weber, C. M. Suchindran, and S. M. Lemon, "Risk factors for horizontal transmission of hepatitis B virus in a rural district in Ghana," *American Journal of Epidemiology*, vol. 147, no. 5, pp. 478–487, 1998.

[36] H. Whittle, H. Inskip, A. K. Bradley et al., "The pattern of childhood hepatitis B infection in two Gambian villages," *Journal of Infectious Diseases*, vol. 161, no. 6, pp. 1112–1115, 1990.

[37] S. S. A. Karim, R. Thejpal, and H. M. Coovadia, "Household clustering and intra-household transmission patterns of hepatitis B virus infection in South Africa," *International Journal of Epidemiology*, vol. 20, no. 2, pp. 495–503, 1991.

[38] A. T. Urbanus, T. J. Van De Laar, I. G. Stolte et al., "Hepatitis C virus infections among HIV-infected men who have sex with men: an expanding epidemic," *AIDS*, vol. 23, no. 12, pp. F1–F7, 2009.

[39] C. Vandelli, F. Renzo, L. Romanò et al., "Lack of evidence of sexual transmission of hepatitis C among monogamous couples: results of a 10-year prospective follow-up study," *American Journal of Gastroenterology*, vol. 99, no. 5, pp. 855–859, 2004.

[40] F. M. Shebl, S. S. El-Kamary, D. A. Saleh et al., "Prospective cohort study of mother-to-infant infection and clearance of hepatitis C in rural Egyptian villages," *Journal of Medical Virology*, vol. 81, no. 6, pp. 1024–1031, 2009.

2

Liver Injury Induced by Anticancer Chemotherapy and Radiation Therapy

Y. Maor[1] and S. Malnick[2]

[1] *Department of Gastroenterology and Hepatology, Sheba Medical Center, 52621 Tel-Hashomer, Israel*
[2] *Department of Internal Medicine C, Kaplan Medical Center, The Hebrew University of Jerusalem, 76100 Rehovot, Israel*

Correspondence should be addressed to Y. Maor; halishy@netvision.net.il

Academic Editor: Matthias Bahr

Cytotoxic chemotherapy prolongs survival of patients with advanced and metastatic tumors. This is, however, a double-edged sword with many adverse effects. Since the liver has a rich blood supply and plays an active role in the metabolism of medications, it is not surprising that there can be hepatic injury related to chemotherapy. In addition, radioembolization may affect the parenchyma of normal and cirrhotic livers. We review chemotherapy-associated liver injury in patients with colorectal liver metastases, including downsizing chemotherapy and neoadjuvant chemotherapy. We discuss the mechanism of the hepatic injury, secondary to reactive oxygen species, and the spectrum of hepatic injury including, steatosis, steatohepatitis, hepatic sinusoidal injury and highlight the pharmacogenomics of such liver insults. Methods for reducing and treating the hepatotoxicity are discussed for specific agents including tamxifen and the newly introduced targeted antibodies.

1. Introduction

Over the last few decades many novel cytotoxic chemotherapeutic agents have been developed which prolong survival of patients with advanced and metastatic tumors., More recently, specifically targeted antibodies and other biological agents have been introduced in various combinations with chemotherapy to further increase life expectancy. For some tumors, for example, colorectal cancer (CRC), preoperative treatment may "downsize" liver metastases to make them compatible with complete resection with a curative intent. External radiation therapy has been an integral part of the armamentarium against primary or metastatic liver tumors. Currently, radiation may be directly targeted at liver tumors with the radioembolization technique. This increased availability of beneficial treatment modalities does not come without a price. Administration of chemotherapy has always been complicated with many adverse effects. In this review we will focus on the effects of chemotherapy and radiotherapy on the liver. The liver may be affected by various pathological manifestations, some culminating in severe liver injury and even liver failure. Chemotherapy-induced liver injury may also bear on the morbidity and mortality after hepatic resection. Radioembolization, although relatively safe, may affect the parenchyma of normal and cirrhotic livers.

2. Chemotherapy-Associated Liver Injury in Patients with Colorectal Liver Metastases

In the absence of any treatment, the prognosis of patients with liver metastases from CRC is dismal [1]. In those patients with resectable disease, liver surgery with complete resection of the metastases has markedly improved long-term survival [2]. The most significant advance regarding CRC over the past decade has been the introduction of several effective cytotoxic chemotherapeutic agents mainly 5-Fluorouracil (5-FU), oxaliplatin, and irinotecan [3]. Further benefits were achieved by the addition of monoclonal antibodies directed against epidermal growth factor receptor (EGFR) or against vascular endothelial growth factor (VEGF), for example, bevacizumab [4]. In patients with metastatic CRC treated in a palliative intention, the combination of oxaliplatin- or irinotecan-based chemotherapy with an antibody increased the median overall survival from 20 to 22 months [4].

Advances in systemic therapy for metastatic CRC have led to more patients being treated with chemotherapy before hepatic resection. For patients with initially unresectable metastases, preoperative therapy can lead to a decrease in the size of metastases and render these patients resectable—referred to as "downsizing chemotherapy" [5, 6]. For patients with initially resectable metastases, progression free survival improves with perioperative chemotherapy compared with surgery alone—this is termed "neoadjuvant chemotherapy." There is less evidence, however, on the beneficial effect of neoadjuvant chemotherapy alone on survival [7]. Potential disadvantages of preoperative chemotherapy are the risk of disease progression before surgery and liver toxicity. Chemotherapy induces various histological changes of the liver parenchyma including steatosis, chemotherapy-associated steatohepatitis (CASH), or sinusoidal injury sinusoidal obstruction syndrome (SOS) [8–10]. Agreement exists on a link between the chemotherapy-associated changes and poor postoperative outcomes. Hepatic parenchymal injury is regimen specific. For example, irinotecan-based regimens are associated with steatohepatitis (number needed to harm 12; 95% CI 7.8–26) whereas oxaliplatin-based regimens being can result in grade 2 or greater sinusoidal injury (number needed to harm 8; 95% confidence interval [CI] 6.4–13.6) [11].

3. Mechanism

The mechanism of chemotherapy-induced hepatic injury is thought to be secondary to production of reactive oxygen species (ROS), intended to induce tumor cell apoptosis [12]. Previously steatotic livers were thought to be most susceptible to chemotherapy-induced injury due to impaired regenerative capability and abnormal innate immunity [13–15].

4. Clinical-Pathological Modes of Liver Injury

4.1. Nonalcoholic Fatty Liver Disease. The epidemic of obesity, insulin resistance, and the resulting metabolic syndrome has led to an increased prevalence of nonalcoholic fatty liver disease. This has been estimated to be present in more than 20% of patients planned for hepatectomy [16]. Steatotic liver is more vulnerable to injury from general anesthesia and ischemia/reperfusion [17]. Protective mechanisms against oxidative stress are significantly impaired in steatosis [18], and impaired energy homeostasis further sensitizes steatotic livers to surgical stress [16]. Regeneration is delayed in steatotic livers [16, 19], with a resulting prolongation of liver dysfunction [16].

4.2. Steatosis. The effect of mild to moderate steatosis without associated inflammation on postoperative outcome is likely to be small. Kooby and colleagues [20] found that, in patients with steatosis who underwent major liver resection, steatosis was associated with infection-related complications but not with major complications or postoperative mortality. However, many patients with steatosis have other comorbid conditions, such as obesity and diabetes that can increase the risk of complications. In a study of patients who had major hepatectomy, patients with steatosis had increased blood loss, more postoperative complications, and a longer mean intensive-care-unit stay per patient as compared with matched control patients with healthy livers [21]. Fluorouracil (5-FU), which remains the backbone of modern chemotherapy, has been linked to the development of steatosis. Reports indicate the development of steatosis in 30 to 47% of patients after 5-FU therapy, although some changes may be reversible [22–24].

4.3. Steatohepatitis. Irinotecan is clearly associated with steatohepatitis, with a rate of 20.2% seen in patients administered this drug, compared with 4.4% in those not having chemotherapy [25–27]. This effect was exacerbated by baseline obesity [28]. Steatohepatitis was found in 24.6% in those with a BMI of $25\,kg/m^2$ or more who were administered irinotecan, but only 12.1% in irinotecan treated patients with a BMI less than $25\,kg/m^2$ [26]. Steatohepatitis increases the risk of liver failure [28, 29] and postoperative complications [18] following major hepatectomy. Primarily because of its effect on regeneration, steatohepatitis is also associated with increased overall postoperative mortality [26]. An almost 10-fold-increased 90-day mortality following hepatectomy in patients with steatohepatitis (mortality 14.7% versus 1.6%) with a six-fold higher risk of death from postoperative liver failure (5.8% versus 0.8%) has been reported [26]. Major hepatic resection should probably be avoided in patients with known steatohepatitis, as should irinotecan in patients with known steatosis or steatohepatitis in whom major hepatic resection is planned.

4.4. Hepatic Sinusoidal Injury. Sinusoidal injury ranges from sinusoidal dilation to hepatic sinusoidal obstruction syndrome, also termed venoocclusive disease, which can progress to regenerative nodular hyperplasia [30]. Injury to the sinusoidal endothelial cells lining the sinusoids, the initial event, leads to subintimal thickening and extravasation of erythrocytes into the subendothelial space of Disse (perisinusoidal space). Sinusoidal endothelial cells and erythrocytes embolize in sinusoids and block venous outflow, resulting in hepatic congestion and sinusoidal dilatation. At later stages, a fibrotic reaction in the sinusoids can lead to obliteration of central venules, leading to hepatic sinusoidal obstruction syndrome. Rates of injury are universally higher in patients receiving oxaliplatin-based chemotherapy. Oxaliplatin was associated with a 10-fold increase in sinusoidal dilation compared with no chemotherapy (18.9% versus 1.9%) [26]. In the European Organisation for Research and Treatment of Cancer EORTC-4098336 study involving administration of chemotherapy, high-grade injuries were much more prominent in the group administered chemotherapy (41%) compared to the control group (0%) [31]. Sinusoidal changes may normalize with time after cessation of chemotherapy, and delaying surgery for several months might be a useful option in patients with diagnosed or suspected sinusoidal injury [32]. Oxaliplatin and other platinum compounds lead to the generation of ROS and could result in depletion of glutathione from sinusoidal endothelial cells (SECs)

[33, 34]. Cisplatin has been shown to cause actin dissociation, which can upregulate matrix-metalloproteinases-9 (MMP-9) activity [35]. Morbidity following hepatectomy is significantly higher in patients with evidence of sinusoidal obstruction syndrome, although there is no increase in mortality [36]. Sinusoidal injury also significantly increases hospital stay [32]. Oxaliplatin is associated with an increased transfusion requirement compared to patients receiving 5 FU/leucovorin or no chemotherapy [37]. It has been suggested that increased blood loss is directly attributable to these vascular lesions. Transfusion is associated with an adverse outcome after hepatectomy and a requirement for red cell transfusion is independently associated with overall morbidity [38]. Mortality was increased from 1.2%, when transfused 2 units of blood or less following hepatectomy, to 11.1% for those requiring more than 2 units [38].

5. Pharmacogenomics

It is increasingly recognized that pharmacogenomics can play a key role in determining the susceptibility of the individual to the toxic effects of chemotherapy. Recently, a randomised trial showed that patients given an irinotecan dose modified on the basis of CYP3A enzymatic activity had reduced interindividual pharmacokinetic variability for irinotecan and its active metabolite, SN-38, and a decreased incidence of severe neutropenia [39]. SN-38 is also inactivated by glucuronidation, which is metabolised by the UGT1A1 enzyme. A polymorphism in the promoter of the gene encoding UGT1A1 results in lower rates of SN-38 glucuronidation, leading to worse diarrhea and neutropenia associated with irinotecan [40]. Similarly, oxaliplatin toxicity is affected by mutations in genes involved in DNA damage repair and conjugation of its metabolites to glutathione [41].

6. Diagnosis

CT is the most widely used imaging technique to investigate CRC liver metastases and is useful for detecting moderate to severe steatosis (hepatic fat content of more than 30%) [42]. MRI was more accurate than noncontrast CT in the diagnosis of steatosis, particularly in patients with BMI of 30 kg/m^2 or more [43]. However, available imaging techniques cannot differentiate steatohepatitis from steatosis or identify sinusoidal injury. Biopsy is the definitive method for the diagnosis of chemotherapy-induced liver injury. Some investigators have advocated staging laparoscopy to visually inspect and sample liver parenchyma prior to performing hepatic resection [8]. This approach, however, may be difficult to apply in routine clinical practice.

7. Prevention and Treatment

Postoperative morbidity was related to the duration of preoperative chemotherapy, with higher morbidity rates among patients who received at least six cycles or more compared with those who received fewer than six cycles [36]. The optimum duration of preoperative chemotherapy, to maximize therapeutic benefit while avoiding hepatotoxicity, is likely to be 4 months [26]. Several studies show that a longer interval between chemotherapy and hepatic resection reduces hepatotoxicity and surgical complications. However, this interval should be balanced with the risk of tumor progression during the treatment-free interval. An interval of 5 weeks is recommended to minimize postoperative complications while avoiding a long delay in treatment [44, 45]. Patients with suspected chemotherapy-associated liver injury who need major hepatic resection should have assessment of their functional future liver remnant to minimize postoperative complications. Methods to predict the function of the expected remnant liver include biochemical tests for hepatic clearance of compounds, such as indocyanine green, and measurement of the future liver remnant measured with CT. In patients with normal liver function, a minimum of 20% is needed to prevent complications after major hepatectomy. In patients with substantial chemotherapy-induced liver damage, a future liver remnant of 30% has been proposed as the minimum volume needed before major hepatic resection. When the future liver remnant is predicted to be insufficient for safe hepatic resection, portal-vein embolization of the part of the liver to be resected can induce hypertrophy of the future liver remnant. Liver remnant hypertrophy of less than 5% is associated with increased postoperative morbidity [46]. Patients with substantial chemotherapy-associated liver injury who have inadequate liver hypertrophy after a portal-vein embolization are not candidates for a major liver resection. Hepatic pedicle clamping (Pringle manoeuvre) to limit blood loss is an integral component of major hepatectomies but may deliver an ischaemic/reperfusion injury to the remnant liver [47]. Adding the anti-VEGF antibody bevacizumab may have a protective effect against oxaliplatin-induced sinusoidal injury. Bevacizumab lowered the incidence of sinusoidal dilatation in patients receiving oxaliplatin and become reduced to less than a third that of severe (grade 2-3) sinusoidal dilatation (8 versus 28%) [48]. However, the overall complication rate was not significantly different between those who received oxaliplatin-based neoadjuvant chemotherapy with or without bevacizumab [49].

8. Tamoxifen-Induced Nonalcoholic Steatohepatitis and Injury Inflicted by Other Hormonal Agents

Tamoxifen is an estrogen-receptor antagonist and at a dose of 20 mg/day is the adjuvant hormonal treatment of choice in women with estrogen-receptor-positive breast cancer [50]. Severe side effects are unusual with tamoxifen, but it is associated with the development of nonalcoholic fatty liver disease (NAFLD) and non alcoholic steatohepatitis (NASH) [50]. NASH is the most prevalent form of progressive liver disease and it is suggested that NAFLD affects 10–39% of the global population. Drugs account for less than 2% of the causes of NASH. Drugs known to be capable of inducing steatosis and steatohepatitis can be divided into three broad groups: those that cause steatosis and steatohepatitis independently (e.g., amiodarone, perhexiline maleate); drugs that can precipitate latent NASH (e.g., tamoxifen); and drugs that induce sporadic events of steatosis/steatohepatitis (e.g., carbamazepine) [51]. An Italian multicentre trial [52] enrolled 5408 healthy women who had hysterectomies, in which half of the women were prospectively assigned to tamoxifen 20 mg daily and the other half to placebo for 5 years. This study showed that the major risk factors for the development of tamoxifen-induced NASH were obesity (central), hyperlipidaemia, and diabetes. The incidence of tamoxifen-induced NAFLD was estimated to be about 40% at 1 year. Overall, tamoxifen was associated with an increased risk of developing NAFLD (hazard ratio: 2.0, 95% confidence interval [CI]: 1.1–3.5), but the association was restricted to overweight women. The increased risk was limited to the first two years of treatment. Mild to moderate non-alcoholic steatohepatitis, when recognized at the onset, seemed to be indolent in the long term, and no progression to cirrhosis was observed after a median followup of 8.7 years [52]. In a large registry of 1105 patients with breast cancer [53], NASH was documented in 2.2%. Seventeen patients (1.5%) developed NASH after their diagnosis of breast cancer. Multivariate logistic regression analysis indicated that age, BMI, and tamoxifen were significant factors associated with NASH. The odds of developing NASH increased 8.2-fold when patients were treated with tamoxifen. The median time from the start of tamoxifen to documented NASH was 22 months. NASH improved after tamoxifen was stopped. Only 2 patients had biopsy-documented cirrhosis in 806 patients who took tamoxifen [53]. Therefore, cirrhosis is considered a rare complication of tamoxifen therapy. Tamoxifen was shown to increase hepatic fat content, through blocking the role of estrogen in maintaining hepatic lipid homeostasis by supporting the expression of genes involved in lipid β-oxidation. In addition, tamoxifen has been shown to increase serum triglyceride and lower low-density lipoprotein and cholesterol levels. It was suggested that fatty liver is vulnerable to oxidants and progresses to steatohepatitis when a second agent (such as tamoxifen) generates liver cell death, inflammation, and activation of stellate cells with production of fibrosis (multiple hit hypothesis) [54, 55]. Increased TNF-α, mitochondrial β-oxidation rates and the production of large amounts of reactive oxygen species play a major role in drug-induced steatohepatitis [56]. Interestingly, the difference in the distribution of CYP genotypes between patients may increase the individual susceptibility for tamoxifen-induced NASH [57]. In addition, serum leptin levels were found to be significantly elevated in patients with hepatic steatosis after tamoxifen treatment [58]. Risk factor management is the most important step in the treatment of NASH. In case of severe NASH, tamoxifen should be stopped and one of the aromatase inhibitors can be started.

Anastrozole is a selective aromatase inhibitor approved for the treatment of postmenopausal hormone-sensitive breast cancer. Few cases of acute hepatitis occurring during treatment with anastrozole have been reported [59, 60]. In one report [60] liver biopsy revealed diffuse liver cell necrosis in acinar zone 3, the preferred location of most drug-metabolizing P450 isoenzymes. These findings are compatible with a metabolically mediated hepatocellular liver injury. A genetic polymorphism of any enzyme involved in drug detoxification could cause an accumulation of the parental drug or its metabolites, predisposing to anastrozole-induced liver toxicity. Liver function parameters rapidly improved after drug withdrawal in the reported cases.

9. Hepatotoxicity of Specific-Targeted Antibodies

9.1. Lapatinib-Induced Hepatitis. Lapatinib is an inhibitor of the tyrosine kinases of human epidermal growth factor receptor type 2 (HER2) and epidermal growth factor receptor type 1. A number of studies have shown that lapatinib has clinical activity in patients with HER2-positive breast cancer, with a significant reduction in the risk of disease progression [61]. In a phase II trial, grade 3 and 4 liver toxicity were uncommon after single agent lapatinib [61]. In one report [62] a women with advanced breast cancer who had been treated with lapatinib for 14 days developed severe hepatitis. Liver biopsy showed portal-to-portal and portal-to-central bridging necrosis, foci of severe hemorrhage, and hepatocellular dropout around the centrilobular areas. Eosinophil infiltrate was seen in many portal spaces. These findings are all consistent with drug-induced hepatitis. Bilirubin and liver enzymes returned to normal within three months of lapatinib discontinuation. A recent study [63] has identified and confirmed associations between lapatinib-associated liver injury and the highly correlated MHC class II alleles *HLA-DQA1∗02:01*, *DRB1∗07:01*, and *DQB1∗02:02* plus an SNP in the same genomic locus, *TNXB* (rs12153855).

9.2. Inflammatory Hepatotoxicity of CTLA-4 Antibody Therapy. The cytotoxic T-lymphocyte (CTLA-4) receptor binds molecules of the B7-family which leads to a suppression of T cells. Specific CTLA-4 antibodies induce an unrestrained T-cell activation. Treatment with the CTLA-4 antibodies ipilimumab and tremelimumab has been approved for metastatic melanoma [64]. A unique set of adverse effects may occur, termed immune-related adverse events. These include rashes and colitis, usually mild to moderate. Less frequent manifestations such as, hypophysitis, hepatitis, pancreatitis, iridocyclitis, lymphadenopathy, neuropathies, and nephritis have also been reported [64]. Immune-related hepatotoxicity was observed in 3% to 9% of patients receiving anti-CTLA-4 antibodies [65, 66] manifested as an asymptomatic increase of aminotransferases and bilirubin, although some patients also had fevers and malaise. A waxing and waning picture may be seen. Biopsies showed a diffuse T-cell infiltrate consistent with immune-related hepatitis. It has been recommended that for grades 3 to 4 hepatotoxicity, one should use high-dose intravenous glucocorticosteroids. If the condition persists, immunosuppressant therapy with mycophenolate mofetil may also be considered. Infliximab, because of its potential for hepatotoxicity, should be avoided in this setting [64].

10. Radiation-Induced Liver Disease

10.1. Liver Injury from External Beam Radiation. Radiation induced liver disease (RILD) after conventionally fractionated radiotherapy was first described several decades ago, and it was soon thereafter recognized to have the histopathologic features of sinusoidal of venoocclusive disease (VOD), currently termed sinusoid obstructive syndrome (SOS) [67, 68]. The clinical scenario commonly called "classic" radiation induced liver disease (RILD) occurs typically within 4 months after hepatic radiation therapy. It is characterized by anicteric ascites and hepatomegaly and an isolated elevation in alkaline phosphatase disproportionate to that of other liver enzymes. "Classic" RILD is unlikely to occur after a mean liver dose of approximately 30 Gy in conventional fractionation. Patients with underlying chronic hepatic disease may present with liver function abnormalities that do not match the criteria described previously, including jaundice and/or Markedly elevated serum transaminases (more than 5 times the upper limit of normal) within 3 months of completion of hepatic radiation therapy [69–71]. All these hepatic toxicities have been included under the umbrella label of "nonclassic RILD." It was postulated that radiation injury to sinusoidal endothelial cells and central vein endothelium initiates activation of the coagulation cascade, leading to accumulation of fibrin and formation of clots in the central veins and hepatic sinusoids [72]. The ensuing hypoxic milieu presumably results in the death of centrilobular hepatocytes and atrophy of the inner hepatic plate, producing the hepatic dysfunction. By maintaining a low mean liver dose and sparing a "critical volume" of liver from radiation, stereotactic delivery techniques allow for the safe administration of higher tumor doses. Caution must be exercised for patients with hepatocellular carcinoma or preexisting liver disease (e.g., Child-Pugh score of B or C) because they are more susceptible to RILD that can manifest in a nonclassic pattern. No pharmacologic interventions have yet been proven to mitigate or treat RILD.

10.2. Radioembolization-Induced Liver Injury. Selective internal radiation therapy (SIRT) [73] with 90yttrium microspheres is a relatively new clinical modality for treating nonresectable malignant liver tumors. This interventional radiology technique employs percutaneous microcatheterisation of the hepatic arterial vasculature to selectively deliver radioembolic microspheres into neoplastic tissue. SIRT results in measurable tumor responses or delayed disease progression in the majority of eligible patients with hepatocellular carcinoma or hepatic metastases arising from CRC. It has also been successfully used as palliative therapy for noncolorectal malignancies metastatic to the liver. Side effects are not common after radioembolization. A postembolization syndrome like the one that appears after TACE is not seen. Radioembolization is safe in patients with portal vein thrombosis [74] in whom TACE may lead to complications such as liver abscess or decompensation of cirrhosis [75]. Results from a small series suggest that it could also be safe in asymptomatic patients with lobar or segmental biliary tract obstruction but normal or near-normal bilirubin [76]. Safety in these special situations is probably the result of the lack of significant ischemia [77]. However, radioembolization may produce relevant toxic effects as a result of radiation of nontarget organs including, cholecystitis, gastrointestinal ulceration, pneumonitis, and most importantly for HCC patients, liver toxicity. Two consequences of cirrhosis may affect radioembolization in the cirrhotic liver. On one hand, the usual distribution of microspheres can be profoundly altered by the vascular changes and the presence of anatomical arterioportal and arteriovenous shunts. This may modify the radiation dose absorbed by the tumor and the nontumoral liver and therefore affect treatment tolerance and effectiveness. On the other hand, the cirrhotic liver has a reduced functional reserve that produces an increased risk of liver failure after liver insults including external irradiation [78]. A direct liver cell injury and a further compromise of liver blood supply produced by radiation-mediated blood vessel damage could all result in a higher risk of clinically relevant liver toxicity after radioembolization in comparison with noncirrhotic livers. Microspheres are often distributed in a heterogeneous way and not infrequently form clusters. This may explain the lack of a clear dose-event relationship in liver tolerance, as happens with tumor response. The general agreement is that the dose absorbed by the nontumoral liver tissue should be kept below 50 Gy for patients with cirrhosis [79]. In non-cirrhotic patients, a form of sinusoidal obstruction syndrome appearing 4–8 weeks after radioembolization as jaundice, mild ascites, and a moderate increase in GGTP and alkaline phosphatase has been described as radioembolization-induced liver disease (REILD) [80]. The actual incidence of this complication in cirrhotics and noncirrhotics is difficult to establish because most published series report on changes in individual laboratory values along different periods of time. In those populations with a predominance of cirrhotic patients, abnormal liver function tests are frequently present at baseline and liver failure may develop as a result of the progression of the chronic liver disease. Thus, differences in reporting criteria may disturb the estimation of the incidence of REILD. In the two largest series ever published [81, 82], grade 3 or higher CTCAE bilirubin levels (a hallmark of REILD) were observed within 3 months after therapy in 14% and 6% of patients treated with glass or resin spheres, respectively. Although a causal relationship with radioembolization could only be confirmed in a controlled clinical, it is very likely that the increased bilirubin levels reflect some kind of REILD.

11. Summary and Outlook

Liver injury secondary to cytotoxic chemotherapy as well as novel molecular targeted and biological agents is one of the most serious adverse effects of anticancer treatment. Liver damage can assume diverse clinical and histological forms that are specific to the offending agent for most cases. Not only can hepatotoxicity culminate in liver failure and death, but it may also result in a postponement of scheduled treatment or complicate hepatic resection with curative intent. Our knowledge about the deleterious effects of chemotherapeutic drugs and innovative radiation treatment is far from complete. We need to fill this gap by several methods, for example, employing basic laboratory methods on animal models of liver injury induced by chemotherapy and multicenter registration of all cases of hepatotoxicity that include detailed clinical and laboratory data for each case. Finally, we have to initiate studies on modes to prevent or mitigate liver injury. Hepatologists and oncologists have to cooperate closely in this underappreciated topic.

References

[1] J. S. Wagner, M. A. Adson, and J. A. Van Heerden, "The natural history of hepatic metastases from colorectal cancer. A comparison with resective treatment," *Annals of Surgery*, vol. 199, no. 5, pp. 502–508, 1984.

[2] J. Figueras, J. Torras, C. Valls et al., "Surgical resection of colorectal liver metastases in patients with expanded indications: a single-center experience with 501 patients," *Diseases of the Colon and Rectum*, vol. 50, no. 4, pp. 478–488, 2007.

[3] M. L. Chen, C. H. Fang, L. S. Liang, L. H. Dai, and X. K. Wang, "A meta-analysis of chemotherapy regimen Fluorouracil/Leucovorin/Oxaliplatin Compared with Fluorouracil/Leucovorin in treating advanced colorectal cancer," *Surgical Oncology*, vol. 19, no. 1, pp. 38–45, 2010.

[4] L. B. Saltz, S. Clarke, E. Diaz-Rubio et al., "Bevacizumab in combination with oxaliplatin-based chemotherapy as first-line therapy in metastatic colorectal cancer: a randomized phase III study," *Journal of Clinical Oncology*, vol. 26, no. 12, pp. 2013–2019, 2008.

[5] P.-A. Clavien, H. Petrowsky, M. L. DeOliveira, and R. Graf, "Strategies for safer liver surgery and partial liver transplantation," *The New England Journal of Medicine*, vol. 356, no. 15, pp. 1545–1559, 2007.

[6] R. Adam, A. Laurent, D. Azoulay et al., "Two-stage hepatectomy: a planned strategy to treat irresectable liver tumors," *Annals of Surgery*, vol. 232, no. 6, pp. 777–785, 2000.

[7] K. Lehmann, A. Rickenbacher, A. Weber et al., "Chemotherapy before liver resection of clorectal metastases: friend or foe?" *Annals of Surgery*, vol. 254, no. 5, pp. 1–11, 2011.

[8] D. Zorzi, A. Laurent, T. M. Pawlik, G. Y. Lauwers, J.-N. Vauthey, and E. K. Abdalla, "Chemotherapy-associated hepatotoxicity and surgery for colorectal liver metastases," *British Journal of Surgery*, vol. 94, no. 3, pp. 274–286, 2007.

[9] G. Morris-Stiff, Y.-M. Tan, and J. N. Vauthey, "Hepatic complications following preoperative chemotherapy with oxaliplatin or irinotecan for hepatic colorectal metastases," *European Journal of Surgical Oncology*, vol. 34, no. 6, pp. 609–614, 2008.

[10] Y. Fong and D. J. Bentrem, "CASH (chemotherapy-associated steatohepatitis) costs," *Annals of Surgery*, vol. 243, no. 1, pp. 8–9, 2006.

[11] S. M. Robinson, C. H. Wilson, A. D. Burt et al., "Chemotherapy-associated liver injury in patients with colorectal liver metastases: a systematic review and meta-analysis," *Annals of Surgical Oncology*, vol. 19, no. 13, pp. 4287–4299, 2012.

[12] S.-C. Lim, J. E. Choi, H. S. Kang, and H. Si, "Ursodeoxycholic acid switches oxaliplatin-induced necrosis to apoptosis by inhibiting reactive oxygen species production and activating p53-caspase 8 pathway in HepG2 hepatocellular carcinoma," *International Journal of Cancer*, vol. 126, no. 7, pp. 1582–1595, 2010.

[13] Z. Li, H. Lin, S. Yang, and A. M. Diehl, "Murine leptin deficiency alters Kupffer cell production of cytokines that regulate the innate immune system," *Gastroenterology*, vol. 123, no. 4, pp. 1304–1310, 2002.

[14] M. A. E. Anna Diehl, "Nonalcoholic steatosis and steatohepatitis IV. Nonalcoholic fatty liver disease abnormalities in macrophage function and cytokines," *American Journal of Physiology*, vol. 282, no. 1, pp. G1–G5, 2002.

[15] R. Veteläinen, A. K. van Vliet, and T. M. van Gulik, "Severe steatosis increases hepatocellular injury and impairs liver regeneration in a rat model of partial hepatectomy," *Annals of Surgery*, vol. 245, no. 1, pp. 44–50, 2007.

[16] R. Veteläinen, A. Van Vliet, D. J. Gouma, and T. M. Van Gulik, "Steatosis as a risk factor in liver surgery," *Annals of Surgery*, vol. 245, no. 1, pp. 20–30, 2007.

[17] J. Belghiti, K. Hiramatsu, S. Benoist, P. P. Massault, A. Sauvanet, and O. Farges, "Seven hundred forty-seven hepatectomies in the 1990s: an update to evaluate the actual risk of liver resection," *Journal of the American College of Surgeons*, vol. 191, no. 1, pp. 38–46, 2000.

[18] A. J. Bilchik, G. Poston, S. A. Curley et al., "Neoadjuvant chemotherapy for metastatic colon cancer: a cautionary note," *Journal of Clinical Oncology*, vol. 23, no. 36, pp. 9073–9078, 2005.

[19] G. Garcea and G. J. Maddern, "Liver failure after major hepatic resection," *Journal of Hepato-Biliary-Pancreatic Surgery*, vol. 16, no. 2, pp. 145–155, 2009.

[20] D. A. Kooby, Y. Fong, A. Suriawinata et al., "Impact of steatosis on perioperative outcome following hepatic resection," *Journal of Gastrointestinal Surgery*, vol. 7, no. 8, pp. 1034–1044, 2003.

[21] L. McCormack, H. Petrowsky, W. Jochum, K. Furrer, and P.-A. Clavien, "Hepatic steatosis is a risk factor for postoperative complications after major hepatectomy: a matched case-control study," *Annals of Surgery*, vol. 245, no. 6, pp. 923–930, 2007.

[22] C. G. Moertel, T. R. Fleming, J. S. Macdonald, D. G. Haller, and J. A. Laurie, "Hepatic toxicity associated with fluorouracil plus levamisole adjuvant therapy," *Journal of Clinical Oncology*, vol. 11, no. 12, pp. 2386–2390, 1993.

[23] P. D. Peppercorn, R. H. Reznek, P. Wilson, M. L. Slevin, and R. K. Gupta, "Demonstration of hepatic steatosis by computerized tomography in patients receiving 5-fluorouracil-based therapy for advanced colorectal cancer," *British Journal of Cancer*, vol. 77, no. 11, pp. 2008–2011, 1998.

[24] P. Sorensen, A. L. Edal, E. L. Madsen et al., "Reversible hepatic steatosis in patients treated with interferon alfa-2a and 5-fluorouracil," *Cancer*, vol. 75, no. 10, pp. 2592–2596, 1995.

[25] T. M. Pawlik, K. Olino, A. L. Gleisner, M. Torbenson, R. Schulick, and M. A. Choti, "Preoperative chemotherapy for colorectal liver metastases: impact on hepatic histology and postoperative outcome," *Journal of Gastrointestinal Surgery*, vol. 11, no. 7, pp. 860–868, 2007.

[26] J.-N. Vauthey, T. M. Pawlik, D. Ribero et al., "Chemotherapy regimen predicts steatohepatitis and an increase in 90-day mortality after surgery for hepatic colorectal metastases," *Journal of Clinical Oncology*, vol. 24, no. 13, pp. 2065–2072, 2006.

[27] U. V. Gentilucci, D. Santini, B. Vincenzi, E. Fiori, A. Picardi, and G. Tonini, "Chemotherapy-induced steatohepatitis in colorectal cancer patients," *Journal of Clinical Oncology*, vol. 24, no. 34, p. 5467, 2006.

[28] A. Sahajpal, C. M. Vollmer Jr., E. Dixon et al., "Chemotherapy for colorectal cancer prior to liver resection for colorectal cancer hepatic metastases does not adversely affect peri-operative outcomes," *Journal of Surgical Oncology*, vol. 95, no. 1, pp. 22–27, 2007.

[29] F. G. Fernandez, J. Ritter, J. W. Goodwin, D. C. Linehan, W. G. Hawkins, and S. M. Strasberg, "Effect of steatohepatitis associated with irinotecan or oxaliplatin pretreatment on

resectability of hepatic colorectal metastases," *Journal of the American College of Surgeons*, vol. 200, no. 6, pp. 845–853, 2005.

[30] L. D. DeLeve, H. M. Shulman, and G. B. McDonald, "Toxic injury to hepatic sinusoids: sinusoidal obstruction syndrome (veno-occlusive disease)," *Seminars in Liver Disease*, vol. 22, no. 1, pp. 27–41, 2002.

[31] C. Julie, M. Lutz, D. Aust et al., "Pathological analysis of hepatic injury after oxaliplatin-based neoadjuvant chemotherapy of colorectal cancer liver metastases: results of the EORTC Intergroup phase III study 40983," *Journal of Clinical Oncology*, vol. 25, abstract 241, 2007.

[32] H. Nakano, E. Oussoultzoglou, E. Rosso et al., "Sinusoidal injury increases morbidity after major hepatectomy in patients with colorectal liver metastases receiving preoperative chemotherapy," *Annals of Surgery*, vol. 247, no. 1, pp. 118–124, 2008.

[33] A. Laurent, C. Nicco, C. Chéreau et al., "Controlling tumor growth by modulating endogenous production of reactive oxygen species," *Cancer Research*, vol. 65, no. 3, pp. 948–956, 2005.

[34] J. Alexandre, C. Nicco, C. Chéreau et al., "Improvement of the therapeutic index of anticancer drugs by the superoxide dismutase mimic mangafodipir," *Journal of the National Cancer Institute*, vol. 98, no. 4, pp. 236–244, 2006.

[35] H. H. Zeng, J. F. Lu, and K. Wang, "The effect of cisplatin and transplatin on the conformation and association of F-actin," *Cell Biology International*, vol. 19, no. 6, pp. 491–497, 1995.

[36] M. Karoui, C. Penna, M. Amin-Hashem et al., "Influence of preoperative chemotherapy on the risk of major hepatectomy for colorectal liver metastases," *Annals of Surgery*, vol. 243, no. 1, pp. 1–7, 2006.

[37] T. Aloia, M. Sebagh, M. Plasse et al., "Liver histology and surgical outcomes after preoperative chemotherapy with fluorouracil plus oxaliplatin in colorectal cancer liver metastases," *Journal of Clinical Oncology*, vol. 24, no. 31, pp. 4983–4990, 2006.

[38] D. A. Kooby, J. Stockman, L. Ben-Porat et al., "Influence of transfusions on perioperative and long-term outcome in patients following hepatic resection for colorectal metastases," *Annals of Surgery*, vol. 237, no. 6, pp. 860–870, 2003.

[39] J. M. Van Der Bol, R. H. Mathijssen, J. Verweij et al., "CYP3A phenotype-based individualized dosing of irinotecan to reduce interindividual variability in pharmacokinetics and toxicity: result from a randomized trial," *Journal of Clinical Oncology*, vol. 26, abstract 2506, 2008.

[40] L. Iyer, S. Das, L. Janisch et al., "UGT1A1∗28 polymorphism as a determinant of irinotecan disposition and toxicity," *Pharmacogenomics Journal*, vol. 2, no. 1, pp. 43–47, 2002.

[41] D. M. Kweekel, H. Gelderblom, and H.-J. Guchelaar, "Pharmacology of oxaliplatin and the use of pharmacogenomics to individualize therapy," *Cancer Treatment Reviews*, vol. 31, no. 2, pp. 90–105, 2005.

[42] Y. Kodama, C. S. Ng, T. T. Wu et al., "Comparison of CT methods for determining the fat content of the liver," *American Journal of Roentgenology*, vol. 188, no. 5, pp. 1307–1312, 2007.

[43] C. S. Cho, S. Curran, L. H. Schwartz et al., "Preoperative radiographic assessment of hepatic steatosis with histologic correlation," *Journal of the American College of Surgeons*, vol. 206, no. 3, pp. 480–488, 2008.

[44] S. Kopetz and J.-N. Vauthey, "Perioperative chemotherapy for resectable hepatic metastases," *The Lancet*, vol. 371, no. 9617, pp. 963–965, 2008.

[45] F. K. S. Welsh, H. S. Tilney, P. P. Tekkis, T. G. John, and M. Rees, "Safe liver resection following chemotherapy for colorectal metastases is a matter of timing," *British Journal of Cancer*, vol. 96, no. 7, pp. 1037–1042, 2007.

[46] D. Ribero, E. K. Abdalla, D. C. Madoff, M. Donadon, E. M. Loyer, and J.-N. Vauthey, "Portal vein embolization before major hepatectomy and its effects on regeneration, resectability and outcome," *British Journal of Surgery*, vol. 94, no. 11, pp. 1386–1394, 2007.

[47] G. Morris-Stiff, Y.-M. Tan, and J. N. Vauthey, "Hepatic complications following preoperative chemotherapy with oxaliplatin or irinotecan for hepatic colorectal metastases," *European Journal of Surgical Oncology*, vol. 34, no. 6, pp. 609–614, 2008.

[48] L. Rubbia-Brandt, G. Y. Lauwers, H. Wang et al., "Sinusoidal obstruction syndrome and nodular regenerative hyperplasia are frequent oxaliplatin-associated liver lesions and partially prevented by bevacizumab in patients with hepatic colorectal metastasis," *Histopathology*, vol. 56, no. 4, pp. 430–439, 2010.

[49] A. E. M. van der Pool, H. A. Marsman, J. Verheij et al., "Effect of bevacizumab added preoperatively to oxaliplatin on liver injury and complications after resection of colorectal liver metastases," *Journal of Surgical Oncology*, vol. 106, no. 7, pp. 892–897, 2012.

[50] D. S. Pratt, T. A. Knox, and J. Erban, "Tamoxifen-induced steatohepatitis," *Annals of Internal Medicine*, vol. 123, no. 3, p. 236, 1995.

[51] A. Grieco, A. Forgione, L. Miele et al., "Fatty liver and drugs," *European Review for Medical and Pharmacological Sciences*, vol. 9, no. 5, pp. 261–263, 2005.

[52] S. Bruno, P. Maisonneuve, P. Castellana et al., "Incidence and risk factors for non-alcoholic steatohepatitis: prospective study of 5408 women enrolled in Italian tamoxifen chemoprevention trial," *British Medical Journal*, vol. 330, no. 7497, pp. 932–935, 2005.

[53] T. Saphner, S. Triest-Robertson, H. Li, and P. Holzman, "The association of nonalcoholic steatohepatitis and tamoxifen in patients with breast cancer," *Cancer*, vol. 115, no. 14, pp. 3189–3195, 2009.

[54] M. H. Ahmed and C. D. Byrne, "Non-alcoholic steatoheptatitis," in *Metabolic Syndrome*, C. D. Byrne and S. Wild, Eds., pp. 279–303, John Wiley & Sons, London, UK, 2005.

[55] M. H. Ahmed and K. A. Osman, "Tamoxifen induced-non-alcoholic steatohepatitis (NASH): has the time come for the oncologist to be diabetologist," *Breast Cancer Research and Treatment*, vol. 97, no. 2, pp. 223–224, 2006.

[56] D. Pessayre, B. Fromenty, and A. Mansouri, "Mitochondrial injury in steatohepatitis," *European Journal of Gastroenterology and Hepatology*, vol. 16, no. 11, pp. 1095–1105, 2004.

[57] T. Ohnishi, Y. Ogawa, T. Saibara et al., "CYP17 polymorphism and tamoxifen-induced hepatic steatosis," *Hepatology Research*, vol. 33, no. 2, pp. 178–180, 2005.

[58] N. Günel, U. Coşkun, F. B. Toruner et al., "Serum leptin levels are associated with tamoxifen-induced hepatic steatosis," *Current Medical Research and Opinion*, vol. 19, no. 1, pp. 47–50, 2003.

[59] A. Inno, M. Basso, F. M. Vecchio et al., "Anastrozole-related acute hepatitis with autoimmune features: a case report," *BMC Gastroenterology*, vol. 31, no. 11, p. 32, 2011.

[60] L. de la Cruz, J. Romero-Vazquez, M. Jiménez-Sáenz, J. R. A. Padron, and J. M. Herrerias-Gutierrez, "Severe acute hepatitis in a patient treated with anastrozole," *The Lancet*, vol. 369, no. 9555, pp. 23–24, 2007.

[61] N. U. Lin, L. A. Carey, M. C. Liu et al., "Phase II trial of lapatinib for brain metastases in patients with human epidermal growth factor receptor 2-positive breast cancer," *Journal of Clinical Oncology*, vol. 26, no. 12, pp. 1993–1999, 2008.

[62] S. Peroukides, T. Makatsoris, A. Koutras et al., "Lapatinib-induced hepatitis: a case report," *World Journal of Gastroenterology*, vol. 17, no. 18, pp. 2349–2352, 2011.

[63] C. F. Spraggs, L. R. Budde, L. P. Briley et al., "HLA-DQA1*02:01 is a major risk factor for lapatinib-induced hepatotoxicity in women with advanced breast cancer," *Journal of Clinical Oncology*, vol. 29, no. 6, pp. 667–673, 2011.

[64] J. S. Weber, K. C. Kähler, and A. Hauschild, "Management of immune-related adverse events and kinetics of response with ipilimumab," *Journal of Clinical Oncology*, vol. 30, no. 21, pp. 2691–2997, 2012.

[65] C. Robert, L. Thomas, I. Bondarenko et al., "Ipilimumab plus dacarbazine for previously untreated metastatic melanoma," *The New England Journal of Medicine*, vol. 364, no. 26, pp. 2517–2526, 2011.

[66] J. D. Wolchok, B. Neyns, G. Linette et al., "Ipilimumab monotherapy in patients with pretreated advanced melanoma: a randomised, double-blind, multicentre, phase 2, dose-ranging study," *The Lancet Oncology*, vol. 11, no. 2, pp. 155–164, 2010.

[67] C. Guha and B. D. Kavanagh, "Hepatic radiation toxicity: avoidance and amelioration," *Seminars in Radiation Oncology*, vol. 21, no. 4, pp. 256–263, 2011.

[68] G. B. Reed Jr. and A. J. Cox Jr., "The human liver after radiation injury. A form of veno-occlusive disease," *American Journal of Pathology*, vol. 48, no. 4, pp. 597–611, 1966.

[69] S.-X. Liang, X.-D. Zhu, Z.-Y. Xu et al., "Radiation-induced liver disease in three-dimensional conformal radiation therapy for primary liver carcinoma: the risk factors and hepatic radiation tolerance," *International Journal of Radiation Oncology Biology Physics*, vol. 65, no. 2, pp. 426–434, 2006.

[70] Z.-Y. Xu, S.-X. Liang, J. Zhu et al., "Prediction of radiation-induced liver disease by Lyman normal-tissue complication probability model in three-dimensional conformal radiation therapy for primary liver carcinoma," *International Journal of Radiation Oncology Biology Physics*, vol. 65, no. 1, pp. 189–195, 2006.

[71] J. C.-H. Cheng, J.-K. Wu, C.-M. Huang et al., "Radiation-induced liver disease after three-dimensional conformal radiotherapy for patients with hepatocellular carcinoma: dosimetric analysis and implication," *International Journal of Radiation Oncology Biology Physics*, vol. 54, no. 1, pp. 156–162, 2002.

[72] T. S. Lawrence, "Hepatic toxicity resulting from cancer treatment," *International Journal of Radiation Oncology Biology Physics*, vol. 31, no. 5, pp. 1237–1248, 1995.

[73] B. Sangro, M. Iñarrairaegui, and J. I. Bilbao, "Radioembolization for hepatocellular carcinoma," *Journal of Hepatology*, vol. 56, no. 2, pp. 464–473, 2012.

[74] M. Iarrairaegui, K. G. Thurston, J. I. Bilbao et al., "Radioembolization with use of yttrium-90 resin microspheres in patients with hepatocellular carcinoma and portal vein thrombosis," *Journal of Vascular and Interventional Radiology*, vol. 21, no. 8, pp. 1205–1212, 2010.

[75] A. O. Chan, M.-F. Yuen, C.-K. Hui, W.-K. Tso, and C.-L. Lai, "A prospective study regarding the complications of transcatheter intraarterial lipiodol chemoembolization in patients with hepatocellular carcinoma," *Cancer*, vol. 94, no. 6, pp. 1747–1752, 2002.

[76] R. C. Gaba, A. Riaz, R. J. Lewandowski et al., "Safety of yttrium-90 microsphere radioembolization in patients with biliary obstruction," *Journal of Vascular and Interventional Radiology*, vol. 21, no. 8, pp. 1213–1218, 2010.

[77] J. I. Bilbao, A. De Martino, E. De Luis et al., "Biocompatibility, inflammatory response, and recannalization characteristics of nonradioactive resin microspheres: histological findings," *CardioVascular and Interventional Radiology*, vol. 32, no. 4, pp. 727–736, 2009.

[78] J. Furuse, H. Ishii, M. Nagase, M. Kawashima, T. Ogino, and M. Yoshino, "Adverse hepatic events caused by radiotherapy for advanced hepatocellular carcinoma," *Journal of Gastroenterology and Hepatology*, vol. 20, no. 10, pp. 1512–1518, 2005.

[79] W.-Y. Lau, A. S. Kennedy, Y. H. Kim et al., "Patient selection and activity planning guide for selective internal radiotherapy with yttrium-90 resin microspheres," *International Journal of Radiation Oncology Biology Physics*, vol. 82, no. 1, pp. 401–407, 2012.

[80] B. Sangro, B. Gil-Alzugaray, J. Rodriguez et al., "Liver disease induced by radioembolization of liver tumors: description and possible risk factors," *Cancer*, vol. 112, no. 7, pp. 1538–1546, 2008.

[81] R. Salem, R. J. Lewandowski, M. F. Mulcahy et al., "Radioembolization for hepatocellular carcinoma using yttrium-90 microspheres: a comprehensive report of long-term outcomes," *Gastroenterology*, vol. 138, no. 1, pp. 52–64, 2010.

[82] B. Sangro, L. Carpanese, R. Cianni et al., "Survival after Yttrium-90 resin microsphere radioembolization of hepatocellular carcinoma across Barcelona clinic liver cancer stages: a European evaluation," *Hepatology*, vol. 54, no. 3, pp. 868–878, 2011.

3

Fructose Induced Endotoxemia in Pediatric Nonalcoholic Fatty Liver Disease

Ran Jin,[1] Andrew Willment,[1] Shivani S. Patel,[2] Xiaoyan Sun,[3] Ming Song,[4] Yanci O. Mannery,[4] Astrid Kosters,[1] Craig J. McClain,[4,5] and Miriam B. Vos[1,6]

[1] *Department of Pediatrics, School of Medicine, Emory University, 2015 Uppergate Drive NE, Atlanta, GA 30322, USA*
[2] *Medical University of South Carolina, Charleston, SC 29425, USA*
[3] *Department of Statistics, Emory University, Atlanta, GA 30322, USA*
[4] *School of Medicine, University of Louisville, Louisville, KY 40202, USA*
[5] *Robley Rex Louisville VAMC, Louisville, KY 40206, USA*
[6] *Children's Healthcare of Atlanta, Atlanta, GA 30329, USA*

Correspondence should be addressed to Miriam B. Vos; mvos@emory.edu

Academic Editor: Matthias Bahr

In preclinical studies of fructose-induced NAFLD, endotoxin appears to play an important role. We retrospectively examined samples from three pediatric cohorts (1) to investigate whether endotoxemia is associated with the presence of hepatic steatosis; (2) to evaluate postprandial endotoxin levels in response to fructose beverage in an acute 24-hour feeding challenge, and (3) to determine the change of fasting endotoxin amounts in a 4-week randomized controlled trial comparing fructose to glucose beverages in NAFLD. We found that adolescents with hepatic steatosis had elevated endotoxin levels compared to obese controls and that the endotoxin level correlated with insulin resistance and several inflammatory cytokines. In a 24-hour feeding study, endotoxin levels in NAFLD adolescents increased after fructose beverages (consumed with meals) as compared to healthy children. Similarly, endotoxin was significantly increased after adolescents consumed fructose beverages for 2 weeks and remained high although not significantly at 4 weeks. In conclusion, these data provide support for the concept of low level endotoxemia contributing to pediatric NAFLD and the possible role of fructose in this process. Further studies are needed to determine if manipulation of the microbiome or other methods of endotoxin reduction would be useful as a therapy for pediatric NAFLD.

1. Introduction

Nonalcoholic fatty liver disease (NAFLD) is a leading cause of chronic liver disease and is estimated to affect 40% of obese adolescents in the United States [1]. In adults with NAFLD, circulating endotoxin (lipopolysaccharide or LPS) has been reported to be elevated [2, 3]. Endogenous antibodies against endotoxin are also increased in adults with biopsy-proven nonalcoholic steatohepatitis (NASH), suggesting chronic exposure [4]. However, studies in the pediatric population remain scarce and it is less clear whether or not endotoxin is an important mediator of NAFLD in the early forms of the disease as seen in children. A study by Alisi et al. found increased endotoxin levels among children with NAFLD compared to healthy weight controls [5], but endotoxin could also be associated with obesity *per se* [6, 7], thus warranting further examination.

Animal models have demonstrated that a high-fructose regimen causes increased portal blood endotoxin levels and hepatic steatosis [8, 9]. In mice, reduction of endotoxin using oral antibiotics improved both hepatic steatosis and inflammation [9]. In spite of the growing body of evidence associating fructose with endotoxemia and the metabolic syndrome from preclinical studies, data from human studies on fructose and endotoxin are scarce. In particular, adolescents are an important group to focus on because of their high intake of fructose [10] and the increased prevalence of NAFLD [1].

In the current study, we utilized stored samples from three separate cohorts and sought to answer two distinct questions: (1) are endotoxin levels increased in adolescents with NAFLD (as shown in adults)? (2) Is there a link between fructose consumption and endotoxin levels in adolescents with NAFLD?

2. Methods

2.1. Subjects and Study Design. This analysis utilized data and samples from a cross-sectional study and two prospective studies of fructose consumption in adolescents with and without NAFLD. The primary outcomes have been previously reported by our research group [11, 12]; however, endotoxin levels have not been evaluated and associated with NAFLD. All studies were approved by the Emory University and Children's Healthcare of Atlanta IRB, and written informed consent (parental consent obtained for subjects <18 years) and assent (when applicable) were obtained for each subject prior to initiation of the study.

Cohort 1 was comprised of 43 Hispanic, obese (BMI z-score ≥ 95th percentile for age and gender) adolescents (aged 11–18 years), who had self-reported high consumption of sweet beverages (at least 3 servings of 12 fl oz per day on average). Because both Hispanic ethnicity [13] and high intake of sweet beverages [14] have been reported to be risk factors for hepatic steatosis, we were able to recruit a group of adolescents in this cohort who were likely to have increased risk of significant steatosis but who had not been previously diagnosed or treated for NAFLD. The subjects and exclusion criteria were carefully described in a previously published article [12]. All recruited participants underwent magnetic resonance spectroscopy (MRS) to quantify their hepatic fat. Subjects with hepatic fat > 5% were considered as having steatosis [15] ($n = 32$), or they were classified as obese controls ($n = 11$) if MRS-documented hepatic fat < 5%.

Cohort 2 included a total of 15 adolescents, with 8 being biopsy-proven NAFLD (7 were NASH) and 7 being matched healthy controls. The study design was described elsewhere in detail [11]. Briefly, it was a 24-hour, randomized, crossover feeding study and participants were randomized to either glucose or fructose beverages at visit 1 and the other sugar beverage at visit 2. For each of two visits, subjects arrived at the inpatient research unit after overnight fasting (>12 hours) and consecutively consumed three study-provided standardized meals (containing 50% carbohydrates, 30% fat, and 20% protein) for breakfast (0800 h), lunch (1200 h), and dinner (1600 h), along with either high fructose or glucose (33% of total estimated daily calories) beverages. Their blood samples were drawn at 0800 h (baseline) before feeding, 1 h after breakfast, and, subsequently, every 2 h until the following morning except at 0400 h to allow the adolescents to sleep. Subjects with nonhemolyzed baseline samples and sufficient postprandial samples were included for the analysis of endotoxin.

Cohort 3 was a subgroup of adolescents from cohort 1 who had elevated hepatic fat (>8% by MRS) and consented to participate in a 4-week calorie-matched, randomized, controlled trial. Randomization and study design in detail can be retrieved at clinicaltrials.gov, NCT01188083, and from our previous publication [12]. In brief, subjects were randomly assigned to study-provided fructose or glucose beverages (3 servings of 12 fl oz bottles each day) to replace their usual consumption of sweet beverages. These beverages contained 33 grams of sugar (standard amount of sugar in a typical soda) in the form of either glucose or fructose, matched for color and flavoring (Power Brands, Beverly Hills, CA). Follow-up visits were scheduled at 2 and 4 weeks after the initiation of randomization to monitor body weight and hepatic fat. Fasting blood samples were also collected for the evaluation of metabolic parameters. At the time of the endotoxin study, a total of 16 subjects had sufficient, nonhemolyzed blood samples available from baseline, 2 and 4 weeks.

2.2. Measurement of Hepatic Fat. Hepatic fat was assessed by MRS using a rapid 15 sec acquisition technique obtained during a single breath hold [16]. The sequence is constructed from five concatenated echoes using a fixed set of echo times (TE) (12, 24, 36, 48, and 72 ms), with each echo having a repetition time (TR) = 3000 ms, voxel = $3 \times 3 \times 3\,\text{cm}^3$, 1024 points, and 1200 Hz bandwidth. Data were exported off-line for automatic processing with in-house software (Matlab, MathWorks, Natick, MA). Water and lipid magnitude spectra were analyzed by determining the area under the curve (AUC) corresponding to a user-defined frequency range surrounding the corresponding water/lipid peaks (water peak: 4.6 ppm; lipid peak: 1.3, 2.0 ppm). The integrated magnitude signals at each TE were fit to exponential $T2$ decay curves, whereby the equilibrium signal (M0) and the relaxation rate ($R2 = 1/T2$) were determined by least-squares regression approximation. Using M0 for water and lipid, the $T2$-corrected hepatic lipid fraction was calculated from % hepatic lipid = M0lipid/(M0lipid + M0water).

2.3. Laboratory Measurement. Serum alanine aminotransferase (ALT) and aspartate aminotransferase (AST) were examined by the Emory University Hospital clinical laboratory. Plasma glucose, insulin, and high sensitivity C-reactive protein (hs-CRP) were measured with immunoturbidimetric methods (Sekisui Diagnostics, Exton, PA) using AU480 chemistry analyzer (Beckman Coulter), by the Emory Lipid Research Laboratory. Plasma tumor necrosis factor-α (TNF-α) and monocyte chemoattractant protein-1 (MCP-1) were determined with multianalyte chemiluminescence detection using Luminex xMap technology (Millipore Corporation, St. Louis, MO). Endotoxin levels were evaluated by colorimetric assay. Plasma samples were diluted 2-fold in pyrogen-free water, mixed, and heated at 75°C for 10 min to remove nonspecific inhibitors of endotoxin. Samples were allowed to cool to room temperature before the colorimetric assay using the limulus amoebocyte lysate (LAL) kit (Lonza Walkersville, MD). Standards and samples were incubated with LAL for 10 min at 37°C followed by 6 min incubation with colorimetric substrate. The reaction was stopped with 25% acetic acid, and the absorbance was read at 405 nm.

2.4. Insulin Resistance Index. Insulin resistance was assessed by the homeostasis model of assessment—insulin resistance (HOMA-IR), which was calculated by glucose (mmol/L) × insulin (mU/L)/22.5 at fasting state.

2.5. Statistical Analyses. Statistical analyses were performed using SAS 9.1. Results in tables were expressed as mean (SD) unless indicated otherwise. Data were examined for normality and equal variance prior to any analyses. Independent two sample t-tests or alternatively Mann-Whitney tests (if not normally distributed) were used for comparison between adolescents with and without hepatic steatosis and between adolescents randomized to glucose or fructose beverage groups. Multiple linear regression models were performed to adjust metabolic parameters including BMI z-score, HOMA-IR, and hs-CRP. Paired t-tests were conducted to determine the significance of percent change in endotoxin levels at weeks 2 and 4, as compared to baseline. The correlations of endotoxin were examined using bivariate correlation tests. In the feeding study, the 9-hour (9-h) and 23-hour (23-h) incremental areas under the curve (IAUC) were calculated for endotoxin by using the trapezoidal method, and independent comparisons were performed for each single time point between NAFLD and non-NAFLD subjects.

3. Results

3.1. Cross-Sectional Comparison of Fasting Endotoxin Level (Cohort 1). Anthropometrics and laboratory parameters for the 32 obese adolescents with hepatic steatosis and the 11 obese adolescents without hepatic steatosis are reported in Table 1. There were no significant differences in age, gender, body weight, BMI z-score, and hs-CRP between the two groups. Adolescents with hepatic steatosis (>5% by MRS) had increased ALT ($P = 0.021$), AST ($P < 0.001$), fasting insulin ($P = 0.010$), and insulin resistance as assessed by HOMA-IR ($P = 0.013$) compared with obese control adolescents. The plasma concentration of endotoxin in obese adolescents without hepatic steatosis averaged 1.22 ± 0.30 EU/mL (mean ± SD, ranging from 0.64 to 1.61 EU/mL), while in participants with steatosis, the mean endotoxin level was significantly increased to 1.54 ± 0.52 EU/mL (mean ± SD, ranging from 0.85 to 2.83 EU/mL) ($P = 0.019$) (Figure 1(a)). In multiple linear regression models, we found that the difference in endotoxin levels between subjects with and without steatosis remained significant after adjusting for BMI z-score ($P = 0.036$) and for hs-CRP ($P = 0.042$), respectively, but was blunted after the adjustment for HOMA-IR ($P = 0.068$) and for the cluster of HOMA-IR, BMI z-score, and hs-CRP ($P = 0.056$).

We further examined TNF-α and MCP-1 levels on a subgroup of subjects who had sufficient blood samples available. We found that adolescents with steatosis had a trend towards higher TNF-α (mean ± SD: 5.46 ± 1.89 versus 4.42±2.28 pg/mL, $P = 0.18$) and significantly increased MCP-1 (mean ± SD: 150 ± 46.4 versus 126 ± 18.5 pg/mL, $P = 0.034$) compared to their obese controls (Figures 1(b) and 1(c)) and that plasma endotoxin amount was positively correlated with TNF-α ($r = 0.471, P = 0.006$), MCP-1 ($r = 0.337, P = 0.047$), and HOMA-IR ($r = 0.381, P = 0.013$).

3.2. Endotoxin Response to Acute Feeding Challenge (Cohort 2). Next, we evaluated postprandial endotoxin levels in samples from a group of 15 adolescents, 8 of whom had histologically confirmed NAFLD and 7 matched healthy adolescents. Their baseline characteristics are summarized in Table 2. In response to fructose beverages (consumed with meals), adolescents with NAFLD had an acute increase of plasma endotoxin levels after 1, 3, and 5 hours ($P < 0.05$ for all) comparing to non-NAFLD subjects. This resulted in an elevation of 9-h IAUC of postprandial endotoxin in NAFLD compared to their healthy controls (mean ± SE: 6.85 ± 1.49 versus 2.50 ± 0.87, $P = 0.026$). The biggest differences were seen after breakfast and lunch and less variation was seen overnight; thus their 23-h IAUC comparison (mean ± SE: 15.11 ± 3.83 versus 10.19 ± 4.23, $P = 0.23$) did not reach statistical significance (Figure 2(a)). In contrast, no significant difference of postprandial endotoxin in response to glucose beverages (consumed with meals) was observed between adolescents with and without NAFLD (Figure 2(b)).

3.3. Endotoxin Response to 4-Week Beverage Trial (Cohort 3). Finally, we measured endotoxin in samples from adolescents with NAFLD who participated in a 4-week study of fructose beverages compared to glucose beverages. The baseline characteristics of the 16 adolescents with hepatic steatosis who participated in the 4-week beverage trial are presented in Table 3. There were no significant differences in age, gender, weight, glycemic status, and lipid profile between the two groups. Compared to baseline, after drinking 3 study-provided fructose beverages per day, participants had significantly increased fasting plasma endotoxin levels at 2 weeks (mean ± SD: 1.21 ± 0.29 versus 1.45 ± 0.50 EU/mL, $P = 0.018$) and a trend for increased endotoxin at 4 weeks (mean ± SD: 1.21±0.29 versus 1.47±0.53 EU/mL, $P = 0.088$), while adolescents who consumed glucose beverages did not have increased endotoxin levels (mean ± SD: 1.61 ± 0.69, 1.39 ± 0.38, and 1.55 ± 0.55 EU/mL at weeks 0, 2, and 4, resp.) (Figure 3).

4. Discussion

Children and adolescents are an important group in which one can study the mechanisms leading to NAFLD because they have an early, possibly more aggressive form of the disease [17]. In addition, they are less likely to have other chronic diseases which could alter gut permeability as well as endotoxin transfer and/or clearance. Through these analyses, we found that obese adolescents with elevated hepatic steatosis had increased plasma endotoxin levels compared to those with normal hepatic fat (<5% by MRS) even after multiple adjustments for metabolic markers, suggesting a possible role for endotoxin in the mechanism of pediatric NAFLD. Second, we observed that adolescents with NAFLD (mostly NASH) had elevated postprandial endotoxin compared to healthy individuals. Finally, in a 4-week randomized controlled trial,

TABLE 1: Anthropometrics and laboratory parameters of the 32 adolescents with hepatic steatosis and the 11 obese controls at fasting state: study cohort 1.

Parameters, mean (SD)	Obese controls (<5% by MRS, $n = 11$)	Subjects with steatosis (>5% by MRS, $n = 32$)	P value
Age, years	14.3 (1.85)	13.7 (2.65)	0.443
Male (n, %)	4 (36.4)	13 (40.6)	0.803
Weight (kg)	82.9 (21.5)	80.5 (14.9)	0.967
BMI z-score	2.00 (0.22)	2.17 (0.37)	0.129
ALT (U/L)	17.8 (7.60)	49.7 (89.5)	0.021
AST (U/L)	21.9 (3.99)	68.2 (180)	<0.001
Hepatic fat (%)	3.87 (0.62)	11.2 (5.27)	<0.001
Glucose (mmol/L)	5.13 (0.89)	5.18 (0.90)	0.978
Insulin (mU/L)	18.2 (6.69)	36.2 (30.5)	0.010
HOMA-IR	4.06 (1.31)	8.79 (9.13)	0.013
hs-CRP (mg/L)	3.17 (3.44)	4.98 (5.92)	0.278

BMI: body mass index; ALT: alanine aminotransferase; AST: aspartate aminotransferase; HOMA-IR: homeostatic model assessment for insulin resistance, calculated as fasting glucose (mmol/L) × insulin (mU/L)/22.5; hs-CRP: high sensitivity C-reactive protein.

TABLE 2: Baseline characteristics of the 8 adolescents with biopsy-proven NAFLD and the 7 healthy controls: study cohort 2.

Parameters, mean (SD)	non-NAFLD ($n = 7$)	NAFLD ($n = 8$)	P value
Age, years	13.7 (2.22)	13.0 (2.73)	0.315
Male, n (%)	5 (71.4)	8 (100)	0.104
BMI z-score	0.18 (0.65)	2.29 (0.38)	0.001
Hepatic fat, %	1.02 (1.18)	22.0 (6.16)	0.001
ALT (U/L)	14.6 (2.51)	130 (63.2)	0.001
AST (U/L)	23.4 (4.30)	79.6 (40.6)	0.001
Glucose (mmol/L)	5.53 (0.40)	5.32 (1.06)	0.487
Insulin (mU/L)	9.67 (12.4)	42.7 (27.7)	0.005
HOMA-IR	2.27 (2.70)	10.2 (6.99)	0.016
hs-CRP (mg/L)	0.25 (0.49)	2.95 (3.33)	0.004

BMI: body mass index; ALT: alanine aminotransferase; AST: aspartate aminotransferase; HOMA-IR: homeostatic model assessment for insulin resistance, calculated as fasting glucose (mmol/L) × insulin (mU/L)/22.5; hs-CRP: high sensitivity C-reactive protein.

TABLE 3: Baseline characteristics of participants enrolled in the 4-week beverage trial: study cohort 3.

Parameters, mean (SD)	Fructose ($n = 8$)	Glucose ($n = 8$)	P value
Age (years)	14.6 (2.50)	13.3 (2.32)	0.273
Male, n (%)	3 (37.5)	4 (50.0)	0.614
Body weight (kg)	86.1 (13.3)	81.3 (15.9)	0.521
BMI z-score	2.32 (0.56)	2.01 (0.26)	0.184
Hepatic fat (%)	14.5 (5.73)	12.1 (4.82)	0.382
ALT (U/L)	35.1 (20.5)	31.3 (18.6)	0.698
AST (U/L)	32.1 (9.76)	32.9 (7.45)	0.865
Triglycerides (mmol/L)	161 (111)	175 (58.5)	0.768
Cholesterol (mmol/L)	166 (28.8)	170 (48.8)	0.836
LDL (mmol/L)	106 (32.5)	105 (38.6)	0.967
HDL (mmol/L)	45.1 (9.84)	45.0 (9.83)	0.986
FFA (mmol/L)	0.97 (0.24)	1.16 (0.51)	0.342
Glucose (mmol/L)	5.46 (0.85)	4.97 (1.59)	0.461
Insulin (mU/L)	30.0 (13.7)	31.4 (30.5)	0.906
HOMA-IR	7.17 (3.03)	7.23 (8.28)	0.985
hs-CRP (mg/L)	4.22 (3.03)	3.16 (2.54)	0.242

ALT: alanine aminotransferase; AST: aspartate aminotransferase; LDL: low-density lipoprotein; HDL: high-density lipoprotein; FFA: free fatty acid; HOMA-IR: homeostatic model assessment for insulin resistance index, calculated as fasting glucose (mg/dL) × insulin (μU/L)/405; hs-CRP: high sensitivity C-reactive protein.

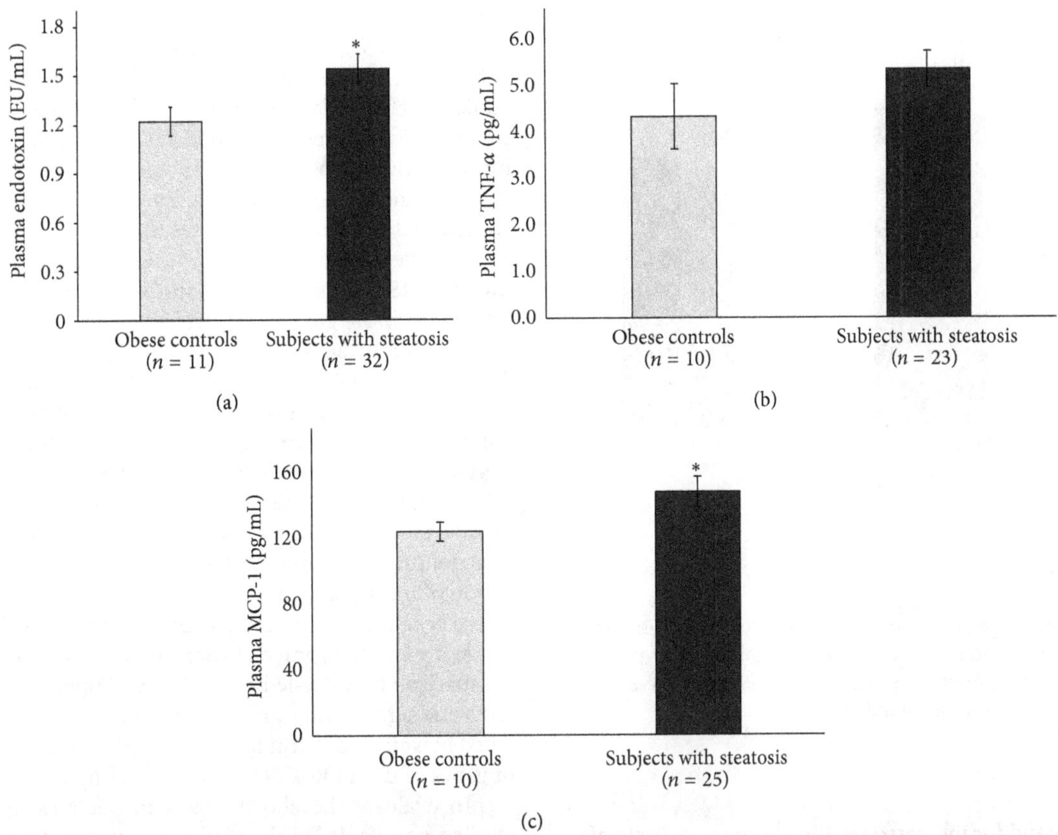

FIGURE 1: Obese adolescents with hepatic steatosis (>5% by MRS) had increased (a) plasma endotoxin levels, (b) plasma TNF-α levels, and (c) plasma MCP-1 levels as compared to obese adolescents without significant steatosis (hepatic fat < 5% by MRS); $^{*}P < 0.05$.

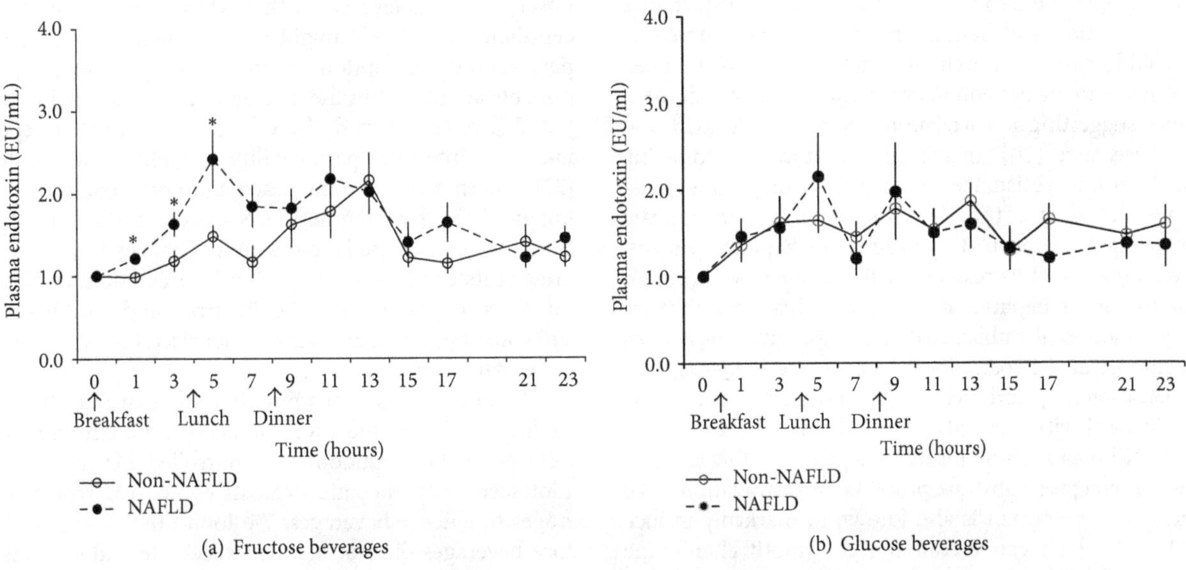

FIGURE 2: Postprandial plasma endotoxin levels in response to (a) fructose and (b) glucose beverages given with breakfast, lunch, and dinner. The solid line represents 7 children without NAFLD and the dashed line shows the response in 8 children with biopsy-proven NAFLD. Baseline values were set as reference (1.0) and the following time points represent the ratio to baseline. $^{*}P < 0.05$ when comparing NAFLD and non-NAFLD subjects at given time point.

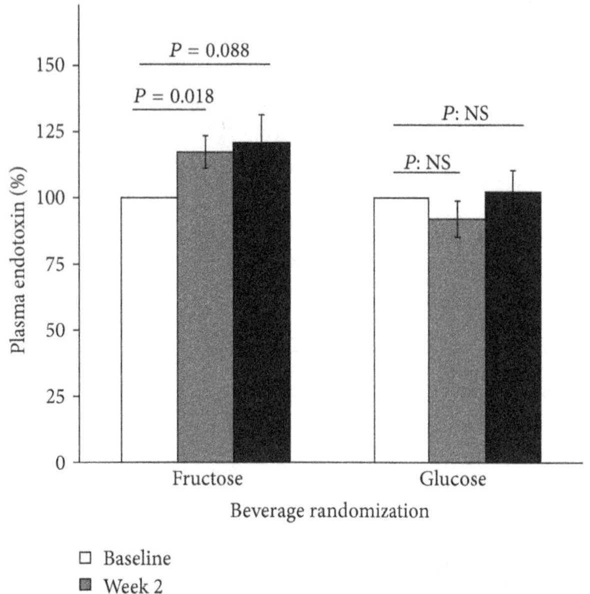

FIGURE 3: Percentage change of plasma endotoxin level in adolescents with NAFLD after 2- and 4-week ingestion of study-provided fructose or glucose-only beverages. Baseline values were set as reference (100%). Error bars stand for SE.

we found a trend for increased fasting plasma endotoxin after exposure to fructose drinks.

A previous study by Alisi et al. suggested that endotoxin levels were increased in pediatric NAFLD compared to healthy weight subjects [5]. We compared endotoxin levels in a weight and ethnicity matched cohort because obesity has been indicated to be associated with dysfunction/disturbance of the gastrointestinal barrier and consequently increased entry of endotoxin into the circulation [18, 19]. It has also been shown that diabetic patients appear to have higher endotoxin amounts suggesting a correlation between endotoxin and insulin resistance [20]. In the current study, by adjusting for BMI, insulin resistance, and inflammatory marker hs-CRP, we found that the elevation of endotoxin appears to be strongly related to the presence of hepatic steatosis. Both endotoxin and its resultant inflammatory perturbation appear to trigger hepatic and peripheral insulin resistance [21]. Agwunobi et al. published data using euglycemic clamps that demonstrated hepatic insulin resistance following LPS administration [22], and Mehta et al. reported a 35% decrease in insulin sensitivity induced by endotoxemia [23]. Cytokines such as TNF-α can inhibit insulin receptor signaling and target insulin receptor substrate proteins for degradation [24]. Furthermore, endotoxin is also known to markedly induce MCP-1 [25] which can recruit the C-C motif chemokine receptor-2 (CCR2)-expressing monocytes in adipose tissue, and CCR2 associates adipose tissue inflammation and systemic insulin resistance [26]. However, given the fact that NAFLD (particularly in its advanced form NASH) has a nearly universal interrelationship with obesity, insulin resistance, and inflammation, it is difficult to distinguish between the effects of endotoxemia on hepatic fat (NAFLD) and its coexisting metabolic morbidities.

The idea that fructose induced endotoxin might contribute to NAFLD has been studied in animal models and adults, but little data were previously available in children. In a fructose fed mouse model, antibiotics reduced fructose induced endotoxin in the portal blood and improved hepatic steatosis and inflammation [9]. Subsequent studies demonstrated that endotoxin stimulates the innate immune system via toll-like receptor 4 (TLR4) to increase inflammation in the liver [8]. In mechanism studies, increased endotoxin release from the gut can activate TLR4 to stimulate myeloid differentiation factor 88 (MyD88) [27]. This interaction of TLR4 and MyD88 triggers the downstream signaling cascade leading to the activation of the nuclear factor κB (NF-κB) pathway, further releasing inflammatory cytokines such as TNF-α and IL-6, which, in turn, can result in liver injury [27]. Furthermore, animals with NAFLD have been shown to have partial loss of the tight junction protein, occluden-1, contributing to increased intestinal permeability and translocation of intestinal endotoxin [28]. Fructose could make this worse because tight junction proteins have been shown to be markedly lower in mice chronically exposed to fructose in comparison to water-fed controls [29]. Supporting this, mice fed with significantly greater amounts of fructose had elevated plasma endotoxin levels and higher hepatic expression of genes of the TLR-4-dependent signaling cascade [30].

To evaluate the above effects in pediatric NAFLD, we studied endotoxin levels in two situations: after acute consumption of fructose and after weeks of fructose beverages. Both NAFLD and non-NAFLD subjects had an acute elevation of postprandial endotoxin concentrations after fructose beverages (consumed with meals) in the 24-hour acute feeding challenge, but there was a significantly higher response observed in adolescents with NAFLD. This increased susceptibility in NAFLD might be explained by increased gut permeability, disruption of intestinal tight junctions, and possible alterations in the microbiome as indicated in adults [28, 31]. A recent study by Giorgio et al. further reported increased intestinal permeability in children with NAFLD [32]. Alternatively, the increased endotoxin could be due to impaired Kupffer cell function. Normally, endotoxin released from the gut is cleared rapidly on first pass by Kupffer cells to prevent its escape into the systemic circulation. In NAFLD, this hepatic clearance may be disturbed and insufficient [33] and could be responsible for the increased level of circulating endotoxin.

Because we saw postprandial increases in the acute feeding challenge study, we evaluated endotoxin in a longer, calorie-matched, randomized controlled beverage trial in adolescents with hepatic steatosis comparing fructose beverages to glucose beverages. We found that 4 weeks of glucose beverages did not further exacerbate endotoxin levels, while continuous provision of fructose beverages resulted in elevation of endotoxin after just 2 weeks with a trend towards an increase at 4 weeks (no longer significant because of subject variability). A pilot study in adults also showed a decrease in endotoxin in response to fructose reduction, although over 6 months. In that study, subjects with NAFLD who consumed 50% less fructose compared to baseline had significantly lower levels of endotoxin as well as hepatic lipid contents [34]. However, causality could not be proven because the subjects also lost weight. In our trial, the body weights remained stable from baseline to the end of the intervention. Putting our data together with the previous studies, it appears possible that when subjects are chronically exposed to a high fructose environment, endotoxemia and subsequent activation of inflammatory cytokines occur and promote insulin resistance in the liver thus contributing to NAFLD.

Strengths of our studies include (1) the well-matched cohorts allowing us to isolate the effect of NAFLD and examine its associations; (2) the precise measurement of hepatic steatosis by MRS; and (3) the utilization of an inpatient feeding study methodology conducted in a metabolic unit. Importantly, in both cohorts 2 and 3, the experiments were randomized, controlled tests of fructose administration in comparison to a calorically matched beverage (glucose drinks). This methodology provides the strongest evidence that fructose is possibly causing the differences seen.

There were several limitations in these studies. Our subjects in cohort 1 are Hispanic-American adolescents; thus our findings may not be generalizable to other racial and ethnic groups, particularly African-American children, who develop NAFLD less often. In our acute feeding challenge study (cohort 2), endotoxemia peaked rapidly after meals and normalized overnight. Because we measured blood every two hours, we may have missed the true peak level(s) of endotoxin. Further, we were unable to determine if endotoxin was elevated because of slower clearance or increased translocation into the bloodstream and whether this increase of endotoxin was caused by the presence of hepatic steatosis or its closely associated metabolic perturbations. In the 4-week randomized controlled trial (cohort 3), it is possible that participants made other changes to their diets in response to the research beverages even though they were requested to keep their diet pattern. Finally, the study did not include stool so we were unable to assess if the endotoxin changes seen were secondary to a change in the microbiota.

In conclusion, we demonstrated that exposure to high fructose both acutely (postprandial) and chronically (2 weeks) is associated with an increase of circulating endotoxin in adolescents with NAFLD, and we also demonstrated correlations of endotoxin with markers of insulin resistance and inflammation. Fructose reduction is a feasible side-effect-free strategy for patients with NAFLD to prevent disease progression. However, further studies will be necessary to prove the therapeutic and possibly preventive benefits of fructose reduction.

Acknowledgments

The authors thank all of the patients and their families for generously giving their time. In addition, these studies would not have been possible without the tireless dedication of the research coordinators, Nicholas Raviele, Xiomara Hinson, Rebecca Cleeton, and Jessica Cruz. This work is supported by the National Institutes of Health (NIH)/National Institute of Diabetes and Digestive and Kidney Diseases Grant K23 DK080953 (Vos); NIH: RO1AA018016, 1R01AA018869, 1U01AA021901, 1U01AA021893-01 (McClain); VA: BX000350 Merit Award (McClain); University of Louisville Clinical and Translational Sciences Pilot Grant Program (McClain). The authors' responsibilities are as follows: Miriam B. Vos designed research, supervised study, wrote parts of the paper, and has primary responsibility for final content; Ran Jin performed part of laboratory measurements, analyzed and interpreted the data, and wrote parts of the paper; Andrew Willment, Ming Song, and Yanci O. Mannery performed part of laboratory measurements; Shivani S. Patel contributed to data analyses; Xiaoyan Sun performed and examined the statistical analyses; Astrid Kosters and Craig J. McClain assisted with data interpretation and contributed to the development of the paper.

References

[1] J. A. Welsh, S. Karpen, and M. B. Vos, "Increasing prevalence of nonalcoholic fatty liver disease among united states adolescents, 1988–1994 to 2007–2010," *Journal of Pediatrics*, vol. 162, no. 3, pp. 496.e1-500.e1, 2013.

[2] A. L. Harte, N. F. Da Silva, S. J. Creely et al., "Elevated endotoxin levels in non-alcoholic fatty liver disease," *Journal of Inflammation*, vol. 7, article 15, 2010.

[3] S. Thuy, R. Ladurner, V. Volynets et al., "Nonalcoholic fatty liver disease in humans is associated with increased plasma endotoxin and plasminogen activator inhibitor 1 concentrations and with fructose intake," *Journal of Nutrition*, vol. 138, no. 8, pp. 1452–1455, 2008.

[4] F. J. Verdam, S. S. Rensen, A. Driessen, J. W. Greve, and W. A. Buurman, "Novel evidence for chronic exposure to endotoxin in human nonalcoholic steatohepatitis," *Journal of Clinical Gastroenterology*, vol. 45, no. 2, pp. 149–152, 2011.

[5] A. Alisi, M. Manco, R. Devito, F. Piemonte, and V. Nobili, "Endotoxin and plasminogen activator inhibitor-1 serum levels associated with nonalcoholic steatohepatitis in children," *Journal of Pediatric Gastroenterology and Nutrition*, vol. 50, no. 6, pp. 645–649, 2010.

[6] M. I. Lassenius, K. H. Pietiläinen, K. Kaartinen et al., "Bacterial endotoxin activity in human serum is associated with dyslipidemia, insulin resistance, obesity, and chronic inflammation," *Diabetes Care*, vol. 34, no. 8, pp. 1809–1815, 2011.

[7] T. F. Teixeira, M. C. Collado, C. L. L. F. Ferreira, J. Bressan, and M. D. C. G. Peluzio, "Potential mechanisms for the emerging link between obesity and increased intestinal permeability," *Nutrition Research*, vol. 32, no. 9, pp. 637–647, 2012.

[8] A. Spruss, G. Kanuri, S. Wagnerberger, S. Haub, S. C. Bischoff, and I. Bergheim, "Toll-like receptor 4 is involved in the development of fructose-induced hepatic steatosis in mice," *Hepatology*, vol. 50, no. 4, pp. 1094–1104, 2009.

[9] I. Bergheim, S. Weber, M. Vos et al., "Antibiotics protect against fructose-induced hepatic lipid accumulation in mice: role of endotoxin," *Journal of Hepatology*, vol. 48, no. 6, pp. 983–992, 2008.

[10] M. B. Vos, J. E. Kimmons, C. Gillespie, J. Welsh, and H. M. Blank, "Dietary fructose consumption among US children and adults: the Third National Health and Nutrition Examination Survey," *MedGenMed Medscape General Medicine*, vol. 10, no. 7, article 160, 2008.

[11] R. Jin, N.-A. Le, S. Liu et al., "Children with NAFLD are more sensitive to the adverse metabolic effects of fructose beverages than children without NAFLD," *Journal of Clinical Endocrinology and Metabolism*, vol. 97, no. 7, pp. E1088–E1098, 2012.

[12] R. Jin, J. A. Welsh, N. A. Le et al., "Dietary fructose reduction improves markers of cardiovascular disease risk in Hispanic-American adolescents with NAFLD," *Nutrients*, vol. 6, pp. 3187–3201, 2014.

[13] J. D. Browning, L. S. Szczepaniak, R. Dobbins et al., "Prevalence of hepatic steatosis in an urban population in the United States: impact of ethnicity," *Hepatology*, vol. 40, no. 6, pp. 1387–1395, 2004.

[14] M. B. Vos and J. E. Lavine, "Dietary fructose in nonalcoholic fatty liver disease," *Hepatology*, vol. 57, no. 6, pp. 2525–2531, 2013.

[15] C. M. Leevy, "Fatty liver: a study of 270 patients with biopsy proven fatty liver and review of the literature," *Medicine*, vol. 41, pp. 249–276, 1962.

[16] N. Pineda, P. Sharma, Q. Xu, X. Hu, M. Vos, and D. R. Martin, "Measurement of hepatic lipid: High-speed T2-corrected multi-echo acquisition at 1H MR spectroscopy—a rapid and accurate technique," *Radiology*, vol. 252, no. 2, pp. 568–576, 2009.

[17] A.-X. L. Holterman, G. Guzman, G. Fantuzzi et al., "Nonalcoholic fatty liver disease in severely obese adolescent and adult patients," *Obesity*, vol. 21, no. 3, pp. 591–597, 2013.

[18] T. H. Frazier, J. K. DiBaise, and C. J. McClain, "Gut microbiota, intestinal permeability, obesity-induced inflammation, and liver injury," *Journal of Parenteral and Enteral Nutrition*, vol. 35, no. 5, supplement, pp. 14S–20S, 2011.

[19] P. Brun, I. Castagliuolo, V. Di Leo et al., "Increased intestinal permeability in obese mice: new evidence in the pathogenesis of nonalcoholic steatohepatitis," *The American Journal of Physiology—Gastrointestinal and Liver Physiology*, vol. 292, no. 2, pp. G518–G525, 2007.

[20] S. J. Creely, P. G. McTernan, C. M. Kusminski et al., "Lipopolysaccharide activates an innate immune system response in human adipose tissue in obesity and type 2 diabetes," *The American Journal of Physiology: Endocrinology and Metabolism*, vol. 292, no. 3, pp. E740–E747, 2007.

[21] S. N. van der Crabben, R. M. E. Blümer, M. E. Stegenga et al., "Early endotoxemia increases peripheral and hepatic insulin sensitivity in healthy humans," *The Journal of Clinical Endocrinology & Metabolism*, vol. 94, no. 2, pp. 463–468, 2009.

[22] A. O. Agwunobi, C. Reid, P. Maycock, R. A. Little, and G. L. Carlson, "Insulin resistance mid substrate utilization in human endotoxemia," *Journal of Clinical Endocrinology and Metabolism*, vol. 85, no. 10, pp. 3770–3778, 2000.

[23] N. N. Mehta, F. C. McGillicuddy, P. D. Anderson et al., "Experimental endotoxemia induces adipose inflammation and insulin resistance in humans," *Diabetes*, vol. 59, no. 1, pp. 172–181, 2010.

[24] K. Ueki, T. Kondo, and C. R. Kahn, "Suppressor of cytokine signaling 1 (SOCS-1) and SOCS-3 cause insulin resistance through inhibition of tyrosine phosphorylation of insulin receptor substrate proteins by discrete mechanisms," *Molecular and Cellular Biology*, vol. 24, no. 12, pp. 5434–5446, 2004.

[25] H. Shi, L. Dong, X. Dang et al., "Effect of chlorogenic acid on LPS-induced proinflammatory signaling in hepatic stellate cells," *Inflammation Research*, vol. 62, no. 6, pp. 581–587, 2013.

[26] S. P. Weisberg, D. Hunter, R. Huber et al., "CCR2 modulates inflammatory and metabolic effects of high-fat feeding," *The Journal of Clinical Investigation*, vol. 116, no. 1, pp. 115–124, 2006.

[27] C. Zuany-Amorim, J. Hastewell, and C. Walker, "Toll-like receptors as potential therapeutic targets for multiple diseases," *Nature Reviews Drug Discovery*, vol. 1, no. 10, pp. 797–807, 2002.

[28] L. Miele, V. Valenza, G. La Torre et al., "Increased intestinal permeability and tight junction alterations in nonalcoholic fatty liver disease," *Hepatology*, vol. 49, no. 6, pp. 1877–1887, 2009.

[29] S. Wagnerberger, A. Spruss, G. Kanuri et al., "Toll-like receptors 1-9 are elevated in livers with fructose-induced hepatic steatosis," *British Journal of Nutrition*, vol. 107, no. 12, pp. 1727–1738, 2012.

[30] A. Spruss, G. Kanuri, C. Stahl, S. C. Bischoff, and I. Bergheim, "Metformin protects against the development of fructose-induced steatosis in mice: role of the intestinal barrier function," *Laboratory Investigation*, vol. 92, no. 7, pp. 1020–1032, 2012.

[31] V. Volynets, M. A. Küper, S. Strahl et al., "Nutrition, intestinal permeability, and blood ethanol levels are altered in patients with nonalcoholic fatty liver disease (NAFLD)," *Digestive Diseases and Sciences*, vol. 57, no. 7, pp. 1932–1941, 2012.

[32] V. Giorgio, L. Miele, L. Principessa et al., "Intestinal permeability is increased in children with non-alcoholic fatty liver disease, and correlates with liver disease severity," *Digestive and Liver Disease*, 2014.

[33] G. Baffy, "Kupffer cells in non-alcoholic fatty liver disease: the emerging view," *Journal of Hepatology*, vol. 51, no. 1, pp. 212–223, 2009.

[34] V. Volynets, J. Machann, M. A. Küper et al., "A moderate weight reduction through dietary intervention decreases hepatic fat content in patients with non-alcoholic fatty liver disease (NAFLD): a pilot study," *European Journal of Nutrition*, vol. 52, no. 2, pp. 527–535, 2013.

4

Management of Bleeding in Extrahepatic Portal Venous Obstruction

N. Chaudhary, S. Mehrotra, M. Srivastava, and S. Nundy

Department of Surgical Gastroenterology and Liver Transplantation, Sir Ganga Ram Hospital, Rajinder Nagar, Room No. 2222, SSR Block, New Delhi 110060, India

Correspondence should be addressed to S. Mehrotra; siddharthmehrotra04@gmail.com

Academic Editor: Matthias Bahr

Extrahepatic portal venous obstruction, although rare in the western world, is a common cause of major and life threatening upper gastrointestinal bleeding among the poor in developing countries. Patients have large spleens and stunted growth. The diagnosis is easily confirmed by Doppler ultrasonography. Endoscopy sclerotherapy is the best option for the control of acute variceal bleeding. For secondary prophylaxis of bleeding, the choice lies between repeated sclerotherapy and a portosystemic shunt. We believe that due consideration should be given to performing a splenectomy and a lienorenal shunt. Performed by experienced surgeons, it carries a low operative mortality of 1%, a rebleeding rate of about 10%, removes the large spleen, reverses hypersplenism, and is not followed by portosystemic encephalopathy. Most importantly, it is a onetime procedure particularly suited to those who have little access to blood transfusion and sophisticated medical facilities.

1. Introduction

Extrahepatic portal venous obstruction (EHPVO) is accompanied by replacement of the extrahepatic portal vein by a cavernoma with or without thrombosis of the intrahepatic portal, splenic, or superior mesenteric veins. In developing countries, EHPVO has been reported to be the most common cause of upper gastrointestinal bleeding (UGIB) in children (70% in some reports) and is also a common cause of variceal bleeding in adults [1]. In western countries, EHPVO is second only to cirrhosis as a cause of portal hypertension, but its relative incidence is much lower compared with that in the developing countries. Its aetiology is still not clear but has been attributed to umbilical sepsis after birth with thrombosis extending to the portal system via the patent umbilical vein or portal pyaemia following intra-abdominal sepsis. However, notwithstanding a lack of knowledge about its cause, most children and adults with EHPVO are generally from the so-called lower economic strata [2].

Variceal bleeding in EHPVO usually occurs in the first or second decade of life [15].

However, the outcome after a bleed is better compared to bleeding in cirrhotics (if adequate blood replacement facilities are at hand), because patients with EHPVO have normal liver function (and histology) which helps them to sustain bleeding episodes without decompensation [16]. However mortality rates of between 5 and 30% have been reported for a single bleeding episode because of the large volumes of blood lost in patients who do not have access to sophisticated medical facilities including blood transfusion [17].

Till the middle of the 20th century, surgery was the only treatment available for these patients. However, with the advent of endoscopic therapy, this soon became the predominant treatment modality for the control of acute bleeding and also an important method for the prevention of a repeated bleeding episode. The main disadvantages of endotherapy are that it requires multiple sessions and a long-term followup with a recurrence rate of up to 40% in some studies [18]. Because the prevalence of EHPVO is the highest in developing countries and the condition affects mainly the poor [2, 19], most of whom do not have access to blood transfusion facilities and are not treatment compliant, the benefits of using a less invasive procedure like endoscopic therapy must be weighed against surgery which, in the best centres carries an operative mortality of 1%, is

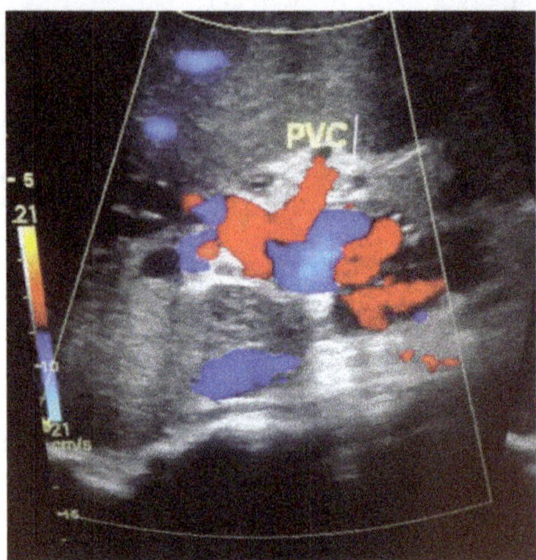

FIGURE 1: USG Doppler showing cavernous transformation of portal vein. PVC—portal vein cavernoma.

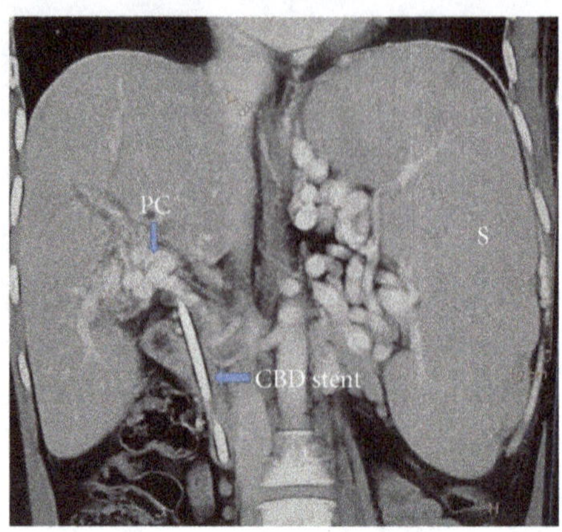

FIGURE 2: CT arterial portogram showing portal vein replaced by multiple collaterals, that is, cavernomatous transformation of the portal vein also known as a Portal Cavernoma (PC), grossly enlarged spleen (S), and CBD stent in situ for portal biliopathy in a patient with EHPVO.

a onetime treatment, is not associated with encephalopathy and followed by rebleeding rates of less than 10%. Moreover, operations like a splenectomy and proximal lienorenal shunt eliminate a large painful spleen and hypersplenism and restore a normal growth pattern in children. Thus, any new treatment for EHPVO must be compared with the results of shunt surgery which have stood the test of time especially if it has been performed by an experienced surgeon.

2. Diagnosis

A history of major upper gastrointestinal bleeding in a child who has oesophagogastric varices in endoscopy and normal liver function tests should raise the suspicion of extrahepatic portal venous obstruction. Although a similar picture can also be present in well compensated Child A, cirrhosis EHPVO is much more common in children especially in the developing world. Investigations to confirm the diagnosis are usually simple and readily available at most centres.

Massive splenomegaly is present in 90% of patients, and a complete blood count may reveal a low haemoglobin level and decreased total leukocyte and platelet counts due to hypersplenism in 50%. Liver function tests are nearly always normal, unlike in cirrhotics, but in the long-term the prothrombin time and albumin levels may be deranged due to the prolonged decreased portal blood flow and hence decreased synthetic function [20].

Ultrasonic Doppler (USG Doppler) examination of the upper abdomen should be the first radiological investigation performed to confirm the diagnosis as it has a sensitivity of 70–90% and a specificity of 99% in diagnosing EHPVO [21]. The characteristic findings are the replacement of portal vein by multiple tortuous vessels, also known as cavernous transformation, with hepatopetal blood flow in the collaterals (Figure 1). The liver echotexture is usually normal.

Upper gastrointestinal endoscopy (UGIE) is done to confirm the presence of varices and to grade their size. It can also identify gastric varices, portal hypertensive gastropathy, and duodenal varices.

Splenoportovenography by splenic puncture or selective coeliac/superior mesenteric angiography provides excellent imaging of the portal venous system but is invasive and has largely been replaced with computed tomography and magnetic resonance angiography.

CT arterial portography is highly accurate, not operator dependent, and useful in circumstances when bowel gas obscures the findings on ultrasound examination.

However, its high cost, exposure to radiation, and the systemic toxicity of the contrast agents used are its main disadvantages (Figure 2).

MR angiography is noninvasive and has a diagnostic accuracy that is similar to CT scans. However, it has limited availability and also has a high cost. With newer MR techniques, a clear portal venogram can be obtained and the direction and velocity of blood flow in the portal system can be determined.

Liver biopsy is usually not required for diagnosing EHPVO. It should be done only if a patient presents with abnormal LFTs or has hepatic dysfunction [20] due possibly to coincident hepatitis following repeated blood transfusions for previous bleeding episodes.

3. Tests to Establish the Aetiopathogenesis of EHPVO

In spite of many years of familiarity with the disease, the causal factors have not been established. Umbilical sepsis at birth, portal pyaemia, and thrombosis, and so forth are rare clinical features. Larroche in his landmark paper in 1970 described portal vein thrombosis occurring after umbilical vein catheterization, but most of these resolved within short period of time and did not progress to EHPVO [22]. However, there seems to be a strong association with levels of hygiene and poverty as the disease seems to affect the socially disadvantaged and has all but disappeared in most western countries and Japan [19] where it was more common in the late nineteenth century. There have been occasional reports of tests for dysmorphic megakaryocytes and endogenous erythroid colony assessment as being sensitive in distinguishing these patients from a normal population [16], but these are not readily available and therefore not commonly used. Tests for venous thromboembolism such as the presence of factor V Leiden, protein C, S and antithrombin III levels, and prothrombin gene mutation may also be positive in certain adult patients [23, 24] but have not had a high yield in the Indian scenario [25].

4. Treatment

Variceal bleeding being the most common and most serious presentation of EHPVO [17], it remains the most common indication for treatment which should be tailored depending on the patient's social circumstances and his or her access to medical facilities. Before the 1980s, conservative medical management was recommended [26–29] which included bed rest and blood transfusions as it was thought that these children would eventually "grow out" of their disease possibly by forming more collaterals to decompress the raised portal venous pressure [30]. However, when it was realized that a single episode of variceal bleeding could carry a mortality rate of up to 30% in western countries [17], most physicians now follow a more active approach. In India, Basu followed 25 patients with EHPVO for five years who had not had any intervention and reported that all had died [31]. The main treatment options available today, as with other forms of variceal bleeding, are pharmacotherapy with beta blockers, endoscopy, and surgery.

4.1. Pharmacotherapy. Prevention of a first episode of variceal bleeding with drugs has been well studied in adults with cirrhosis. In children with Child A cirrhosis and portal hypertension, Ozsoylu et al. [32] found propranolol to be effective. However this has not been studied in those with EHPVO. One of the most probable reasons may be that these patients usually present with bleeding as their first symptom (rather than splenomegaly), and hence primary prevention is difficult to study. Further studies are required to assess the role of drugs for primary prevention of variceal bleeding in EHPVO.

Secondary prophylaxis with beta blockers has been shown to be effective in reducing presinusoidal portal hypertension in animals and humans, but their efficacy in preventing variceal bleeding in EHPVO has not been proved [33].

4.2. Endoscopic Therapy

4.2.1. In Acute Bleeding. Excellent results have been achieved using endoscopic therapy in the control of acute bleeding, and this has now become the therapeutic modality of choice [1] in this situation with injection sclerotherapy and elastic band ligation being effective in 90% of cases. In those few patients who continue to bleed or are bleeding so massively that endoscopic control is not a possible surgical treatment in the form of portosystemic shunts or oesophagogastric devascularisation, it has been shown to be effective [34–36] but carries mortality rates ranging from 10–30% [37].

4.2.2. In Primary Prophylaxis. Endoscopy has also been used for primary prevention of a bleeding episode. Gonçalves et al. in a prospective randomized study including both cirrhotic and noncirrhotic children with portal hypertension found that 42% of patients with oesophageal varices who had no intervention presented with bleeding as compared to 24% patients in whom sclerotherapy was used for primary prevention [38]. However, there was no difference in survival and patients with sclerotherapy had more bleeding episodes from ectopic sites after the procedure. But since few EHPVO patients in the developing world present before a bleeding episode, endoscopic therapy for primary prophylaxis has not become an established mode of treatment.

4.2.3. In Secondary Prophylaxis. Complete eradication of varices with endoscopic sclerotherapy (EST) and variceal band ligation (EVL) occurs in 80–90% of patients with EHPVO. At present, endoscopic variceal eradication therapy is mainly indicated if

(i) it is used as a primary treatment modality,

(ii) the vessels are too small for anastomosis,

(iii) extensive thrombosis of the portal venous system which means there are no veins available for shunting, and

(iv) in those patients who cannot tolerate the surgical procedure due to underlying comorbidities.

However it must be remembered that endotherapy does not relieve the underlying portal hypertension and may result in an increased incidence of gastric and ectopic varices [39].

EST is associated with higher rates of ulcer and stricture formation than EVL which has the additional advantages of eradicating varices in fewer sessions. A randomized study by Zargar et al. has shown superiority of EVL over EST [40], but others have found that EVL alone may be associated with increased risk of recurrence of varices (40% in one study) [41]. Poddar et al. in 2005 showed that EVL + EST compared to EST alone was a better method in treatment of oesophageal varices in children with EHPVO because of fewer treatment sessions and fewer complications [42]. They achieved a 100% eradication with EVL + EST with no postprocedure esophageal stricture. Variceal recurrence rates were low in both the groups over a followup of 27 months (6.6% in EVL + EST group as compared to 10% in the EST group). Similar results have been shown by the same author in another study [43]. Further studies are, however, needed to establish the superior efficacy of EVL + EST over EST or EVL alone. However, EST is still favoured over EVL in many places due to its low cost.

Long-Term Follow-up Results with Endoscopic Therapy (Table 1). Zargar et al. have shown 88% success with injection sclerotherapy in a followup of 15 yrs [6]. Most of their patients had recurrent bleeding in the first 4 yrs after variceal

Table 1: Followup results with endoscopic variceal eradication therapy.

Author (yr)	No. of patients	Eradication (%)	Rebleed (%)	Recurrence (%)	Followup period
Howard et al. (1988) [3]	33	100	9	6	35 months
Chawla et al. (1990) [4]	122	91	16	6	24 months
Stringer and Howard (1994) [5]	32	100	31	16	8.7 years
Zargar et al. (2004) [6]	69	91	12	14	15 years
Thomas et al. (2009) [7]	198	100	17	19	20 years

eradication which was also managed by endoscopic therapy, and therefore the authors recommended annual endoscopy for the first 4 yrs after variceal eradication. In contrast, a similar study from King's College Hospital in London, UK, had previously shown that after a mean followup of 8.7 yrs, recurrent bleeding occurred in 31% [5].

4.3. Surgical Management. Surgery is the definitive treatment modality for EHPVO. We believe that it should be recommended as the treatment of choice for secondary prophylaxis in developing countries where the disease is more common and the accessibility to health care resources is poor.

Surgical intervention in variceal bleeding in EHPVO is indicated if there is

(i) failure of endoscopic management in acute variceal bleeding,

(ii) bleeding not amenable to endoscopic treatment such as portal hypertensive gastropathy and ectopic varices,

(iii) as a onetime treatment for secondary prophylaxis in those who have difficult access to specialized centres

(iv) for associated complications like portal biliopathy, growth retardation, hypersplenism, and massive splenomegaly leading to poor quality of life.

The surgical options include portosystemic shunts (PSS) and ablative procedures.

4.3.1. Portosystemic Shunts. These procedures divert blood flow from the high pressure portal circulation to low pressure systemic circulation by creation of an anastomosis between a tributary of the portal vein (splenic, superior mesenteric, and left gastric, left gastroepiploic) and a systemic vein (renal, inferior vena cava, and adrenal). The shunts may be selective (i.e., only decompressing the varices) or nonselective (decompressing the entire portal venous system). The main requirement for shunt procedure is the presence of a vessel free of thrombus and of sufficient size. For shunt to be effective and remain patent, it should be at least 10 mm in diameter although Bismuth et al. [44] and Prasad et al. [9] have had patency rates ranging from 84 to 96% after anastomosing veins of down to 4 mm in diameter.

(A) *Nonselective Shunts.* These are the most commonly performed procedures and include proximal splenorenal (PSRS), mesocaval, and portacaval shunts. The initial results with nonselective shunts were not promising since shunt thrombosis and rebleed and encephalopathy occurred in a large proportion of patients [29, 45]. But recent series have shown rebleed rates of 2–11%, a mortality rate of <2%, and no postshunt encephalopathy [9, 10]. Orloff et al. in 1994 found similar results with proximal side-side splenorenal shunts with or without splenectomy and end-side cavomesenteric shunts. They showed survival rates of >96% after 10 years and shunt thrombosis rates of <2% over a 15 yr followup [10].

A PSRS is the most commonly performed shunt along with a splenectomy. It is advantageous in that, along with diversion of blood flow to decrease portal pressure and control bleeding, it also relieves the patient from symptomatic enlarged spleen and the effects of hypersplenism. PSRS has shown good long-term results. In a study by Prasad et al., the 15 yr survival was 95% in 160 patients of EHPVO treated with PSRS with a rebleeding rate of 11% [9]. The long-term outcomes with shunts are shown below (Table 2).

The rebleeding rates after shunts are also lower than that after endoscopic therapy. In a recent prospective randomized study by Wani et al. in which the authors compared endoscopic sclerotherapy and shunt surgery revealed that rebleeding rates were significantly lower in the shunt surgery group (3.3% versus 22.6%) [46]. Treatment failure rates were also much less in the surgery group (6.7% versus 19.4%). Shunt procedures may also result in an improved quality of life (QOL). A study by Krishna et al. evaluating QOL after endoscopic or surgical treatment of EHPVO showed that endoscopic variceal eradication had no significant effect on QOL, but the postsurgery group had improvement in physical, psychosocial, and total QOL scores. However, the differences were not statistically significant [47].

The risks of overwhelming postsplenectomy infection have been described, but many studies including those from India and Mexico have shown low rates of postsplenectomy sepsis [9, 48, 49]. Other disadvantage is rebleeding due to shunt thrombosis. Rates of shunt thrombosis vary from 4–16% [8–11], and rebleeding in these patients is usually easily controlled by endoscopic therapy.

Surgical shunts in cirrhotics have been shown to be associated with neurological disturbances. In EHPVO, however this complication is rare, but there have been occasional reports of abnormal findings on electroencephalography, late CNS side effects, and emotional disorders even after 20 yrs [26]. Minimum hepatic encephalopathy (MHE) rates were higher in surgically shunted patients as compared to nonshunted children (but the difference was not significant) [50]. However, most studies have shown no postshunt encephalopathy [8–11].

TABLE 2: Outcomes of different shunt surgeries in EHPVO.

Author (yr)	Type of shunt performed	No. of patients	Shunt patency (%)	Rebleed (%)	Encephalopathy (%)	Operative mortality (%)	Follow up period	Survival
Mitra et al. (1993) [8]	Side-side lienorenal shunt (SSLR)	81	84	11	Nil	Nil	54 months	100%
Prasad et al. (1994) [9]	Proximal splenorenal shunt (PSRS)	160	NA	11	Nil	1.9	Up to 15 yrs	95% at 15 yrs
Orloff et al. (1994) [10]	PSRS, SSLR, and mesocaval shunt	162	98	2	Nil	Nil	Up to 35 yrs	96% at 10 yr
Rao et al. (2004) [11]	SSLR, PSRS	20	95	Nil	Nil	NA	3–5 yrs	95%
Warren et al. (1988) [12]	Distal splenorenal shunt	25	96	12	Nil	Nil	60 months	96%
Superina et al. (2006) [13]	Rex shunt	34	95	NA	Nil	NA	Up to 7 yrs	100%
Sharif et al. (2010) [14]	Rex shunt	24	96	2	NA	Nil	5.3–8.8 yrs	NA

NA: not available.

Shunt procedures, however, are not popular in the emergency setting because they are (i) time consuming, (ii) need technical expertise and associated with (iii) high rates of shunt thrombosis, and encephalopathy. However, the rate of shunt thrombosis depends on the experience of surgeon. A study by Orloff et al. showed shunt thrombosis rates of 0.5% in emergencies [51].

(B) *Selective Shunts.* Selective shunts aim to decompress only the gastrosplenic circulation leaving the blood flow to the liver intact, therefore, theoretically at least decreasing the rebleeding risk from oesophagogastric varices whilst preserving hepatopetal flow. The distal splenorenal shunt (Warren shunt) is the most commonly performed selective shunt although other shunts also have been described like the left gastroepiploic to left renal vein and left gastric to left renal vein shunts. Warren et al. reported a 5 yr followup of patients treated with distal splenorenal shunts. The patency rates were 92%, rebleeding rates of 12%, shunt dysfunction occurred in 25%, and encephalopathy in none of their patients [12]. These good results have been validated by others [52].

The main disadvantages are the need for surgical expertise and increased operation time. Such shunts cannot be performed in patients with thrombosis of the splenic vein or those who have a history of splenectomy.

Rex Shunt. Superina et al. in a study of 34 patients showed that mesenterico left portal vein bypass (MLPVB) or Rex shunt was successful in 91%, and they concluded that it was a more physiological shunt for EHPVO [13]. They claim that the shunt results in liver growth and normalization of coagulation parameters. But it requires the presence of a patent superior mesenteric vein, intrahepatic left portal vein, and internal jugular vein. However, it is still not popular in developing countries.

4.3.2. Variceal Ablative Procedures. These include splenectomy either alone or in combination with oesophagogastric devascularisation. These procedures are indicated if (i) performed as salvage therapy in variceal bleeding not controlled with endoscopic measures, (ii) a suitable size vein is not available for a shunt procedure, (iii) surgical expertise for a shunt procedure is not available. Splenectomy alone is not recommended since it does not decompress the portal circulation and also leads to thrombosis of splenic vein which thereafter cannot be used for shunting later.

Mathur et al. evaluated the role of oesophagogastric devascularisation with or without gastro-oesophageal stapling in acute variceal bleeding [34]. In their study, 20 patients had EHPVO and the operative mortality was 5%; recurrent varices occurred in 5% with rebleeding in 11%. None of their patients had encephalopathy. In a retrospective study of 24 patients with EHPVO undergoing salvage surgery for variceal bleeding (13 had devascularisation procedures; 11 had proximal splenorenal shunts), they achieved control of bleeding in 96%. One patient who had continued to bleed after surgery died [35]. Goyal et al. retrospectively reported a four-year followup of 22 patients with noncirrhotic portal hypertension in whom the bleeding was not controlled with endoscopic therapy. In their study, the rebleeding rate was 10% and overall survival was 95% [36].

Summary. EHPVO more commonly involves children from the lower socioeconomic strata in developing countries. Variceal bleeding is the most common presentation. Endoscopy is the established treatment for acute control of bleeding. Salvage surgery after failure of endoscopy has also shown good results. Both endoscopy and shunt surgeries have shown good long-term results in secondary prophylaxis. However, treatment should take into account the socioeconomic status of the patient and facilities available locally. Splenectomy and proximal lienorenal shunt being a one-time procedure with, if performed by experienced surgeons, low mortality and occlusion rates and an absence of postprocedure encephalopathy should be considered as the main treatment in patients with difficult access to sophisticated medical facilities. The role of shunt surgery has expanded since it is also effective in correcting portal biliopathy, hypersplenism, and growth retardation and may improve the quality of life.

References

[1] S. K. Sarin, J. D. Sollano, Y. K. Chawla et al., "Consensus on extra-hepatic portal vein obstruction," *Liver International*, vol. 26, no. 5, pp. 512–519, 2006.

[2] N. K. Arora and M. K. Das, *Extra Hepatic Portal Venous Obstruction in Children*, The INCLEN Trust International, New Delhi, India.

[3] E. R. Howard, M. D. Stringer, and A. P. Mowat, "Assessment of injection sclerotherapy in the management of 152 children with oesophageal varices," *The British Journal of Surgery*, vol. 75, no. 5, pp. 404–408, 1988.

[4] Y. K. Chawla, J. B. Dilawari, G. N. Ramesh, U. Kaur, S. K. Mitra, and B. N. S. Walia, "Sclerotherapy in extrahepatic portal venous obstruction," *Gut*, vol. 31, no. 2, pp. 213-216, 1990.

[5] M. D. Stringer and E. R. Howard, "Long term outcome after injection sclerotherapy for oesophageal varices in children with extrahepatic portal hypertension," *Gut*, vol. 35, no. 2, pp. 257–259, 1994.

[6] S. A. Zargar, G. N. Yattoo, G. Javid et al., "Fifteen-year follow up of endoscopic injection sclerotherapy in children with extra-hepatic portal venous obstruction," *Journal of Gastroenterology and Hepatology*, vol. 19, no. 2, pp. 139–145, 2004.

[7] V. Thomas, T. Jose, and S. Kumar, "Natural history of bleeding after esophageal variceal eradication in patients with extrahepatic portal venous obstruction; a 20-year follow-up," *Indian Journal of Gastroenterology*, vol. 28, no. 6, pp. 206–211, 2009.

[8] S. K. Mitra, K. L. N. Rao, K. L. Narasimhan et al., "Side-to-side lienorenal shunt without splenectomy in noncirrhotic portal hypertension in children," *Journal of Pediatric Surgery*, vol. 28, no. 3, pp. 398–402, 1993.

[9] A. S. Prasad, S. Gupta, V. Kohli, G. K. Pande, P. Sahni, and S. Nundy, "Proximal splenorenal shunts for extrahepatic portal venous obstruction in children," *Annals of Surgery*, vol. 219, no. 2, pp. 193–196, 1994.

[10] M. J. Orloff, M. S. Orloff, and M. Rambotti, "Treatment of bleeding esophagogastric varices due to extrahepatic portal hypertension: results of portal-systemic shunts during 35 years," *Journal of Pediatric Surgery*, vol. 29, no. 2, pp. 142–154, 1994.

[11] K. L. N. Rao, A. Goyal, P. Menon et al., "Extrahepatic portal hypertension in children: observations on three surgical procedures," *Pediatric Surgery International*, vol. 20, no. 9, pp. 679–684, 2004.

[12] W. D. Warren, J. M. Henderson, W. J. Millikan, J. T. Galambos, and F. C. Bryan, "Management of variceal bleeding in patients with noncirrhotic portal vein thrombosis," *Annals of Surgery*, vol. 207, no. 5, pp. 623–634, 1988.

[13] R. Superina, D. A. Bambini, J. Lokar, C. Rigsby, and P. F. Whitington, "Correction of extrahepatic portal vein thrombosis by the mesenteric to left portal vein bypass," *Annals of Surgery*, vol. 243, no. 4, pp. 515–521, 2006.

[14] K. Sharif, P. Mckiernan, and J. de Ville de Goyet, "Mesoportal bypass for extrahepatic portal vein obstruction in children: close to a cure for most!," *Journal of Pediatric Surgery*, vol. 45, no. 1, pp. 272–276, 2010.

[15] B. Weiss, E. Shteyer, A. Vivante et al., "Etiology and long-term outcome of extrahepatic portal vein obstruction in children," *World Journal of Gastroenterology*, vol. 16, no. 39, pp. 4968–4972, 2010.

[16] S. K. Sarin, A. Kumar, Y. K. Chawla et al., "Noncirrhotic portal fibrosis/idiopathic portal hypertension: APASL recommendations for diagnosis and treatment," *Hepatology International*, vol. 1, no. 3, pp. 398–413, 2007.

[17] A. P. Mowat, "Prevention of variceal bleeding," *Journal of Pediatric Gastroenterology and Nutrition*, vol. 5, no. 5, pp. 679–687, 1986.

[18] S. Itha and S. K. Yachha, "Endoscopic outcome beyond esophageal variceal eradication in children with extrahepatic portal venous obstruction," *Journal of Pediatric Gastroenterology and Nutrition*, vol. 42, no. 2, pp. 196–200, 2006.

[19] M. Okudaira, M. Ohbu, and K. Okuda, "Idiopathic portal hypertension and its pathology," *Seminars in Liver Disease*, vol. 22, no. 1, pp. 59–71, 2002.

[20] M. Rangari, R. Gupta, M. Jain, V. Malhotra, and S. K. Sarin, "Hepatic dysfunction in patients with extrahepatic portal venous obstruction," *Liver International*, vol. 23, no. 6, pp. 434–439, 2003.

[21] T. Nyandak, P. Prakash, U. Das et al., "Portal vein thrombosis—clinical profile," *Journal of Indian Academy of Clinical Medicine*, vol. 12, no. 2, pp. 134–140, 2011.

[22] J. C. Larroche, "Umbilical catheterization: its complications," *Biology of the Neonate*, vol. 16, no. 1, pp. 101–116, 1970.

[23] M. Primignani, I. Martinelli, P. Bucciarelli et al., "Risk factors for thrombophilia in extrahepatic portal vein obstruction," *Hepatology*, vol. 41, no. 3, pp. 603–608, 2005.

[24] D. Valla, N. Casadevall, M. G. Huisse et al., "Etiology of portal vein thrombosis in adults. A prospective evaluation of primary myeloproliferative disorders," *Gastroenterology*, vol. 94, no. 4, pp. 1063–1069, 1988.

[25] S. Sharma, S. I. Kumar, U. Poddar, S. K. Yachha, and R. Aggarwal, "Factor V Leiden and prothrombin gene G20210A mutations are uncommon in portal vein thrombosis in India," *Indian Journal of Gastroenterology*, vol. 25, no. 5, pp. 236–239, 2006.

[26] A. B. Voorhees and J. B. Price, "Extrahepatic portal hypertension. A retrospective analysis of 127 cases and associated clinical implications," *Archives of Surgery*, vol. 108, no. 3, pp. 338–341, 1974.

[27] E. W. Fonkalsrud, N. A. Myers, and M. J. Robinson, "Management of extrahepatic portal hypertension in children," *Annals of Surgery*, vol. 180, no. 4, pp. 487–493, 1974.

[28] H. W. Clatworthy and E. T. Boles, "Extrahepatic portal bed block in children: pathogenesis and treatment," *Annals of Surgery*, vol. 150, no. 3, pp. 371–383, 1959.

[29] L. J. Webb and S. Sherlock, "The aetiology, presentation and natural history of extra-hepatic portal venous obstruction," *Quarterly Journal of Medicine*, vol. 48, no. 192, pp. 627–639, 1979.

[30] D. Y. Hsia and S. S. Gellis, "Portal hypertension in infants and children," *AMA American Journal of Diseases of Children*, vol. 90, no. 3, pp. 290–291, 1955.

[31] A. K. Basu, "Surgical management of juvenile portal hypertension," in *Proceedings of the 37th International Paediatric Congress*, New Delhi, India, December 1977.

[32] S. Ozsoylu, N. Kocak, and A. Yuce, "Propranolol therapy for portal hypertension in children," *Journal of Pediatrics*, vol. 106, no. 2, pp. 317–321, 1985.

[33] A. Braillon, R. Moreau, A. Hadengue, D. Roulot, R. Sayegh, and D. Lebrec, "Hyperkinetic circulatory syndrome in patients with presinusoidal portal hypertension. Effect of propranolol," *Journal of Hepatology*, vol. 9, no. 3, pp. 312–318, 1989.

[34] S. K. Mathur, S. R. Shah, Z. F. Soonawala et al., "Transabdominal extensive oesophagogastric devascularization with gastro-oesophageal stapling in the management of acute variceal bleeding," *The British Journal of Surgery*, vol. 84, no. 3, pp. 413–417, 1997.

[35] A. Sharma, P. Vijayaraghavan, R. Lal et al., "Salvage surgery in variceal bleeding due to portal hypertension," *Indian Journal of Gastroenterology*, vol. 26, no. 1, pp. 14–17, 2007.

[36] N. Goyal, D. Singhal, S. Gupta, A. S. Soin, and S. Nundy, "Transabdominal gastroesophageal devascularization without transection for bleeding varices: results and indicators of prognosis," *Journal of Gastroenterology and Hepatology*, vol. 22, no. 1, pp. 47–50, 2007.

[37] S. K. Mitra, V. Kumar, D. V. Datta et al., "Extrahepatic portal hypertension: a review of 70 cases," *Journal of Pediatric Surgery*, vol. 13, no. 1, pp. 51–54, 1978.

[38] M. E. P. Gonçalves, S. R. Cardoso, and J. G. Maksoud, "Prophylactic sclerotherapy in children with esophageal varices: long-term results of a controlled prospective randomized trial," *Journal of Pediatric Surgery*, vol. 35, no. 3, pp. 401–405, 2000.

[39] U. Poddar, B. R. Thapa, and K. Singh, "Frequency of gastropathy and gastric varices in children with extrahepatic portal venous obstruction treated with sclerotherapy," *Journal of Gastroenterology and Hepatology*, vol. 19, no. 11, pp. 1253–1256, 2004.

[40] S. A. Zargar, G. Javid, B. A. Khan et al., "Endoscopic ligation compared with sclerotherapy for bleeding esophageal varices in children with extrahepatic portal venous obstruction," *Hepatology*, vol. 36, no. 3, pp. 666–672, 2002.

[41] P. J. McKiernan, S. V. Beath, and S. M. Davison, "A prospective study of endoscopic esophageal variceal ligation using a multiband ligator," *Journal of Pediatric Gastroenterology and Nutrition*, vol. 34, no. 2, pp. 207–211, 2002.

[42] U. Poddar, B. R. Thapa, and K. Singh, "Band ligation plus sclerotherapy versus sclerotherapy alone in children with extrahepatic portal venous obstruction," *Journal of Clinical Gastroenterology*, vol. 39, no. 7, pp. 626–629, 2005.

[43] U. Poddar, S. Bhatnagar, and S. K. Yachha, "Endoscopic band ligation followed by sclerotherapy: is it superior to sclerotherapy in children with extrahepatic portal venous obstruction?" *Journal of Gastroenterology and Hepatology*, vol. 26, no. 2, pp. 255–259, 2011.

[44] H. Bismuth, D. Franco, and J. Hepp, "Portal systemic shunt in hepatic cirrhosis: does the type of shunt decisively influence the clinical result?" *Annals of Surgery*, vol. 179, no. 2, pp. 209–218, 1974.

[45] E. W. Fonkalsrud, "Surgical management of portal hypertension in childhood. Long-term results," *Archives of Surgery*, vol. 115, no. 9, pp. 1042–1045, 1980.

[46] A. H. Wani, O. J. Shah, and S. A. Zargar, "Management of variceal hemorrhage in children with extrahepatic portal venous obstruction-shunt surgery versus endoscopic sclerotherapy," *Indian Journal of Surgery*, vol. 73, no. 6, pp. 409–413, 2011.

[47] Y. R. Krishna, S. K. Yachha, A. Srivastava, D. Negi, R. Lal, and U. Poddar, "Quality of life in children managed for extrahepatic portal venous obstruction," *Journal of Pediatric Gastroenterology and Nutrition*, vol. 50, no. 5, pp. 531–536, 2010.

[48] H. Orozco, T. Takahashi, M. A. Mercado, G. Garcia-Tsao, and J. Hernandez-Ortiz, "The Sugiura procedure for patients with hemorrhagic portal hypertension secondary to extrahepatic portal vein thrombosis," *Surgery Gynecology and Obstetrics*, vol. 173, no. 1, pp. 45–48, 1991.

[49] A. K. Sharma, H. K. Rangam, and R. P. Choubey, "Splenectomy and lieno-renal shunt for extra hepatic portal venous obstruction," *Indian Pediatrics*, vol. 37, no. 4, pp. 422–425, 2000.

[50] A. Srivastava, S. K. Yadav, R. Lal et al., "Effect of surgical portosystemic shunt on prevalence of minimal hepatic encephalopathy in children with extrahepatic portal venous obstruction: assessment by magnetic resonance imaging and psychometry," *Journal of Pediatric Gastroenterology and Nutrition*, vol. 51, no. 6, pp. 766–772, 2010.

[51] M. J. Orloff, M. S. Orloff, S. L. Orloff, M. Rambotti, and B. Girard, "Three decades of experience with emergency portacaval shunt for acutely bleeding esophageal varices in 400 unselected patients with cirrhosis of the liver," *Journal of the American College of Surgeons*, vol. 180, no. 3, pp. 257–272, 1995.

[52] J. M. Henderson, W. J. Millikan, J. T. Galambos, and W. D. Warren, "Selective variceal decompression in portal vein thrombosis," *The British Journal of Surgery*, vol. 71, no. 10, pp. 745–749, 1984.

5

Cholangiocarcinoma with respect to IgG4 Reaction

Kenichi Harada[1] and Yasuni Nakanuma[1,2]

[1] *Department of Human Pathology, Kanazawa University School of Medicine, Kanazawa 920-8640, Japan*
[2] *Department of Pathology, Shizuoka Cancer Center, Shizuoka 411-8777, Japan*

Correspondence should be addressed to Kenichi Harada; kenichih@med.kanazawa-u.ac.jp

Academic Editor: Valérie Paradis

IgG4 reactions marked by infiltration of IgG4-positive plasma cells in affected organs occur in cancer patients and in patients with IgG4-related diseases. Extrahepatic cholangiocarcinomas including gall bladder cancer are often accompanied by significant IgG4 reactions; these reactions show a negative correlation with CD8-positive cytotoxic T cells, suggesting that the evasion of immune surveillance is associated with cytotoxic T cells. The regulatory cytokine IL-10 may induce IgG4-positive plasma cell differentiation or promote B cell switching to IgG4 in the presence of IL-4. Cholangiocarcinoma cells may function as nonprofessional antigen presenting cells that indirectly induce IgG4 reactions via the IL-10-producing cells and/or these may act as Foxp3-positive and IL-10-producing cells that directly induce IgG4 reactions. Moreover, IgG4-related disease is a high-risk factor for cancer development; IgG4-related sclerosing cholangitis (IgG4-SC) cases associated with cholangiocarcinoma or its precursor lesion biliary intraepithelial neoplasia (BilIN) have been reported. IgG4-positive cell infiltration is an important finding of IgG4-SC but is not a histological hallmark of IgG4-SC. For the diagnosis of IgG4-SC, its differentiation from cholangiocarcinoma remains important.

1. Introduction

Inflammatory biliary diseases with periductal fibrosis are categorized as sclerosing cholangitis. In addition to the prototype of sclerosing cholangitis, primary sclerosing cholangitis (PSC), IgG4-related sclerosing cholangitis (IgG4-SC) is categorized as sclerosing cholangitis. Although IgG4-SC is characterized by the infiltration of numerous IgG4-positive cells in the wall of bile ducts, this IgG4 reaction is also found in PSC, hepatolithiasis, and cholangiocarcinoma. In particular, the differentiation between IgG4-SC and cholangiocarcinoma is an important clinical issue. Moreover, carcinogenesis in IgG4-related diseases has been noted [1] and a few cholangiocarcinoma cases arising from IgG4-SC have also been reported [2, 3]. In this review, we focus on the IgG4 reaction in cholangiocarcinoma and the pathological IgG4-SC-induced carcinogenic features of cholangiocarcinoma.

2. IgG4-Related Diseases and Clinicopathological Issues

IgG4 is a minor immunoglobulin subtype that does not activate complement and comprises only 3–6% of all circulating IgG in adults [4]. Elevated serum IgG4 levels and abundant IgG4-positive plasma cell infiltration in affected organs mark IgG4-related diseases [4–6]. The physiological and pathological significance of IgG4 remains unknown in both healthy individuals and IgG4-related disease patients. However, IgG4 responses occur at various levels in diseases not related to IgG4 including PSC [7, 8]. Moreover, IgG4-SC and type I autoimmune pancreatitis are characterized by sclerosing lesions (storiform fibrosis). Setting an upper normal limit for serum IgG4 to be 135 mg/dL, Hamano et al. [4] reported diagnostic sensitivity of 95% and specificity of 97% (versus pancreatic cancer) for autoimmune pancreatitis. Raina et al. [9] reported that as many as 7% of pancreatic cancer patients have serum IgG4 levels >135 mg/dL and concluded that, for patients with pancreatic mass lesions and suspected cancer, an IgG4 level between 135 and 200 mg/dL should be cautiously interpreted and rejected as the diagnostic criterion for autoimmune pancreatitis without further evaluation. Therefore, a pathological examination is necessary to differentiate IgG4-related diseases from tumors in other organs. IgG4 reactions characterized by an increase in the number of IgG4-positive cells are speculated to be nonspecific during pathological conditions including cancer and the presence of IgG4-positive cells is not a histological hallmark of IgG4-related diseases. An IgG4 reaction may simply be the result of an immunoreaction within a certain cytokine milieu and may have limited pathological significance in affected organs. Moreover, storiform-type sclerosing fibrosis is a characteristic feature of IgG4-related diseases including IgG4-SC, but cholangiocarcinomas and pancreatic cancer usually accompany some degree of desmoplastic change.

3. IgG4 Reaction and Its Distribution in Biliary Tract Cancers

Biliary tract cancers can be anatomically divided into intrahepatic and extrahepatic cholangiocarcinomas; the latter includes hepatic hilar cancer, common bile duct cancer, gall bladder cancer, and cancer of the papilla of Vater. The biological behavior and carcinogenicity of each cancer differ, but the histology of most biliary tract cancers is the same as that of ordinary adenocarcinomas. In addition to neoplastic lesions, several types of cholangitis causing biliary stenosis are important in the differential diagnosis of biliary diseases. PSC and IgG4-SC clinicopathologically mimic extrahepatic cholangiocarcinomas. In particular, the clinicopathological differentiation of IgG4-related diseases from neoplasms is important because desmoplastic change and, rarely, mass formation as well as marked IgG4-positive cell infiltration are found. Moreover, the IgG4 reaction often occurs in malignant neoplasms including pancreatic cancer [9–12] and the relation between cancer-related immunity and IgG4 reaction has been speculated. We surveyed the IgG4 reaction in biliary tract cancers and demonstrated that the IgG4 reaction occurs at various degrees in most cholangiocarcinomas located in the hepatic hilus, common bile ducts, papilla of Vater, and gall bladder cancers (Figures 1(a) and 1(b)) but very rarely in cholangiocarcinoma of the liver (intrahepatic cholangiocarcinoma, ICC). In addition, IgG4-SC mainly affects bile ducts in the hepatic hilus, common bile ducts, and gall bladder [13–15], indicating anatomical similarities between organs affected by IgG4-SC and biliary tract cancers with the IgG4 reaction. In biliary tract cancers, except ICC, 43% cases exhibited >10 IgG4-positive plasma cells/hpf, clinical diagnostic criteria of IgG4-SC 2012 [16], and 9% cases exhibited marked infiltration of IgG4-positive cells over 50/hpf. Moreover, Resheq et al. [17] recently showed that six out of 19 (32%) patients with hilar cholangiocarcinoma were IgG4-positive (≥20 IgG4-positive plasma cells/hpf). However, the authors concluded that IgG4-positive plasma cells in combination with clinical parameters as criteria to distinguish hilar cholangiocarcinoma from IgG4-SC had limited utility and may be misleading under conditions when malignancy is not diagnosed.

The IgG4 reaction is scattered within and around cancerous nests. IgG4-positive cells are particularly prominent around nests, invasive areas facing noncancerous biliary walls, and fibroadipose tissue and are interspersed with other inflammatory cells. Moreover, in biliary tract cancer with a marked IgG4 reaction, the surrounding nonneoplastic biliary mucosa and the carcinoma area are often accompanied with an IgG4 reaction (Figures 1(c) and 1(d)). One characteristic feature of IgG4-related diseases, the perineural infiltration of IgG4-positive cells (also a characteristic feature of IgG4-SC), is mostly found in cases with the IgG4 reaction, suggesting neurotropic IgG4-positive cells irrespective of IgG4-SC and biliary tract cancer with the IgG4 reaction. However the significance and mechanism of perineural infiltration of IgG4-positive cells are unknown. Obliterative phlebitis caused by IgG4-positive cells and storiform-type fibrosis are characteristic features of IgG4-SC. However, these findings have to be differentiated from vascular invasion by cancer cells and desmoplastic change in extrahepatic cholangiocarcinomas.

In the advanced cholangiocarcinoma cases, the presence of the cholangiocarcinoma arising from IgG4-SC is speculated, but it is pathologically hard to differentiate between cholangiocarcinoma with IgG4 reaction and cholangiocarcinoma arising from IgG4-SC. However, the presence of IgG4-SC cases accompanying biliary precancerous lesion indicates the possibility of biliary carcinogenesis arising from IgG4-SC.

4. Pathological Significance of the IgG4 Reaction in Biliary Tract Cancer

Some pancreatic cancer cases accompanied by the IgG4 reaction and/or elevated serum IgG4 levels [9–12] in addition to cases with pancreatic cancer or cholangiocarcinoma result from IgG4-related autoimmune pancreatitis or IgG4-SC, respectively [3, 18], suggesting an association between cancer-related immunity and the IgG4 reaction. During the carcinogenesis of pancreatic cancer, the number of Foxp3-positive regulatory T cells (Treg cells) increases, whereas that of cytotoxic CD8-positive cells decreases, suggesting that Treg cells are involved in immune response control against pancreatic cancers that evade tumor-associated immune surveillance [19]. Treg cells inhibit anticancer immunity via the production of regulatory cytokines, such as IL-10 and TGF-β. High Treg cell frequency is speculated to reflect a poor prognosis in pancreatic and colon cancer patients [19, 20]. In addition, Treg cells play an important role in the histogenesis of IgG4 reaction in IgG4-related diseases [21–25], suggesting that these cells perform a similar function in the pathogenesis of IgG4-SC and carcinoma. We studied the association of the IgG4 reaction versus Treg and CD8-positive T cells in biliary tract cancers and demonstrated that numerous Treg cells accompanied cases with a marked IgG4 reaction. CD8-positive cytotoxic T cells (CTLs) were scattered to various degrees, irrespective of their location within or around cancer nests. CTLs mark immune activity against

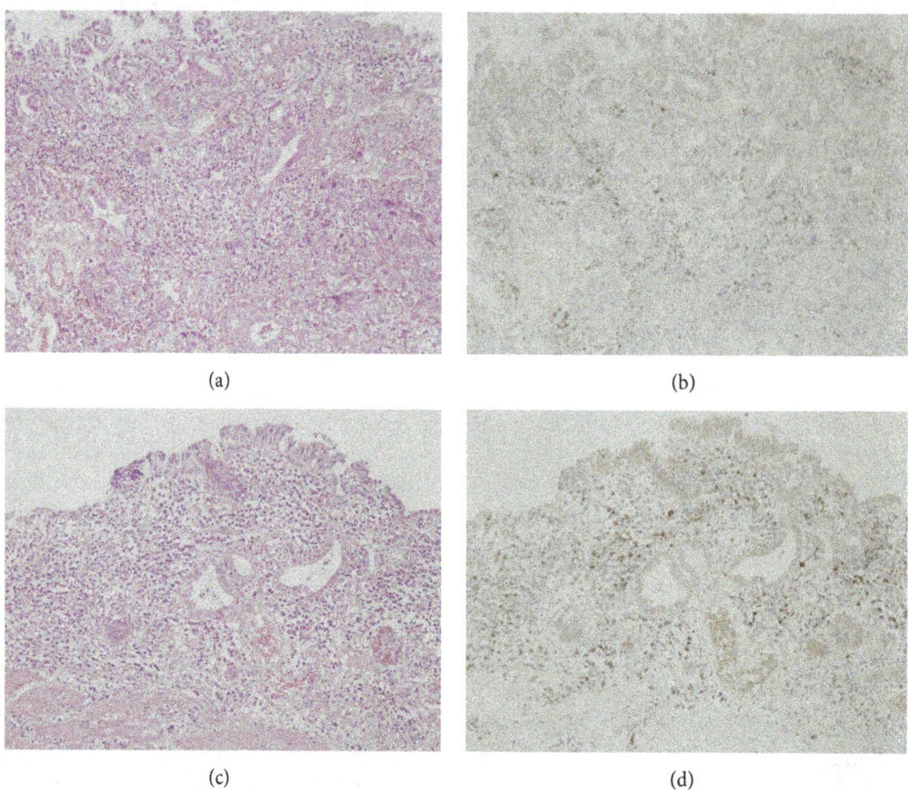

FIGURE 1: Carcinoma ((a) and (b)) and nonneoplastic ((c) and (d)) areas at the mucosal surface of gall bladder cancer. Severe inflammation ((a) and (c)) and many IgG4-positive cells ((b) and (d)) were found in both neoplastic and nonneoplastic areas. (a) and (c) hematoxylin and eosin stain (HE); (b) and (d) IgG4 immunohistochemistry.

cancers and invade cancerous nests resembling intraepithelial lymphocytes (IELs) that are found in nonneoplastic biliary epithelial layers of biliary diseases such as primary biliary cirrhosis [26]. Consequently, patients with many CD8-positive CTLs resembling IELs showed scant IgG4 reactions (IgG4-poor cases, Figure 2). In contrast, IgG4-rich cases have few CD8-positive CTLs and a poor prognosis compared with IgG4-poor cases [27]. In other words, it is suggested that the IgG4 reaction showed positive and negative correlation with Treg cells and CTLs, respectively, signifying that immune surveillance evasion was associated with CTLs through Treg cell regulatory function.

5. Mechanisms of the IgG4 Reaction in Biliary Tract Cancers

Th2-type cytokines, IL-4 and IL-10, are important in the pathogenesis of IgG4-related diseases including IgG4-SC. Treg cells are characterized by the production of IL-10 and TGF-β and are involved in the IgG4 reaction [22, 25, 28]. In particular, IL-10 (a regulatory cytokine mainly produced by Treg cells), Th2 cells, and IL-10-producing regulatory T cells could be thought to induce the differentiation of IgG4-positive plasma cells or promote B cell switching to IgG4 in the presence of IL-4 [28, 29]. Several carcinoma tissues and cultured cancer cell lines demonstrate the expression of Foxp3 and IL-10, suggesting that cancer cells induce the Treg cell-like immunoregulatory milieu to evade immunosurveillance [30–33]. We describe two mechanisms where cholangiocarcinoma cells directly participate in the histogenesis of IgG4 reactions via cytokine milieu of IL-10 (Figure 3).

6. Cholangiocarcinoma Cells as Nonprofessional Antigen Presenting Cells (APCs)

Professional APCs such as dendritic cells expressing both MHC class II and the costimulatory molecules CD80 (B7-1) and CD86 (B7-2) present antigens with costimulatory molecules to CD4-positive T cells and differentiate from CD4-positive cells into Th1, Th2, TH17, or Treg cells depending on cytokine milieu. However, MHC class II-positive cells lacking costimulatory molecules induce anergy in native T cells. T regulatory type 1 cells (Tr1 cells) are characterized by the production of IL-10 and are induced by immature dendritic cells [34]. Moreover, costimulation-dependent T cell clones stimulated without the costimulatory signal do not proliferate but instead differentiate into IL-10-producing anergic T cells in primary biliary cirrhosis [35]. Immunocompetent cells like dendritic cells and nonimmunocompetent cells including carcinoma and normal epithelial cells express MHC class II and may present antigens. However, MHC class II-positive epithelial cells (also referred to as nonprofessional

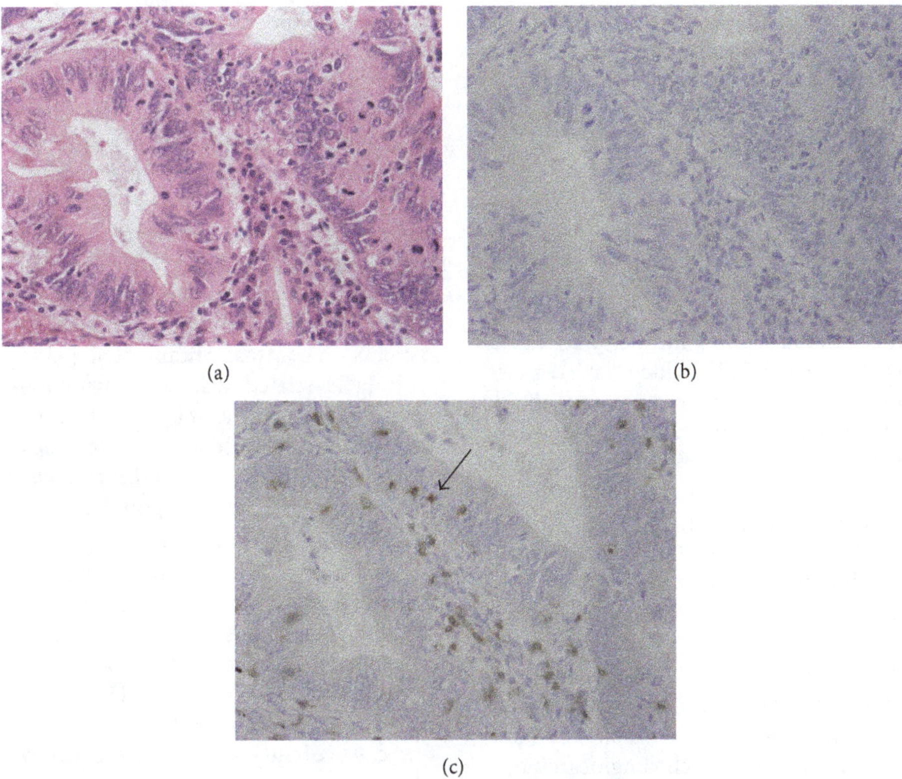

FIGURE 2: Extrahepatic cholangiocarcinoma with scant IgG4 reactions. Hematoxylin and eosin stain of inflammatory cells in the stroma of adenocarcinoma (a). Immunohistochemistry identified no IgG4-positive cells (b), but CD8-positive T cells were scattered throughout the stroma and cancerous nests (arrows, (c)).

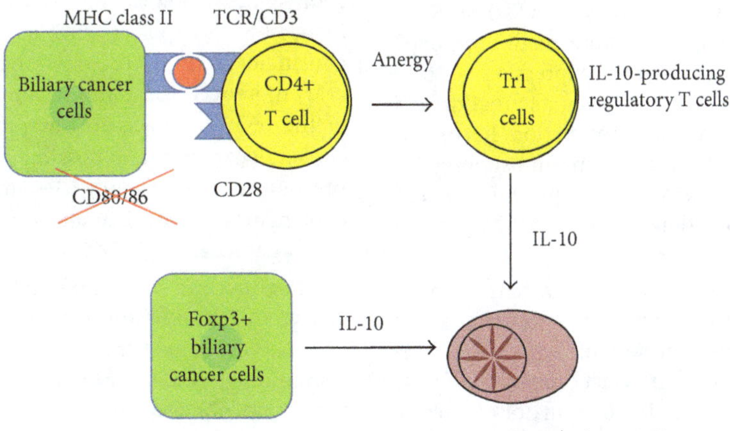

FIGURE 3: Proposed mechanisms for the induction of IgG4-positive plasma cells in cholangiocarcinoma.

APCs) differ from professional APCs such as dendritic cells. MHC class II-positive cells that do not express the costimulatory molecules CD80 (B7-1) and CD86 (B7-2) induce IL-10-producing anergic T cells or Tr1 cells from native T cells [34, 35]. Several studies suggest that antigen presentation by MHC class II-positive epithelial cells that lack costimulation signals, for example, keratinocytes and pancreatic islet cells, promotes anergic T cells generation [36–38]. In biliary tract cancers, carcinoma cases expressing MHC class II but lacking costimulatory molecules (CD80 and CD86) are found in 54% (Figure 4(a)). These biliary tract cancer cells could act as nonprofessional APCs by generating IL-10-producing regulatory T cells (anergy T cells). Furthermore, an IL-10-predominant cytokine milieu could cause the induction of

IgG4-positive cells [28, 29]. In these phenotypic cases, the number of IgG4-positive cells infiltrating carcinoma tissues was higher than that in MHC class II-negative cases.

7. Cholangiocarcinoma Cells as Regulatory Cells

Treg cells, Th2 cells, and IL-10-producing regulatory T cells mainly produce IL-10. Although Foxp3 is a master transcription factor for Treg cells, Foxp3 and IL-10 are expressed in several carcinoma tissues and cultured cancer cell lines, suggesting that cancer cells induce the Treg cell-like immunoregulatory milieu to evade immunosurveillance [30–33]. To validate the hypothesis that cholangiocarcinoma cells themselves function in immunosuppression similar to Treg cells, we examined the expression of Foxp3 in biliary tract cancer. The antibody reacting with the N-terminus of Foxp3 highlighted carcinoma cells and Treg cells in 39% of biliary tract cancers while the antibody reacting with the C-terminus of Foxp3 detects only the mononuclear cells that correspond to Treg cells (Figure 4(b)). Moreover, the number of IgG4-positive cells is significantly higher in Foxp3-positive than Foxp3-negative cases. This discrepancy between antibodies against different antigenic sites of Foxp3 suggests the presence of Foxp3 splice variants in cholangiocarcinoma cells. RT-PCR demonstrated that the cholangiocarcinoma cell line HuCCT1 expresses Foxp3 mRNA. Further examination of cholangiocarcinoma cells with four primer sets revealed a Foxp3 splice variant lacking exon 3 that caused a frameshift at the C-terminus creating a novel amino acid, which has been reported in a melanoma cell line [32]. Furthermore, RT-PCR and ELISA revealed that HuCCT1 cells express IL-10 mRNA and secrete IL-10 protein into the culture medium. Foxp3 expression is closely correlated with the expression of IL-10 in all Foxp3-positive cell lines [33]; however, its function as a transcription factor requires further investigation. In conclusion, cholangiocarcinoma cells perform immunosuppressive functions similar to Treg cells via IL-10 production and possibly induce the differentiation of IgG4-positive plasma cells in biliary tract cancers.

As mentioned above, cholangiocarcinoma cells are non-professional APCs and/or regulatory cells that directly induce IgG4 reactions in an IL-10-predominant cytokine milieu. Although the IgG4 reaction in biliary tract cancers and IgG4-SC are closely associated with the IL-10 regulatory cytokine milieu, it is possible that both mechanisms are specific for cancer tissues but different from IgG4-related pathogenesis.

8. Carcinogenesis in Patients with IgG4-SC

Patients with autoimmune pancreatitis occasionally have other types of cancer including pancreatic cancer [39–41] and bile duct cancer [3]. These patients are at an increased risk for various cancers and it is suggested that autoimmune pancreatitis may develop as a paraneoplastic syndrome in some patients [1, 42]. Pancreatic and biliary cancers have been reported in IgG4-related diseases [3, 11, 18], although the cause-and-effect relationship between IgG4 reactions and cancer is unknown. A study by Shiokawa et al. [1] reported that 18 cancers in various organs were found in 15 out of 108 autoimmune pancreatitis patients (13.9%), during a median follow-up period of 3.3 years. The relative risk of cancer was 4.9 for the autoimmune pancreatitis patients on diagnosis. Before autoimmune pancreatitis patients initiated corticosteroid therapy, numerous IgG4-positive plasma cells were observed in the cancer stroma; no patient had an autoimmune pancreatitis relapse after successful cancer treatment. Therefore, it was concluded that autoimmune pancreatitis may have developed as a paraneoplastic syndrome in some patients. In contrast, Hirano et al. [43] surveyed 113 patients with IgG4-related disease in whom malignancy was not diagnosed at the time of IgG4-RD onset and revealed that the incidence of the observed malignancies was not significant, compared with the expected incidence in an age- and sex-matched general Japanese population.

PSC and IgG4-SC target large bile ducts such as the hepatic hilar bile duct and extrahepatic bile ducts. Both diseases exhibit similar clinicopathological behaviors, that is, bile duct stenosis and biliary obstruction. PSC often develops into cholangiocarcinoma (incidence 7–15%, annual incidence of 0.5–1.5%) [44, 45]. The relationship between cholangiocarcinoma and IgG4-SC is unclear, although a few cases of IgG4-SC are associated with cholangiocarcinoma or its precursor lesion [2, 46]. The World Health Organization (WHO) defines biliary intraepithelial neoplasia (BilIN) as a cholangiocarcinoma precursor that is classified according to morphological atypia into the three subtypes BilIN1, BilIN2, and BilIN3 [47]. BilIN3 *in situ* carcinoma directly contributes to the progression of overt invasive cholangiocarcinomas. BilIN3 as well as BilIN1-2 is found in IgG4-SC as well as PSC, suggesting a risk for invasive cholangiocarcinoma progression in IgG4-SC. In the IgG4-SC case, moreover, the BilIN lesion expressed a mutated form of the p53 tumor suppressor protein [46], suggesting that cholangiocarcinoma is possibly associated with IgG4-SC as precursors of malignancy. Therefore, note the possibility that cholangiocarcinoma is associated with IgG4-SC during IgG4-SC diagnosis and IgG4-SC treatment.

Two mechanisms are possible regarding cooccurrence of cancer and autoimmunity: (1) sustained inflammation in the presence of an autoimmune disease is considered to create immunological environments favorable for cancer development and (2) cancers may induce autoimmune diseases as a paraneoplastic syndrome [1]. Although it is unknown whether IgG4-related diseases including IgG4-SC are true autoimmune diseases, an immune dysfunction including autoimmunity is surely associated with the pathogenesis of IgG4-related diseases. As mentioned above, the regulatory cytokine IL-10 induces the differentiation of IgG4-positive plasma cells, promotes the conversion of B cells into IgG4 in the presence of IL-4 [28, 29], and closely associates with the pathogenesis of IgG4-related diseases [25, 48]. IL-10 is a regulatory cytokine that broadly functions as an immune inhibitory cytokine to support tumor growth. This suggests that Treg cells play a role in the progression and metastasis of various malignant tumors, particularly for controlling

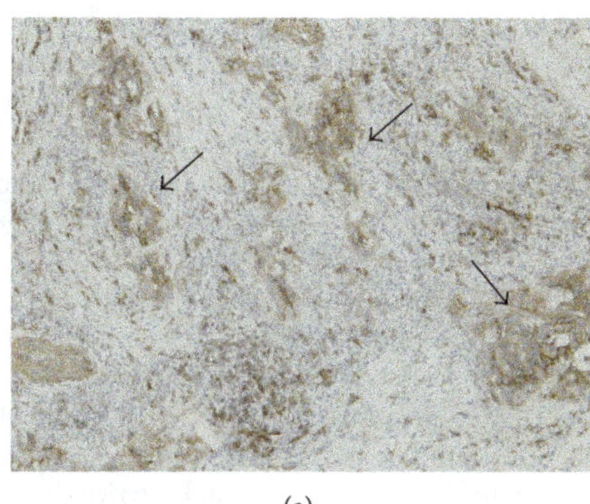

(a)

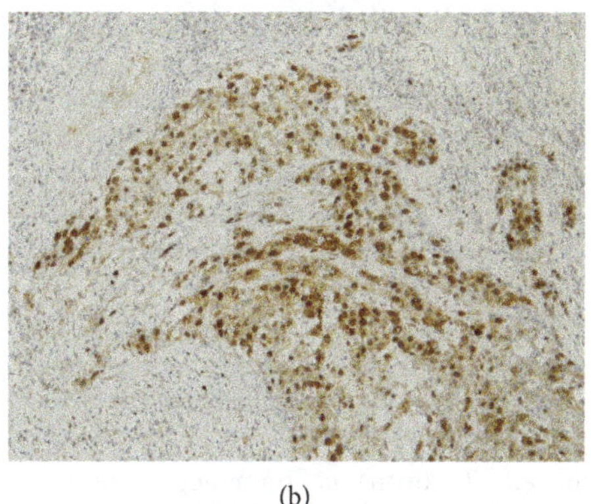

(b)

FIGURE 4: Immunohistochemistry for MHC class II (HLA-DR) (a) and the N-terminus of Foxp3 (b) in biliary tract cancers. In addition to infiltrating mononuclear cells, carcinoma cells are positive for HLA-DR ((a), arrows). The antibody reacting with the N-terminus of Foxp3 (b) highlights the nucleus and cytoplasm of cholangiocarcinoma cells.

the immune responses against carcinomas from the pre-malignant stage until established cancer [19, 49]. Therefore, in IgG4-SC, an IL-10-related cytokine milieu initiates the IgG4 reaction and also suppresses tumor-reactive T cells, suggesting that IgG4-SC may accelerate cholangiocarcinoma development. In conclusion, IL-10-based regulatory cytokine networks evade host immune responses in cancer patients with IgG4-related diseases and further suggest an association with cholangiocarcinoma.

9. Differential Diagnosis

IgG4-SC complicated autoimmune pancreatitis can be differentiated by the same diagnostic criteria as autoimmune pancreatitis, such as serum IgG4 levels and lesion distribution. However, differentiating IgG4-SC cases without pancreatic and other organs involvement from conditions such as PSC and cholangiocarcinoma is challenging. Moreover, the mean IgG4 serum level is relatively lower in IgG4-SC cases without autoimmune pancreatitis than in cases with autoimmune pancreatitis. Furthermore, hilar hepatic lesions that resemble hepatic hilar cholangiocarcinoma frequently accompany IgG4-SC cases without autoimmune pancreatitis [50, 51]. Bile duct biopsy and cytological examination are particularly important to exclude malignancies. At present, >40% IgG-positive plasma cells and >10 cells/hpf of biopsy samples are comprehensive histological diagnostic criteria for IgG4-related diseases (2011 and 2012) [16, 52–54]. However, these criteria should be applied only if malignant neoplasms are denied. Cholangiocarcinoma cases in which an inflammatory reaction is characterized by large numbers of IgG4-positive plasma cells within or around the tumors exist in addition to cholangiocarcinoma cases and BilIN lesions that are preceded by IgG4-SC. Moreover, other histological features of IgG4-SC, storiform fibrosis and obliterative phlebitis, can be differentiated from cholangiocarcinoma and PSC but are not located at the superficial biliary mucosa. Therefore, it is difficult to identify histological findings from small biopsies of the superficial bile duct mucosa and impossible to completely exclude cholangiocarcinoma during IgG4-SC diagnosis by biopsy and cytology. Multiple biopsies and specimens from the same site may be needed to identify cancerous or atypical cells [4]. Moreover, biopsies from the papilla of Vater [55] and liver [56] are useful for IgG4-SC diagnosis.

10. Concluding Remarks

In this review, we described the IgG4 reaction in cholangiocarcinoma. Correlations between IgG4 and malignant neoplasms are noted; however, their cause-and-effect relationship needs further clarification. Furthermore, a prospective study is needed to elucidate the role of IgG4-related diseases in carcinogenesis. At this moment, the most important procedure is ruling out cancer in the diagnosis of IgG4-SC. We, pathologists, have to know the IgG4 reaction in cholangiocarcinoma from the aspect of the presence of IgG4-positive cells, its density, and its distribution in order to avoid the rapid diagnosis that the presence of IgG4-positive cells in biliary mucosa is of help as evidence of IgG4-SC.

References

[1] M. Shiokawa, Y. Kodama, K. Yoshimura et al., "Risk of cancer in patients with autoimmune pancreatitis," *American Journal of Gastroenterology*, vol. 108, no. 4, pp. 610–617, 2013.

[2] B. K. Straub, I. Esposito, D. Gotthardt et al., "IgG4-associated cholangitis with cholangiocarcinoma," *Virchows Archiv*, vol. 458, no. 6, pp. 761–765, 2011.

[3] C. H. Oh, J. G. Kim, J. W. Kim et al., "Early bile duct cancer in a background of sclerosing cholangitis and autoimmune pancreatitis," *Internal Medicine*, vol. 47, no. 23, pp. 2025–2028, 2008.

[4] H. Hamano, S. Kawa, A. Horiuchi et al., "High serum IgG4 concentrations in patients with sclerosing pancreatitis," *The*

New England Journal of Medicine, vol. 344, no. 10, pp. 732–738, 2001.

[5] H. Hamano, S. Kawa, Y. Ochi et al., "Hydronephrosis associated with retroperitoneal fibrosis and sclerosing pancreatitis," *The Lancet*, vol. 359, no. 9315, pp. 1403–1404, 2002.

[6] Y. Zen and Y. Nakanuma, "IgG4-related disease: a cross-sectional study of 114 cases," *American Journal of Surgical Pathology*, vol. 34, no. 12, pp. 1812–1819, 2010.

[7] M. Koyabu, K. Uchida, N. Fukata et al., "Primary sclerosing cholangitis with elevated serum IgG4 levels and/or infiltration of abundant IgG4-positive plasma cells," *Journal of Gastroenterology*, vol. 45, no. 1, pp. 122–129, 2010.

[8] Y. Zen, A. Quaglia, and B. Portmann, "Immunoglobulin G4-positive plasma cell infiltration in explanted livers for primary sclerosing cholangitis," *Histopathology*, vol. 58, no. 3, pp. 414–422, 2011.

[9] A. Raina, A. M. Krasinskas, J. B. Greer et al., "Serum immunoglobulin G fraction 4 levels in pancreatic cancer: elevations not associated with autoimmune pancreatitis," *Archives of Pathology & Laboratory Medicine*, vol. 132, no. 1, pp. 48–53, 2008.

[10] A. Ghazale, S. T. Chari, T. C. Smyrk et al., "Value of serum IgG4 in the diagnosis of autoimmune pancreatitis and in distinguishing it from pancreatic cancer," *American Journal of Gastroenterology*, vol. 102, no. 8, pp. 1646–1653, 2007.

[11] T. Kamisawa, P. Y. Chen, Y. Tu et al., "Pancreatic cancer with a high serum IgG4 concentration," *World Journal of Gastroenterology*, vol. 12, no. 38, pp. 6225–6228, 2006.

[12] D. Dhall, A. A. Suriawinata, L. H. Tang, J. Shia, and D. S. Klimstra, "Use of immunohistochemistry for IgG4 in the distinction of autoimmune pancreatitis from peritumoral pancreatitis," *Human Pathology*, vol. 41, no. 5, pp. 643–652, 2010.

[13] M. D. Leise, T. C. Smyrk, N. Takahashi, S. R. Sweetser, S. S. Vege, and S. T. Chari, "IgG4-associated cholecystitis: another clue in the diagnosis of autoimmune pancreatitis," *Digestive Diseases and Sciences*, vol. 56, no. 5, pp. 1290–1294, 2011.

[14] S. C. Abraham, M. Cruz-Correa, P. Argani, E. E. Furth, R. H. Hruban, and J. K. Boitnott, "Lymphoplasmacytic chronic cholecystitis and biliary tract disease in patients with lymphoplasmacytic sclerosing pancreatitis," *The American Journal of Surgical Pathology*, vol. 27, no. 4, pp. 441–451, 2003.

[15] T. Kamisawa, Y. Tu, H. Nakajima et al., "Sclerosing cholecystitis associated with autoimmune pancreatitis," *World Journal of Gastroenterology*, vol. 12, no. 23, pp. 3736–3739, 2006.

[16] H. Ohara, K. Okazaki, H. Tsubouchi et al., "Clinical diagnostic criteria of IgG4-related sclerosing cholangitis 2012," *Journal of Hepato-Biliary-Pancreatic Sciences*, vol. 19, no. 5, pp. 536–542, 2012.

[17] Y. J. Resheq, A. Quaas, D. von Renteln, C. Schramm, A. W. Lohse, and S. Lüth, "Infiltration of peritumoural but tumour-free parenchyma with IgG4-positive plasma cells in hilar cholangiocarcinoma and pancreatic adenocarcinoma," *Digestive and Liver Disease*, vol. 45, no. 10, pp. 859–865, 2013.

[18] U. Motosugi, T. Ichikawa, H. Yamaguchi et al., "Small invasive ductal adenocarcinoma of the pancreas associated with lymphoplasmacytic sclerosing pancreatitis: case Report," *Pathology International*, vol. 59, no. 10, pp. 744–747, 2009.

[19] N. Hiraoka, K. Onozato, T. Kosuge, and S. Hirohashi, "Prevalence of $FOXP3^+$ regulatory T cells increases during the progression of pancreatic ductal adenocarcinoma and its premalignant lesions," *Clinical Cancer Research*, vol. 12, no. 18, pp. 5423–5434, 2006.

[20] H. Suzuki, N. Chikazawa, T. Tasaka et al., "Intratumoral $CD8^+$ T/$FOXP_3^+$ cell ratio is a predictive marker for survival in patients with colorectal cancer," *Cancer Immunology, Immunotherapy*, vol. 59, no. 5, pp. 653–661, 2010.

[21] H. Miyoshi, K. Uchida, T. Taniguchi et al., "Circulating naïve and CD4+CD25high regulatory T cells in patients with autoimmune pancreatitis," *Pancreas*, vol. 36, no. 2, pp. 133–140, 2008.

[22] M. Koyabu, K. Uchida, H. Miyoshi et al., "Analysis of regulatory T cells and IgG4-positive plasma cells among patients of IgG4-related sclerosing cholangitis and autoimmune liver diseases," *Journal of Gastroenterology*, vol. 45, no. 7, pp. 732–741, 2010.

[23] T. Kusuda, K. Uchida, H. Miyoshi et al., "Involvement of inducible costimulator- and interleukin 10-positive regulatory T cells in the development of IgG4-related autoimmune pancreatitis," *Pancreas*, vol. 40, no. 7, pp. 1120–1130, 2011.

[24] Y. Fukui, K. Uchida, K. Sumimoto et al., "The similarity of Type 1 autoimmune pancreatitis to pancreatic ductal adenocarcinoma with significant IgG4-positive plasma cell infiltration," *Journal of Gastroenterology*, vol. 48, no. 6, pp. 751–761, 2013.

[25] Y. Zen, T. Fujii, K. Harada et al., "Th2 and regulatory immune reactions are increased in immunoglobin G4-related sclerosing pancreatitis and cholangitis," *Hepatology*, vol. 45, no. 6, pp. 1538–1546, 2007.

[26] K. Isse, K. Harada, Y. Sato, and Y. Nakanuma, "Characterization of biliary intra-epithelial lymphocytes at different anatomical levels of intrahepatic bile ducts under normal and pathological conditions: numbers of $CD4^+CD28^-$ intra-epithelial lymphocytes are increased in primary biliary cirrhosis," *Pathology International*, vol. 56, no. 1, pp. 17–24, 2006.

[27] Y. Kimura, K. Harada, and Y. Nakanuma, "Pathologic significance of immunoglobulin G4-positive plasma cells in extrahepatic cholangiocarcinoma," *Human Pathology*, vol. 43, no. 12, pp. 2149–2156, 2012.

[28] P. Jeannin, S. Lecoanet, Y. Delneste, J. F. Gauchat, and J. Y. Bonnefoy, "IgE versus IgG4 production can be differentially regulated by IL-10," *Journal of Immunology*, vol. 160, no. 7, pp. 3555–3561, 1998.

[29] D. S. Robinson, M. Larché, and S. R. Durham, "Tregs and allergic disease," *The Journal of Clinical Investigation*, vol. 114, no. 10, pp. 1389–1397, 2004.

[30] S. Hinz, L. Pagerols-Raluy, H. Oberg et al., "Foxp3 expression in pancreatic carcinoma cells as a novel mechanism of immune evasion in cancer," *Cancer Research*, vol. 67, no. 17, pp. 8344–8350, 2007.

[31] W. H. Wang, C. L. Jiang, W. Yan et al., "FOXP3 expression and clinical characteristics of hepatocellular carcinoma," *World Journal of Gastroenterology*, vol. 16, no. 43, pp. 5502–5509, 2010.

[32] L. M. Ebert, B. S. Tan, J. Browning et al., "The regulatory T cell-associated transcription factor FoxP3 is expressed by tumor cells," *Cancer Research*, vol. 68, no. 8, pp. 3001–3009, 2008.

[33] V. Karanikas, M. Speletas, M. Zamanakou et al., "Foxp3 expression in human cancer cells," *Journal of Translational Medicine*, vol. 6, article 19, 2008.

[34] M. Battaglia, C. Gianfrani, S. Gregori, and M. G. Roncarolo, "IL-10-producing T regulatory type 1 cells and oral tolerance," *Annals of the New York Academy of Sciences*, vol. 1029, pp. 142–153, 2004.

[35] S. Shimoda, F. Ishikawa, T. Kamihira et al., "Autoreactive T-cell responses in primary biliary cirrhosis are proinflammatory whereas those of controls are regulatory," *Gastroenterology*, vol. 131, no. 2, pp. 606–618, 2006.

[36] V. Bal, A. McIndoe, G. Denton et al., "Antigen presentation by keratinocytes induces tolerance in human T cells," *European Journal of Immunology*, vol. 20, no. 9, pp. 1893–1897, 1990.

[37] J. Markmann, D. Lo, A. Naji, R. D. Palmiter, R. L. Brinster, and E. Heber-Katz, "Antigen presenting function of class II MHC expressing pancreatic beta cells," *Nature*, vol. 336, no. 6198, pp. 476–479, 1988.

[38] G. Lombardi, K. Arnold, J. Uren et al., "Antigen presentation by interferon-γ-treated thyroid follicular cells inhibits interleukin-2 (IL-2) and supports IL-4 production by B7-dependent human T cells," *European Journal of Immunology*, vol. 27, no. 1, pp. 62–71, 1997.

[39] H. Inoue, H. Miyatani, Y. Sawada, and Y. Yoshida, "A case of pancreas cancer with autoimmune pancreatitis," *Pancreas*, vol. 33, no. 2, pp. 208–209, 2006.

[40] M. Loos, I. Esposito, D. M. Hedderich et al., "Autoimmune pancreatitis complicated by carcinoma of the pancreatobiliary system: a case report and review of the literature," *Pancreas*, vol. 40, no. 1, pp. 151–154, 2011.

[41] R. Pezzilli, S. Vecchiarelli, M. C. Di Marco et al., "Pancreatic ductal adenocarcinoma associated with autoimmune pancreatitis," *Case Reports in Gastroenterology*, vol. 5, no. 2, pp. 378–385, 2011.

[42] M. Yamamoto, H. Takahashi, T. Tabeya et al., "Risk of malignancies in IgG4-related disease," *Modern Rheumatology*, vol. 22, no. 3, pp. 414–418, 2012.

[43] K. Hirano, M. Tada, N. Sasahira et al., "Incidence of malignancies in patients with IgG4-related disease," *Internal Medicine*, vol. 53, no. 3, pp. 171–176, 2014.

[44] F. Mendes and K. D. Lindor, "Primary sclerosing cholangitis: overview and update," *Nature Reviews Gastroenterology and Hepatology*, vol. 7, no. 11, pp. 611–619, 2010.

[45] A. Tanaka, S. Tazuma, K. Okazaki, H. Tsubouchi, K. Inui, and H. Takikawa, "Nationwide survey for primary sclerosing cholangitis and IgG4-related sclerosing cholangitis in Japan," *Journal of Hepato-Biliary-Pancreatic Sciences*, vol. 21, no. 1, pp. 43–50, 2014.

[46] H. Ohtani, H. Ishida, Y. Ito, T. Yamaguchi, and M. Koizumi, "Autoimmune pancreatitis and biliary intraepithelial neoplasia of the common bile duct: a case with diagnostically challenging but pathogenetically significant association," *Pathology International*, vol. 61, no. 8, pp. 481–485, 2011.

[47] Y. Nakanuma, M.-P. Curado, S. Franceschi et al., "Intrahepatic cholangiocarcinoma," in *WHO Classification of Tumors of the Digestive System; World Health Organization of Tumors*, F. T. Bosman, F. Carneiro, R. H. Hruban, and N. D. Theise, Eds., pp. 217–224, IARC, Lyon, France, 2010.

[48] M. Takeuchi, Y. Sato, K. Ohno et al., "T helper 2 and regulatory T-cell cytokine production by mast cells: a key factor in the pathogenesis of IgG4-related disease," *Modern Pathology*, 2014.

[49] T. Tanikawa, C. M. Wilke, I. Kryczek et al., "Interleukin-10 ablation promotes tumor development, growth, and metastasis," *Cancer Research*, vol. 72, no. 2, pp. 420–429, 2012.

[50] K. Harada and Y. Nakanuma, "Pathological differences between IgG4-related sclerosing cholangitis with and without autoimmune pancreatitis (the 102nd USCAP annual meeting abstracts)," *Modern Pathology*, vol. 26, supplement 2, p. 403A, 2013.

[51] H. Hamano, S. Kawa, T. Uehara et al., "Immunoglobulin G4-related lymphoplasmacytic sclerosing cholangitis that mimics infiltrating hilar cholangiocarcinoma: part of a spectrum of autoimmune pancreatitis?" *Gastrointestinal Endoscopy*, vol. 62, no. 1, pp. 152–157, 2005.

[52] H. Umehara, K. Okazaki, Y. Masaki et al., "Comprehensive diagnostic criteria for IgG4-related disease (IgG4-RD), 2011," *Modern Rheumatology*, vol. 22, no. 1, pp. 21–30, 2012.

[53] A. Ghazale, S. T. Chari, L. Zhang et al., "Immunoglobulin G4-associated cholangitis: clinical profile and response to therapy," *Gastroenterology*, vol. 134, no. 3, pp. 706–715, 2008.

[54] S. T. Chari, T. C. Smyrk, M. J. Levy et al., "Diagnosis of autoimmune pancreatitis: the mayo clinic experience," *Clinical Gastroenterology and Hepatology*, vol. 4, no. 8, pp. 1010–1016, 2006.

[55] H. Kawakami, Y. Zen, M. Kuwatani et al., "IgG4-related sclerosing cholangitis and autoimmune pancreatitis: histological assessment of biopsies from Vater's ampulla and the bile duct," *Journal of Gastroenterology and Hepatology*, vol. 25, no. 10, pp. 1648–1655, 2010.

[56] T. Umemura, Y. Zen, H. Hamano, S. Kawa, Y. Nakanuma, and K. Kiyosawa, "Immunoglobin G4-hepatopathy: association of immunoglobin G4-bearing plasma cells in liver with autoimmune pancreatitis," *Hepatology*, vol. 46, no. 2, pp. 463–471, 2007.

6

Pathological Diagnosis of Hepatocellular Cellular Adenoma according to the Clinical Context

Paulette Bioulac-Sage,[1,2] Christine Sempoux,[3] Laurent Possenti,[4] Nora Frulio,[5] Hervé Laumonier,[5] Christophe Laurent,[6] Laurence Chiche,[7] Jean Frédéric Blanc,[2,4] Jean Saric,[6] Hervé Trillaud,[5] Brigitte Le Bail,[1,2] and Charles Balabaud[2]

[1] *Service d'Anatomie Pathologique, Hôpital Pellegrin, CHU Bordeaux, 33076 Bordeaux, France*
[2] *U1053 Université Bordeaux 2, 33076 Bordeaux, France*
[3] *Service d'Anatomie Pathologique, Cliniques Universitaires Saint Luc, Université Catholique de Louvain, 1200 Brussels, Belgium*
[4] *Service d'Hépatologie, Gastroenterologie, Hôpital St André CHU Bordeaux, 33000 Bordeaux, France*
[5] *Service de Radiologie, Hôpital St André CHU Bordeaux, 33000 Bordeaux, France*
[6] *Service de Chirurgie Digestive, Hôpital St André CHU Bordeaux, 33000 Bordeaux, France*
[7] *Service Hépatobiliare et Pancréatique, Hôpital Haut Lévêque CHU Bordeaux, 33604 Pessac, France*

Correspondence should be addressed to Paulette Bioulac-Sage; paulette.bioulac-sage@chu-bordeaux.fr

Academic Editor: Türkan Terkivatan

In Europe and North America, hepatocellular adenomas (HCA) occur, classically, in middle-aged woman taking oral contraceptives. Twenty percent of women, however, are not exposed to oral contraceptives; HCA can more rarely occur in men, children, and women over 65 years. HCA have been observed in many pathological conditions such as glycogenosis, familial adenomatous polyposis, MODY3, after male hormone administration, and in vascular diseases. Obesity is frequent particularly in inflammatory HCA. The background liver is often normal, but steatosis is a frequent finding particularly in inflammatory HCA. The diagnosis of HCA is more difficult when the background liver is fibrotic, notably in vascular diseases. HCA can be solitary, or multiple or in great number (adenomatosis). When nodules are multiple, they are usually of the same subtype. HNF1α-inactivated HCA occur almost exclusively in woman. The most important point of the classification is the identification of β-catenin mutated HCA, a strong argument to identify patients at risk of malignant transformation. Some HCA already present criteria indicating malignant transformation. When the whole nodule is a hepatocellular carcinoma, it is extremely difficult to prove that it is the consequence of a former HCA. It is occasionally difficult to identify HCA remodeled by necrosis or hemorrhage.

1. Introduction

The diagnosis of hepatocellular adenomas (HCA) may occasionally be difficult for the following reasons.

(i) The nodule is discovered in a context different to what we are used to see, such as in men, in women not exposed to oral contraceptives (OC), in older persons, or in children.

(ii) The tumor *per se* may be difficult to identify due to the partial necrosis or to the major remodeling of the tumor leading to the presence of criteria seen mostly in focal nodular hyperplasia (FNH) and/or to difficulties in differentiation from hepatocellular carcinoma (HCC).

(iii) The presence of an underlying liver disease such as nonalcoholic steatohepatitis (NASH), vascular disorder, and fibrosis.

(iv) HCA, HCC, and FNH or different HCA subtypes can be present in the same patient, some more prone

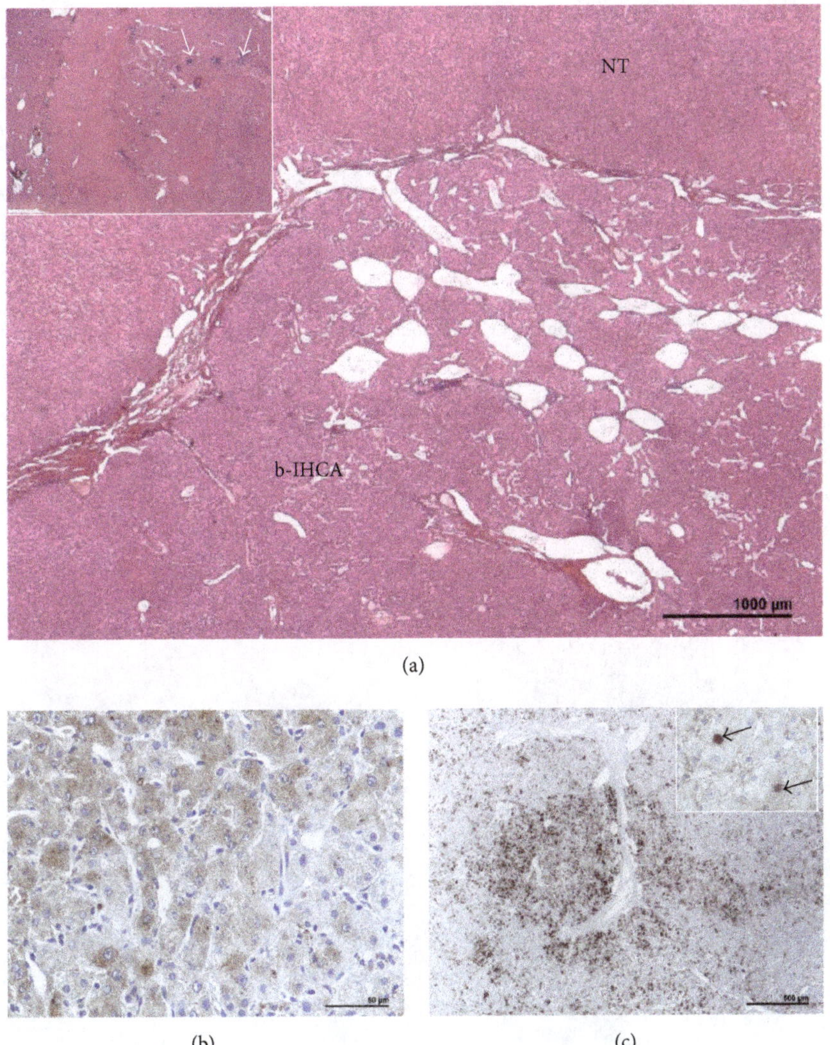

(a)

(b) (c)

Figure 1: b-IHCA (with discovery of an HCC 12 years later). A woman born in 1959. Discovery of a nodule 17 cm. Oral contraceptives 4 years, BMI 21.5. Surgery 1984: right hepatectomy but incomplete resection. Followup refused by the patient: 2 pregnancies. Patient seen 12 years later with numerous liver nodules of a well-differentiated HCC. Death occurred few months later. (a) H&E—proliferation of hepatocytes with some atypia (not visible at this magnification) and numerous dilated vessels; no arguments for overt malignancy; inset: a few inflammatory infiltrates (arrows). (b) Moderate expression of SAA by adenomatous hepatocytes. (c) Heterogenous, patchy expression of GS; inset: aberrant expression of a few hepatocytic nuclei (arrows).

to HCC transformation, with the difficult task, in some cases, to differentiate HCA from HCC.

(v) Finally, HCA can be discovered unexpectedly in patients treated for other liver tumors or developed in the context of diseases affecting the liver or other organs.

In this paper, we review the clinical/epidemiological context of HCA, based on our experience (personal cases and consult cases); all these cases being classified according to the pathomolecular classification into four groups, as previously published are HNF1α-inactivated HCA (H-HCA), inflammatory HCA (IHCA), β-catenin activated HCA (b-HCA and b-IHCA) and unclassified HCA (UHCA).

2. HCA: Age, Gender, and Oral Contraceptives

(1) The great majority of HCA occurs in middle age women genitally active, taking OC (at least in many Northern European countries and in North America) [1]. The magnitude of the risk of HCA in OC users is yet defined but is considered to be dose and time dependent. The difference in the incidence of HCA between countries among women taking OC has not been evaluated but seems real. Our experience is presented in Table 1. The incidence seems higher in France than in the US. A possible explanation could be the youngest age of the women exposed to the contraceptive pills in France compared to the US. Less than 20% of women with HCA are not exposed to OC or are exposed for very short periods of time.

Table 1: Hepatocellular adenomas: Bordeaux cases.

	Total	H-HCA	IHCA	b-IHCA	b-HCA	UHCA
n	184*	66	68	13	14	22
Mean age (extreme)	40 (14–66)	41 (14–65)	41 (25–59)	35 (18–59)	35 (14–66)	36.5 (22–52)
n W	163	62	59	8	11	22
Mean age (extreme)	40 (21–66)	41 (23–60)	40 (25–54)	35.5 (26–46)	35 (21–66)	36.5 (22–52)
n W (OC)	146	52	54	7	11	21
n W BMI > 25	52	13	24	0	2	12
n M	19	3**	9	5	2	0

n: number; W: adult women; M: adult men; BMI: body mass index; OC: oral contraceptives; *includes 2 children; **2 patients with MODY3.

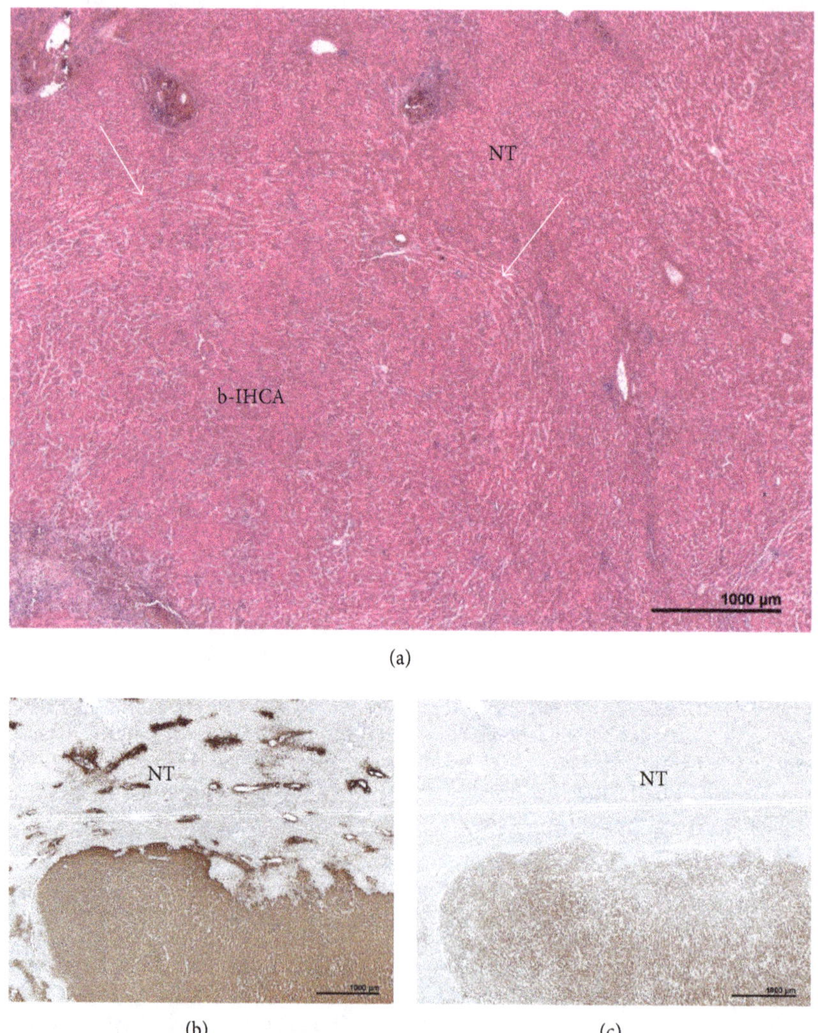

Figure 2: b-IHCA in the context of a FAP. A man born in 1966. Familial adenomatous polyposis (surgery in 1990 and 1996). Liver nodule discovered by chance, 9 cm. BMI 32.3. Segmentectomies V and VI. (a) H&E: HCA with ill-defined border (arrows). (b) Strong and diffuse expression of GS, contrasting with normal GS staining limited to a few centrolobular hepatocytes in the nontumoral liver (NT). (c) Diffuse expression of SAA in adenomatous hepatocytes with sharp demarcation from the surrounding NT.

If the role of OC in the development of HCA is certain, the individual susceptibility to the risk is of paramount importance. No particular HCA subtypes have been observed in women; however, HCA in very young women (in their twenties) taking or not OC without specific etiology are rare and found, in our experience, mainly in the b-HCA and UHCA subgroups.

(2) HCA in men are rare [2–8]. To the exception of HCA cases related to MODY3 (H-HCA) and male hormone administration (b-HCA), the immense majority are found

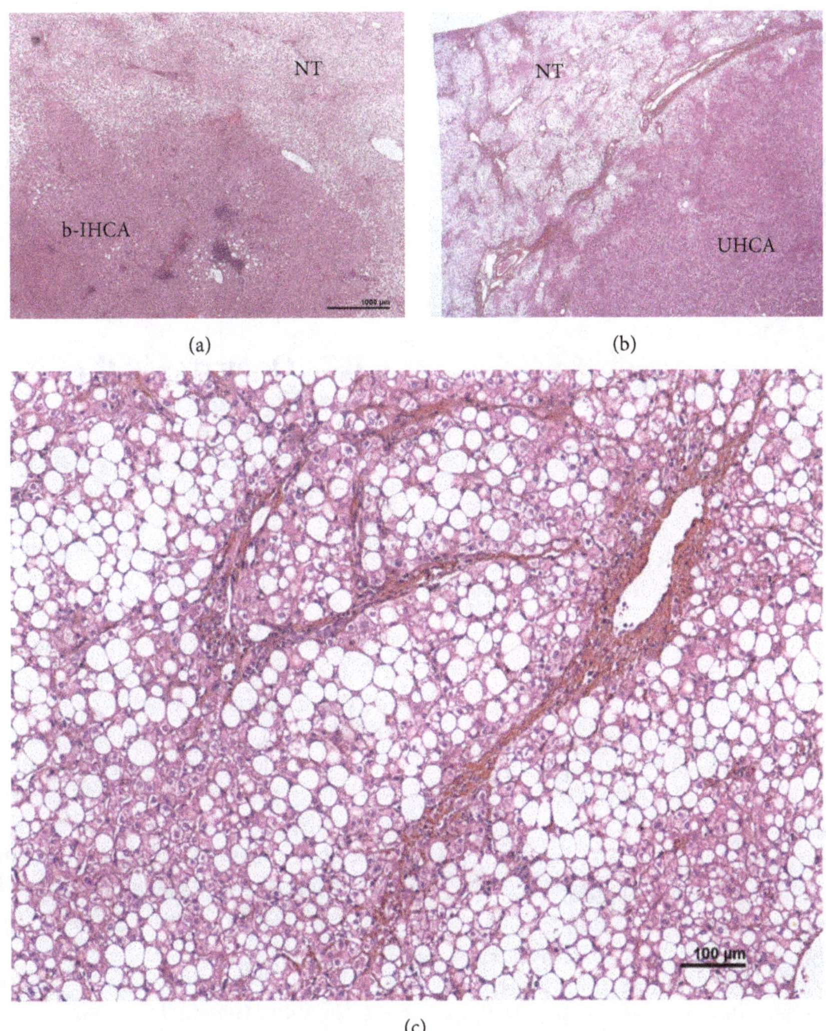

FIGURE 3: HCA on the background of NASH. (a) A woman born in 1956. Several nodules in the liver, largest 8 cm. Oral contraceptives for 31 years; BMI 24.6. Surgery in 2007 (several tumorectomies and segmentectomies). H&E: IHCA (typical expression of SAA and CRP—not shown), very mild steatosis, contrasting with highly steatotic (60%) nontumoral liver (NT): NASH with mild activity, without fibrosis. (b-c) Woman born in 1973, metabolic syndrome (noninsulin-dependant diabetes, hypercholesterolemia, hypertriglyceridemia). Oral contraceptives 15 years, BMI 31.6. Two liver nodules, largest 26 mm in segment IV. Segmentectomy IVB plus radio frequency of the other nodule (1 cm) in segment VIII. (b) H&E: nonsteatotic HCA (without immunohistochemical characteristics), classified as UHCA; its limit contrast with severe steatotic non tumoral liver (NT). (c) H&E: nontumoral liver: NASH with severe steatosis (80%), mild activity, and septal fibrosis (stage 3).

in the IHCA and b-IHCA subgroups. They are usually solitary. Patients are often overweight with one or several features of the metabolic syndrome. As the risk of HCC is important, resection of the nodule is recommended even for nodules smaller than 5 cm [9, 10].

(3) HCA occurring in infants, adolescents, or young adults are mainly related to specific etiology such as vascular disorders, familial adenomatous polyposis (FAP), or MODY 3.

(4) HCA in patients over 65 are rare. We have observed 4 H-HCA cases, all in women.

(5) In addition to age, gender, OC, and background liver diseases (see below), the biological and radiological parameters are also good indicators of HCA subgroups. Radiologists are now able to identify with confidence typical H-HCA and IHCA. Furthermore, a raised CRP level in the blood is a strong argument to identify IHCA.

3. HCA and HCC

It is well admitted that HCA may transform into HCC [11–25]. However, the risk of malignant transformation of HCA cannot be reliably quantified yet. Several series are concordant to show that approximately 5% of patients, whom HCA has been resected, had pathological evidence of HCC within their HCA. This figure, however, does not take into account fully transformed HCA where evidence of the preexisting benign lesion might have disappeared. The risk

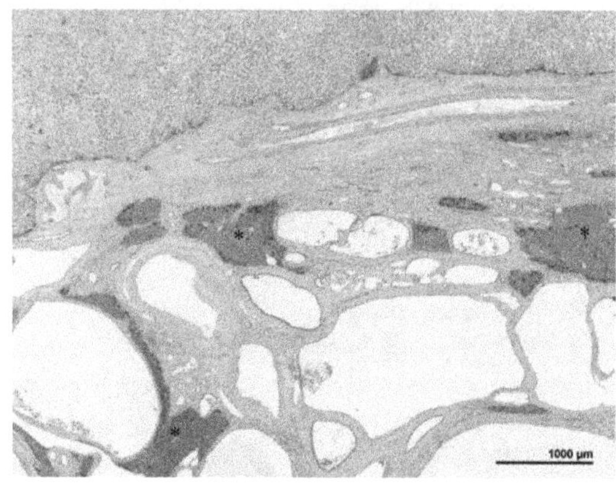

Figure 4: H-HCA associated with polycystic disease. Woman born in 1954. In 1991: kidney transplantation for polycystic kidney disease. In 2000: left hepatectomy for a 11 cm liver nodule. On oral contraceptives for 2 years, BMI 21.2. LFABP immunostaining: numerous biliary cysts with some areas of liver normally expressing LFABP (asterisk), contrasting with a portion of the H-HCA (upper) where LFABP is sharply decreased.

of malignant transformation is correlated with the b-catenin mutated subtype, and with the size of the HCA. HCA malignant transformation is unusual for nodules <5 cm. These results suggest that small HCA occurring in women could be safely observed, as they are also at low risk of bleeding.

HCC that developed on HCA are typically well differentiated without vascular extension or satellite nodules. AFP measurement is not reliable as it is usually normal. The prognosis is—compared to HCC in cirrhotic patients—relatively good if we consider that tumors are usually large tumors (>5 cm).

Prevalence of malignancy within HCA is 10 times more frequent in men than in women and management of HCA should primarily be based on gender. In addition to men, reported cases of HCC on HCA concern rare etiologies such as glycogenosis, male hormone administration, and vascular diseases. Metabolic syndrome also appears as an emerging condition associated with malignant transformation of HCA particularly in men and is the likely most frequent predisposing condition for HCC in this setting. For the pathologists, there are different degrees of difficulties to make the diagnosis of HCA transformation into HCC (see article Balabaud et al. in this issue).

(1) The tumor is definitively an HCC: malignant transformation of an HCA is likely when the HCC occurs in a specific context such as glycogenosis, male hormone administration, or when the diagnosis of HCA has been established several years before. The link exists but cannot be demonstrated when the cause of the putative HCA is not well documented (i.e., in patient exposed to anticonvulsive drugs), or when there are areas in the tumor, particularly at the border, looking benign but that could correspond to a very well-differentiated HCC.

(2) The tumor is benign but there are foci with cytological/architectural criteria in favor of premalignant changes (i.e., rosette formation, increased CD34 staining, irregular/decreased reticulin network).

(3) The tumor is possibly malignant, at least in part (i.e., areas with loss of reticulin, diffuse CD34 staining positivity, GPC3 even mild and focal, etc.). In many occasions, the diagnosis of true malignancy remains impossible to assert and the term "borderline tumor HCA/HCC" can be used. In our own series, we observed 17 cases of HCC possibly linked to HCA with 2 deaths (Figure 1).

4. HCA Occurring in the Context of Specific Etiology

4.1. Vascular Diseases. Many different types of hepatocellular nodules ranging from nodular regenerative hyperplasia (NRH), focal nodular hyperplasia (FNH), and macroregenerative nodule (MRN)/FNH-like, to HCA and HCC have been described in different types of vascular disorders [26–42] such as Budd Chiari syndrome [26–31], hereditary hemorrhagic telangiectasia [32], agenesis of the portal vein, intrahepatic shunts (congenital or acquired) [33–40], and the Fontan procedure [41, 42]. Unfortunately there is today no reliable data using modern techniques of identification of these nodules (imaging, histopathology, molecular biology). Recent data suggest that the majority of nodules are MRN/FNH-like and in addition, different HCA subtypes have been observed with possible malignant transformation [31]. In our personal experience (including consults), we have observed 4 cases (2 with HCC).

4.2. HCA and Genetic Disorders

4.2.1. Glycogenosis. In a large series of 43 patients published in 1997, 51.8% of patients with type 1 and 25% of patients with type 3 glycogen storage disease had HCA at the time of the study. The male to female ratio was 2 to 1 in type 1, and no female had adenomas in type 3 [43]. In a retrospective chart review performed in 117 patients with glycogenosis 1a, it was shown that metabolic control measured on the basis of serum triglyceride concentration may be related to HCA formation [44]. Immunohistochemistry (IHC) has been described in 2 large series of type 1 glycogenosis [45, 46]. IHCA was the main subtype; b-HCA has been also observed but not H-HCA [46]. In our series, we observed in 2 cases different HCA subtypes: IHCA, b-HCA, and b-IHCA. One male patient with type 3 glycogenosis and hepatic nodules detected at the age of 3 died at the age of 27 of HCC in our unit; the diagnosis of HCA and HCC was based on radiological criteria. HCC is a rare but major complication of glycogenosis [17].

4.2.2. Familial Adenomatous Polyposis. HCA in patients with FAP have been reported previously [15, 47–50] with inactivation of HNF1α [48] as well as biallelic inactivation of the APC gene [49, 50]. Malignant transformation has also been described [15]. In our series we have observed 2 cases of b-IHCA associated with FAP (Figure 2).

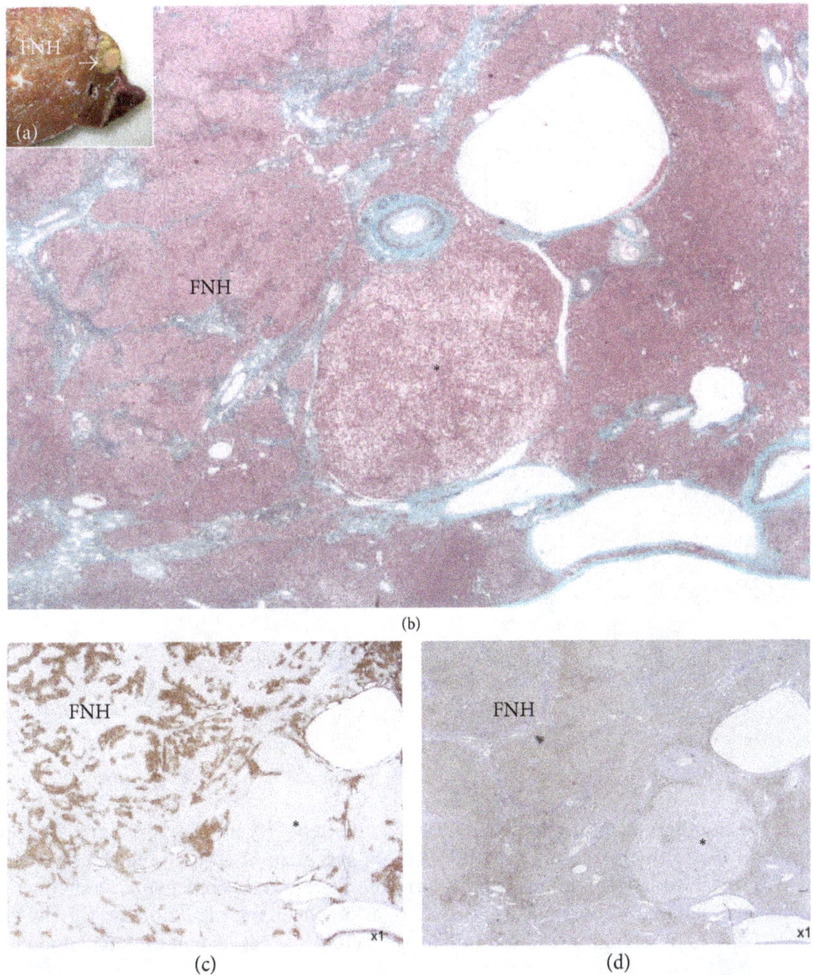

FIGURE 5: FNH associated with H-HCA. Woman born in 1966. Three FNH, largest 10 cm. Surgery in 2008 (segments V and VI). Discovery on the resected specimen of several small H-HCA. (a) Fresh specimen: typical FNH closed to a small yellow nodule (arrow). (b) Masson's trichrome: typical aspect of FNH, nearby a small steatotic nodule (asterisk). (c) GS staining is negative in the nodule, contrasting with map-like positivity in FNH. (d) LFABP is lacking in the small nodule, whereas it is normally expressed in FNH (as in nontumoral liver, not shown).

4.2.3. MODY3. The discovery of H-HCA in MODY3 is a great success of molecular biology with important clinical consequences [51–55]. The diagnosis of MODY3 should be evoked in H-HCA in the following circumstances: young age of the patient, adenomatosis, history of familial HCA, and diabetes in young age. H-HCA in men are observed only in MODY3 patients. We have confirmed the diagnosis of H-HCA due to MODY3 in 2 families [53, 55].

4.2.4. Tyrosinemia. Cases of HCA have been reported in tyrosinemia [1]. The diagnosis of HCA, in cirrhotic patients, remains very difficult to establish.

4.3. Drugs. HCA and HCC have been reported in patients taking male hormones for medical purposes, that is, Danazol [56–59], or to increase their muscular mass such as body builders [60, 61]. We had at least 2 cases of women taking OC and exposed also to Danazol; both were b-HCA. In one case there were multiple nodules, the largest one shrunk massively after stopping Danazol and all nodules presented features of involute HCC. The link between HCA and the long-term exposition to antiepileptic drugs is not well established [62–66]. We saw 3 such cases possibly linked to antiepileptic drugs.

4.4. Overweight/Obesity. The number of HCA noticeably increased faster in the 2001–2011 period compared to the 1990–2000 period. This phenomenon concurred with an increasing number of patients overweight or obese [67–69]. More overweight patients are found to harbor IHCA than H-HCA. Females still represent the great majority of overweight/obese patients with HCA. Overweight/obese male or female patients constitute a new entity in the IHCA and β-catenin activated IHCA subgroups. Overweight/obesity may soon represent a major risk of malignant transformation of HCA, possibly because of the activation of the IL-6 pathway. In HCA, the nontumoral liver is usually normal

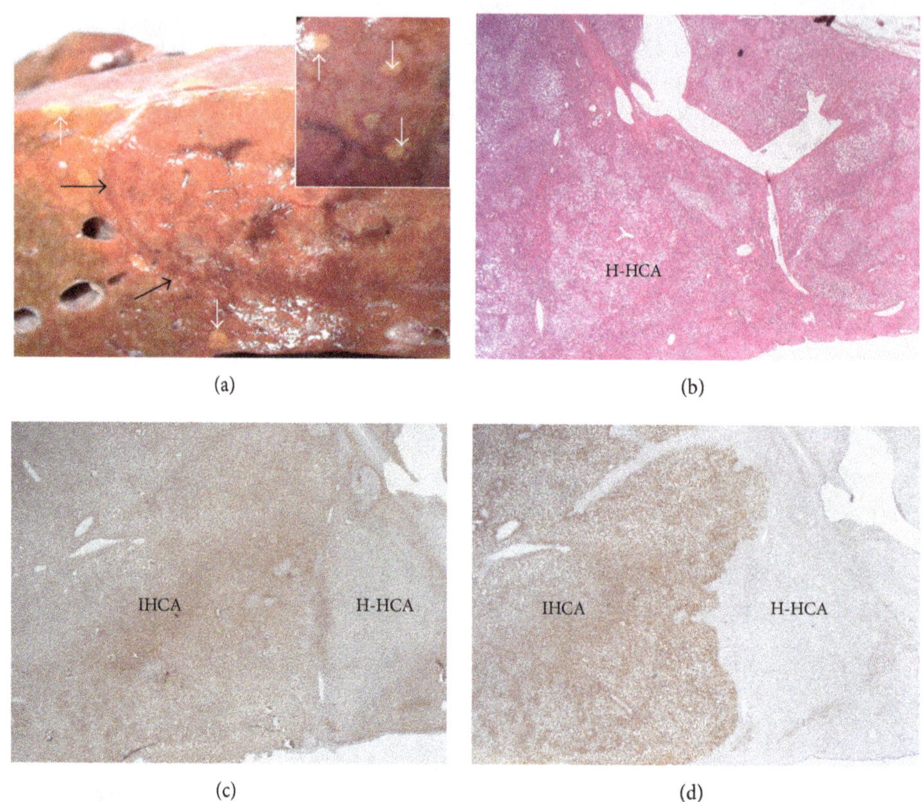

FIGURE 6: H-HCA and IHCA. Woman born in 1965. Abnormal liver function tests. Hypertriglyceridemia. Multiple nodules largest 9.5 cm. BMI 21.5. 18-year oral contraceptives. Left hepatectomy in 2011. (a) Fresh specimen—the large reddish nodule is not well limited (black arrows), associated with numerous yellowish small nodules in the surrounding resected parenchyma, sometimes visible under the Glisson's capsule (white arrows). (b) The small nodules are steatotic. (c) LFABP is lacking in all the small nodules (H-HCA), contrasting with normal expression in the nearby IHCA. (d) CRP is strongly expressed in IHCA, whereas it is negative in the small nodule of H-HCA.

or subnormal. Steatosis (mild to severe) is quite often observed in overweight/obese patients with or without metabolic syndrome; NASH is rare [70]. Most of the time, there is a clear difference on gross pathology or under the microscope between the tumoral and nontumoral liver (Figure 3). The distinction may be difficult at first glance when the nontumoral liver is steatotic as well as the tumor. Steatosis in the nontumoral liver can also be observed in other instances such as in alcoholic liver disease, glycogenosis, or the Fanconi anemia.

4.5. Anemia. (1) *Fanconi anemia.* The Fanconi anemia is an autosomal recessive disease, causing secondary aplastic anemia and congenital abnormalities, associated with an increased risk of tumors [56, 71, 72]. In patients with the Fanconi anemia, androgen therapy and iron overload may contribute to the development of HCA and HCC; the latter may occur as a transformation of HCA. With prolongation of survival, continued development of liver tumors can be expected. Routine detection should therefore be considered in these patients.

(2) *beta thalassemia.* Hepatocellular adenoma has been reported [1].

(3) *Anemia of chronic disease.* In 2002, severe anemia of chronic disease was described in an unusual group of patients with glycogen storage disease type 1a. The anemia was directly related to the presence of large hepatic adenomas that inappropriately produced hepcidin [73, 74]. A similar mechanism was described in another case not related to glycogenosis [75]. In our experience at least 2 patients were investigated during several years for the diagnosis of inflammatory anemias without any clues until one or several liver nodules were discovered. The anemia was cured after resection of the IHCA [76]. In patients with IHCA, it is not rare to observe biological criteria of inflammatory anemia [10].

4.6. Endocrine Disorders. (1) *Polycystic ovary syndrome.* A case of a young woman with HCA in a context of polycystic ovary syndrome, associated with high levels of androgens and following a high dose hormonal therapy, has been described [77]. We observed a similar case (IHCA).

(2) *Cushing's syndrome.* To our knowledge no case of HCA has been reported yet in Cushing syndrome patients. In our file, one b-HCA occurring in a patient with a Cushing syndrome became malignant years later; however, this old case was poorly documented.

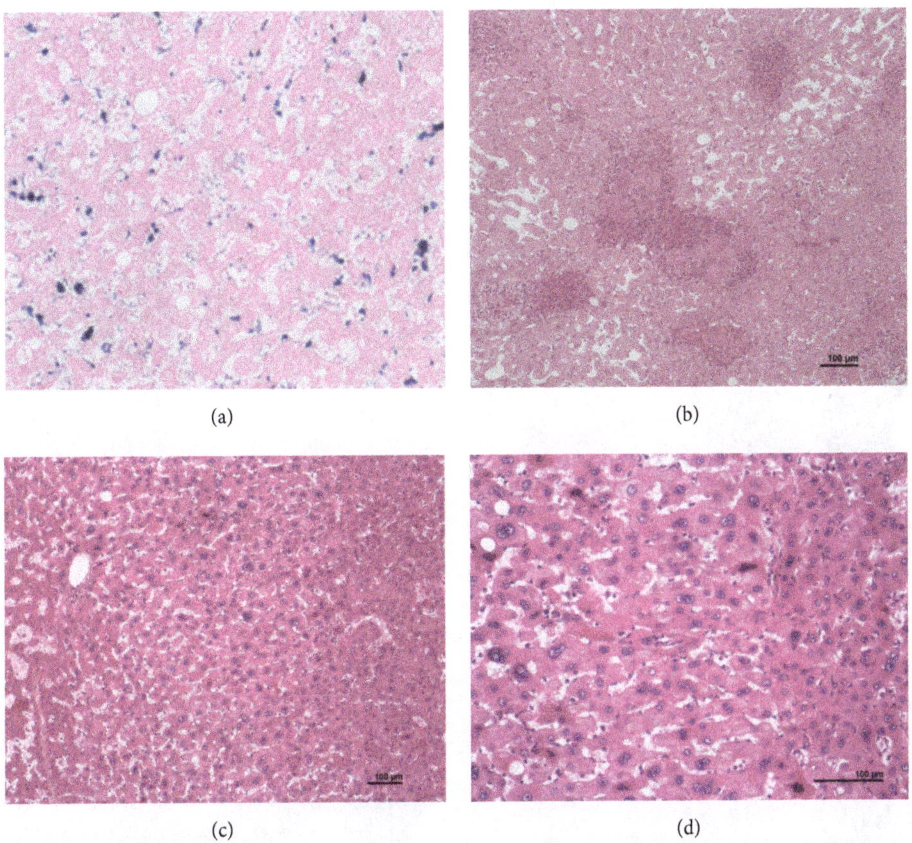

FIGURE 7: Rare, misleading cytological findings. (a) Woman born in 1964. Abnormal liver tests and anemia. No oral contraceptives, BMI 40.4. Alcohol (30 to 40 g per day), hypercholesterolemia, and type 2 diabetes. Biopsy: IHCA. Right hepatectomy 2006: IHCA. The anemia corrected several months after surgery. Perls staining: positivity in sinusoidal cells of the IHCA. (b) Woman born in 1936. Oral contraceptives 21 years. Several liver nodules. Tumorectomies in 1989. H&E: numerous epithelioid granulomas are widespread within the IHCA. (c-d): Woman born in 1947. Massive bleeding. No oral contraceptives, BMI 21.5. Right hepatectomy 2000. Massive liver necrosis. Pathological diagnosis: IHCA. H&E: areas with cytological abnormalities: dystrophic nuclei (irregular, hyperchromatic), nearby necrotic/hemorrhagic zones of the IHCA.

4.7. Fibrotic Background Liver. In severe fibrosis/cirrhosis, the diagnosis of HCA was not reported until recently in alcoholic patients [78]. Here the difficulty is to differentiate an IHCA from a MRN/FNH-like expressing inflammatory proteins. In our experience MRN and MRN-FNH-like, which are frequently observed in cirrhotic background, can express CRP. Molecular data are necessary to identify with certainty HCA in cirrhotic patients.

5. Association of HCA with Other Tumors

5.1. Association of HCA with HCC and Nonhepatocellular Tumors. We have observed HCA associated with other tumors occurring elsewhere in the liver. In all these cases, HCA were in the H-HCA subgroup, associated with an HCC, an angiomyolipoma, and a mucinous cystadenoma, and one was associated with cysts in the context of a kidney polycystic disease (Figure 4). These associations are possibly fortuitous in the 2 first observations. We cannot, however, rule out the possibility of a common genetic parameter, at least in the last observation.

5.2. Association between Different Benign Hepatocellular Tumors

(i) *Association of HCA and FNH.* The association is probably not fortuitous. FNH are particularly frequent in adenomatosis, and it is not rare that small H-HCA could be fortuitously discovered on the resected specimen (Figure 5). It is well known that liver vascular diseases are prone to the development of FNH. As such they may also play a role in the development of HCA [79].

(ii) *Association of different HCA subtypes.* H-HCA and IHCA are rarely associated in the same liver; we have observed, however, a few cases presenting such association (Figure 6). This association supports the concept of an individual susceptibility to develop HCA, common to several subtypes.

(iii) *Association of IHCA and b-IHCA.* In cases with multiple IHCA, some nodules can be in addition b-catenin activated indicating that b-catenin mutation could be a late event in the development of

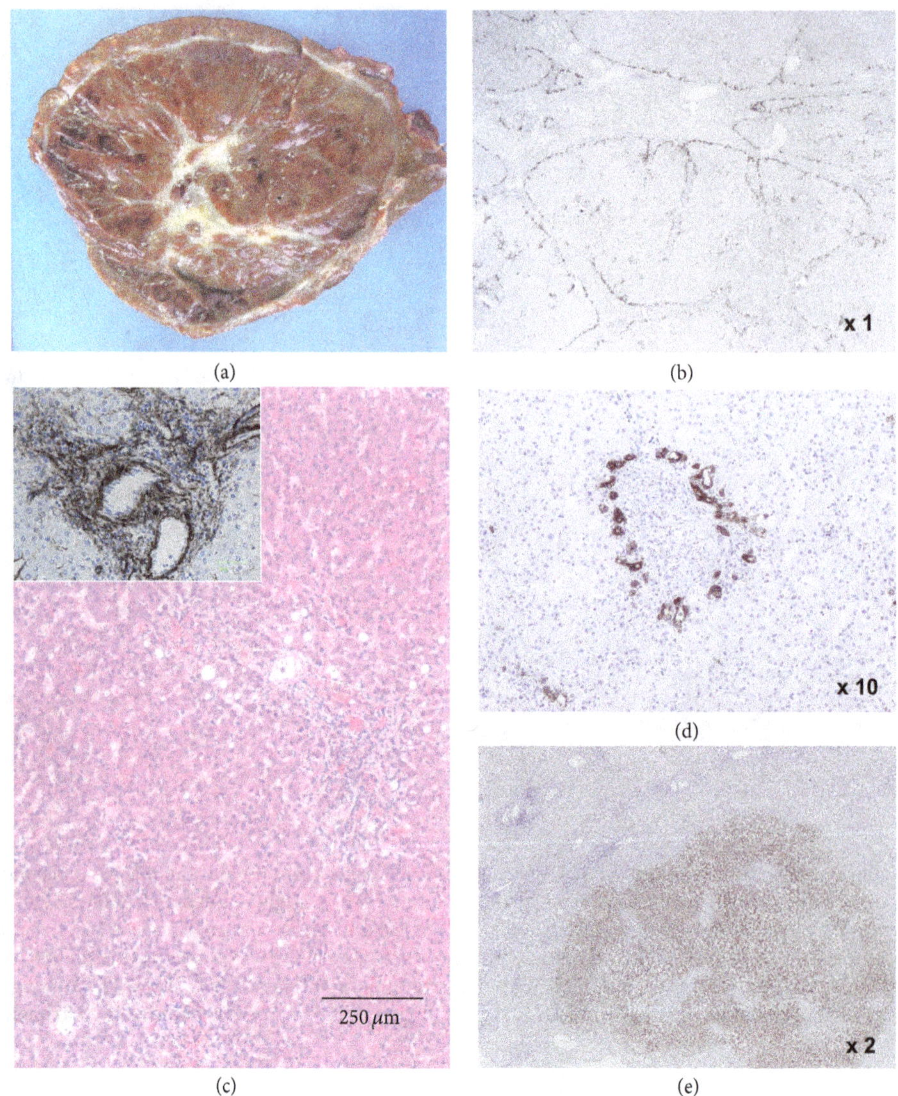

Figure 8: HCA looking like FNH. Same as patient 7A. (a) Fresh specimen: large subcapsular reddish tumor, with a white stellate area of loose fibrosis in the center. (b) CK7 is expressed at the border of fibrotic bands delineating nodules. (c) H&E (αSMA insert). The overall aspect is in favor of an IHCA. (d) Ductular reaction around inflammatory pseudo-portal tracts. (e) CRP is diffusely expressed in the nodule. The diagnosis of IHCA was reinforced by the disappearance of the chronic anemia after resection of the nodule.

the nodule; indeed, in such cases large nodules were b-IHCA whereas the small ones were IHCA.

5.3. Association of HCA with Extra Hepatic Tumors. (1) In 1989, Wanless et al. reported 13 cases with multiple FNH associated with other lesions such as hemangioma of liver meningioma, astrocytoma, telangiectasia of the brain, berry aneurysm, dysplastic systemic arteries, and portal vein atresia [80]. In the same paper, Wanless described the so-called "telangiectatic subtype of FNH" which occurs in this syndrome as well as in a minority of patients with solitary FNH. Today we know that the so-called telangiectatic FNH are IHCA [81, 82]. FNH with major sinusoidal dilatation, however, does exist [83]. We still have to clarify the association between the above brain tumors and benign hepatocellular nodules.

(2) HCA are so rare that patients with cancer (breast, colon, etc.) and a nodule in the liver are thought to have, *a priori*, a metastasis. We have encountered 3 patients already treated by chemotherapy where HCA were discovered by chance during the followup.

6. HCA with Rare or Misleading Features

6.1. Rare Findings in HCA. Iron [74] or other pigments such as lipofuscin granules, Dubin Johnson pigment [7, 8, 16, 84], hematopoiesis, calcifications [85], and inflammatory granulomas [86–88] are occasionally observed in HCA. Iron is located in hepatocytes in the Fanconi anemia. Surprisingly no iron was observed in HCA with chronic anemia related to hepcidin production. In our experience, among our cases of HCA associated with chronic anemia, we did not observe iron

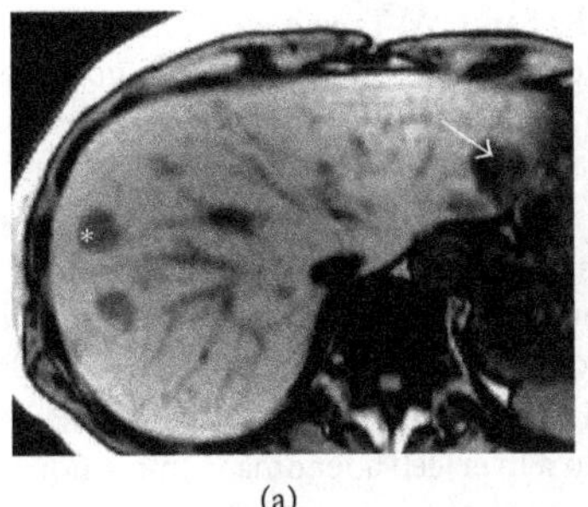
(a)

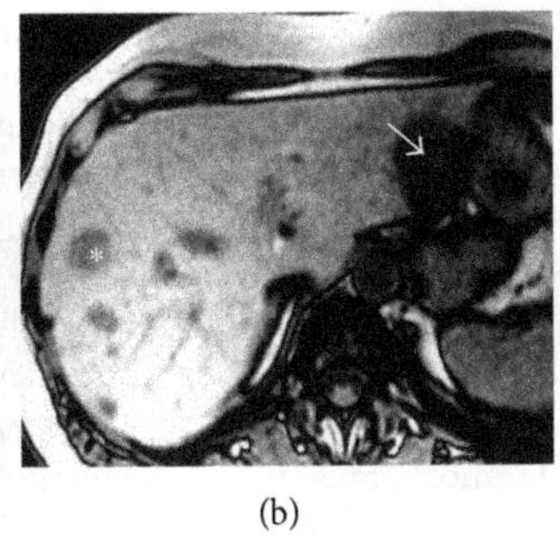
(b)

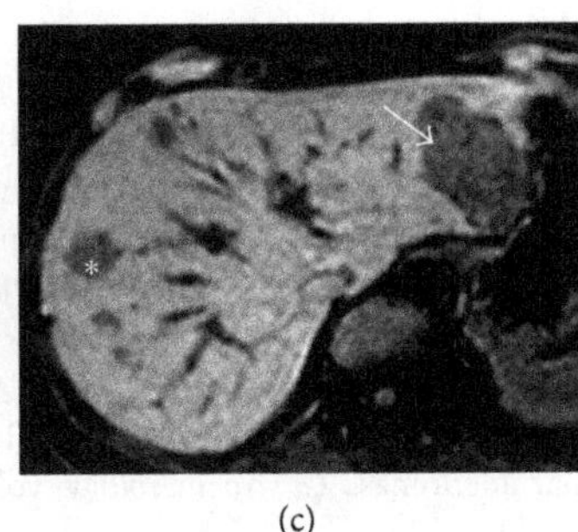
(c)

FIGURE 9: H-HCA size increment. Woman born in 1952. Abnormal liver function tests. Oral contraceptives 13 years, BMI 25.4 MRI adenomatosis, largest nodule 6 cm. Segmentectomies IV and VI 2001. Follow-up: increase size of one nodule Segmentectomy III, 2010. (a–c) Phased-opposed T1 weighted MR images in 2001 (a), 2007 (b), and 2010 (c) showing multiple hepatocellular adenomas showing hypointense because of the massive fat component. The nodule located in segment II (arrow) gradually increases in diameter between 2001 and 2010. As the 13 mm nodule located in segment VIII (asterisk), other nodules did not change their size.

overload except in 2 cases where iron was almost exclusively found in Kupffer cells (Figure 7(a)).

6.2. Cytological/Architectural Abnormalities Not Linked to Malignancy Transformation. Abnormalities such as mainly dystrophic nuclei or 2-3 cells thick hepatocytic plates are often seen when HCA exhibits large hemorrhagic/necrotic areas (Figure 7(b)). These misleading features are probably linked to a secondary regenerative process.

6.3. HCA Presenting Features of FNH. HCA can also be remodeled following necrosis/hemorrhage. Fibrotic bands and even scars can form so that HCA look like FNH; these changes are more frequently seen in IHCA subtypes (Figure 8). The arguments to favor one diagnosis over the other rely mainly on clinical, biological, and IHC data; this may not represent, however, strong enough arguments in some difficult cases.

6.4. HCA Number and Size Variation. HCA are solitary or multiple (from few to many). Many HCA defined the so-called entity adenomatosis (arbitrarily more than 10 nodules). For surgeons, adenomatosis is defined also by the number of nodules whose size raises therapeutic decision. Therefore, we have to distinguish cases with a single large nodule accompanied by myriads of small millimetric nodules from cases with multiple large nodules. Adenomatosis is more frequently observed in H-HCA and to a lesser extent in IHCA [10]. Apart from metabolic disorders, adenomatosis is rare in b-HCA and UHCA. Interestingly enough in the immense majority of cases, HCA when detected seems to be already at their maximum size (for those not resected). During followup (and after OC stopped), size remains stable or decrease. The impression, that needs to be confirmed, is that H-HCA remains stable and that IHCA tends to decrease. It is necessary to remember that in HNF1α-inactivated adenomatosis, there are myriads of small HCA that tend to aggregates to form larger nodules [89]. We have observed 2 HNF1α adenomatosis where such large nodules were interpreted as increasing in size, requiring reintervention (Figure 9). It is not known if the hemorrhagic risk is linked to the apparent global size of the nodule or not.

7. Recommendations and Conclusion

If it is tempting to publish rare cases, such as HCA with unusual cytological abnormalities, HCA in rare pathological context (beta thalassemia, tyrosinemia, etc.), HCA associated with rare hepatic or extrahepatic tumors, HCA have to be classified in subgroups with the help of IHC, to understand the pathophysiology of the disease and, in the long term, to better diagnose liver tumors and adapt the management of the patients. Not all HCA can be correctly classified with histological tools only. To prevent this limitation, it is recommended to freeze tissue, in order to perform molecular studies, that are particularly important to understand unusual and unclassified HCA cases. It is hoped that the pathomolecular classification of hepatocellular adenomas developed on normal as well as on fibrotic liver will help us to make progress in this field.

References

[1] "Hepatocellular Adenoma," *eMedicine Gastroenterology*, http://emedicine.medscape.com/article/170205-overview.

[2] T. P. Theruvath, B. Izar, J. McGillicuddy, E. Stewar, A. Reuben, and K. D. Chavin, "Hepatocellular adenoma in men: a rare cause for liver resection," *The American Surgeon*, vol. 77, pp. 373–376, 2011.

[3] T. Monchal, L. Barbier, E. Hornez et al., "Ruptured liver cell adenoma in man: great fortune in misfortune," *Acta Chirurgica Belgica*, vol. 110, no. 5, pp. 555–557, 2010.

[4] Y. Goudard, D. Rouquie, C. Bertocchi et al., "Malignant transformation of hepatocellular adenoma in men," *Gastroenterologie Clinique et Biologique*, vol. 34, no. 3, pp. 168–170, 2010.

[5] E. A. Psatha, R. C. Semelka, D. Armao, J. T. Woosley, Z. Firat, and G. Schneider, "Hepatocellular adenomas in men: MRI findings in four patients," *Journal of Magnetic Resonance Imaging*, vol. 22, no. 2, pp. 258–264, 2005.

[6] Y. Mamada, M. Onda, T. Tajiri et al., "Liver cell adenoma in a 26-year-old man," *Journal of Nippon Medical School*, vol. 68, no. 6, pp. 516–519, 2001.

[7] P. H. Bernard, J. F. Blanc, C. Paulusma et al., "Multiple black hepatocellular adenomas in a male patient," *European Journal of Gastroenterology and Hepatology*, vol. 12, no. 11, pp. 1253–1257, 2000.

[8] N. Hasan, M. Coutts, and B. Portmann, "Pigmented liver cell adenoma in two male patients," *The American Journal of Surgical Pathology*, vol. 24, no. 10, pp. 1429–1432, 2000.

[9] S. Dokmak, V. Paradis, V. Vilgrain et al., "A single-center surgical experience of 122 patients with single and multiple hepatocellular adenomas," *Gastroenterology*, vol. 137, no. 5, pp. 1698–1705, 2009.

[10] P. Bioulac-Sage, H. Laumonier, G. Couchy et al., "Hepatocellular adenoma management and phenotypic classification: the Bordeaux experience," *Hepatology*, vol. 50, no. 2, pp. 481–489, 2009.

[11] O. Farges, N. Ferreira, S. Dokmak, J. Belghiti, P. Bedossa, and V. Paradis, "Changing trends in malignant transformation of hepatocellular adenoma," *Gut*, vol. 60, no. 1, pp. 85–89, 2011.

[12] O. Farges and S. Dokmak, "Malignant transformation of liver adenoma: an analysis of the literature," *Digestive Surgery*, vol. 27, no. 1, pp. 32–38, 2010.

[13] J. H. Stoot, R. J. Coelen, M. C. De Jong, and C. H. Dejong, "Malignant transformation of hepatocellular adenomas into hepatocellular carcinomas: a systematic review including more than 1600 adenoma cases," *HPB*, vol. 12, no. 8, pp. 509–522, 2010.

[14] V. Paradis, S. Zalisnski, E. Chelbi et al., "Hepatocellular carcinomas in patients with metabolic syndrome often develop without significant liverfibrosis: a pathological analysis," *Hepatology*, vol. 49, no. 3, pp. 851–859, 2009.

[15] Y. Toiyama, Y. Inoue, H. Yasuda et al., "Hepatocellular adenoma containing hepatocellular carcinoma in a male patient with familial adenomatous polyposis coli: report of a case," *Surgery Today*, vol. 41, pp. 1442–1446, 2011.

[16] J. F. Hechtman, M. Raoufi, M. I. Fiel et al., "Hepatocellular carcinoma arising in a pigmented telangiectatic adenoma with nuclear β-catenin and glutamine synthetase positivity: case report and review of the literature," *The American Journal of Surgical Pathology*, vol. 35, no. 6, pp. 927–932, 2011.

[17] D. Cassiman, L. Libbrecht, C. Verslype et al., "An adult male patient with multiple adenomas and a hepatocellular carcinoma: mild glycogen storage disease type Ia," *Journal of Hepatology*, vol. 53, no. 1, pp. 213–217, 2010.

[18] J. L. Deneve, T. M. Pawlik, S. Cunningham et al., "Liver cell adenoma: a multicenter analysis of risk factors for rupture and malignancy," *Annals of Surgical Oncology*, vol. 16, no. 3, pp. 640–648, 2009.

[19] S. T. L. Micchelli, P. Vivekanandan, J. K. Boitnott, T. M. Pawlik, M. A. Choti, and M. Torbenson, "Malignant transformation of hepatic adenomas," *Modern Pathology*, vol. 21, no. 4, pp. 491–497, 2008.

[20] P. Gorayski, C. H. Thompson, H. S. Subhash, and A. C. Thomas, "Hepatocellular carcinoma associated with recreational anabolic steroid use," *British Journal of Sports Medicine*, vol. 42, no. 1, pp. 74–75, 2008.

[21] P. Gorayski, C. H. Thompson, H. S. Subhash, and A. C. Thomas, "Erratum: hepatocellular carcinoma associated with recreational anabolic steroid use, British Journal of Sports Medicine, 42(1):74–75, 2008," *British Journal of Sports Medicine*, vol. 44, article e5, 2009.

[22] R. Colovic, N. Grubor, M. Micev, and V. Radak, "Hepatocellular adenoma with malignant alteration," *Hepato-Gastroenterology*, vol. 54, no. 74, pp. 386–388, 2007.

[23] Y. Seyama, K. Sano, W. Tang et al., "Simultaneous resection of liver cell adenomas and an intrahepatic portosystemic venous shunt with elevation of serum PIVKA-II level," *Journal of Gastroenterology*, vol. 41, no. 9, pp. 909–912, 2006.

[24] N. Arvind, D. Duraimurugan, and J. S. Rajkumar, "Hepatic adenomatosis—a rare double complication of multiple adenoma rupture and malignant transformation," *Indian Journal of Gastroenterology*, vol. 25, no. 4, pp. 209–210, 2006.

[25] E. Burri, M. Steuerwald, G. Cathomas et al., "Hepatocellular carcinoma in a liver-cell adenoma within a non-cirrhotic liver," *European Journal of Gastroenterology and Hepatology*, vol. 18, no. 4, pp. 437–441, 2006.

[26] R. Moucari, P. E. Rautou, D. Cazals-Hatem et al., "Hepatocellular carcinoma in Budd-Chiari syndrome: characteristics and risk factors," *Gut*, vol. 57, pp. 828–835, 2008.

[27] D. Cazals-Hatem, V. Vilgrain, P. Genin et al., "Arterial and portal circulation and parenchymal changes in Budd-Chiari syndrome: a study in 17 explanted livers," *Hepatology*, vol. 37, no. 3, pp. 510–519, 2003.

[28] M. Tanaka and I. R. Wanless, "Pathology of the liver in Budd-Chiari syndrome: portal vein thrombosis and the histogenesis of veno-centric cirrhosis, veno-portal cirrhosis, and large regenerative nodules," *Hepatology*, vol. 27, no. 2, pp. 488–496, 1998.

[29] E. C. Oliveira, A. G. E. Duarte, I. F. S. F. Boin, J. R. S. Almeida, and C. A. F. Escanhoela, "Large benign hepatocellular nodules in cirrhosis due to chronic venous outflow obstruction: diagnostic confusion with hepatocellular carcinoma," *Transplantation Proceedings*, vol. 42, no. 10, pp. 4116–4118, 2010.

[30] N. Flor, M. Zuin, F. Brovelli et al., "Regenerative nodules in patients with chronic Budd-Chiari syndrome: a longitudinal study using multiphase contrast-enhanced multidetector CT," *European Journal of Radiology*, vol. 73, no. 3, pp. 588–593, 2010.

[31] P. Bioulac-Sage, C. Sempoux, V. Paradis et al., "Characterization of liver nodules in patients with Budd Chiari syndrome (BCS) and portal vein agenesis (PVA)," *Hepatology*, vol. 56, supplement 1, article 460A, 2012.

[32] R. Brenard, X. Chapaux, P. Deltenre et al., "Large spectrum of liver vascular lesions including high prevalence of focal nodular hyperplasia in patients with hereditary haemorrhagic telangiectasia: the Belgian Registry based on 30 patients," *European Journal of Gastroenterology and Hepatology*, vol. 22, no. 10, pp. 1253–1259, 2010.

[33] E. Alonso-Gamarra, M. Parrón, A. Pérez, C. Prieto, L. Hierro, and M. López-Santamaría, "Clinical and radiologic manifestations of congenital extrahepatic portosystemic shunts: a comprehensive review," *Radiographics*, vol. 31, pp. 707–722, 2011.

[34] Y. Tanaka, M. Takayanagi, Y. Shiratori et al., "Congenital absence of portal vein with multiple hyperplastic nodular lesions in the liver," *Journal of Gastroenterology*, vol. 38, no. 3, pp. 288–294, 2003.

[35] A. S. Glatard, S. Hillaire, G. d'Assignies et al., "Obliterative portal venopathy: findings at CT imaging," *Radiology*, vol. 263, pp. 741–750, 2012.

[36] S. Kobayashi, O. Matsui, T. Gabata et al., "Radiological and histopathological manifestations of hepatocellular nodular lesions concomitant with various congenital and acquired hepatic hemodynamic abnormalities," *Japanese Journal of Radiology*, vol. 27, no. 2, pp. 53–68, 2009.

[37] D. Zeitoun, G. Brancatelli, M. Colombat et al., "Congenital hepatic fibrosis: CT findings in 18 adults," *Radiology*, vol. 231, no. 1, pp. 109–116, 2004.

[38] F. Kondo, Y. Koshima, and M. Ebara, "Nodular lesions associated with abnormal liver circulation," *Intervirology*, vol. 47, no. 3–5, pp. 277–287, 2004.

[39] M. Kawakatsu, V. Vilgrain, J. Belghiti, J. F. Flejou, and H. Nahum, "Association of multiple liver cell adenomas with spontaneous intrahepatic portohepatic shunt," *Abdominal Imaging*, vol. 19, no. 5, pp. 438–440, 1994.

[40] V. Dhalluin-Venier, M. Fabre, E. Jacquemin, A. S. Rangheard, G. Pelletier, and C. Buffet, "Liver cell adenomas and portosystemic shunt," *Gastroenterologie Clinique et Biologique*, vol. 32, no. 2, pp. 164–166, 2008.

[41] K. Babaoglu, F. K. Binnetoglu, A. Aydoğan et al., "Hepatic adenomatosis in a 7-year-old child treated earlier with a Fontan procedure," *Pediatric Cardiology*, vol. 31, pp. 861–864, 2010.

[42] A. A. Ghaferi and G. M. Hutchins, "Progression of liver pathology in patients undergoing the Fontan procedure: chronic passive congestion, cardiac cirrhosis, hepatic adenoma, and hepatocellular carcinoma," *Journal of Thoracic and Cardiovascular Surgery*, vol. 129, no. 6, pp. 1348–1352, 2005.

[43] P. Labrune, P. Trioche, I. Duvaltier, P. Chevalier, and M. Odièvre, "Hepatocellular adenomas in glycogen storage disease type I and III: a series of 43 patients and review of the literature," *Journal of Pediatric Gastroenterology and Nutrition*, vol. 24, no. 3, pp. 276–279, 1997.

[44] D. Q. Wang, L. M. Fiske, C. T. Carreras, and D. A. Weinstein, "Natural history of hepatocellular adenoma formation in glycogen storage disease type I," *Journal of Pediatrics*, vol. 159, pp. 442–446, 2011.

[45] S. Sakellariou, H. Al-Hussaini, A. Scalori et al., "Hepatocellular adenoma in glycogen storage disorder type I: a clinicopathological and molecular study," *Histopathology*, vol. 60, pp. E58–E65, 2012.

[46] J. Calderaro, P. Labrune, G. Morcrette et al., "Molecular characterization of hepatocellular adenomas developed in patients with glycogen storage disease type I," *Journal of Hepatology*, vol. 58, no. 2, pp. 350–357, 2012.

[47] Y. Okamura, A. Maeda, K. Matsunaga et al., "Hepatocellular adenoma in a male with familial adenomatous polyposis coli," *Journal of Hepato-Biliary-Pancreatic Surgery*, vol. 16, pp. 571–574, 2009.

[48] E. Jeannot, D. Wendum, F. Paye et al., "Hepatocellular adenoma displaying a HNF1α inactivation in a patient with familial adenomatous polyposis coli," *Journal of Hepatology*, vol. 45, no. 6, pp. 883–886, 2006.

[49] S. Bala, P. H. Wunsch, and W. G. Ballhausen, "Childhood hepatocellular adenoma in familial adenomatous polyposis: mutations in adenomatous polyposis coli gene and p53," *Gastroenterology*, vol. 112, no. 3, pp. 919–922, 1997.

[50] H. Bläker, C. Sutter, M. Kadmon et al., "Analysis of somatic APC mutations in rare extracolonic tumors of patients with familial adenomatous polyposis coli," *Genes Chromosomes and Cancer*, vol. 41, no. 2, pp. 93–98, 2004.

[51] O. Bluteau, E. Jeannot, P. Bioulac-Sage et al., "Bi-allelic inactivation of TCF1 in hepatic adenomas," *Nature Genetics*, vol. 32, no. 2, pp. 312–315, 2002.

[52] Y. Reznik, T. Dao, R. Coutant et al., "Hepatocyte nuclear factor-1α gene inactivation: cosegregation between liver adenomatosis and diabetes phenotypes in two maturity-onset diabetes of the young (MODY)3 families," *Journal of Clinical Endocrinology and Metabolism*, vol. 89, no. 3, pp. 1476–1480, 2004.

[53] Y. Bacq, E. Jacquemin, C. Balabaud et al., "Familial liver adenomatosis associated with hepatocyte nuclear factor 1alpha inactivation," *Gastroenterology*, vol. 125, no. 5, pp. 1470–1475, 2003.

[54] E. Jeannot, L. Mellottee, P. Bioulac-Sage et al., "Spectrum of HNF1A somatic mutations in hepatocellular adenoma differs from that in patients with MODY3 and suggests genotoxic damage," *Diabetes*, vol. 59, no. 7, pp. 1836–1844, 2010.

[55] E. Jeannot, G. Lacape, H. Gin et al., "Double heterozygous germline HNF1A mutations in a patient with liver adenomatosis," *Diabetes Care*, vol. 35, article e35, 2012.

[56] I. Velazquez and B. P. Alter, "Androgens and liver tumors: Fanconi's anemia and non-Fanconi's conditions," *American Journal of Hematology*, vol. 77, pp. 257–267, 2004.

[57] K. Bork and V. Schneiders, "Danazol-induced hepatocellular adenoma in patients with hereditary angio-oedema," *Journal of Hepatology*, vol. 36, pp. 707–709, 2002.

[58] K. Bork, M. Pitton, P. Harten, and P. Koch, "Hepatocellular adenomas in patients taking danazol for hereditary angio-oedema," *The Lancet*, vol. 353, no. 9158, pp. 1066–1067, 1999.

[59] H. Kahn, C. Manzarbeitia, N. Theise, M. Schwartz, C. Miller, and S. N. Thung, "Danazol-induced hepatocellular adenomas: a case report and review of the literature," *Archives of Pathology and Laboratory Medicine*, vol. 115, no. 10, pp. 1054–1057, 1991.

[60] L. Socas, M. Zumbado, O. Pérez-Luzardo et al., "Hepatocellular adenomas associated with anabolic androgenic steroid abuse in bodybuilders: a report of two cases and a review of the literature," *British Journal of Sports Medicine*, vol. 39, no. 5, p. e27, 2005.

[61] S. Bagia, P. M. Hewitt, and D. L. Morris, "Anabolic steroid-induced hepatic adenomas with spontaneous haemorrhage in a bodybuilder," *Australian and New Zealand Journal of Surgery*, vol. 70, no. 9, pp. 686–687, 2000.

[62] A. Seki, T. Inoue, Y. Maegaki et al., "Polycystic ovary syndrome and hepatocellular adenoma related to long-term use of sodium valproate in a young woman," *No To Hattatsu*, vol. 38, no. 3, pp. 205–208, 2006.

[63] A. Ferko, J. Bedrna, and J. Nozicka, "Pigmented hepatocellular adenoma of the liver caused by long-term use of phenobarbital," *Rozhledy v Chirurgii*, vol. 82, no. 4, pp. 192–195, 2003.

[64] J. J. Vazquez and M. A. Marigil, "Liver-cell adenoma in an epileptic man on barbiturates," *Histology and Histopathology*, vol. 4, no. 3, pp. 301–303, 1989.

[65] T. B. Lautz, M. J. Finegold, A. C. Chin, and R. A. Superina, "Giant hepatic adenoma with atypical features in a patient on oxcarbazepine therapy," *Journal of Pediatric Surgery*, vol. 43, no. 4, pp. 751–754, 2008.

[66] K. Tazawa, M. Yasuda, Y. Ohtani, H. Makuuchi, and R. Y. Osamura, "Multiple hepatocellular adenomas associated with long-term carbamazepine," *Histopathology*, vol. 35, no. 1, pp. 92–94, 1999.

[67] P. Bioulac-Sage, S. Taouji, L. Possenti, and C. Balabaud, "Hepatocellular adenoma subtypes: the impact of overweight and obesity," *Liver International*, vol. 32, no. 8, pp. 1217–1221, 2012.

[68] C. Bunchorntavakul, R. Bahirwani, D. Drazek et al., "Clinical features and natural history of hepatocellular adenomas: the impact of obesity," *Alimentary Pharmacology & Therapeutics*, vol. 34, pp. 664–674, 2011.

[69] V. Paradis, A. Champault, M. Ronot et al., "Telangiectatic adenoma: an entity associated with increased body mass index and inflammation," *Hepatology*, vol. 46, no. 1, pp. 140–146, 2007.

[70] J. Watkins, C. Balabaud, P. Bioulac-Sage, D. Sharma, and A. Dhillon, "Hepatocellular adenoma in advanced-stage fatty liver

disease," *European Journal of Gastroenterology and Hepatology*, vol. 21, no. 8, pp. 932–936, 2009.

[71] V. Ozenne, V. Paradis, M. P. Vullierme et al., "Liver tumours in patients with Fanconi anaemia: a report of three cases," *European Journal of Gastroenterology and Hepatology*, vol. 20, pp. 1036–1039, 2008.

[72] C. Masserot-Lureau, N. Adoui, F. Degos et al., "Incidence of liver abnormalities in Fanconi anemia patients," *American Journal of Hematology*, vol. 87, pp. 547–549, 2012.

[73] C. N. Roy, D. A. Weinstein, and N. C. Andrews, "2002 E. Mead Johnson Award for research in pediatrics lecture: the molecular biology of the anemia of chronic disease: a hypothesis," *Pediatric Research*, vol. 53, no. 3, pp. 507–512, 2003.

[74] D. A. Weinstein, C. N. Roy, M. D. Fleming, M. F. Loda, J. I. Wolfsdorf, and N. C. Andrews, "Inappropriate expression of hepcidin is associated with iron refractory anemia: implications for the anemia of chronic disease," *Blood*, vol. 100, no. 10, pp. 3776–3781, 2002.

[75] A. Y. F. Chung, K. W. Leo, G. C. Wong, K. L. Chuah, J. W. Ren, and C. G. L. Lee, "Giant hepatocellular adenoma presenting with chronic iron deficiency anemia," *American Journal of Gastroenterology*, vol. 101, no. 9, pp. 2160–2162, 2006.

[76] A. Sa Cunha, J. F. Blanc, E. Lazaro et al., "Inflammatory syndrome with liver adenomatosis: the beneficial effects of surgical management," *Gut*, vol. 56, no. 2, pp. 307–309, 2007.

[77] C. Toso, L. Rubbia-Brandt, F. Negro, P. Morel, and G. Mentha, "Hepatocellular adenoma polycystic ovary syndrome," *Liver International*, vol. 23, no. 1, pp. 35–37, 2003.

[78] M. Sasaki, N. Yoneda, S. Kitamura, Y. Sato, and Y. Nakanuma, "A serum amyloid A-positive hepatocellular neoplasm arising in alcoholic cirrhosis: a previously unrecognized type of inflammatory hepatocellular tumor," *Modern Pathology*, vol. 25, no. 12, pp. 1584–1593, 2012.

[79] C. Laurent, H. Trillaud, S. Lepreux, C. Balabaud, and P. Bioulac-Sage, "Association of adenoma and focal nodular hyperplasia: experience of a single French academic center," *Comparative Hepatology*, vol. 2, article 6, 2003.

[80] I. R. Wanless, S. Albrecht, J. Bilbao et al., "Multiple focal nodular hyperplasia of the liver associated with vascular malformations of various organs and neoplasia of the brain: a new syndrome," *Modern Pathology*, vol. 2, no. 5, pp. 456–462, 1989.

[81] P. Bioulac-Sage, S. Rebouissou, A. Sa Cunha et al., "Clinical, morphologic, and molecular features defining so-called telangiectatic focal nodular hyperplasias of the liver," *Gastroenterology*, vol. 128, no. 5, pp. 1211–1218, 2005.

[82] V. Paradis, A. Benzekri, D. Dargére et al., "Telangiectatic focal nodular hyperplasia: a variant of hepatocellular adenoma," *Gastroenterology*, vol. 126, no. 5, pp. 1323–1329, 2004.

[83] H. Laumonier, N. Frulio, C. Laurent, C. Balabaud, J. Zucman-Rossi, and P. Bioulac-Sage, "Focal nodular hyperplasia with major sinusoidal dilatation: a misleading entity," *BMJ Case Reports*, 2010.

[84] T. Masuda, T. Beppu, K. Ikeda et al., "Pigmented hepatocellular adenoma: report of a case," *Surgery Today*, vol. 41, no. 6, pp. 881–883, 2011.

[85] T. Ichikawa, M. P. Federle, L. Grazioli, and M. Nalesnik, "Hepatocellular adenoma: multiphasic CT and histopathologic findings in 25 patients," *Radiology*, vol. 214, no. 3, pp. 861–868, 2000.

[86] B. Le Bail, H. Jouhanole, Y. Deugnier et al., "Liver adenomatosis with granulomas in two patients on long-term oral contraceptives," *The American Journal of Surgical Pathology*, vol. 16, no. 10, pp. 982–987, 1992.

[87] K. C. Kazi, R. Deshpande, R. Soman, M. Lala, and S. Shah, "Liver cell adenoma with co-existing hepatic granulomas in an HIV-positive patient," *Indian Journal of Gastroenterology*, vol. 24, no. 6, pp. 274–275, 2005.

[88] M. Bieze, P. Bioulac-Sage, J. Verheij, C. Balabaud, C. Laurent, and T. M. van Gulik, "Hepatocellular adenomas associated with hepatic granulomas: experience in five cases," *Case Reports in Gastroenterology*, vol. 6, pp. 677–683, 2012.

[89] S. Lepreux, C. Laurent, J. F. Blanc et al., "The identification of small nodules in liver adenomatosis," *Journal of Hepatology*, vol. 39, no. 1, pp. 77–85, 2003.

7

Mystery of Hepatitis E Virus: Recent Advances in Its Diagnosis and Management

Aftab Ahmed,[1] Ijlal Akbar Ali,[1] Hira Ghazal,[2] Javid Fazili,[3] and Salman Nusrat[3]

[1] *Department of Internal Medicine, Oklahoma University Health Sciences Center, Williams Pavilion 1130, P.O. Box 26901, Oklahoma City, OK 73104, USA*
[2] *Dow Medical College, Mission Road, Karachi 74200, Pakistan*
[3] *Section of Digestive Diseases and Nutrition, Oklahoma University Health Sciences Center, Williams Pavilion 1345, 920 SL Young Boulevard, Oklahoma City, OK 73104, USA*

Correspondence should be addressed to Salman Nusrat; salman-nusrat@ouhsc.edu

Academic Editor: Maria Buti

Mysterious aspects of the long presumed to be well-known hepatitis E virus (HEV) have recently surfaced that distinguish it from other hepatotropic viruses. It is a cause of chronic hepatitis in immunosuppressed patients. It has human to human transmission through blood and mantains high seroprevalence in blood donors. HEV has also been found to occur more frequently in the West in those without a history of travel to endemic countries. It has varied extrahepatic manifestations and has multiple non-human reservoirs including pigs and rats. Considering these recent discoveries, it appears odd that HEV is not sought more frequently when working up acute and chronic hepatitis patients. The disease is particularly severe among pregnant women and has a high attack rate in young adults. What adds to its ambiguity is the absence of a well-established diagnostic criteria for its detection and that there is no specific antiviral drug for hepatitis E, except for isolated cases where ribavirin or pegylated interferon alpha has been used with occasional success. This review paper discusses the recent advances in the knowledge of the virus itself, its epidemiology, diagnostic approach and prevention, and the treatment options available.

1. Introduction

In 1978 the existence of a non-A, non-B hepatitis virus, likely hepatitis E virus (HEV) was suggested during an outbreak of acute hepatitis in Kashmir [1–3]. However, it was not truly identified until 1983 when a researcher investigating an outbreak of unexplained hepatitis in Soviet soldiers in Afghanistan ingested fecal extract from affected military personnel and developed acute hepatitis and small viral particles were identified in his stool [3]. Recently, mysterious aspects of this once presumed to be well known virus have surfaced. Over the last few years our practices and understanding pertaining to its prevalence, mode of infection, clinical manifestations, diagnostic tests, treatment options, and role of vaccination have evolved tremendously. There is now good evidence that HEV infection is neither rare nor limited to developing countries and no clinical presentation is limited to acute infection (Table 2). Lack of knowledge among physicians and absence of standardized tests result in failure to diagnose and therefore can lead to an increase in morbidity and mortality. All this underscores the importance of HEV as a virus that might have taken us off guard.

2. Virology and Taxonomic Status

HEV is a small (27–34 nm) nonenveloped virus. The viral genome consists of a single-stranded, positive-sense RNA molecule organized into three open reading frames (ORF1, ORF2, and ORF3) (Figure 1). ORF1 is involved in viral replication and protein processing through RNA-dependent RNA polymerase. ORF2 encodes the viral capsid protein, which is involved in attachment to host cells and induction of neutralizing antibodies. Finally, ORF3 encodes for a small immunogenic phosphorylated protein (pORF3) involved in virion morphogenesis and release [4].

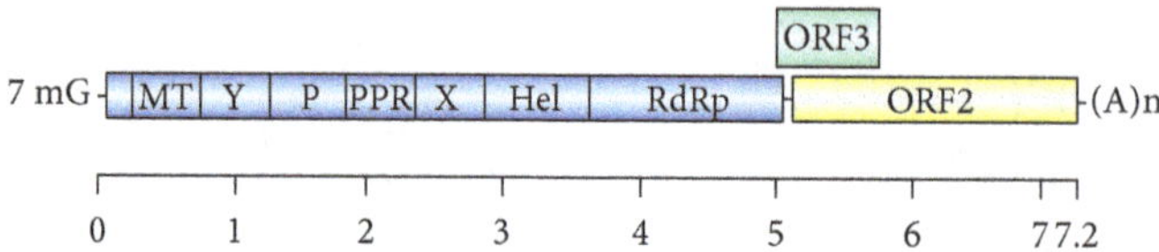

FIGURE 1: The structure of the hepatitis E virus genome. RNA length: 7.2 kb. It has short 5 and 3 noncoding regions and three overlapping open reading frames (ORFs). ORF1 encodes the nonstructural proteins, including a methyl transferase (MT), cysteine protease (P), helicase (Hel), and RNA polymerase (RdRp), as well as three regions of unknown function (Y, PPR, and X). The 5 end of the RNA genome is capped with 7-methylguanosine (7 mG), and the 3 end is polyadenylated (poly A).

It belongs to the Hepeviridae family and is the sole member of genus *Hepevirus* [5]. HEV genotypes are further classified into subtypes: genotype 1, five (1a–1e); genotype 2, two (2a and 2b); genotype 3, ten (3a–3j); and genotype 4, seven (4a–4g) [4]. Genotype 2 appears to be exclusively anthroponotic, while genotype 1 infects mainly humans but has also been detected in pigs [4, 6]. Genotypes 3 and 4 also infect other animals, particularly pigs (Table 1).

3. Epidemiology

HEV is one of the leading causes of hepatitis worldwide. Human infection with HEV is not only prevalent in developing countries but is also common in western nations and based on geographical distribution there are two distinct epidemiological patterns [3, 7].

3.1. Infection in Developing Countries. Hepatitis E has long been considered a disease of developing countries. Although lack of routinely available diagnostics tests and dual infection with HAV makes it difficult to estimate its true prevalence, some have reported a prevalence as high as 50% [8]. Outbreak is more common during summer. For unclear reasons it predominantly affects males between the ages of 15 and 30 years and is uncommon in children younger than 10 years [3]. Genotype 1 tends to be more common in Southern and Central Asia; similarly others are more prevalent in other geographical locations (Table 1). HEV1 is prevalent in Southern and Central Asia, the Far East, North Africa, and the Caribbean. HEV2 is predominant in Mexico (probably subtype 2a) and West Africa (subtype 2b). HEV3 infections are found to occur worldwide, including America, Europe, China, and Japan and HEV4 predominates in China whilst also being detected in swine livestock from India and Indonesia and recently in Central Europe [1, 3, 6, 7, 9, 10]. Increasing the complexity of the HEV epidemiology, HEV is occasionally associated with hepatitis A virus outbreaks in developing regions in the form of dual infection [6]. These waterborne outbreaks have been exclusively associated with genotypes 1 and 2 strains [6]. Due to the lesser stability of its particle, HEV is less prevalent in the population than HAV [9].

3.2. Infection in Developed Countries. In developed countries, HEV infection has traditionally been recognized among travelers returning from endemic countries. However, during the past decade, sporadic autochthonous (locally acquired) cases of HEV genotypes 3 and 4 infection have also been reported without recent travel history to endemic countries [3, 11], with a predilection for middle-aged elderly males aged over 40 (mean age 60 years; male/female ratio = 3 : 1) [3]. In contrast to prevalence in developing parts of the world, in non-endemic countries hepatitis E represents about 1% of the acute viral hepatitis [7, 12]. As exposure appears to be unrelated to age or sex, it seems unconventional [13] and puzzling that older men are more often exposed to HEV and implies that host factors could be important [3]. HEV strains responsible for autochthonous infections have been isolated from various animal species including wild and domestic swine, deer, chicken, rats, rabbit [6], and camels [14], slurry lagoons, rivers, the sea, shellfish, and soft fruits [13]. Phylogenetic studies have proven the relationship between HEV strains circulating in pigs and human beings, thus promoting the notion of autochthonous zoonotic transmission [3].

4. Mode of Transmission

The fecooral route is the primary and most well documented mode of transmission. It is more prevalent with HEV-1 and -2 and explains the endemicity and frequent outbreaks of HEV-1 and -2 in developing countries [7, 15, 16]. Genotype 3 has been detected in pig liver in grocery stores and thus may partially account for HEV exposure in the United States [17].

In developed countries, some cases of vertical transmissions of HEV have been reported [4]. However, transmission through breast milk has not been described [6].

Recently transmission via blood transfusions has become a concern. Seroprevalence rates as high as 50% have been reported among asymptomatic individuals in nonendemic countries. Although not representative of active infection or carrier state, such high seropositive states in asymptomatic individuals raise concerns about the spread of infection during periods of infectivity particularly in the absence of standardized screening tests [4, 6].

HEV has recently been reported in homosexual men, which supports its sexual transmission [18, 19]. Direct animal transmission is also a possibility as studies have shown that veterinarians and swine handlers have more chances to be anti-HEV IgG positive than the general population [3].

5. Clinical Presentation

Hepatitis E has variable clinical presentations and ranges from asymptomatic carriers to fulminant hepatitis. As one

TABLE 1: Epidemiology and clinical features of hepatitis E virus [3, 6, 10, 20, 21].

Genotype	1	2	3	4
Host	Human; also isolated from pig	Human exclusively	Human, pigs, and other mammalian species	
Route of transmission	Fecal-oral; vertical transmission; zoonotic (genotype 1)		Zoonotic (usually swine, with humans being accidental hosts); environmental (shellfish, river); blood transfusion	
Geographical distribution	Mainly Asia and Latin America (Cuba, Venezuela, and Uruguay)	Mexico and West Africa	Worldwide	China, East Asia, Central Europe, and America
Epidemiological features	Causes epidemic outbreaks and sporadic cases in developing countries; occasionally in travelers returning from developing countries	Causes epidemic outbreaks and sporadic cases in developing countries	Causes sporadic autochthonous cases in developed countries	
Seasonality	Yes (outbreaks in flooding/monsoon)		No	
Clinical presentation	Mostly asymptomatic; acute self-limited hepatitis	Mostly asymptomatic; acute self-limited hepatitis	Varies from asymptomatic to acute self-limited hepatitis and may lead to chronicity in immunosuppressed cases (HEV3)	
Age	Adolescents and young (15–30 y)		Middle-aged and elderly (>50 y)	
Gender (M : F)	2 : 1		>3 : 1	
Prognosis	High mortality in pregnancy and in patients with underlying chronic liver disease	Fulminant hepatitis has not been noted in HEV2	Higher overall mortality rate relative to genotype 1; higher mortality among older adults	
Chronic infection	No		Yes	Yes

TABLE 2: Individuals at higher risk of acute liver failure from HEV infection [1, 3, 6, 7, 12, 22–24].

Pregnant women
Individuals with preexisting liver disease
Hepatitis B virus carriers
Individuals with drug induced liver injuries
Active alcohol abusers

would expect clinical manifestations to some extent depend on the predominant genotype. In endemic areas where genotypes 1 and 2 are most prevalent it primarily manifests as acute hepatitis. On the other hand in developed countries genotypes 3 and 4 are more prevalent and patients are mostly asymptomatic [25]. This notion was supported by Kumar et al. who identified that all the acute cases resulted from subtype Ia and that the fulminant cases were secondary to subtype Ic [16]. However, Smith and Simmonds [26] in their study suggested that it is the host-specific factors rather than virus genotype that dictate the risk of fulminant hepatitis.

In acute HEV, the incubation period is 3–8 weeks followed by a short prodromal phase. The symptomatic phase can last anywhere from days to several weeks (mean 4–6 weeks) [27]. As with acute hepatitis from other etiologies patients present with jaundice, right upper quadrant pain, and nondescript symptoms such as fever, asthenia, nausea, vomiting, and joint pains [1, 28, 29]. Recent data has shown that it is not uncommon that patients with acute hepatitis from HEV are misdiagnosed as having drug-induced liver injury [22]. HEV at times can infect patient with chronic liver disease; however a similar clinical picture makes diagnosis difficult and challenging [7, 13, 23, 30]. This is particularly important as prognosis is grim in patients with preexisting chronic liver disease and some studies report a mortality rate as high as 70% [3]. Other risk factors for acute liver failure are noted in Table 1.

A wide range of extrahepatic manifestations have been attributed to HEV. Those associated with acute illness include rash and arthralgia [24], Guillain-Barre syndrome [31, 32], myasthenia gravis [33], bilateral brachial neuritis, peripheral neuralgia with meningitis, seizures, nerve palsies, and pseudotumor cerebri.

5.1. Chronic Hepatitis. Chronic HEV infection by definition requires elevated aminotransferase levels, positive serum HEV RNA, and suggestive histologic findings for at least 3 months [3]. It is usually caused by genotype 3 and chronic infection secondary to genotypes 1 and 2 has not been documented [4]. One case of chronic HEV infection by genotype 4 has been reported in the literature [20]. Risk factors include immunosuppression, solid organ transplantation, HIV infection, hemodialysis, and hematological malignancies [1, 3, 4, 17, 34–40].

The route of transmission is not different from that seen in acute infection [3]. Most patients are either asymptomatic or present with vague symptoms. Extraintestinal manifestations neuralgic amyotrophy [41], peripheral neuropathies, encephalitis [32, 42], encephalopathy [32, 43], Parsonage-Turner syndrome [42], paroxysmal myopathy, and bilateral pyramidal syndromes are known to occur [1].

Presence of chronic infection in immunocompromised patients carries a bad prognosis which if left untreated rapidly progresses to cirrhosis (10% in 2 years) and end-stage liver disease (ESLD) [1, 13].

5.2. HEV Infection during Pregnancy. HEV infection during pregnancy is associated with increased risk of prematurity, abortion, low birth weight, perinatal mortality, fulminant hepatitis, and maternal mortality [6]. Maternal mortality rates are highest during the third trimester and have been reported to be as high as 25% [3]. Interestingly, in some countries such as Egypt, HEV infection during pregnancy is not associated with increased mortality. This phenomenon can likely be explained by the fact that the predominant genotype is less virulent [3].

6. Diagnosis

Clinical signs, symptoms, and laboratory findings often overlap with hepatitis from other etiologies and make confirmation of diagnosis difficult. Some experts suggest that testing for hepatitis E should be part of the diagnostic algorithm for all patients with acute or chronic hepatitis that cannot be explained by other causes [8].

Diagnostic methods are broadly classified into two types: direct and indirect. The direct methods detect the virus, viral proteins, or nucleic acids in blood and stool samples by immune-electron microscopy and RT-PCR. The indirect methods detect the anti-HEV IgM and IgG antibodies [1].

Detection of anti-HEV IgM is considered diagnostic for acute infection. The presence of IgG antibodies points out to previous exposure to HEV [4]. Anti-HEV IgM is detectable 4 days after the onset of jaundice and persists for up to 3–5 months [6]. Shortly after the appearance of IgM, IgG antibodies develop and peak at about 4 weeks after the onset of symptoms and persist for a variable period of 1 to 14 years after infection [6].

The detection of HEV RNA in biologic specimen (serum and/or stools) is the "gold standard" for the confirmation of acute HEV infection [9]. HEV RNA can be detected in stools 1 week before and up to 6 weeks after the onset of symptoms and in serum for 3-4 weeks from the onset of illness [4, 7].

The sensitivity of molecular tests for the detection of HEV RNA is dependent on how early the patient presents, timely collection of specimens along with its rapid transport, processing, and viral genotype inclusivity. Therefore, undetectable HEV RNA does not rule out recent infection [4].

PCR assays published so far have a high degree of performance variability. Therefore, World Health Organization (WHO) has recommended an international standard for HEV RNA detection and quantification that uses genotype 3a due to its worldwide distribution and its detection in chronic infections [3, 4, 6]. Another nucleic acid amplification technique, the loop-mediated isothermal amplification (LAMP) assay, has been developed for the detection of HEV RNA. The LAMP assay is quicker than real-time PCR and does not need special equipment, making it ideal for resource limited areas [3].

Insensitive and unspecific diagnostic tests for anti-HEV antibodies have made diagnosis challenging. In a study, in only 13.3% of the samples, anti-HEV IgM serology correlated to HEV polymerase chain reaction (PCR) positivity. This demonstrates an extremely low level of correlation with PCR-confirmed HEV infections [6]. Furthermore, false reactivity for anti-HEV IgM with Epstein-Barr virus (EBV) and cytomegalovirus (CMV), 33.3% and 24.2%, respectively, has been expressed in a study [6]. This is a clinically important consideration because these viruses form the differential diagnosis for acute non-A, non-B hepatitis. Nonetheless, recently developed "point-of-care" assays for anti-HIV IgM are simple, rapid, highly sensitive, and specific, ideal for resource-limited areas [3, 44]. Recently, novel efficient cell cultures have been generated for HEV3(4) and HEV4(3) that permitted the propagation of HEV in fecal and serum samples [3]. This discovery will be indispensable for extracting the infectivity titers of inocula in the future [3].

Anti-HEV-IgG and -IgM are fairly reliable methods of diagnosis in immune-competent hosts. However, they are frequently false-negative in immunocompromised host, which imposes a diagnostic challenge. RT-PCR is recommended to diagnose HEV infection in this subset of patients. In this setting, HEV RNA detection and quantification also has a role in monitoring response to antiviral therapy and determining the genotype of HEV involved [4, 5, 7, 9]. Nucleic acid amplification technology methods by RT-PCR have been demonstrated as having a higher sensitivity when compared to HEV IGM and HEV antigen. They are therefore better screening tests [45].

7. Treatment

Acute hepatitis E usually does not require treatment in immune-competent individuals. Data on treatment of HEV in immunocompromised, frequently chronic hepatitis is sparse, and, therefore, patient tailored therapy is the best option.

If HEV RNA persists for 3 months, then the patient is very unlikely to achieve spontaneous viral clearance without therapeutic intervention [3]. The most important step that should be considered is whether immunosuppression can be reduced. A study reports 25% HEV clearance rates by this strategy [46]. However, chances of transplant organ rejection greatly increase when immunosuppression is reduced. So, it can be rightly called a double-edged sword. Additionally, pegylated interferons have been used fairly successfully at times but are associated with significant side effects. They are better options in transplant recipients where reducing immunosuppression is not an option. Another somewhat promising option is ribavirin therapy. Ribavirin has been used to successfully treat severe acute hepatitis E patients with compromised immune systems [47]. Although there is no convincing data on it yet to make it a standardized option of HEV treatment, two French studies have shown virologic responses in 2 out of 2 and 4 out of 6 patients, respectively [48, 49]. However ribavirin is contraindicated in pregnancy. Liver transplant is the only option in patients who get fulminant hepatic failure.

8. Vaccination

Should one be infected by hepatitis E and recover, he or she will get protective immunity, with the courtesy of CD4 and CD8 T cells. Another way to induce immunity is via vaccination [50]. The HEV vaccine which is in the most advanced stages of development is HEV 239. It is a Chinese manufactured vaccine that has a 94–100% efficacy in a phase III trial conducted on more than 100,000 Chinese soldiers. Although it is based on the type 1 genotype, it works even against genotypes 1 and 4. Response to genotype 3 is not known. It is still in the development stage to be used worldwide but has been approved for use in China [51].

9. Conclusion

Keeping in view the history of identification of HEV, that is, a water-borne epidemic of acute hepatitis in a developing country, today, hardly few decades from its diagnosis, we can hardly limit it to "acute," "hepatic," "water-borne," "epidemic," or "developing" settings.

Recent identification of chronic HEV in immunosuppressed cases and its extrahepatic presentation manifests how limited our knowledge about HEV has been. One cannot stop wondering, "Do we know all about Hepatitis E?" We can no longer underestimate the importance of further research on the virus that had taken us off guard.

The fact that HEV is a common cause of acute hepatitis worldwide and recent appearance of many cases of acute hepatitis caused by HEV being misdiagnosed for causes such as drug-induced hepatitis, HEV testing should be considered among the first line when evaluating acute liver injury.

High mortality in pregnant females due to HEV and chronic HEV hepatitis in immunosuppressed cases and in those with underlying chronic liver disease expresses the urgent need of appropriate measures aimed at improving the current state of diagnosis and treatment of HEV.

Also, unexpectedly high seroprevalence in blood donors proclaims that emphasis be laid on consideration of screening of HEV in blood donors. And probably the first step would be to call attention to development of standardized diagnostic tests that have higher sensitivity and specificity and are cost-effective and commercially available.

References

[1] S. Fujiwara, Y. Yokokawa, K. Morino, K. Hayasaka, M. Kawabata, and T. Shimizu, "Chronic hepatitis E: a review of the literature," *Journal of Viral Hepatitis*, vol. 21, no. 2, pp. 78–89, 2014.

[2] C. Féray, J.-M. Pawlotsky, A.-M. Roque-Afonso, D. Samuel, and D. Dhumeaux, "Should we screen blood products for hepatitis e virus RNA?" *The Lancet*, vol. 383, no. 9913, p. 218, 2014.

[3] N. Kamar, H. R. Dalton, F. Abravanel, and J. Izopet, "Hepatitis E virus infection," *Clinical Microbiology Reviews*, vol. 27, no. 1, pp. 116–138, 2014.

[4] J. E. Arends, V. Ghisetti, W. Irving et al., "Hepatitis E: an emerging infection in high income countries," *Journal of Clinical Virology*, vol. 59, no. 2, pp. 81–88, 2014.

[5] N. Kamar, R. Bendall, F. Legrand-Abravanel et al., "Hepatitis E," *The Lancet*, vol. 379, pp. 2477–2488, 2012.

[6] S. Mirazo, N. Ramos, V. Mainardi, S. Gerona, and J. Arbiza, "Transmission, diagnosis, and management of hepatitis E: an update," *Journal of Hepatic Medicine: Evidence and Research*, vol. 6, pp. 45–59, 2014.

[7] M. T. Pérez-Gracia, B. Suay, and M. L. Mateos-Lindemann, "Hepatitis E: an emerging disease," *Infection, Genetics and Evolution*, vol. 22, pp. 40–59, 2014.

[8] S. Pischke and H. Wedemeyer, "Hepatitis E virus infection: multiple faces of an underestimated problem," *Journal of Hepatology*, vol. 58, no. 5, pp. 1045–1046, 2013.

[9] J.-M. Echevarría, "Light and darkness: prevalence of hepatitis E virus infection among the general population," *Scientifica*, vol. 2014, Article ID 481016, 14 pages, 2014.

[10] N. Kamar, R. Bendall, F. Legrand-Abravanel et al., "Hepatitis E," *The Lancet*, vol. 379, no. 9835, pp. 2477–2488, 2012.

[11] H. R. Dalton, J. G. Hunter, and R. Bendall, "Autochthonous hepatitis e in developed countries and HEV/HIV coinfection," *Seminars in Liver Disease*, vol. 33, no. 1, pp. 50–61, 2013.

[12] P. Colson, P. Borentain, B. Queyriaux et al., "Pig liver sausage as a source of hepatitis e virus transmission to humans," *The Journal of Infectious Diseases*, vol. 202, no. 6, pp. 825–834, 2010.

[13] H. R. Dalton, "Hepatitis E: the 'new kid on the block' or an old friend?" *Transfusion Medicine and Hemotherapy*, vol. 41, no. 1, pp. 6–9, 2014.

[14] P. C. Y. Woo, S. K. P. Lau, J. L. L. Teng et al., "New hepatitis E virus genotype in camels, the Middle East," *Emerging Infectious Diseases*, vol. 20, no. 6, pp. 1044–1048, 2014.

[15] C. Alvarado-Esquivel, L. F. Sanchez-Anguiano, and J. Hernandez-Tinoco, "Seroepidemiology of hepatitis E virus infection in general population in rural durango, Mexico," *Hepatitis Monthly*, vol. 14, no. 6, Article ID e16876, 2014.

[16] S. Kumar, S. Subhadra, B. Singh, and B. K. Panda, "Hepatitis E virus: the current scenario," *International Journal of Infectious Diseases*, vol. 17, no. 4, pp. e228–e233, 2013.

[17] T. M. Pavri, D. A. Herbst, and K. R. Reddy, "Chronic hepatitis E virus infection: challenges in diagnosis and recognition in the United States," *Journal of Clinical Gastroenterology*, vol. 49, no. 1, pp. 86–88, 2014.

[18] F. Montella, G. Reza, F. di Sora, P. Pezotti, and O. Recchia, "Association between hepatitis E virus and HIV infection in homosexual men," *The Lancet*, vol. 344, no. 8934, p. 1433, 1994.

[19] B. A. I. Payne, M. Medhi, S. Ijaz et al., "Hepatitis E virus seroprevalence among men who have sex with men, United Kingdom," *Emerging Infectious Diseases*, vol. 19, no. 2, pp. 333–335, 2013.

[20] Y. Geng, H. Zhang, W. Huang et al., "Persistent hepatitis E virus genotype 4 infection in a child with acute lymphoblastic leukemia," *Hepatitis Monthly*, vol. 14, no. 1, Article ID e15618, 2014.

[21] J. H. Hoofnagle, K. E. Nelson, and R. H. Purcell, "Current concept hepatitis E," *The New England Journal of Medicine*, vol. 367, pp. 1237–1244, 2012.

[22] C. L. Crossan, K. J. Simpson, D. G. Craig et al., "Hepatitis E virus in patients with acute severe liver injury," *World Journal of Hepatology*, vol. 6, no. 6, pp. 426–434, 2014.

[23] S. Haim-Boukobza, A. Coilly, M. Sebagh et al., "Hepatitis E infection in patients with severe acute alcoholic hepatitis," *Liver International*, 2014.

[24] I. Al-Shukri, E. Davidson, A. Tan et al., "Rash and arthralgia caused by hepatitis E," *The Lancet*, vol. 382, no. 9907, p. 1856, 2013.

[25] J. Price, "An update on hepatitis B, D, and E viruses," *Topics in Antiviral Medicine*, vol. 21, no. 5, pp. 157–163, 2013.

[26] D. B. Smith and P. Simmonds, "Hepatitis E virus and fulminant hepatitis—a virus or host-specific pathology?" *Liver International*, 2014.

[27] J. H. Hoofnagle, K. E. Nelson, and R. H. Purcell, "Hepatitis E," *The New England Journal of Medicine*, vol. 367, no. 13, pp. 1237–1244, 2012.

[28] R. Aggarwal Jr., "Epidemiologic concerns and advances in knowledge on hepatitis E," *Gastroenterology & Hepatology*, vol. 9, no. 3, pp. 173–175, 2013.

[29] I. Masood, A. Rafiq, and Z. Majid, "Hepatitis E presenting with thrombocytopaenia," *Tropical Doctor*, vol. 44, no. 4, pp. 219–220, 2014.

[30] S.-J. Huang, X.-H. Liu, J. Zhang, and M.-H. Ng, "Protective immunity against HEV," *Current Opinion in Virology*, vol. 5, pp. 1–6, 2014.

[31] T. Comont, D. Bonnet, N. Sigur, A. Gerdelat, F. Legrand-Abravanel, N. Kamar et al., "Acute hepatitis E infection associated with Guillain-Barré syndrome in an immunocompetent patient," *La Revue de Medecine Interne*, vol. 35, no. 5, pp. 333–336, 2014.

[32] X. Wu, K. Liu, and H. L. Zhang, "Guillain–Barré syndrome and encephalitis/encephalopathy associated with acute severe hepatitis E infection," *Neurological Sciences*, 2014.

[33] A. Belbezier, A. Deroux, F. Sarrot-Reynauld, S. Larrat, and L. Bouillet, "Myasthenia gravis associated with acute hepatitis E infection in immunocompetent woman," *Emerging Infectious Diseases*, vol. 20, no. 5, pp. 908–910, 2014.

[34] N. Kamar, J. Selves, J.-M. Mansuy et al., "Hepatitis E virus and chronic hepatitis in organ-transplant recipients," *The New England Journal of Medicine*, vol. 358, no. 8, pp. 811–817, 2008.

[35] X. Zhou, R. A. de Man, R. J. de Knegt, H. J. Metselaar, M. P. Peppelenbosch, and Q. Pan, "Epidemiology and management of chronic hepatitis E infection in solid organ transplantation: a comprehensive literature review," *Reviews in Medical Virology*, vol. 23, no. 5, pp. 295–304, 2013.

[36] H. R. Dalton, R. P. Bendall, F. E. Keane, R. S. Tedder, and S. Ijaz, "Persistent carriage of hepatitis E virus in patients with HIV infection," *The New England Journal of Medicine*, vol. 361, no. 10, pp. 1025–1027, 2009.

[37] Z. Abbas and R. Afzal, "Hepatitis E: when to treat and how to treat," *Antiviral Therapy*, vol. 19, no. 2, pp. 125–131, 2014.

[38] M. T. Giordani, P. Fabris, E. Brunetti, S. Goblirsch, and L. Romanò, "Hepatitis E and lymphocytic leukemia in man, Italy," *Emerging Infectious Diseases*, vol. 19, no. 12, pp. 2054–2056, 2013.

[39] Y. Wang, H. J. Metselaar, M. P. Peppelenbosch, and Q. Pan, "Chronic hepatitis E in solid-organ transplantation: the key implications of immunosuppressants," *Current Opinion in Infectious Diseases*, vol. 27, no. 4, pp. 303–308, 2014.

[40] N. Kamar and J. Izopet, "Does chronic hepatitis E virus infection exist in immunocompetent patients?" *Hepatology*, vol. 60, no. 1, p. 427, 2014.

[41] J. J. van Eijk, R. G. Madden, A. A. van der Eijk et al., "Neuralgic amyotrophy and hepatitis E virus infection," *Neurology*, vol. 82, no. 6, pp. 498–503, 2014.

[42] A. Deroux, J. P. Brion, L. Hyerle et al., "Association between hepatitis E and neurological disorders: two case studies and literature review," *Journal of Clinical Virology*, vol. 60, no. 1, pp. 60–62, 2014.

[43] M. A. de Vries, J. P. A. Samijn, R. de Man, and J. M. M. Boots, "Hepatitis E-associated encephalopathy in a renal transplant recipient," *BMJ Case Reports*, 2014.

[44] D. J. Seo, H. Tahk, K. B. Lee et al., "Detecting hepatitis E virus with a reverse transcription polymerase chain reaction enzyme-linked immunosorbent assay," *Food and Environmental Virology*, vol. 4, no. 1, pp. 14–20, 2012.

[45] T. Vollmer, C. Knabbe, and J. Dreier, "Comparison of real-time PCR and antigen assays for detection of hepatitis e virus in blood donors," *Journal of Clinical Microbiology*, vol. 52, no. 6, pp. 2150–2156, 2014.

[46] N. Kamar, F. Abravanel, J. Selves et al., "Influence of immunosuppressive therapy on the natural history of genotype 3 hepatitis-e virus infection after organ transplantation," *Transplantation*, vol. 89, no. 3, pp. 353–360, 2010.

[47] A. Robbins, D. Lambert, F. Ehrhard et al., "Severe acute hepatitis E in an HIV infected patient: successful treatment with ribavirin," *Journal of Clinical Virology*, vol. 60, no. 4, pp. 422–423, 2014.

[48] N. Kamar, L. Rostaing, F. Abravanel et al., "Ribavirin therapy inhibits viral replication on patients with chronic hepatitis E virus infection," *Gastroenterology*, vol. 139, no. 5, pp. 1612–1618, 2010.

[49] V. Mallet, E. Nicand, P. Sultanik et al., "Brief communication: case reports of ribavirin treatment for chronic hepatitis E," *Annals of Internal Medicine*, vol. 153, no. 2, pp. 85–89, 2010.

[50] H. Wedemeyer, S. Pischke, and M. P. Manns, "Pathogenesis and treatment of hepatitis E virus infection," *Gastroenterology*, vol. 142, no. 6, pp. 1388.e1–1397.e1, 2012.

[51] F.-C. Zhu, J. Zhang, X.-F. Zhang et al., "Efficacy and safety of a recombinant hepatitis e vaccine in healthy adults: a large-scale, randomised, double-blind placebo-controlled, phase 3 trial," *The Lancet*, vol. 376, no. 9744, pp. 895–902, 2010.

8

Serum Cytokeratin-18 Is Associated with NOX2-Generated Oxidative Stress in Patients with Nonalcoholic Fatty Liver

M. Del Ben,[1] L. Polimeni,[1] F. Baratta,[1] S. Bartimoccia,[1] R. Carnevale,[1] L. Loffredo,[1] P. Pignatelli,[1] F. Violi,[1] and F. Angelico[1,2]

[1] *Department of Internal Medicine and Medical Specialities, Sapienza University, Rome, Italy*
[2] *Department of Public Health and Infectious Disease, Sapienza University, Rome, Italy*

Correspondence should be addressed to F. Angelico; francesco.angelico@uniroma1.it

Academic Editor: Claus Hellerbrand

Background & Aims. Hepatocyte apoptosis may play a role in progression of nonalcoholic fatty liver and oxidative stress seems one of the key mechanisms responsible for liver damage. The aim was to determine the association of oxidative stress with cytokeratin-18 M30 fragment levels, a marker of hepatocyte apoptosis. *Methods.* Steatosis severity was defined according to Hamaguchi's echographic criteria in 209 patients with nonalcoholic fatty liver. Serum cytokeratin-18, urinary 8-iso-prostaglandin F2α, soluble NOX2-derived peptide, and adiponectin were measured. *Results.* Serum cytokeratin-18 progressively increased with steatosis severity (from 169.5 (129.3/183.8) to 176 (140/190) and 180 (169.5/192.5) μIU/mL in mild, moderate, and severe steatosis, respectively; $P < 0.01$). After stratification by cytokeratin-18 tertiles, a significant progression of body mass index, HOMA-IR, triglycerides, urinary 8-iso-PGF2α, soluble NOX2-derived peptide, and of the prevalence of diabetes and severe steatosis was found, while HDL-cholesterol and adiponectin progressively decreased. A positive correlation between cytokeratin-18 and body mass index, HOMA-IR, Hamaguchi's score, urinary 8-iso-PGF2α, and soluble NOX2-derived peptide and a negative correlation between cytokeratin-18 and HDL-cholesterol and adiponectin were found. Body mass index, adiponectin, and soluble NOX2-derived peptide were independent predictors of serum cytokeratin-18 levels (adjusted $R^2 = 0.36$). *Conclusion.* We support an association between oxidative stress and severity of liver damage in patients with nonalcoholic fatty liver.

1. Introduction

Nonalcoholic fatty liver disease (NAFLD) represents the most common and emerging form of chronic liver disease worldwide. Indeed, NAFLD reached epidemic proportions and the general prevalence of this condition is reported to be ranging between 20–30% and 70–90% in patients with severe obesity or with type 2 diabetes mellitus [1–4].

NAFLD includes a wide spectrum of liver diseases ranging from simple fatty liver to nonalcoholic steatohepatitis (NASH), which may progress to fibrosis and even cirrhosis and hepatocellular carcinoma. Simple steatosis generally represents a benign condition following a nonprogressive clinical course. On the contrary, a subset of patients with NASH, in particular those with a more severe fibrosis, is at higher risk for progressing to liver disease complications such as decompensated cirrhosis and hepatocellular carcinoma [5].

Several lines of evidence suggest that chronic oxidative stress is one of the key mechanisms responsible for liver damage and disease progression in NAFLD [6]. In particular, according to the "two-hit" theory, oxidative stress is a major player triggering the progression of steatosis to NASH as the result of an imbalance between pro-oxidant and antioxidant chemicals that lead to liver cell damage. Consistent with the above theory, in a previous study, we demonstrated an increased systemic oxidative stress in subjects with NAFLD, which was associated with severity of liver steatosis (submitted).

Recently, it has been reported that blood levels of Cytokeratin-18 (CK-18) fragments, the major intermediate filament protein in the liver, may predict histological NASH and severity of liver damage in patients with NAFLD, [7] representing a marker of hepatocyte apoptosis. Indeed, cell repair, inflammation, regeneration, and fibrosis typical of NASH may be triggered by hepatocyte apoptosis. A link between hepatocyte apoptosis and liver fibrogenesis in fact is supported by both experimental and human studies [8], and data suggest that apoptosis is prominent in NASH but not in simple steatosis [9]. However, very limited information is available regarding the possible role of oxidative stress in triggering hepatocyte apoptosis in this setting.

Notably, no study has documented the relationship between novel and validated markers of oxidative stress such as urinary 8-iso-prostaglandin F2α (8-iso-PGF2α) or soluble NOX2-derived peptide (sNOX2-dp) and CK-18 serum levels.

The aim of this study was to determine the predictors of CK-18 levels to elucidate the possible role of oxidative stress in the severity of liver disease in a population of NAFLD patients.

2. Patients and Methods

2.1. Study Patients. The study was performed in 209 consecutive patients referred to our metabolic outpatient clinic for suspected metabolic disease, who had a liver ultrasonographic scanning (US) positive for NAFLD performed as part of routine clinical examination.

To be eligible for the study, patients had to have fulfilled the following criteria: no history of current or past excessive alcohol drinking as defined by an average daily consumption of alcohol >20 g; negative tests for the presence of hepatitis B surface antigen and antibody to hepatitis C virus; absence of history and clinical, biochemical, and US findings consistent with cirrhosis and other chronic liver diseases. None of the subjects was taking amiodarone and other drugs known to promote fatty liver disease.

Subjects underwent routine clinical and biochemical evaluation. Waist circumference, height, and weight were recorded and body mass index (BMI) was calculated as weight (Kg) divided by height^2. Blood pressure was recorded following standard procedures. Diabetes was diagnosed according to the WHO criteria [10]. Subjects taking insulin or oral antidiabetic drugs were considered to have diabetes. According to the modified criteria of the ATP III Expert Panel of the US National Cholesterol Education Program [11], MetS was diagnosed on the concomitant presence of at least three of the following five clinical features: waist circumference (central obesity) ≥102 cm in men and ≥88 cm in women, fasting blood glucose ≥100 mg/dL, triglycerides ≥150 mg/dL, HDL-cholesterol <40 mg/dL in men and <50 mg/dL in women, and arterial systolic/diastolic blood pressure ≥130/≥85 mm/Hg. A metabolic score was calculated for each patient based on the number of the discrete components of MetS. NAFLD fibrosis score (NFS) based on age, BMI, hyperglycemia, platelet count, albumin, and AST/ALT ratio, was calculated for each patient according to Angulo et al. [12].

Written informed consent was obtained from all patients before the study.The study was approved by the hospital ethics committee and conforms to the ethical guidelines of the 1975 Declaration of Helsinki.

2.2. Assessment of Steatosis. Liver US scanning was performed to assess the degree of steatosis. All US were performed by the same operator who was blinded to laboratory values using a GE VividS6 apparatus equipped with a convex 3, 5 MHz probe. Liver steatosis was defined according to Hamaguchi criteria based on the presence of abnormally intense, high level echoes arising from the hepatic parenchyma, liver-kidney difference in echo amplitude, echo penetration into deep portion of the liver, and clarity of liver blood vessel structure [13, 14]. Steatosis was assessed semiquantitatively on a scale of 0–6 : 0, absent; 1, 2 mild; 3, 4 moderate; and 5, 6 severe.

The splenic diameter was calculated as the maximum length of the spleen after visualizing the organ in a plane passing through the splenic hilum.

2.3. Laboratory Measurements. Serum total cholesterol, HDL-cholesterol, and triglycerides were measured by an Olympus AN 560 apparatus using an enzymatic colorimetric method. LDL-cholesterol levels were calculated according to the Friedewald formula. Plasma insulin levels were assayed by commercially available radioimmunoassay. The homeostasis model of insulin resistance (HOMA-IR), based on serum fasting glucose and insulin levels, was used as a measure of insulin resistance [15]. Serum levels of Cytokeratin 18-M30 (CK-18) were measured as markers of liver damage with a commercial immunoassay (Tema Ricerca, Italy) and expressed as mL U/mL. Intraassay and inter-assay coefficients were 6% and 7%, respectively. Urinary 8-iso-prostaglandin F2α (8-iso-PGF2α), as marker of whole body oxidative stress, was measured by a previously described and validated enzyme immunoassay method [16]. Intra-assay and inter-assay coefficients of variation were 2.1% and 4.5%, respectively. Serum levels of soluble NOX2-derived peptide (sNOX2-dp) were detected by ELISA method as previously described [17]; intra-assay and inter-assay coefficients of variation were 5.2% and 6%, respectively. Adiponectin (APN) serum levels were measured with a commercial immunoassay (Tema Ricerca, Italy). Intra-assay and inter-assay coefficients of variation were 6 and 8%, respectively.

2.4. Statistical Analysis. Statistical analysis was performed by using the SPSS statistical software version 20.0 for Windows (SPSS, Inc., Chicago, IL). Proportions and categorical variables were tested by the χ^2-test and by the 2-tailed Fisher's exact method when appropriate. Distribution of continuous variables was tested for normality using a Kolmogorov-Smirnov test. Data are expressed as median followed by 25th and 75th centiles for nonnormally distributed data and as mean ± SD for normally distributed variables. Group comparisons for nonnormally distributed variables were tested by the Mann-Whitney test and Kruskall-Wallis test. Instead, normally distributed variables were analyzed by the use of analysis of variance (ANOVA) and unpaired Student's t-test

Table 1: Clinical and biochemical characteristics of 209 subjects with NAFLD.

Variables	
Age (ys)	54.3 ± 12.0
Male (%)	64.6
Body mass index (kg/m^2)	31.6 ± 5.6
Waist circumference (cm)	108 (101/118)
Total cholesterol (mg/dL)	199.9 ± 39.4
HDL cholesterol (mg/dL)	46 (39/55)
Urinary 8-iso-PGF2α (pg/mg creatinine)	714.4 ± 121.5
Fasting glucose (mg/dL)	99 (92/115)
Fasting insulin (μIU/mL)	13.5 (9.8/19.9)
HOMA-IR	3.4 (2.4/5.7)
Triglycerides (mg/dL)	142 (103/182)
γ-GT (IU/L)	26 (18/43)
AST (IU/L)	21 (18/27)
ALT (IU/L)	28 (20/40)
Adiponectin (ng/mL)	7.5 (5.3/12.0)
Cytokeratin-18 (μIU/mL)	180 (148/190)
sNOX2-dp (pg/mL)	60 (49/67)
Metabolic syndrome (%)	67.6
Diabetes mellitus (%)	31.1

when appropriate. All P values are two-tailed; a P value of less than 0.05 was considered to indicate statistical significance. Stepwise, multivariate, regression analysis was performed to assess the independent predictors of serum CK-18 values. The predictor variables entered were age, BMI, HOMA-IR, serum triglycerides, ALT and APN, urinary 8-iso-PGF2α, sNOX2-dp, Hamaguchi score, and spleen diameter.

3. Results

The study was performed in 209 patients with NAFLD (43 with mild, 87 with moderate, and 79 with severe steatosis, resp.). Median serum CK-18 values progressively increased with NAFLD severity (from 169.5 (129.3/183.8) to 176 (140/190) and 180 (169.5/192.5) μIU/mL in mild, moderate, and severe steatosis, resp.; $P < 0.01$). Clinical and biochemical characteristics of subjects are reported in Table 1.

After stratification of subjects in serum CK-18 tertiles, significant differences of some variables were found. BMI (27.2 ± 3.9 versus 31.6 ± 3.3 versus 36.1 ± 5.4 kg/m^2; $P < 0.001$), HOMA-IR (2.8 (1.9/4.0) versus 3.2 (2.4/5.7) versus 5.3 (3.4/7.3); $P < 0.001$), serum triglycerides (125.5 (85.5/160.3) versus 138 (102.0/180.5) versus 165.0 (125.0/206.0) mg/dL; $P < 0.01$), prevalence of diabetes (20.3% versus 30.1 versus 43.3; $P < 0.05$), prevalence of severe NAFLD (24.6 versus 42.5 versus 46.3; $P < 0.05$), urinary 8-iso-PGF2α (616.7±122.9 versus 727.5±82.1 versus 800.9±82.1 pg/mg creatinine; $P < 0.001$), and sNOX2-dp (49 (40/58.3) versus 60 (50/66) versus 67 (64/71) pg/mL; $P < 0.001$) increased significantly from first to third CK-18 tertile. Instead, serum HDL-cholesterol (50 (43/61) versus 47 (38/54) versus 43 (39/51) mg/dL; $P < 0.05$) and APN (12 (10.4/14.1), versus 7.5 (5.5/10.5) versus 5 (4/7) ng/mL; $P < 0.001$) progressively decreased (Table 2).

Linear bivariate regression showed a positive correlation between serum CK-18 and BMI ($r = 0.58$; $P < 0.001$), HOMA-IR ($r = 0.19$; $P < 0.01$), Hamaguchi's score ($r = 0.19$; $P < 0.01$), urinary 8-iso-PGF2α ($r = 0.61$; $P < 0.001$), sNOX2dp ($r = 0.45$; $P < 0.001$), and NFS (0.30; $P < 0.01$); conversely, a negative correlation between serum CK-18 and serum HDL-cholesterol ($r = -0.15$; $P < 0.05$) and APN ($r = -0.45$; $P < 0.001$) was observed (Table 3).

Stepwise, multiple regression analysis was performed to assess the independent contributors to serum CK-18 levels. In the final equation, BMI, serum APN, and sNOX2-dp were independent predictors of serum CK-18 levels, after controlling for age, HOMA-IR, serum triglycerides, ALT, urinary 8-iso-PGF2α, Hamaguchi score, and spleen diameter (adjusted $R^2 = 0.36$) (Table 4).

4. Discussion

In our study, performed in a large series of subjects with documented NAFLD at US scanning, we have demonstrated a strong and independent association between sNOX2-dp and CK-18 serum levels. Moreover, at univariate analysis, also urinary 8-iso-PGF2α was positively correlated with CK-18 values. To our knowledge, this is the first evidence of an association between two markers of systemic oxidative stress and a marker of apoptosis and liver disease severity in subjects with NAFLD.

To assess oxidative stress *in vivo*, we measured urinary 8-iso-PGF2α and serum levels of sNOX2-dp. Measurement of urinary 8-iso-PGF2α is widely accepted as a reliable indicator of oxidative stress *in vivo* [18, 19]. Soluble NOX2-dp is a marker of NOX2 activation by blood cells, which is a member of the NADPH oxidase family which plays an important role in ROS generation [20, 21]. In previous studies, we have described elevated urinary 8-iso-PGF2α and serum sNOX2-dp levels in a number of chronic inflammatory and metabolic diseases such as metabolic syndrome, hypercholesterolemia, obstructive sleep apnoea syndrome, and obesity [22–25]. Moreover, in a recent study, we demonstrated an increased NOX2 generated oxidative stress also in subjects with NAFLD (submitted); in this clinical setting, oxidative stress was independent from obesity, diabetes, and MetS and increased with the severity of liver steatosis at US.

To assess liver damage and hepatocyte apoptosis, we measured serum CK-18 levels, which have been recently reported to predict histological NASH and severity of liver disease in patients with NAFLD [7, 26]. Indeed, some recent studies investigated circulating levels of CK-18 fragments as novel biomarkers for the presence of NASH in patients with NAFLD, and suggested the potential usefulness of this test in clinical practice. In fact, in a study performed in 44 consecutive patients with suspected NAFLD at the time of liver biopsy, plasma CK-18 fragments were markedly increased in patients with NASH compared with patients with simple steatosis or normal biopsies and independently predicted NASH (OR 1.95; 95% CI 1.18–3.22

Table 2: Clinical and biochemical characteristics of 209 subjects with NAFLD divided by serum cytokeratin-18 tertiles.

	Cytokeratin-18 tertiles			P
	I	II	III	
Males (%)	68.1	63.0	62.7	ns
Age (yrs)	53.8 ± 12.9	54.7 ± 10.9	54.2 ± 12.3	ns
Body mass index (kg/m^2)	27.2 ± 3.9	31.6 ± 3.3	36.1 ± 5.4	<0.001
Urinary 8-iso-PGF2α (pg/mg creatinine)	616.7 ± 122.9	727.5 ± 82.1	800.9 ± 82.1	<0.001
HOMA-IR	2.8 (1.9/4.0)	3.2 (2.4/5.7)	5.3 (3.4/7.3)	<0.001
Total cholesterol (mg/dL)	201.4 ± 38.4	196.9 ± 38.5	201.4 ± 41.5	ns
HDL (mg/dL)	50 (43/61)	47 (38/54)	43 (39/51)	<0.05
Triglycerides (mg/dL)	125.5 (85.5/160.3)	138 (102.0/180.5)	165.0 (125.0/206.0)	<0.01
γ-GT (IU/L)	23 (16.8/36.5)	27 (17.5/44.0)	30 (18/53)	ns
ALT (IU/L)	31 (22.8/40)	28 (20/41.5)	26 (20/40)	ns
AST (IU/L)	22 (18/28)	21 (17/26.5)	21 (17/28)	ns
Adiponectin (ng/mL)	12 (10.4/14.1)	7.5 (5.5/10.5)	5 (4/7)	<0.001
sNOX2-dp (pg/mL)	49 (40/58.3)	60 (50/66)	67 (64/71)	<0.001
Hamaguchi score	3.5 ± 1.3	4.0 ± 1.3	4.3 ± 1.3	<0.01
Metabolic syndrome (%)	49.4	69.0	84.8	<0.001
Diabetes (%)	20.3	30.1	43.3	<0.05

Table 3: Correlations between serum cytokeratin-18 and some clinical and metabolic characteristics.

	Cytokeratin-18	
	r	P
Age (yrs)	0.031	ns
BMI (kg/m^2)	0.577	<0.001
Waist circumference	0.601	<0.001
HOMA-IR	0.191	<0.01
Fasting blood glucose (mg/dL)	0.216	<0.01
Total cholesterol (mg/dL)	0.036	ns
HDL cholesterol (mg/dL)	−0.150	<0.05
Triglycerides (mg/dL)	0.100	ns
γ-GT (IU/l)	0.137	<0.05
AST (IU/l)	−0.078	ns
ALT (UI/l)	−0.039	ns
Serum ferritin (mg/dL)	−0.106	ns
Serum albumin (mg/dL)	−0.207	<0.01
Adiponectin	−0.455	<0.001
Urinary 8-iso-PGF2α (pg/mg creatinine)	0.607	<0.001
sNOX2-dp (pg/mL)	0.451	<0.001
Hamaguchi score	0.194	<0.001
Spleen diameter	0.190	<0.05
NAFLD Fibrosis score	0.299	<0.001
MetS score	0.377	<0.001

for every 50 U/L increase) [26]. Moreover, CK-18 fragment levels were validated as noninvasive biomarkers for NASH also in a multicenter study performed in a large, diverse population of patients with biopsy-proven NAFLD [7].

Consistent with this theory, we found a significant correlation between CK-18 serum levels and NFS, an accurate, noninvasive scoring system based on routinely measured and readily available clinical and laboratory data, that identifies advanced liver fibrosis in patients with NAFLD [27]. Recently, NFS has been validated for predicting death or liver complications in NAFLD patients over long-term follow-up [28]. To our knowledge, this is the first time that the association between serum CK-18 and NFS has been described.

The finding of a strong independent positive association of two reliable markers of oxidative stress with a marker of hepatocyte apoptosis is consistent with the "two-hit" theory based on the prominent role of oxidative stress as a major player triggering the progression of steatosis to NASH. In fact, according to the "two hits hypothesis," the development of NASH requires "two hits" to become manifested. The first one is represented by the development of steatosis, while the second hit is induced by a disbalance between oxidative stress and antioxidant systems, leading to cell injury and inflammation (i.e., steatohepatitis) and lipid peroxidation. In keeping with this theory, hepatocyte apoptosis is likely to be considered a component of the second hit. Accordingly, a working model in which apoptosis and formation of reactive oxygen species are caspase dependent [9], with final release of CK-18 fragments, has been proposed. Indeed, cell repair, inflammation, regeneration, and fibrosis typical of NASH may be triggered by hepatocyte apoptosis. A link between hepatocyte apoptosis and liver fibrogenesis is supported by both experimental and human studies [8].

High serum CK-18 values were associated with high HOMA-IR, high fasting blood glucose and triglycerides, and low HDL cholesterol, that is, the metabolic features of MetS, whose prevalence in patients belonging to the top CK-18 tertile reached 85%.

TABLE 4: Stepwise multiple linear regression analysis of independent predictors of serum cytokeratin-18 levels in 209 subjects with NAFLD.

	B	S.E.	*P*	95.0% C.I. for *B*	
				Lower	Upper
BMI (kg/m^2)	2.145	0.710	0.003	0.743	3.546
Adiponectin (ng/mL)	−2.121	0.892	0.005	−4.282	−0.760
sNOX2-dp (pg/mL)	0.523	0.235	0.027	0.059	0.986

Variables entered in step 1: age, BMI, HOMA-IR, serum triglycerides, ALT and adiponectin, urinary 8-iso-PGF2α, sNOX2-dp, Hamaguchi score, and spleen diameter.

At multivariate analysis, an independent association between low serum APN and increased CK-18 was also observed. APN is lower in central obesity and has powerful antioxidant properties. In a previous study, we have shown that higher APN serum levels are associated with NADPH oxidase down-regulation [29]. Higher levels of APN have been also associated with a more beneficial oxidative stress profile, and higher levels of antioxidants together with lower levels of lipid peroxidation [30]. Moreover, serum APN negatively correlated with urinary isoprostanes raising the possibility that APN may modulate oxidative stress, resulting in a less proinflammatory state [31]. This is in keeping with the observation that lower serum APN levels are associated with more extensive necroinflammation in NAFLD and that they may contribute and even be a potential indicator of the progression from simple steatosis to NASH [32–34].

Our study may have some limitations. First, we detected fatty liver by ultrasound, which is a qualitative method inadequate to quantify less than 30% liver fat content [35]. The gold standard for the diagnosis of NAFLD is liver biopsy, but this is an invasive procedure with potentially serious complications and is therefore not acceptable without clinical indication. We acknowledge that grades of steatosis could have been better determined by magnetic resonance spectroscopy. However, the Hamaguchi score showed 100% specificity and 91.7% sensitivity when compared with liver biopsy in NAFLD patients [14]. Second, although performed in a large series of patients, the study has been carried out in patients recruited in a hospital-based setting and the study design did not contemplate controls. Finally, our study has a cross-sectional design and prospective interventions with antioxidants are needed to demonstrate the causal role of oxidative stress on NAFLD to NASH progression.

In summary, our findings support the concept of an association between oxidative stress and severity of liver damage in patients with NAFLD. Moreover, to the best of our knowledge, this is the first association study that considered urinary 8-iso-PGF2α and serum sNOX2-dp as markers of systemic oxidative stress, and CK-18 for the assessment of hepatocyte apoptosis.

Abbreviations

NAFLD: Nonalcoholic fatty liver disease
NASH: Nonalcoholic steatohepatitis
8-iso-PGF2α: 8-iso-prostaglandin F2α
sNOX2-dp: Soluble NOX2-derived peptide
ALT: Alanine aminotransferase
CK-18: Cytokeratin-18
HOMA-IR: Homeostasis model of insulin resistance
MetS: Metabolic syndrome
US: Ultrasonographic scanning
BMI: Body mass index
APN: Adiponectin.

Authors' Contribution

M. Del Ben contributed to study design and wrote the manuscript. L. Polimeni, R. Carnevale, F. Baratta and S. Bartimoccia, contributed to data collection, analysis and interpretation; L. Loffredo and P. Pignatelli reviewed the manuscript; F. Violi reviewed and edited the manuscript. F. Angelico designed the study and wrote the manuscript; he is the guarantor of this work and, as such, had full access to all the data in the study and takes responsibility for the integrity of the data and the accuracy of the data analysis.

References

[1] J. D. Browning, L. S. Szczepaniak, R. Dobbins et al., "Prevalence of hepatic steatosis in an urban population in the United States: impact of ethnicity," *Hepatology*, vol. 40, no. 6, pp. 1387–1395, 2004.

[2] G. Vernon, A. Baranova, and Z. M. Younossi, "Systematic review: the epidemiology and natural history of non-alcoholic fatty liver disease and non-alcoholic steatohepatitis in adults," *Alimentary Pharmacology and Therapeutics*, vol. 34, no. 3, pp. 274–285, 2011.

[3] N. C. Leite, G. F. Salles, A. L. E. Araujo, C. A. Villela-Nogueira, and C. R. L. Cardoso, "Prevalence and associated factors of non-alcoholic fatty liver disease in patients with type-2 diabetes mellitus," *Liver International*, vol. 29, no. 1, pp. 113–119, 2009.

[4] S. Bellentani, G. Saccoccio, F. Masutti et al., "Prevalence of and risk factors for hepatic steatosis in northern Italy," *Annals of Internal Medicine*, vol. 132, no. 2, pp. 112–117, 2000.

[5] P. Angulo, "Medical progress: nonalcoholic fatty liver disease," *The New England Journal of Medicine*, vol. 346, no. 16, pp. 1221–1231, 2002.

[6] C. P. Day, "Pathogenesis of steatohepatitis," *Bailliere's Best Practice and Research in Clinical Gastroenterology*, vol. 16, no. 5, pp. 663–678, 2002.

[7] A. E. Feldstein, A. Wieckowska, A. R. Lopez, Y.-C. Liu, N. N. Zein, and A. J. McCullough, "Cytokeratin-18 fragment levels as noninvasive biomarkers for nonalcoholic steatohepatitis: a multicenter validation study," *Hepatology*, vol. 50, no. 4, pp. 1072–1078, 2009.

[8] A. Canbay, S. Friedman, and G. J. Gores, "Apoptosis: the nexus of liver injury and fibrosis," *Hepatology*, vol. 39, no. 2, pp. 273–278, 2004.

[9] A. E. Feldstein, A. Canbay, P. Angulo et al., "Hepatocyte apoptosis and Fas expression are prominent features of human nonalcoholic steatohepatitis," *Gastroenterology*, vol. 125, no. 2, pp. 437–443, 2003.

[10] "World Health Organisation Definition diagnosis and classification of diabetes mellitus and its complications," Report of A WHO ConsultAtion, World Health Organisation, Geneva, Switzerland, 1999.

[11] S. M. Grundy, J. I. Cleeman, S. R. Daniels et al., "Diagnosis and management of the metabolic syndrome: an American Heart Association/National Heart, Lung, and Blood Institute scientific statement," *Circulation*, vol. 112, no. 17, pp. 2735–2752, 2005.

[12] P. Angulo, J. M. Hui, G. Marchesini et al., "The NAFLD fibrosis score: a noninvasive system that identifies liver fibrosis in patients with NAFLD," *Hepatology*, vol. 45, no. 4, pp. 846–854, 2007.

[13] S. H. Saverymuttu, A. E. A. Joseph, and J. D. Maxwell, "Ultrasound scanning in the detection of hepatic fibrosis and steatosis," *British Medical Journal*, vol. 292, no. 6512, pp. 13–15, 1986.

[14] M. Hamaguchi, T. Kojima, Y. Itoh et al., "The severity of ultrasonographic findings in nonalcoholic fatty liver disease reflects the metabolic syndrome and visceral fat accumulation," *The American Journal of Gastroenterology*, vol. 102, no. 12, pp. 2708–2715, 2007.

[15] D. R. Matthews, J. P. Hosker, and A. S. Rudenski, "Homeostasis model assessment: insulin resistance and β-cell function from fasting plasma glucose and insulin concentrations in man," *Diabetologia*, vol. 28, no. 7, pp. 412–419, 1985.

[16] P. Pignatelli, R. Carnevale, R. Cangemi et al., "Atorvastatin inhibits gp91phox circulating levels in patients with hypercholesterolemia," *Arteriosclerosis, Thrombosis, and Vascular Biology*, vol. 30, no. 2, pp. 360–367, 2010.

[17] Z. Wang, G. Ciabattoni, C. Creminon et al., "Immunological characterization of urinary 8-epi-prostaglandin F(2α) excretion in man," *Journal of Pharmacology and Experimental Therapeutics*, vol. 275, no. 1, pp. 94–100, 1995.

[18] D. Il'yasova, P. Scarbrough, and I. Spasojevic, "Urinary biomarkers of oxidative status," *Clinica Chimica Acta*, vol. 413, pp. 1446–1453, 2012.

[19] P. Montuschi, P. J. Barnes, and L. J. Roberts II, "Isoprostanes: markers and mediators of oxidative stress," *The FASEB Journal*, vol. 18, no. 15, pp. 1791–1800, 2004.

[20] D. Praticò, "Prostanoid and isoprostanoid pathways in atherogenesis," *Atherosclerosis*, vol. 201, no. 1, pp. 8–16, 2008.

[21] A. C. Cave, A. C. Brewer, A. Narayanapanicker et al., "NADPH oxidases in cardiovascular health and disease," *Antioxidants and Redox Signaling*, vol. 8, no. 5-6, pp. 691–728, 2006.

[22] R. Cangemi, F. Angelico, L. Loffredo et al., "Oxidative stress-mediated arterial dysfunction in patients with metabolic syndrome: effect of ascorbic acid," *Free Radical Biology and Medicine*, vol. 43, no. 5, pp. 853–859, 2007.

[23] F. Angelico, L. Loffredo, P. Pignatelli et al., "Weight loss is associated with improved endothelial dysfunction via NOX2-generated oxidative stress down-regulation in patients with the metabolic syndrome," *Internal and Emergency Medicine*, vol. 7, pp. 219–227, 2012.

[24] L. Loffredo, F. Martino, R. Carnevale et al., "Obesity and hypercholesterolemia are associated with NOX-2 generated oxidative stress and arterial dysfunction," *Journal of Pediatrics*, vol. 161, pp. 1004–1009, 2012.

[25] M. Del Ben, M. Fabiani, L. Loffredo et al., "Oxidative stress mediated arterial dysfunction in patients with obstructive sleep apnoea and the effect of continuous positive airway pressure treatment," *BMC Pulmonary Medicine*, vol. 12, article 36, 2012.

[26] A. Wieckowska, N. N. Zein, L. M. Yerian, A. R. Lopez, A. J. McCullough, and A. E. Feldstein, "In vivo assessment of liver cell apoptosis as a novel biomarker of disease severity in nonalcoholic fatty liver disease," *Hepatology*, vol. 44, no. 1, pp. 27–33, 2006.

[27] P. Angulo, J. M. Hui, G. Marchesini et al., "The NAFLD fibrosis score: a noninvasive system that identifies liver fibrosis in patients with NAFLD," *Hepatology*, vol. 45, no. 4, pp. 846–854, 2007.

[28] S. Treeprasertsuk, E. Björnsson, F. Enders et al., "NAFLD fibrosis score: a prognostic predictor for mortality and liver complications among NAFLD patients," *World Journal of Gastroenterology*, vol. 19, pp. 1219–1229, 2013.

[29] R. Carnevale, P. Pignatelli, S. di Santo et al., "Atorvastatin inhibits oxidative stress via adiponectin-mediated NADPH oxidase down-regulation in hypercholesterolemic patients," *Atherosclerosis*, vol. 213, no. 1, pp. 225–234, 2010.

[30] S. Gustafsson, L. Lind, S. Söderberg et al., "Oxidative stress and inflammatory markers in relation to circulating levels of adiponectin," *Obesity*, vol. 21, no. 7, pp. 1467–1473, 2013.

[31] S. Nakanishi, K. Yamane, N. Kamei, H. Nojima, M. Okubo, and N. Kohno, "A protective effect of adiponectin against oxidative stress in Japanese Americans: the association between adiponectin or leptin and urinary isoprostane," *Metabolism*, vol. 54, no. 2, pp. 194–199, 2005.

[32] V. A. Arvaniti, K. C. Thomopoulos, A. Tsamandas et al., "Serum adiponectin levels in different types of non alcoholic liver disease: correlation with steatosis, necroinflammation and fibrosis," *Acta Gastro-Enterologica Belgica*, vol. 71, no. 4, pp. 355–360, 2008.

[33] M. Lemoine, V. Ratziu, M. Kim et al., "Serum adipokine levels predictive of liver injury in non-alcoholic fatty liver disease," *Liver International*, vol. 29, no. 9, pp. 1431–1438, 2009.

[34] S. A. Polyzos, K. A. Toulis, D. G. Goulis, C. Zavos, and J. Kountouras, "Serum total adiponectin in nonalcoholic fatty liver disease: a systematic review and meta-analysis," *Metabolism*, vol. 60, no. 3, pp. 313–326, 2011.

[35] B. Palmentieri, I. de Sio, V. la Mura et al., "The role of bright liver echo pattern on ultrasound B-mode examination in the diagnosis of liver steatosis," *Digestive and Liver Disease*, vol. 38, no. 7, pp. 485–489, 2006.

9

Patterns of Antimicrobial Resistance in the Causative Organisms of Spontaneous Bacterial Peritonitis: A Single Centre, Six-Year Experience of 1981 Samples

Sara Sheikhbahaei,[1,2] Alireza Abdollahi,[1] Nima Hafezi-Nejad,[1,2] and Elham Zare[1]

[1] *Department of Pathology, Imam Hospital Complex, Tehran University of Medical Sciences (TUMS), P.O. Box 14197-33141, Tehran, Iran*
[2] *Students' Scientific Research Center (SSRC), Tehran University of Medical Sciences (TUMS), P.O. Box 14155-6537, Tehran, Iran*

Correspondence should be addressed to Alireza Abdollahi; dr_p_abdollahi@yahoo.com

Academic Editor: Matthias Bahr

Background/Aims. Spontaneous bacterial peritonitis (SBP) is one of the leading causes of morbidity and mortality in patients with cirrhosis. This study aims to determine the microbial agents of SBP and the pattern of antibiotic resistance, in a large number of ascitic samples. *Methodology.* In a cross-sectional, single center, hospital based study, 1981 consecutive ascitic fluid samples were recruited from 2005 to 2011. Samples were dichotomized into three-year periods, in order to assess the trend of resistance to the first-line empirical antibiotics. *Results.* SBP was found in 482 (24.33%) of samples, of which 314 (65.15%) were culture positive. The most prevalent isolated pathogen was *E. coli* (33.8%), followed by *staphylococcus aureus* (8.9%) and *Enterococcus* (8.6%). No significant changes in the proportion of gram-negative/gram-positive infections occurred during this period. A percentage of resistant strains to cefotaxime (62.5%, 85.7%), ceftazidim (73%, 82.1%), ciprofloxacin (30, 59.8%), ofloxacin (36.8%, 50%), and oxacilin (35%, 51.6%) were significantly increased. *E. coli* was most sensitive to imipenem, piperacillin-tazobactam, amikacin, ceftizoxime, and gentamicin. *Conclusions.* The microbial aetiology of SBP remains relatively constant. However, the resistance rate especially to the first-line recommended antibiotics was significantly increased. This pattern must be watched closely and taken into account in empirical antibiotic treatment.

1. Introduction

Spontaneous bacterial peritonitis (SBP) is one of the leading causes of morbidity and mortality in patients with cirrhosis [1–3]. Unselected hospitalized cirrhotic patients with ascites were estimated to have 10%–30% risk of developing SBP [2, 3]. Early diagnosis and a prompt antibiotic therapy have considerably decreased the mortality rate associated with an episode of SBP from 80% to approximately 20–30% in the last decade [1, 2, 4–6].

SBP is defined as a monomicrobial infection of the ascitic fluid, which is not accompanied by a definite evidence of a surgically treatable origin [1, 3, 4]. The infection occurs following a translocation or haematogenous dissemination of the intestinal flora. Intestinal bacterial overgrowth can also exacerbate the condition [1, 3]. Studies have indicated that gram-negative Enterobacteriaceae such as *Escherichia coli* (*E. coli*) was the most common isolated organisms in SBP [1, 3, 7].

Diagnosis of SBP is established by an elevated ascitic fluid polymorphonuclear leukocyte (PMNL) count (≥250 cells/mm^3) [1, 3, 4]. Some studies suggest that the type and the etiology of SBP have been changing in the recent years. Involvement with gram-positive bacteria and increased frequency of multiple antibiotic resistant bacteria are evidences that support this viewpoint [6, 8, 9].

Based on EASL guidelines, third-generation cephalosporins (including cefotaxime and ceftriaxone) are recommended as the first-line therapy [1–4]. However, knowledge about the local epidemiological pattern of antibiotic resistance would be necessary for an effective treatment [2]. According to the pattern of antibiotic consumption, great differences exist in antibiotic sensitivity and resistance among various countries. Meanwhile, information regarding the spectrum of the involved bacteria and the pattern of antibiotic resistance in developing countries is scarce. The present study aims to determine the current causative agents of SBP and the pattern of antibiotic resistance, in a large number of ascitic samples. The antibiotic susceptibility patterns are delineated by in vitro methods. We further assess the trends of resistance to the first-line empirical antibiotics within a six-year period. The result of this study could be implicated in future management and treatment of patients with SBP in similar settings.

2. Methodology

2.1. Samples. This cross-sectional hospital based study was conducted in Imam Hospital Complex affiliated to the Tehran University of Medical Sciences, Iran. All ascitic fluid samples, referred to the pathology division of the hospital from April 2005 to September 2011, were included. Samples were recruited from cirrhotic patients with new onset grade 2 or 3 ascitic patients hospitalized for worsening of ascites and patients who developed symptoms suggestive of SBP or any complication of cirrhosis [1].

The ascitic fluid analyses include cell counts and differential, culture, and antibiotic susceptibility pattern. Culture-positive SBP was diagnosed in the presence of ascitic fluid PMNL ≥ 250 cells/mm^3 and positive ascitic fluid culture for a single organism. When the ascitic fluid culture results are negative, but the PMNL counts are 250 cells/mm^3 or higher, culture-negative neutrocytic ascites were diagnosed [1, 10]. Samples with polymicrobial infections were excluded from the study.

2.2. Laboratory Investigations. Ascitic fluid cell counts were determined by automated cell blood counter. Specimens were cultured on blood agar mediums. The basal agar mediums were autoclaved and then cooled to the 50 degrees of Celsius in the laboratory environment. After then, defibrinated blood (5–7%) was added to the basal mediums. Prepared blood agar medium was transferred to the sterile plates in order to culture the obtained samples. Hemolysis pattern was visually observed.

2.3. Antimicrobial Susceptibility. Antimicrobial susceptibility testing of isolated bacteria was determined according to the guidelines of the National Committee for Clinical Laboratory Standard's Institutes (CLSI) disk diffusion method. Mueller-Hinton agar was the handled medium. A 0.5 McFarland turbidity standard of the bacterial suspension was adjusted using barium sulphate precipitate. Cultured mediums were stored in laboratory environment for 24 hours. After then, the results were evaluated as sensitive or resistant according to the diffusion radiation. Samples with two or more isolated microorganisms suggestive of secondary peritonitis were excluded. Antibiotic disks used for gram-positive and gram-negative strains were as follows: gentamicin, vancomycin, cefalotin, clindamycin, erythromycin, oxacillin, rifampin, cotrimoxazol, ciprofloxacin, amikacin, imipenem, ceftazidime, ceftriaxone, ampicillin sulbactam, and piperacillin. Antibiotic disks were obtained from HiMedia brand, India, Pakistan, and/or Iran.

This study was carried out in accordance with the principles of the Declaration of Helsinki and was formally approved by the Institutional Ethical Committee.

2.4. Statistical Analysis. The SPSS software v.16 for Windows (Chicago, Illinois, USA) was used for analysis. Variables were described as mean (standard deviation, SD) or proportion. Student's t-test and chi-squared test were used for comparison of the continuous and categorical variables, respectively. Odd ratios (ORs) were derived by cross tabulating the number of favorable conditions. A two-tailed P value < 0.05 was considered statistically significant.

3. Results

The mean age (SD) of the study population is 51 (±9) and the male: female ratio is 1.25. Of the total of 1981 ascitic fluid samples, 482 samples (24.33%) were diagnosed as SBP. Out of these samples, 314 samples (65.15%) were identified as culture-positive SBP and 168 samples (34.85%) were culture-negative neutrocytic ascites. Males significantly had higher prevalence of positive culture (OR (95% CI) = 2.69 (1.08–3.06), $P < 0.01$).

Overall, the causative microorganisms of culture-positive episodes of SBP were mainly gram-negative organisms (62.9%). Gram-positive and nonbacterial organisms were responsible for 28.8% and 8.3% of the culture-positive samples. Of 228 episodes of bacterial SBP, 81.25% were owing to anaerobic fecal bacteria and 18.75% were aerobic.

Table 1 represents different microorganisms isolated from ascitic samples regarding different wards of the hospital. *E. coli* was the most prevalent causative microorganism isolated in all wards. As a whole, 16% of the culture-positive episodes of SBP were owing to skin contamination including the Coagulase-negative *Staphylococcus epidermidis* (6.7%), fungal species (8.3%), and *Stenotrophomonas maltophilia* (1%).

Table 2 represents the antibiotic resistance pattern of the isolated organisms. Overall, resistance to ciprofloxacin and ofloxacin was found in 54.6% and 57.1% of the isolated organisms. However, organisms were most sensitive to vancomycin, chloramphenicol, imipenem, piperacillin-tazobactam, tazobactam, meropenem, gentamicin, and amikacin.

In order to assess the trend of antibiotic resistance over time, samples were dichotomized into three-year periods (Table 3). There were no significant differences in the proportion of culture-positive organism as well as the frequency of gram-negative and gram-positive strains in this period.

Additionally, considering these two time periods, the overall antibiotic resistance rates to cefotaxime (62.5%,

TABLE 1: Profiles of the isolated microorganisms in spontaneous bacterial peritonitis in different wards.

	All	Different wards of the hospital				
		Emergency ward	Internal ward	Surgery ward	ICU ward	Paediatric ward
	N (%)	*N* (%)	*N* (%)	*N* (%)	*N* (%)	*N* (%)
Positive growth	314 (15.85%)	121 (6.10%)	79 (4.00%)	58 (2.90%)	55 (2.80%)	1 (0.05%)
Organism						
E. coli	106 (33.8%)	50 (5.1%)	20 (3.2%)	20 (9.3%)	15 (9.4%)	1 (16.7%)
Staphylococcus aureus	28 (8.9%)	14 (1.4%)	7 (1.1%)	7 (3.3%)	—	—
Enterococcus	27 (8.6%)	6 (0.6%)	12 (1.9%)	4 (1.9%)	—	—
Acinetobacter	25 (8%)	5 (0.5%)	7 (1.1%)	3 (1.4%)	10 (6.2%)	—
Candida	23 (7.3%)	8 (0.8%)	6 (1%)	5 (2.3%)	4 (2.5%)	—
Staphylococcus epidermidis	21 (6.7%)	8 (0.8%)	8 (1.3%)	3 (1.4%)	2 (1%)	—
Klebsiella	17 (5.4%)	7 (0.7%)	3 (0.5%)	6 (2.8%)	1 (0.6%)	—
Citrobacter	16 (5.1%)	6 (0.6%)	2 (0.3%)	1 (0.5%)	7 (4.4%)	—
Pseudomonas	15 (4.8%)	2 (0.2%)	5 (0.8%)	4 (1.9%)	4 (2.5%)	—
Enterobacter	11 (3.3%)	1 (0.1%)	3 (0.5%)	3 (1.4%)	4 (2.5%)	—
Nonhemolytic *Streptococcus*	5 (1.6%)	2 (0.2%)	2 (0.3%)	—	1 (0.6%)	—
Alcaligenes sp.	4 (1.3%)	4 (0.4%)	—	—	—	—
Hemolytic Streptococcus	4 (1.3%)	2 (0.2%)	1 (0.2%)	—	1 (0.6%)	—
Streptococcus group D	4 (1.3%)	4 (0.4%)	—	—	—	—
Proteus	3 (1%)	—	2 (0.3%)	1 (0.5%)	—	—
Stenotrophomonas maltophilia	3 (1%)	1 (0.1%)	1 (0.2%)	1 (0.5%)	—	—
Streptococcus pneumoniae	2 (0.6%)	1 (0.1%)	—	—	1 (0.6%)	—

85.7%), ciprofloxacin (30, 59.8%), amikacin (19.8%, 29%), ceftazidime (73%, 82.1%), ofloxacin (36.8%, 50%), and oxacillin (35%, 51.6%) were increased ($P < 0.01$ for all). However, no changes in rate of ceftriaxone resistant strains were observed (57.8%, 59%, $P = 0.12$).

4. Discussion

There is an apparent lack of data on current spectrum of causative microorganisms of SBP and their antibiotic sensitivity in our region. Herein, the frequency and the patterns of antibiotic resistance among isolated microorganisms from ascitic fluid samples were determined using data collected over six years.

In this study, 24.33% of samples were diagnosed as SBP from which 65.15% were culture positive. The remaining 34.85% were considered as culture-negative neutrocytic ascites. The culture-negative neutrocytic ascites have been estimated to occur in 30 to 60% of patients with SBP [1, 10]. This could also be the result of poor culturing techniques or late-stage resolving infection [10]. Nonetheless, empirical antibiotic therapy should be initiated in all patients with PMNL ≥ 250 cells/mm^3 [1, 10].

Historically, gram-negative bacteria were known as the most prevalent cause of culture-positive samples [2, 3, 7]. However, the etiological pattern of peritonitis varied in different geographical regions [7, 11]. In the present study gram-negative bacteria are among the main etiological agents (62.9%) isolated from ascitic fluid samples and gram-positive bacteria (28.8%) are the next. Our data also indicated that no significant changes in the proportion of gram-negative to gram-positive infections occurred during these 6 years. Although this pattern still holds true in some countries, recent studies suggested an increasing trend in infections caused by gram-positive cocci [8, 9, 12]. In the present study, the most prevalent isolated organisms in a descending order were as follows: *E. coli* (33.8%), *Staphylococcus aureus* (8.9%), *Enterococcus* (8.6%), *Acinetobacter* (8%), *Candida* (7.3%), *Staphylococcus epidermidis* (6.7%), and *Klebsiella* (5.4%). Our result indicated that *E. coli* is still the most common cause of culture-positive SBP, independent of the wards. This corresponds to the data obtained in other investigations [1–3, 7, 11, 13–15].

On the other hand, recent studies suggest an increase in the prevalence of enterococcal SBP [8, 9]. In a 12-year retrospective study in Germany, the frequency of enterococcal infections was increased from 11% to 35% and associated with increased resistance to cephalosporins [16]. Other investigations unveiled the poor prognosis of enterococcal SBP and declared that *Enterococcus* strains were mostly resistant to third-generation cephalosporins range between 77% and 100% [8, 17]. As can be seen, ceftriaxone and ceftazidime were inactive against 100% *Enterococcus* strains in this study. Our results were also consistent with those obtained in Korea indicating that enterococcal SBP was susceptible to ampicillin-gentamicin as well as vancomycin [8].

Furthermore, *Streptococcus pneumoniae* was isolated from 0.6% of ascitic samples, which was noticeably lower than some other reports [7, 11]. This could be explained by

Table 2: Patterns of antibiotic resistance among isolated microorganisms.

	All positive culture	*E. coli*	*Staphylococcus aureus*	*Enterococcus*	*Acinetobacter*	*Staphylococcus epidermidis*	*Klebsiella*	*Citrobacter*	*Enterobacter*	*Pseudomonas*
	Resistance rate %									
Amikacin	17.9%	7.2%	42.9%	50.0%	52.6%	0%	12.5%	22.2%	14.3%	—
Amoxicillin	64.7%	—	—	25%	—	—	—	—	—	—
Ampicillin	45.4%	37.5%	25%	46.7%	—	50%	—	—	—	—
Ampicillin sulbactam	66.6%	50%	—	50%	25%	—	44.4%	27.3%	62.5%	100%
Cefazolin	61.9%	—	33.3%	—	—	16.7%	—	0%	—	—
Cefepime	63.6%	70%	—	—	100%	—	60%		0%	60%
Cefixime	71.3%	67.4%	100%	—	91.7%	—	40%	33.3%	40%	100%
Cefoxitin		—	—	—	100%	20%	—	—	—	—
Cefotaxim	77.3%	72.7%	100%	—	100%	33.3%	66.7%	—	—	100%
Cefoxitin	71.3%	—	45.5%	—	—	100%	—	—	—	—
Ceftazidime	77.3%	75.8%	—	100%	84.6%	—	77.8%	50%	0%	87.5%
Ceftizoxime	70%	8.3%	—	—	4%	—	50%	0%	—	100%
Ceftriaxon	58.2%	56.6%	—	100%	77.8%	—	45.5%	41.7%	66.7%	80%
Chloramphenicol	6.2%	—	33.3%	0%	—	—	—	—	—	—
Ciprofloxacin	45.4%	54.2%	26.3%	42.9%	95%	—	28.6%	44.4%	0%	0%
Clindamycin	50%	0%	44%	100%	100%	—	—	50%	—	—
Cloxacillin	77.8%	—	33.3%	—	100%	—	—	—	—	—
Coamoxiclav	71.3%	—	—	—	100%	—	—	—	—	—
Cotrimoxazol	61.9%	65.9%	28%	61.1%	91.3%	42.9%	77.8%	50%	12.5%	92.3%
Erythromycin	72.7%	—	39.1%	28.6%	—	31.6%	—	0%	—	—
Gentamicin	4.1%	15.6%	54.5%	25%	50%	16.7%	0%	—	33.3%	25%
Imipenem	5.2%	1%	0%	0%	17.4%	0%	0%	0%	0%	13.3%
Ofloxacin	42.9%	—	—	50%	—	—	—	—	—	—
Oxacillin	44%	—	40%	83.3%	—	26.7%	—	50%	—	—
Piperacillin	23.2%	74.4%	0%	—	77.8%	55.6%	—	—	0%	66.7%
Piperacillin-tazobactam	4%	3.7%	0%	—	0%	—	12.5%	0%	0%	0%
Rifampicin	32.4%	—	—	50%	—	14.3%	—	—	—	—
Teicoplanin	63.3%	—	—	50%	—	—	—	—	—	—
Ticarcillin	55.7%	67.5%	—	—	88.9%	—	28.6%	40%	14.3%	20%
Vancomycin	6.7%	—	—	25%	—	0%		0%	0%	—

TABLE 3: Changes in the pattern of causative microorganism and the resistance rate to the first-line recommended antibiotics (2005–2011).

	2005 to 2008	2008 to 2011
Culture positive	15.4%	16.3%
Gram negative	60.2%	64.9%
Gram positive	39.8%	35.1%
	Antibiotic resistance rate %	
Cefotaxime	62.5%	85.7%*
Ceftazidime	73.0%	82.1%*
Ceftriaxone	57.8%	59.0%
Ciprofloxacin	30.0%	59.8%*
Ofloxacin	36.8%	50.0%*
Oxacillin	35%	51.6%*

*$P < 0.01$.

implementing pneumococcal vaccination in patients with cirrhosis. The current guideline [1, 2] recommended initiating empirical antibiotic treatment following the diagnosis of SBP. Since the most frequently isolated microorganisms were gram-negative enteric bacteria, third-generation cephalosporins are suggested as the first-line therapy for SBP. Amoxicillin-clavulanic acid and quinolones (ciprofloxacin, ofloxacin) were also known as effective alternatives [1, 2].

Besides, the antibiotic resistance rates could vary in different region based on the pattern of antibiotic consumption. A number of studies were conducted in different countries to assess the efficacy of the current guideline and help the clinicians to choose the most appropriate antibiotic as first-line treatment. Recent studies notice the emergence of resistance to third-generation cephalosporins. The rates of cephalosporin resistance in patients with SBP were shown to be 21% to 45% [2, 7, 15, 16, 18, 19]. The exposure to systemic antibiotics and nosocomial infections was introduced as independent predictors of resistance to first-line antibiotic regimens [19, 20]. On the contrary, study conducted in Korea declared that cefotaxime could still be the choice of primary empirical antibiotics for the treatment of SBP [7]. Another study in Spain indicated that a short course of ceftriaxone is efficient for resolution of 73% of patients [12].

In this study, overall antibiotic resistance to third-generation cephalosporins and quinolones was as follows: cefotaxime and ceftazidime (77.3%), cefoxitin and cefixime (71.3%), ceftizoxime (70%), cefazolin (61.9%), ceftriaxone (58.2%), ciprofloxacin (45.4%), oxacillin (44%), and ofloxacin (42.9%). In addition, about 71.3% of strains were resistant to coamoxiclav.

Recent study in India also indicated a low response rate to third-generation cephalosporins in patients with SBP. As the sensitivity rates to ceftriaxone were 50%, they suggest that cefoperazone-sulbactam could be a better alternative choice [15]. In the present study, *E. coli*, the predominant isolated pathogen, was most sensitive to imipenem, piperacillin-tazobactam, amikacin, ceftizoxime, and gentamicin, whereas only 20–30% of *E. coli* isolates were sensitive to cefotaxime and ceftazidime and the sensitivity rates to ceftriaxone were 43.4%.

To identify the occurring changes in antibiotic resistance rates of the causative agents, we divided the study period into two 3-year intervals. The resistance rate to cefotaxime, ceftazidime, ciprofloxacin, amikacin, and oxacillin was significantly increased during this time period.

Overall, results of the present study highlight the emergence of resistant strains in our region, as most of the isolated bacteria showed an increased level of resistance to first-line empirical antibiotics. Besides, our rates of cephalosporins resistance are noticeably higher than most of the published literature [2, 7, 14, 18, 19]. Higher resistance rate to the third-generation cephalosporins in this study may be explained by indiscriminate use of these antibiotics during the past decade in our region. In contrary, most of the isolated organisms were sensitive to imipenem, piperacillin-tazobactam, and gentamicin. This may be due to the less frequency of usage of these drugs, as they were usually prescribed in complicated patients.

Precise knowledge about previous SBPs, prior history of antibiotic consumption, and/or use of SBP prophylaxis would be beneficial in explaining the results. Unfortunately, there was little information in this regard in our retrospective database. Nevertheless, as there have been no reports clearly assessing the microbial agents and antibiotic resistance of SBP in our region, our study still declares its critical role in elucidating the situation for the first time in the region.

This study suggests that the current recommended empirical antibiotics need to be reassessed. The empirical treatment of SBP should be adapted to the local epidemiological pattern of antibiotic susceptibility, in order to decrease the morbidity and mortality associated with SBP.

5. Conclusion

Present study indicates that, during 2005–2011 time period, the microbial etiology of SBP remains relatively constant; however, the antibiotic resistance rate especially for third-generation cephalosporins (including cefotaxime and ceftazidime), ciprofloxacin, and ofloxacin increased dramatically. Congruent with these findings, only 10–20% of strains were sensitive to cefotaxime and ceftazidime. This pattern must be watched closely and taken into account in empirical antibiotic treatment.

References

[1] European Association for the Study of the Liver, "EASL clinical practice guidelines on the management of ascites, spontaneous bacterial peritonitis, and hepatorenal syndrome in cirrhosis," *Journal of Hepatology*, vol. 53, no. 3, pp. 397–417, 2010.

[2] S. Ageloni, C. Leboffe, A. Parente et al., "Efficacy of current guidelines for the treatment of spontaneous bacterial peritonitis

in the clinical practice," *World Journal of Gastroenterology*, vol. 14, no. 17, pp. 2757–2762, 2008.

[3] J. M. Lee, K.-H. Han, and S. H. Ahn, "Ascites and spontaneous bacterial peritonitis: an Asian perspective," *Journal of Gastroenterology and Hepatology*, vol. 24, no. 9, pp. 1494–1503, 2009.

[4] G. Garcia-Tsao, "Current management of the complications of cirrhosis and portal hypertension: variceal hemorrhage, ascites, and spontaneous bacterial peritonitis," *Gastroenterology*, vol. 120, no. 3, pp. 726–748, 2001.

[5] R. Terg, S. Cobas, E. Fassio et al., "Oral ciprofloxacin after a short course of intravenous ciprofloxacin in the treatment of spontaneous bacterial peritonitis: results of a multicenter, randomized study," *Journal of Hepatology*, vol. 33, no. 4, pp. 564–569, 2000.

[6] N. Singh, M. M. Wagener, and T. Gayowski, "Changing epidemiology and predictors of mortality in patients with spontaneous bacterial peritonitis at a liver transplant unit," *Clinical Microbiology and Infection*, vol. 9, no. 6, pp. 531–537, 2003.

[7] M. K. Park, J. H. Lee, Y. H. Byun et al., "Changes in the profiles of causative agents and antibiotic resistance rate for spontaneous bacterial peritonitis: an analysis of cultured microorganisms in recent 12 years," *The Korean Journal of Hepatology*, vol. 13, no. 3, pp. 370–377, 2007.

[8] J.-H. Lee, J.-H. Yoon, B. H. Kim et al., "Enterococcus: not an innocent bystander in cirrhotic patients with spontaneous bacterial peritonitis," *European Journal of Clinical Microbiology and Infectious Diseases*, vol. 28, no. 1, pp. 21–26, 2009.

[9] A. Alexopoulou, N. Papadopoulos, D. G. Eliopoulos et al., "Increasing frequency of gram-positive cocci and gram-negative multidrug- resistant bacteria in spontaneous bacterial peritonitis," *Liver International*, vol. 33, no. 7, pp. 975–981, 2013.

[10] J. Lata, O. Stiburek, and M. Kopacova, "Spontaneous bacterial peritonitis: a severe complication of liver cirrhosis," *World Journal of Gastroenterology*, vol. 15, no. 44, pp. 5505–5510, 2009.

[11] L. Piroth, A. Pechinot, A. Minello et al., "Bacterial epidemiology and antimicrobial resistance in ascitic fluid: a 2-year retrospective study," *Scandinavian Journal of Infectious Diseases*, vol. 41, no. 11-12, pp. 847–851, 2009.

[12] J. Fernández, M. Navasa, J. Gómez et al., "Bacterial infections in cirrhosis: epidemiological changes with invasive procedures and norfloxacin prophylaxis," *Hepatology*, vol. 35, no. 1, pp. 140–148, 2002.

[13] H. G. Song, H. C. Lee, Y. H. Joo et al., "Clinical and microbiological characteristics of spontaneous bacterial peritonitis (SBP) in a recent five year period," *Taehan Kan Hakhoe Chi*, vol. 8, no. 1, pp. 61–70, 2002.

[14] A. Umgelter, W. Reindl, M. Miedaner, R. M. Schmid, and W. Huber, "Failure of current antibiotic first-line regimens and mortality in hospitalized patients with spontaneous bacterial peritonitis," *Infection*, vol. 37, no. 1, pp. 2–8, 2009.

[15] G. Bhat, K. E. Vandana, S. Bhatia, D. Suvarna, and C. G. Pai, "Spontaneous ascitic fluid infection in liver cirrhosis: bacteriological profile and response toantibi otic therapy," *Indian Journal of Gastroenterology*, vol. 32, no. 5, pp. 297–301, 2013.

[16] P. A. Reuken, M. W. Pletz, M. Baier, W. Pfister, A. Stallmach, and T. Bruns, "Emergence of spontaneous bacterial peritonitis due to enterococci—risk factors and outcome in a 12-year retrospective study," *Alimentary Pharmacology and Therapeutics*, vol. 35, no. 10, pp. 1199–1208, 2012.

[17] T. Yakar, M. Güçlü, E. Serin, and H. AlIşkan, "A recent evaluation of empirical cephalosporin treatment and antibiotic resistance of changing bacterial profiles in spontaneous bacterial peritonitis," *Digestive Diseases and Sciences*, vol. 55, no. 4, pp. 1149–1154, 2010.

[18] X. Ariza, J. Castellote, J. Lora-Tamayo et al., "Risk factors for resistance to ceftriaxone and its impact on mortality in community, healthcare and nosocomial spontaneous bacterial peritonitis," *Journal of Hepatology*, vol. 56, no. 4, pp. 825–832, 2012.

[19] P. Tandon, A. Delisle, J. E. Topal, and G. Garcia-Tsao, "High prevalence of antibiotic-resistant bacterial infections among patients with cirrhosis at a US liver center," *Clinical Gastroenterology and Hepatology*, vol. 10, no. 11, pp. 1291–1298, 2012.

[20] J. Acevedo, A. Silva, V. Prado, and J. Fernandez, "The new epidemiology of nosocomial bacterial infections in cirrhosis: therapeutical implications," *Hepatology International*, vol. 7, no. 1, pp. 72–79, 2013.

10

Serum Adiponectin, Vitamin D, and Alpha-Fetoprotein in Children with Chronic Hepatitis C: Can They Predict Treatment Response?

Mohamed Ahmed Khedr,[1] Ahmad Mohamed Sira,[1] Magdy Anwar Saber,[1] and Gamal Yousef Raia[2]

[1]*Department of Pediatric Hepatology, National Liver Institute, Menofiya University, Shebin El-koom, Menofiya 32511, Egypt*
[2]*Department of Clinical Pathology, National Liver Institute, Menofiya University, Shebin El-koom, Menofiya 32511, Egypt*

Correspondence should be addressed to Ahmad Mohamed Sira; asira@liver-eg.org

Academic Editor: Pierluigi Toniutto

Background & Aims. The currently available treatment for chronic hepatitis C (CHC) in children is costly and with much toxicity. So, predicting the likelihood of response before starting therapy is important. *Methods.* Serum adiponectin, vitamin D, and alpha-fetoprotein (AFP) were measured before starting pegylated-interferon/ribavirin therapy for 50 children with CHC. Another 21 healthy children were recruited as controls. *Results.* Serum adiponectin, vitamin D, and AFP were higher in the CHC group than healthy controls ($p < 0.0001$, $p = 0.071$, and $p = 0.87$, resp.). In univariate analysis, serum adiponectin was significantly higher in responders than nonresponders ($p < 0.0001$) and at a cutoff value ≥8.04 ng/mL it can predict treatment response by 77.8% sensitivity and 92.9% specificity, while both AFP and viremia were significantly lower in responders than nonresponders, $p < 0.0001$ and $p = 0.0003$, respectively, and at cutoff values ≤3.265 ng/mL and ≤235,384 IU/mL, respectively, they can predict treatment response with a sensitivity of 83.3% for both and specificity of 85.7% and 78.6%, respectively. In multivariate analysis, adiponectin was found to be the only independent predictor of treatment response ($p = 0.044$). *Conclusions.* The pretreatment serum level of adiponectin can predict the likelihood of treatment response, thus avoiding toxicities for those unlikely to respond to therapy.

1. Introduction

Although chronic hepatitis C (CHC) in children is usually asymptomatic, it is often persistent and is a possible cause of morbidity in later life. Moreover, progressive liver disease, including cirrhosis, has been reported during childhood [1]. Although new direct-acting antivirals (DAAs) are now the cornerstones in the treatment of HCV infection in adults, combination therapy with pegylated interferon (Peg-IFN) alpha and ribavirin (RBV) (Peg/RBV therapy) is still the current standard therapy in children [2, 3]. Although this regimen was found to be highly effective in children with genotypes 2 and 3 [4], it has limited efficacy for those with genotype 4 [5, 6], the prevalent genotype in Egypt [7]. Therefore, the ability to predict response to this costly with many side effects antiviral regimen remains an important research goal.

In spite of the extensive researches in this field, knowledge is still defective. On defining predictors of treatment response, many studies concentrated on virus genotype, gender, age, race, and fibrosis stage, among others. Nevertheless, all of these are nonmodifiable factors but only give a prediction about the likelihood of sustained virologic response (SVR). Moreover, some of them are expensive and invasive [8]. On investigating the role of *interleukin-28B* (*IL28B*) polymorphism in pediatric patients with CHC, one study suggested that *IL28B* genotype was not a strong predictor of SVR [9], while other studies have shown usefulness of *IL28B* genotype as a predictor of treatment response [10–12].

Virological responses during therapy, such as rapid virologic response (RVR) and early virologic response (EVR), are widely used for predicting end of treatment response (ETR) and SVR [13]. Nonetheless, it is obvious that predictions made before administration of therapy are more desirable than those done during treatment course.

We aimed to investigate some inexpensive, easy to perform, and noninvasive modifiable (as adiponectin and vitamin D) and nonmodifiable (as alpha-fetoprotein "AFP") factors which may have a relation to treatment response in children with CHC. If we found a significant relation to successful treatment, we can use them not just to predict the likelihood of treatment response but also to improve the SVR rates by modulating the modifiable ones. This knowledge can also constitute a base for later on researches when DAA became approved in pediatric age.

2. Methods

2.1. Study Population. This prospective cohort study included fifty children with CHC recruited from Pediatric Hepatology Department, National Liver Institute (a tertiary level institute), Menofiya University, Egypt, between June 2012 and June 2014. Their mean age was 11.46 ± 3.48 years and thirty three (66%) of them were males. Another 21 healthy children with comparable age (mean; 9.14±3.31 years) and sex (males; 13 "61.9%") to the disease group were enrolled as controls. CHC was diagnosed on the basis of positive anti-HCV antibodies and positive HCV-RNA for more than 6 months duration, together with the pathological picture of CHC [1]. Any case with associated liver disease (either identified by laboratory or histological examination) or out of the inclusion criteria for Peg/RBV therapy, as defined by El Naghi et al. [5], was excluded. A signed informed consent was obtained from parents of all recruited children before enrollment in the study. The study was approved by the Research Ethics Committee of the National Liver Institute, Menofiya University, and conforms to the 1975 Declaration of Helsinki and its later amendments.

2.2. Laboratory Investigations and Ultrasonographic Evaluation. Alanine transaminase (ALT), aspartate transaminase (AST), prothrombin time (PT), complete blood count (CBC), thyroid stimulating hormone (TSH), and serum autoantibodies (anti-nuclear antibodies, anti-smooth muscle antibodies, and liver-kidney microsomal antibodies) were performed for every patient.

Viral markers (anti-HCV, hepatitis B virus (HBV) surface antigen, HBV core immunoglobulin (Ig)M, and IgG antibodies) were performed for all patients using chemiluminescence immunoassay (Roche Diagnostic Inc., Mannheim, Germany). Real-time PCR for HCV-RNA was performed using Abbott m2000 real-time system (Abbott Molecular Inc., Des Plaines, Illinois, USA) for every patient before starting therapy and at week 12 of therapy. For those who continued therapy, PCR was tested at weeks 24 and 48 of treatment and lastly 6 months after the end of treatment. The detection limit was 15 IU/mL.

Abdominal ultrasound was performed using 2–5 MHz curved linear and 4–8 MHz linear transducers (Xario XG; Toshiba, Tokyo, Japan).

2.3. Liver Biopsy and Histopathological Evaluation. An ultrasonographic-guided liver biopsy was performed for all patients using a true-cut needle, size 16 G. Biopsy specimens were fixed in formalin, embedded in paraffin, and finally the slides obtained were stained by hematoxylin and eosin (H&E), perls, and orcein for routine histopathological evaluation.

Histological evaluation of chronic hepatitis was performed using Ishak et al. [14] scoring system. Grades of necroinflammatory activity 1–3 were ascribed as minimal, grades 4–7 as mild, and grades 8–12 as moderate, whereas grades >13 were ascribed as severe chronic hepatitis. Stages of fibrosis of 0-1 indicated absent/minimal fibrosis, stages 2-3 indicated significant fibrosis, and stages 4–6 indicated advanced fibrosis.

2.4. Peg/RBV Therapy. All children with CHC received Peg-IFNα-2b (PegIntron; Schering-Plough, New Jersey, USA) at a dosage of 60 μg/m^2/week subcutaneously and RBV orally at a dosage of 15 mg/kg/day on two divided doses. The duration of therapy for those who completed the course was 48 weeks. Virological responses of therapy were defined as reported by Ghany et al. [6]. Thirty-six (72%) children attained ETR and SVR with no relapses, while 14 (28%) children were nonresponders.

2.5. Serum Adiponectin, Vitamin D, and Alpha-Fetoprotein Assay. Serum samples were collected from every patient before starting Peg/RBV therapy and from healthy controls then stored at −80°C until used. Serum adiponectin level was determined by the Human Adiponectin (Acrp30) enzyme-linked immunosorbent assay (ELISA) kit (Orgenium Laboratories, Vantaa Finland). Serum vitamin D was measured using 25-OH Vitamin D Enzyme-Immunoassay (EIA) Kit (Immundiagnostik, Bensheim and Biomedica, Wien Austria) intended for the quantitative determination of the 25-OH vitamin D in plasma or serum. Lastly, serum AFP was measured by Quantikine, a human AFP EIA kit (R&D Systems Inc., Minneapolis, USA). Serum levels of the three test parameters were expressed as nanograms per milliliter (ng/mL).

2.6. Statistical Analysis. Values were expressed as mean ± standard deviation (range) or number (percentage) of individuals with a condition. For quantitative data, statistical significance was tested by either independent samples t-test or nonparametric Mann-Whitney U test according to the nature of the data. For qualitative data, significance was tested by Chi-square test or Fisher exact test. A multivariate analysis was performed using a binary logistic regression analysis for factors that significantly associated with treatment response on univariate analysis. Correlation was tested by Spearman test. The cutoff values for optimal clinical performance of adiponectin, vitamin D, AFP, and level of HCV-RNA for differentiation between responders and nonresponders were determined from the receiver-operating characteristic (ROC)

TABLE 1: Baseline demographic, laboratory, and histopathological characteristics of the hepatitis C virus-infected group.

Item	All ($n = 50$)	Responders ($n = 36$)	Nonresponders ($n = 14$)	p value
Age (years)	11.46 ± 3.48 (4–18)	11.8 ± 3.6 (4–18)	10.6 ± 3.1 (5–16)	0.237
Sex (male)	33 (66%)	25 (69.4%)	8 (57.1%)	0.41
BMI	18.56 ± 2.79 (14.21–25.36)	18.8 ± 2.9 (14.2–25.4)	17.98 ± 2.4 (14.8–21.1)	0.334
Hemoglobin (g/dL)	11.7 ± 0.76 (10–13.2)	11.6 ± 0.75 (10–13.1)	11.9 ± 0.75 (10.3–13.2)	0.209
White blood cells ($\times 10^3/\mu L$)	7.3 ± 1.8 (4.5–12.3)	7.3 ± 1.6 (4.5–11.8)	7.3 ± 2.2 (4.8–12.3)	0.892
Neutrophils ($\times 10^3/\mu L$)	5.14 ± 1.2 (3.24–8.14)	5.1 ± 1.13 (3.24–8.14)	5.2 ± 1.4 (3.3–7.6)	0.828
Platelets ($\times 10^3/\mu L$)	242 ± 82 (122–431)	238 ± 84 (122–431)	253 ± 76 (123–351)	0.544
ALT (U/L)	56.4 ± 13.6 (40–108)	56.3 ± 12.3 (40–86)	56.6 ± 17.1 (40–108)	0.943
AST (U/L)	62.9 ± 25.7 (35–157)	63 ± 28.1 (35–157)	61.9 ± 19.4 (40–110)	0.665
Stage of fibrosis				0.23
Absent/minimal	29 (58%)	19 (52.8%)	10 (71.4%)	
Significant	21 (42%)	17 (47.2%)	4 (28.6%)	
Grade of activity				0.345
Minimal	7 (14%)	4 (11.1%)	3 (21.4%)	
Mild	43 (86%)	32 (88.9%)	11 (78.6%)	

HCV: hepatitis C virus; BMI: body mass index; ALT: alanine transaminase, AST: aspartate transaminase. p value is for the comparison between responders and nonresponders.

curves. The diagnostic performance was presented as sensitivity, specificity, negative predictive value (NPV), positive predictive value (PPV), and accuracy. Results were considered significant if p value was <0.05. Statistical analysis was performed using SPSS, version 13 (SPSS Inc., Chicago, IL, USA).

3. Results

3.1. Baseline Demographic, Laboratory, and Histopathological Characteristics of the Studied Children. Body mass index of children with CHC was within average with a mean of 18.56± 2.79 kg/m^2. Level of hepatitis C viremia ranged from 8.04×10^3 to 6.23×10^6 with a mean of $6.28 \times 10^5 \pm 1.23 \times 10^6$ IU/mL. Forty-five (90%) patients with CHC showed mild stage of fibrosis and 5 (10%) cases showed moderate fibrosis. Most of (86%) CHC children had mild activity, while 7 (14%) cases had minimal activity. Laboratory parameters are shown in Table 1.

3.2. Serum Adiponectin, Vitamin D and Alpha-Fetoprotein in Both CHC and Control Groups. Serum adiponectin was significantly higher in the CHC group than healthy controls (8.92 ± 2.85 and 6.049 ± 1.04 ng/mL, resp.; $p < 0.0001$). Also, in spite of being insignificant, serum vitamin D and AFP were higher in the CHC group (71.6 ± 49.1 ng/mL and 3.6 ± 2.96 ng/mL, resp.) than healthy controls (46.4 ± 21.8 ng/mL and 3.0 ± 0.39 ng/mL, resp.) (Figure 1).

3.3. Factors Associated with SVR. Pretreatment factors that could be associated with response to peg/RBV therapy were compared between treatment responders (SVR) and treatment nonresponders (Figure 2). It was found that adiponectin was significantly higher in those with SVR (9.79±2.7 versus 6.69±1.77 ng/mL; $p < 0.0001$). On the other hand it was found that both AFP and viremia were significantly lower in the treatment responders (2.84 ± 0.51 ng/mL and $4.18 \times 10^5 \pm 1.03 \times 10^6$ IU/mL, resp.) than in nonresponders (5.69 ± 5.1 ng/mL and $1.16 \times 10^6 \pm 1.57 \times 10^6$ IU/mL, resp.) with $p < 0.0001$ and $p = 0.0003$, respectively. Lastly, vitamin D was found to be higher in the treatment responders (77.2 ± 46.6 ng/mL) than nonresponders (57.2 ± 53.9 ng/mL), with borderline significance, $p = 0.076$. Other studied pretreatment parameters showed no difference between responders and nonresponders (Table 1), while in multivariate analysis adiponectin was shown to be the only significant independent predictor of treatment response ($p = 0.044$) (Table 3).

3.4. Diagnostic Performance of Predictors of Treatment Response. Cutoff points for variables showing significant associations with treatment response were analyzed by the ROC curves (Figure 3). For adiponectin it was found that at a cutoff value of >8.04 ng/mL, it can predict treatment response by 77.8% sensitivity, 92.9% specificity, 96.6% PPV, 61.9% NPV, and 82.3% accuracy, while AFP and HCV-RNA at cutoff values <3.265 ng/mL and <235,384 IU/mL, respectively, can predict treatment response with a sensitivity of 83.3% and 83.3%, specificity of 85.7% and 78.6%, PPV of 93.75% and 90.9%, NPV of 66.7% and 64.7%, and accuracy of 82.36% and 79.38%, respectively.

3.5. Correlation of Predictors of Treatment Response with Other Studied Parameters. Adiponectin was found to be significantly negatively correlated with both AFP ($r = -0.29$ and $p = 0.043$) and level of viremia ($r = -0.39$ and $p = 0.005$), with no significant correlation with other studied parameters. Also, there was no significant correlation between AFP,

TABLE 2: Correlation of predictors of treatment response with other studied parameters.

Item	Adiponectin		Alpha-fetoprotein		HCV-RNA		Vitamin D	
	r	*p*	*r*	*p*	*r*	*p*	*r*	*p*
Alpha-fetoprotein	−0.29	**0.043**						
HCV-RNA	−0.39	**0.005**	0.217	0.13				
Vitamin D	0.124	0.391	−0.09	0.545	−0.06	0.66		
Age	0.055	0.705	0.05	0.731	0.042	0.773	0.203	0.157
BMI	0.045	0.755	0.223	0.119	−0.03	0.812	0.129	0.372
HB	−0.04	0.765	0.04	0.782	−0.02	0.882	0.028	0.85
WBCs	0.096	0.508	−0.14	0.315	0.032	0.823	0.001	0.996
Neutrophils	0.123	0.396	−0.10	0.474	0.067	0.644	−0.01	0.953
Platelets	−0.21	0.142	−0.04	0.795	0.127	0.379	0.027	0.855
ALT	0.06	0.677	−0.06	0.705	−0.06	0.666	−0.04	0.768
AST	0.162	0.262	0.077	0.594	0.153	0.287	−0.06	0.677
Stage of fibrosis	0.189	0.189	−0.09	0.524	0.016	0.911	0.141	0.327
Grade of activity	0.084	0.563	0.166	0.25	0.049	0.737	0.073	0.616

HCV-RNA: hepatitis C virus ribonucleic acid; BMI: body mass index; HB: hemoglobin; WBCs: white blood cells; ALT: alanine transaminase; AST: aspartate transaminase.

TABLE 3: Multiple regression analysis for pretreatment predictors of treatment response.

Item	β	*p* value	95% CI	
			Lower	Upper
HCV-RNA by PCR (IU/mL)	−0.000002	0.119	1.0	1.0
Alpha-fetoprotein (ng/mL)	−8.51	0.056	0.00000003	1.24
Adiponectin (ng/mL)	3.142	0.044	1.095	489.93

B: regression coefficient; CI: confidence interval.

vitamin D, and level of viremia and all other studied parameters (Table 2).

4. Discussion

This study is, to our knowledge, the first to show the predictive value of baseline serum levels of adiponectin, vitamin D, and AFP for the treatment response of CHC in children.

Adiponectin is an adipocytokine secreted by adipocytes. It is a protein hormone that modulates a number of metabolic processes including glucose and fatty acid catabolism. Also it has been suggested that adiponectin has a hepatoprotective role [15]. The anti-inflammatory effects of adiponectin could protect the liver from the development of inflammation and cell injury [16].

In the present work, the significantly higher adiponectin in the CHC group than the control group may be due to an anti-inflammatory role of adiponectin in those with CHC. In previous studies, adiponectin was found to directly affect the inflammatory response by regulating both production and activity of cytokines [16]. In addition, hypoadiponectinemia has been reported to enhance hepatic steatosis, inflammation, fibrosis, and hepatocarcinogenesis in animal models of liver diseases [17–19]. Moreover, nonalcoholic steatohepatitis patients show lower levels of adiponectin with higher grades of inflammation [15].

In this work, the pretreatment serum level of adiponectin was significantly higher in the treatment responders (SVR) than nonresponders, and at a cutoff value of >8.04 ng/mL it can predict the treatment response by a sensitivity of 77.8% and a specificity of 92.9%. Zografos et al. [20] found that lower adiponectin was an independent predictor of no virological response at the end of treatment ($p < 0.001$). This may indicate the benefit of the anti-inflammatory role of adiponectin [16] in those with CHC. Adiponectin administration, in both alcoholic and nonalcoholic fatty liver in mice, was found to suppress hepatic production and the circulating levels of tumor necrosis factor-α and ameliorates hepatic steatosis [21].

Moreover, the significant negative correlation found in this work between serum adiponectin and viremia may indicate an antiviral role of adiponectin. On the other hand, it may suggest that HCV may directly affect adiponectin. This later concept was suggested by the study of Zografos et al. [20] who found a significant increase of adiponectin at the end of HCV treatment for those with ETR.

Abdel Latif et al. [22] found that serum adiponectin levels were lower in HCV-infected patients with steatosis than in those without steatosis and these levels tend to decrease with the increase in the grade of steatosis, the advance in the grade of histological activity, and the stage of fibrosis. In our work, there was no significant correlation between adiponectin and stage of fibrosis or grade of necroinflammatory activity. This difference may relate to the difference in age range and the relatively mild histological affection of our CHC group.

According to the previous results, not only can adiponectin be used as a reliable pretreatment predictor of treatment response in combination with other defined parameters but also it can be tried as an adjuvant therapy with peg/RBV especially for those with pretreatment lower serum levels. To prove this, it needs a well controlled clinical trial.

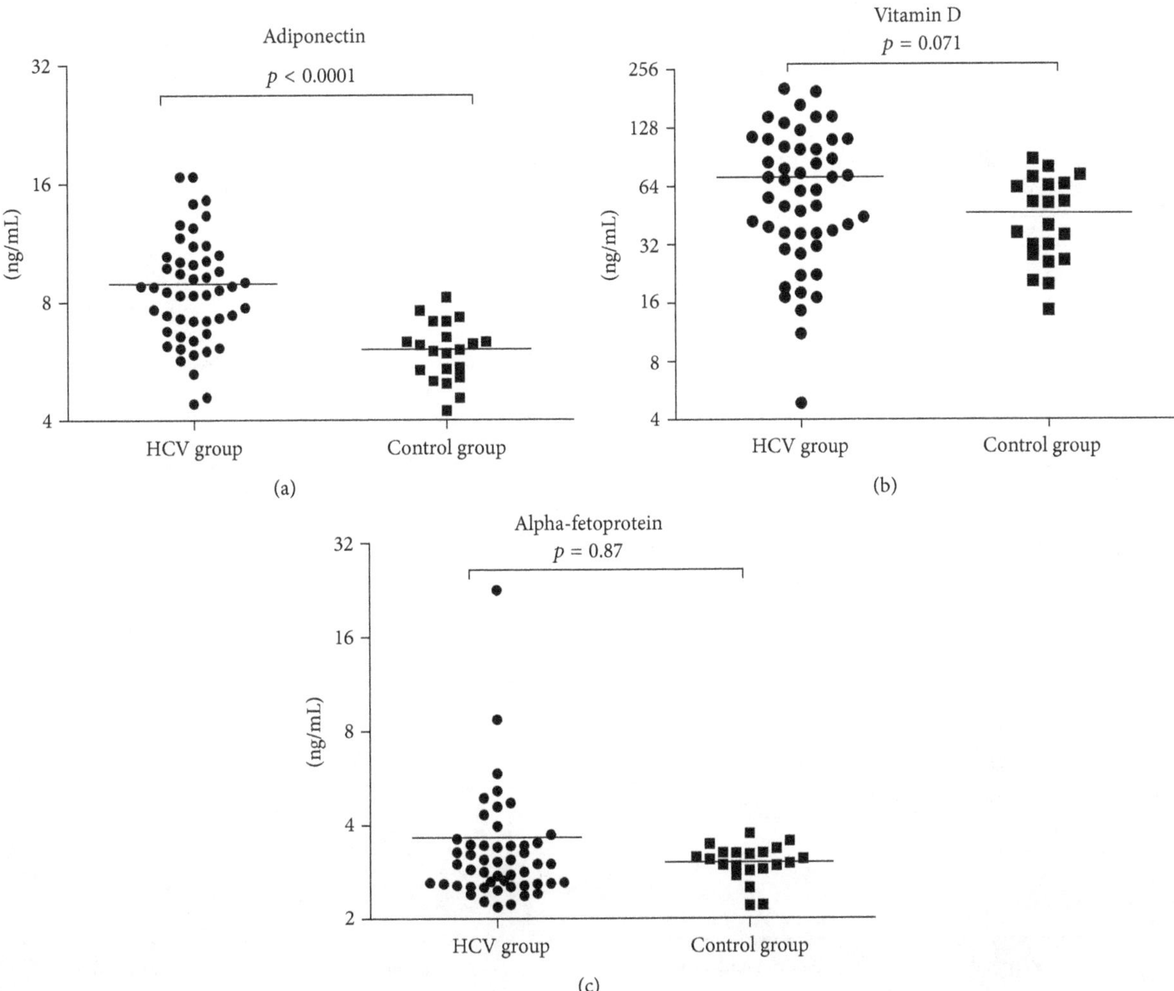

FIGURE 1: Comparison of pretreatment factors between HCV group and control group. (a) Adiponectin was significantly ($p < 0.0001$) higher in HCV group (8.92 ± 2.85 ng/mL, range; 4.4–16.7 ng/mL) than control group (6.049 ± 1.04 ng/mL, range; 4.2–8.2 ng/mL). (b) Vitamin D was insignificantly ($p = 0.071$) higher in HCV group (71.6 ± 49.1 ng/mL, range; 4.87–202 ng/mL) than control group (46.4 ± 21.8 ng/mL, range; 14.7–88 ng/mL). (c) AFP was insignificantly ($p = 0.87$) higher in HCV group (3.6 ± 2.96 ng/mL, range; 2.18–22.6 ng/mL) than control group (3.0 ± 0.39 ng/mL, range; 2.2–3.7 ng/mL).

Beside its action in calcium homeostasis, vitamin D has a significant immunomodulatory action and is an important mediator of innate and adaptive immune systems [23]. In spite of many researches, no strict data are found on the relationship between vitamin D and CHC. Generally, in relation to vitamin D synthesis in the liver, mild to moderate liver dysfunction causes malabsorption of vitamin D. Moreover, liver dysfunction of 90% or more results in inability to make sufficient 25-OH vitamin D [24]. Some researchers showed that adults with CHC have higher incidence of severe 25-OH vitamin D deficiency compared to the normal control [25]. On the contrary, in the present study we found that vitamin D was higher in children with CHC than normal controls with borderline significance ($p = 0.071$). This difference from Lange et al. [25] study may be due to younger age and milder liver affection in our children compared to their adult population. Hypothetically, this reported vitamin D increase in children with CHC reflects a possible antiviral role of vitamin D. This is supported by Matsumura et al. [26] who demonstrated in in vitro study that 25-OH vitamin D is an anti-HCV agent that targets viral particle assembly step.

Petta et al. [27] found that low vitamin D serum level is related to severe fibrosis in adults with CHC. However, we did not find significant correlation between vitamin D and any of the stage of fibrosis or grade of activity or any other studied pretreatment parameter.

Vitamin D concentration has emerged recently as a new predictor of HCV treatment response. This novel predictor is of great interest because it is easily modifiable by supplementation [28]. However, no previous data are available for the pediatric age group.

In the present work, a higher vitamin D level was found in HCV treatment responders than nonresponders but with borderline significance. Similar to our results Petta et al. [27], Bitetto et al. [28], and Nimer and Mouch [29] detected an association between lower vitamin D serum levels and failure

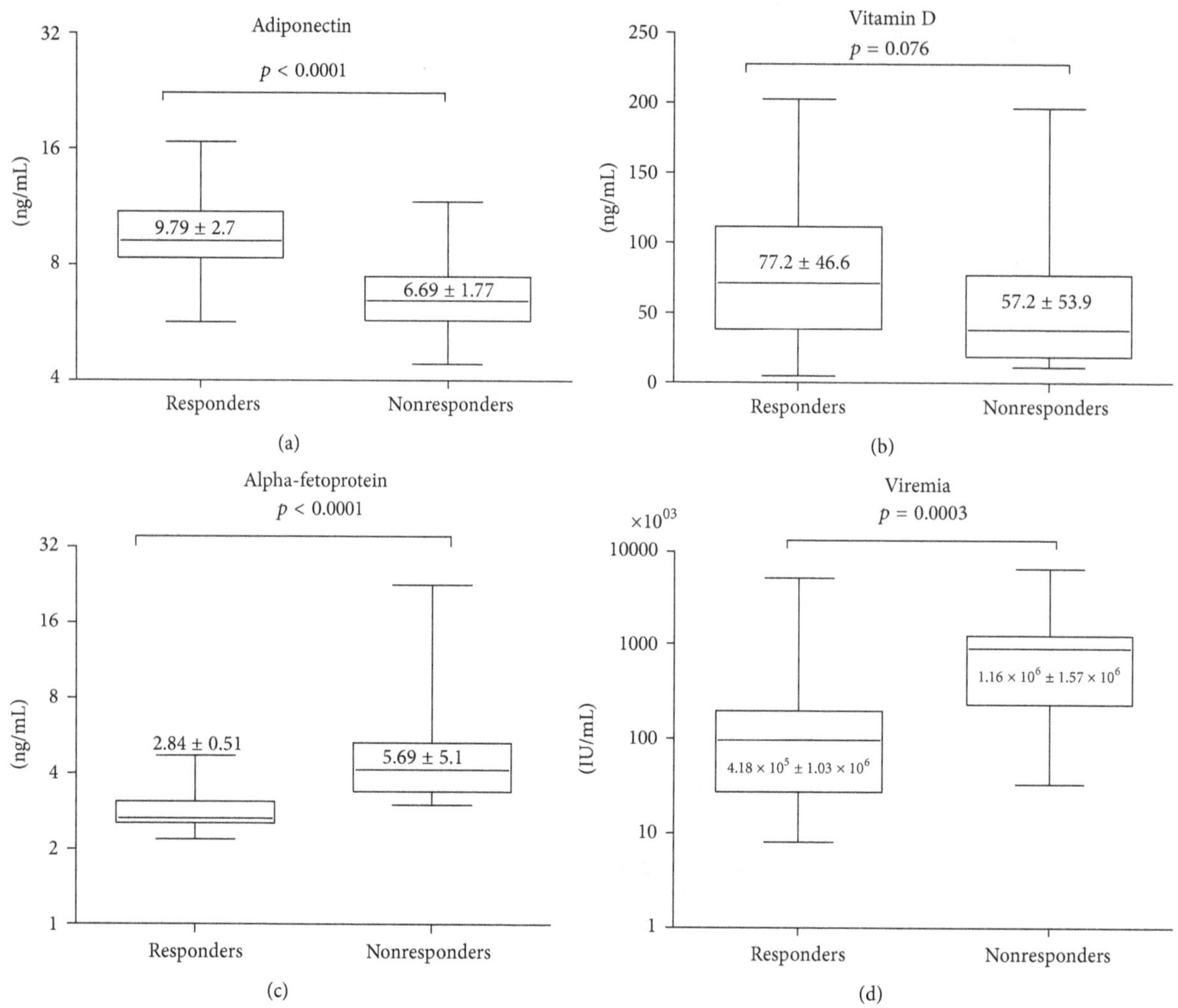

FIGURE 2: Comparison of pretreatment factors between responders and nonresponders. Box-and-whiskers plot for serum adiponectin, vitamin D, and AFP. The number indicated on the box represents mean ± standard deviation. (a) Adiponectin was significantly ($p < 0.0001$) higher in responders (9.79 ± 2.7 ng/mL, range; 5.68–16.68 ng/mL) than nonresponders (6.69 ± 1.77 ng/mL, range; 4.4–11.67 ng/mL). (b) Vitamin D was insignificantly ($p = 0.076$) higher in responders (77.2 ± 46.6 ng/mL, range; 4.9–202.4 ng/mL) than nonresponders (57.2 ± 53.9 ng/mL, range; 11.1–196 ng/mL). (c) AFP was significantly ($p < 0.0001$) lower in responders (2.84 ± 0.51 ng/mL, range; 2.18–4.7 ng/mL) than nonresponders (5.69 ± 5.1 ng/mL, range; 3–22.6 ng/mL). (d) Viremia was significantly ($p = 0.0003$) lower in responders ($4.18 \times 10^5 \pm 1.03 \times 10^6$ IU/mL, range; 8.04×10^3–4.96×10^6 IU/mL) than nonresponders ($1.16 \times 10^6 \pm 1.57 \times 10^6$ IU/mL, range; 3.29×10^4–6.24×10^6 IU/mL).

to achieve SVR in adults with CHC. On the other hand, Lange et al. [25] found that pretreatment serum level of vitamin D is not an optimal predictor of treatment response in HCV genotype 1.

Hypothetically, in the presence of vitamin D deficiency, it might be preferable to correct the deficiency before starting antiviral therapy. Nevertheless, to date there are few published reports on the role of vitamin D supplementation in patients with CHC. Bitetto et al. [30] found that vitamin D supplementation, in adults with recurrent hepatitis C postliver transplant, improves the probability of achieving a SVR. Also, Nimer and Mouch [29] found that adding vitamin D to conventional Peg/RBV therapy for patients with HCV genotypes 2-3 significantly improved viral response.

The reported higher vitamin D among treatment responders in the present study together with the known immunomodulatory action of vitamin D [23] and previous clinical trials of vitamin D supplementation in adults [29, 30] suggest that adding vitamin D to Peg/RBV therapy in children may increase SVR rates without serious adverse events. However, to prove these findings, well designed and large prospective studies are needed.

Serum AFP is a fetal glycoprotein produced by the yolk sac and fetal liver. Following birth, AFP levels decrease rapidly to less than 20 ng/mL and increase significantly in certain pathologic conditions. Serum AFP is a routinely used marker for hepatocellular carcinoma [31]. Yet, significant elevations of AFP are commonly seen in nonhepatic

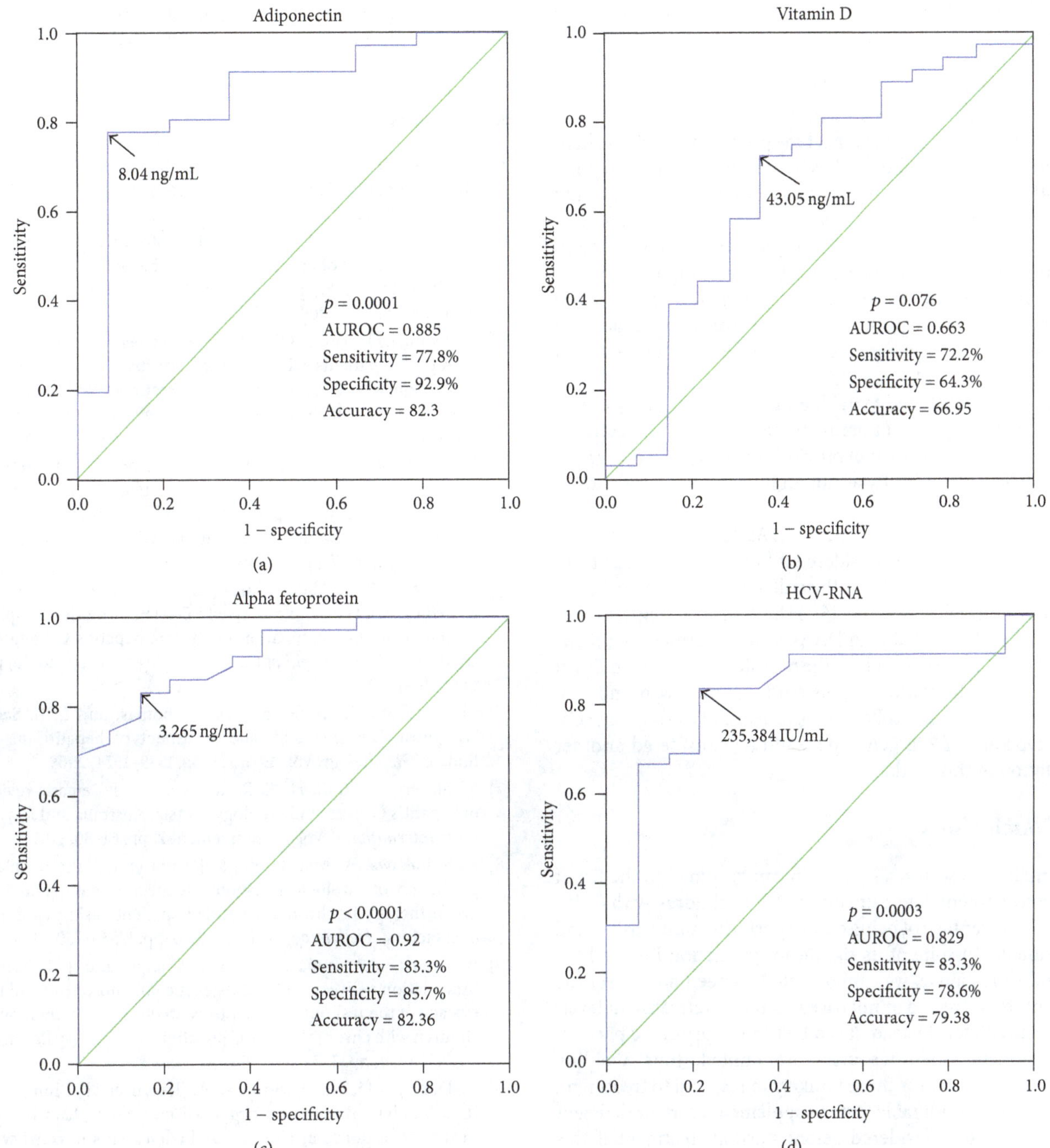

FIGURE 3: Diagnostic performance of pretreatment parameters for differentiation between responders and nonresponders. Receiver-operating characteristic (ROC) curves of (a) adiponectin, (b) vitamin D, (c) AFP, and (d) HCV-RNA level for differentiation between responders and nonresponders. The arrows indicate the cutoff values. AUROC: area under ROC.

malignancies and benign conditions, such as acute and chronic viral hepatitis [32]. Previous studies reported that the prevalence of increased serum AFP varies from 10% to 43% in adult patients with CHC and suggested an association between an increased serum AFP and advanced fibrosis or cirrhosis [33–36].

In agreement with the above reports, we found that AFP was higher in children with CHC than healthy controls with statistically insignificant difference. The absence of a significant correlation between AFP and stage of fibrosis in the present work may be due to the milder liver affection with low stages of fibrosis in reported cases when compared to the adult series.

Some studies found significant correlation of pretreatment low AFP serum level and treatment response in adults with CHC [37–39]. In accordance with the previous studies, we found that lower serum AFP was significantly related to SVR in children with CHC but with borderline significance in multivariate analysis. The SVR was 93.75% among children with AFP below 3.265 ng/mL and 33.3% for children with AFP ≥ 3.265 ng/mL.

The link between AFP and treatment response needs further studies. Increased production of AFP in hepatitis and cirrhosis was first thought to reflect the process of surviving hepatocytes, but this hypothesis has been refuted by other reports [33, 40]. More recent hypothesis ascribes the increased serum AFP to the hepatic damage *per se* with selective transcriptional activation of the AFP gene [32]. In the present study, the reported negative correlation between adiponectin with its known hepatoprotective role [15] and AFP ($p = 0.043$) is supporting this hypothesis and may give an explanation to the link between the baseline serum AFP and the treatment response.

In the present study viral load in univariate analysis was found to be a significant pretreatment predictor of treatment response as it was shown in previous reports [6]. However, in multivariate analysis, it was not an independent predictor of treatment response.

The emergence of the new DAAs for the treatment of CHC [41, 42] may be considered a limitation in the current study. However, peg/RBV is the still approved standard therapy for children with CHC [5, 43]. Moreover, Peg-IFN and RBV are still included with DAAs in the treatment regimens of those with genotype 4 [41], the prevalent genotype in Egypt [7]. A major limitation of this study is the low number of cases and controls enrolled. Also, absence of testing for HCV genotype and *IL28B* genotype could be considered another limitation of this work.

5. Conclusions

In conclusion, serum adiponectin can be added to the list of the pretreatment determinants of SVR in children with CHC, with the advantage of being easy to perform, noninvasive, and modifiable. In spite of its significant prediction for the likelihood of response, we cannot state to screen and select the patients to be treated or not based on their pretreatment levels of this predictor. Instead, it can be used to prioritize patients to treatment when resources are limited, thus avoiding toxicities and cost for those unlikely to respond to treatment. Also as it is a modifiable factor, supplementation for deficient cases could be considered before starting treatment if this could be proved in further studies.

Conflict of Interests

All authors declare that they have no conflict of interests regarding the publication of this paper.

Acknowledgments

The authors acknowledge the National Liver Institute, Menofiya University, for funding this work. They would like to thank the residents and nursing staff of the Pediatric Hepatology Department and all physicians and working staff of the Pathology Department for their contribution. This study was funded by the National Liver Institute, Menofiya University, Egypt, without any particular role in the study design, recruitment of individuals, data analysis, or writing of the report.

References

[1] Z. D. Goodman, H. R. Makhlouf, L. Liu et al., "Pathology of chronic hepatitis C in children: liver biopsy findings in the Peds-C trial," *Hepatology*, vol. 47, no. 3, pp. 836–843, 2008.

[2] P. J. Ruane, D. Ain, R. Stryker et al., "Sofosbuvir plus ribavirin for the treatment of chronic genotype 4 hepatitis C virus infection in patients of Egyptian ancestry," *Journal of Hepatology*, vol. 62, no. 5, pp. 1040–1046, 2015.

[3] P. Mishra, J. Florian, K. Qi et al., "FDA perspective on sofosbuvir therapy for patients with chronic hepatitis C virus genotype 1 infection who did not respond to treatment with pegylated interferon and ribavirin," *Gastroenterology*, vol. 147, no. 6, pp. 1196–1200, 2014.

[4] E. Druyts, K. Thorlund, P. Wu et al., "Efficacy and safety of pegylated interferon Alfa-2a or Alfa-2b plus ribavirin for the treatment of chronic hepatitis C in children and adolescents: a systematic review and meta-analysis," *Clinical Infectious Diseases*, vol. 56, no. 7, pp. 961–967, 2013.

[5] S. El Naghi, T. Y. Abdel-Ghaffar, H. El-Karaksy et al., "Safety and efficacy of Hansenula-derived PEGylated-interferon alpha-2a and ribavirin combination in chronic hepatitis C Egyptian children," *World Journal of Gastroenterology*, vol. 20, no. 16, pp. 4681–4691, 2014.

[6] M. G. Ghany, D. B. Strader, D. L. Thomas, and L. B. Seeff, "Diagnosis, management, and treatment of hepatitis C: an update," *Hepatology*, vol. 49, no. 4, pp. 1335–1374, 2009.

[7] W. Sievert, I. Altraif, H. A. Razavi et al., "A systematic review of hepatitis C virus epidemiology in Asia, Australia and Egypt," *Liver International*, vol. 31, supplement 2, pp. 61–80, 2011.

[8] H. Shirakawa, A. Matsumoto, S. Joshita et al., "Pretreatment prediction of virological response to peginterferon plus ribavirin therapy in chronic hepatitis C patients using viral and host factors," *Hepatology*, vol. 48, no. 6, pp. 1753–1760, 2008.

[9] H. Komatsu, A. Inui, T. Tsunoda, T. Sogo, and T. Fujisawa, "Association between an IL-28B genetic polymorphism and the efficacy of the response-guided pegylated interferon therapy in children with chronic hepatic C infection," *Hepatology Research*, vol. 43, no. 4, pp. 327–338, 2013.

[10] K. Domagalski, M. Pawłowska, A. Tretyn et al., "Impact of IL-28B polymorphisms on pegylated interferon plus ribavirin treatment response in children and adolescents infected with HCV genotypes 1 and 4," *European Journal of Clinical Microbiology & Infectious Diseases*, vol. 32, no. 6, pp. 745–754, 2013.

[11] O. G. Shaker, Y. H. Nassar, Z. A. Nour, and M. El Raziky, "Single-nucleotide polymorphisms of IL-10 and IL-28B as predictors of the response of IFN therapy in HCV genotype 4-infected children," *Journal of Pediatric Gastroenterology and Nutrition*, vol. 57, no. 2, pp. 155–160, 2013.

[12] H. Tajiri, Y. Tanaka, T. Takano et al., "Association of IL28B polymorphisms with virological response to peginterferon and ribavirin therapy in children and adolescents with chronic hepatitis C," *Hepatology Research*, vol. 44, no. 10, pp. E38–E44, 2014.

[13] P. Ferenci, M. W. Fried, M. L. Shiffman et al., "Predicting sustained virological responses in chronic hepatitis C patients treated with peginterferon alfa-2a (40 KD)/ribavirin," *Journal of Hepatology*, vol. 43, no. 3, pp. 425–433, 2005.

[14] K. Ishak, A. Baptista, L. Bianchi et al., "Histological grading and staging of chronic hepatitis," *Journal of Hepatology*, vol. 22, no. 6, pp. 696–699, 1995.

[15] C. Menzaghi, V. Trischitta, and A. Doria, "Genetic influences of adiponectin on insulin resistance, type 2 diabetes, and cardiovascular disease," *Diabetes*, vol. 56, no. 5, pp. 1198–1209, 2007.

[16] N. Ouchi, S. Kihara, Y. Arita et al., "Adiponectin, an adipocyte-derived plasma protein, inhibits endothelial NF-kappaB signaling through a cAMP-dependent pathway," *Circulation*, vol. 102, no. 11, pp. 1296–1301, 2000.

[17] T. Asano, K. Watanabe, N. Kubota et al., "Adiponectin knockout mice on high fat diet develop fibrosing steatohepatitis," *Journal of Gastroenterology and Hepatology*, vol. 24, no. 10, pp. 1669–1676, 2009.

[18] Y. Kamada, H. Matsumoto, S. Tamura et al., "Hypoadiponectinemia accelerates hepatic tumor formation in a nonalcoholic steatohepatitis mouse model," *Journal of Hepatology*, vol. 47, no. 4, pp. 556–564, 2007.

[19] Y. Kamada, S. Tamura, S. Kiso et al., "Enhanced carbon tetrachloride-induced liver fibrosis in mice lacking adiponectin," *Gastroenterology*, vol. 125, no. 6, pp. 1796–1807, 2003.

[20] T. A. Zografos, C. Liaskos, E. I. Rigopoulou et al., "Adiponectin: a new independent predictor of liver steatosis and response to IFN-alpha treatment in chronic hepatitis C," *The American Journal of Gastroenterology*, vol. 103, no. 3, pp. 605–614, 2008.

[21] A. Xu, Y. Wang, H. Keshaw, L. Y. Xu, K. S. L. Lam, and G. J. S. Cooper, "The fat-derived hormone adiponectin alleviates alcoholic and nonalcoholic fatty liver diseases in mice," *The Journal of Clinical Investigation*, vol. 112, no. 1, pp. 91–100, 2003.

[22] H. Abdel Latif, H. S. Assal, M. Mahmoud, and W. I. Rasheed, "Role of serum adiponectin level in the development of liver cirrhosis in patients with hepatitis C virus," *Clinical and Experimental Medicine*, vol. 11, no. 2, pp. 123–129, 2011.

[23] F. Baeke, T. Takiishi, H. Korf, C. Gysemans, and C. Mathieu, "Vitamin D: modulator of the immune system," *Current Opinion in Pharmacology*, vol. 10, no. 4, pp. 482–496, 2010.

[24] M. F. Holick, "Vitamin D deficiency," *The New England Journal of Medicine*, vol. 357, no. 3, pp. 266–281, 2007.

[25] C. M. Lange, J. Bojunga, E. Ramos-Lopez et al., "Vitamin D deficiency and a CYP27B1-1260 promoter polymorphism are associated with chronic hepatitis C and poor response to interferon-alfa based therapy," *Journal of Hepatology*, vol. 54, no. 5, pp. 887–893, 2011.

[26] T. Matsumura, T. Kato, N. Sugiyama et al., "25-Hydroxyvitamin D3 suppresses hepatitis C virus production," *Hepatology*, vol. 56, no. 4, pp. 1231–1239, 2012.

[27] S. Petta, C. Cammà, C. Scazzone et al., "Low vitamin d serum level is related to severe fibrosis and low responsiveness to interferon-based therapy in genotype 1 chronic hepatitis C," *Hepatology*, vol. 51, no. 4, pp. 1158–1167, 2010.

[28] D. Bitetto, G. Fattovich, C. Fabris et al., "Complementary role of vitamin D deficiency and the interleukin-28B rs12979860 C/T polymorphism in predicting antiviral response in chronic hepatitis C," *Hepatology*, vol. 53, no. 4, pp. 1118–1126, 2011.

[29] A. Nimer and A. Mouch, "Vitamin D improves viral response in hepatitis C genotype 2-3 naïve patients," *World Journal of Gastroenterology*, vol. 18, no. 8, pp. 800–805, 2012.

[30] D. Bitetto, C. Fabris, E. Fornasiere et al., "Vitamin D supplementation improves response to antiviral treatment for recurrent hepatitis C," *Transplant International*, vol. 24, no. 1, pp. 43–50, 2011.

[31] S. Gupta, S. Bent, and J. Kohlwes, "Test characteristics of alpha-fetoprotein for detecting hepatocellular carcinoma in patients with hepatitis C. A systematic review and critical analysis," *Annals of Internal Medicine*, vol. 139, no. 1, pp. 46–50, 2003.

[32] K. Taketa, "Alpha-fetoprotein: reevaluation in hepatology," *Hepatology*, vol. 12, no. 6, pp. 1420–1432, 1990.

[33] N. S. Goldstein, D. E. Blue, R. Hankin et al., "Serum alpha-fetoprotein levels in patients with chronic hepatitis C. Relationships with serum alanine aminotransferase values, histologic activity index, and hepatocyte MIB-1 scores," *American Journal of Clinical Pathology*, vol. 111, no. 6, pp. 811–816, 1999.

[34] N. Bayati, A. L. Silverman, and S. C. Gordon, "Serum alpha-fetoprotein levels and liver histology in patients with chronic hepatitis C," *American Journal of Gastroenterology*, vol. 93, no. 12, pp. 2452–2456, 1998.

[35] C.-W. Chu, S.-J. Hwang, J.-C. Luo et al., "Clinical, virologic, and pathologic significance of elevated serum alpha-fetoprotein levels in patients with chronic hepatitis C," *Journal of Clinical Gastroenterology*, vol. 32, no. 3, pp. 240–244, 2001.

[36] K.-Q. Hu, N. L. Kyulo, N. Lim, B. Elhazin, D. J. Hillebrand, and T. Bock, "Clinical significance of elevated alpha-fetoprotein (AFP) in patients with chronic hepatitis C, but not hepatocellular carcinoma," *American Journal of Gastroenterology*, vol. 99, no. 5, pp. 860–865, 2004.

[37] S. Males, R. R. Gad, G. Esmat et al., "Serum alpha-foetoprotein level predicts treatment outcome in chronic hepatitis C," *Antiviral Therapy*, vol. 12, no. 5, pp. 797–803, 2007.

[38] H. Abdoul, V. Mallet, S. Pol, and A. Fontanet, "Serum alpha-fetoprotein predicts treatment outcome in chronic hepatitis C patients regardless of HCV genotype," *PLoS ONE*, vol. 3, no. 6, Article ID e2391, 2008.

[39] M. Abd El Samiee, E. Tharwa, M. A. Obada, A. K. Abou Gabal, and M. Salama, "Gamma-glutamyl transpeptidase and α-fetoprotein," *Egyptian Liver Journal*, vol. 1, no. 1, pp. 18–24, 2011.

[40] E. Alpert and E. R. Feller, "Alpha-Fetoprotein (AFP) in benign liver disease. Evidence that normal liver regeneration does not induce AFP synthesis," *Gastroenterology*, vol. 74, no. 5, pp. 856–858, 1978.

[41] E. Degasperi and A. Aghemo, "Sofosbuvir for the treatment of chronic hepatitis C: between current evidence and future perspectives," *Hepatic Medicine: Evidence and Research*, vol. 6, pp. 25–33, 2014.

[42] B. Lam, L. Henry, and Z. Younossi, "Sofosbuvir (Sovaldi) for the treatment of hepatitis C," *Expert Review of Clinical Pharmacology*, vol. 7, no. 5, pp. 555–566, 2014.

[43] M. Pawlowska, "Pegylated IFN-α-2a and ribavirin in the treatment of hepatitis C infection in children," *Expert Opinion on Drug Safety*, vol. 14, no. 3, pp. 343–348, 2015.

11

Role of FNA and Core Biopsy of Primary and Metastatic Liver Disease

John P. McGahan,[1] John Bishop,[2] John Webb,[1] Lydia Howell,[2] Natalie Torok,[3] Ramit Lamba,[1] and Michael T. Corwin[1]

[1] *Davis Medical Center, Department of Radiology, University of California, 4860 Y Street, Suite 3100, Sacramento, CA 95817, USA*
[2] *Davis Medical Center, Department of Pathology, University of California, 4400 V Street, Path Building, Sacramento, CA 95817, USA*
[3] *Davis Medical Center, Department of Internal Medicine, University of California, 4150 V Street, Suite 3500, Sacramento, CA 95817, USA*

Correspondence should be addressed to John P. McGahan; john.mcgahan@ucdmc.ucdavis.edu

Academic Editor: Fredric D. Gordon

Objective. To examine our experience with cytology and histology biopsy of the liver and to define methods for improvement of diagnosis of primary liver tumors. *Methods.* This include retrospective study of 189 biopsies of 185 liver masses for cytological or histological analysis. Patients were subdivided into two groups. Group 1 consisted of 124 suspected metastasis. Group 2 consisted of 61 suspected primary neoplasms. Biopsies were considered positive or equivocal. In equivocal cases, special stains were performed. In Group 2, cases were classified by contrast CT or MRI as to (I) classic HCC, (II) infiltrated HCC, or (Ill) equivocal. *Results.* Definitive diagnosis was obtained in 117/124 masses (94%) in Group 1, 48/61 masses (79%) in Group 2, and (Ill) equivocal 13 cases in Group II. In two equivocal cases in which special stains were performed, they were reclassified as HCC. In 8/13 cases, CT findings were consistent with HCC. *Conclusion.* Liver biopsies are useful in obtaining a definitive diagnosis of suspected metastatic liver disease. Biopsy results are less reliable in patients with suspected primary liver tumors. In these situations, strategies can include basing treatment on imaging criteria or use of newer special pathological stains. *Advances in Knowledge.* Use of newer special immunological stains improves accuracy in definitive diagnosis of primary liver tumors.

1. Introduction

Percutaneous fine needle aspiration cytology (FNAC) and automated needle core biopsy (NCB) for histological retrieval have been used to diagnose malignancy in abdominal organs for over three decades [1, 2]. These techniques of FNAC and NCB have been useful in obtaining a diagnosis of focal liver masses [3–5]. In the past when previously performing liver biopsies of focal masses the biopsies often were performed for metastatic disease. However, more recently we have noticed an increasing number of biopsies for suspected hepatocellular carcinoma. The epidemiology of hepatocellular carcinoma (HCC) is changing in North America and Europe for several reasons, including the viral hepatitis epidemic and the increasing number of patients diagnosed with nonalcoholic fatty liver disease [6]. In these groups, surveillance is difficult and has included use of serum markers such as alpha feto protein (AFP) and imaging with ultrasound, CT, or MRI. However, definitive diagnosis often requires biopsy of focal masses. We have felt that we had maintained very high rate of specific diagnosis for fine needle aspiration cytology (FNAC) or needle core biopsy (NCB) for focal liver masses for possible metastatic disease but have noticed more equivocal results for FNAC or NCB for patients with suspected primary liver tumors. The image guided biopsy strategies are only effective in achieving the goal of reducing mortality if HCC can be adequately distinguished from regenerating nodules by cytology or histology. Our general impression is that definitive diagnosis of HCC is not as easily made as metastatic carcinoma. Therefore, the purpose of this paper is to examine our experience with cytology and histology to find key aspects for the improvement of diagnosis of primary liver tumors, that may be helpful for physicians that encounter patients with suspected primary liver tumors.

2. Materials and Methods

This is a retrospective study conducted at our institution between July 8, 2005 and December 17, 2009. This has full Institution Review Board approval at our institution. Written informed consent was waived. This data set consisted of 240 consecutive targeted liver biopsies performed at our institution. To qualify for the study, a patient had to be over age 18 years and must have a contrast enhanced cross-sectional imaging, magnetic resonance imaging (MRI), or computed tomography (CT) for evaluation of a suspected liver tumor. Computed Tomography was performed with either a General Electric (16 Detector) high speed (General Electric, Milwaukee, WI) or a Siemens Somotom Definition Dual Source (64 Detector) CT (Siemens Medical Solutions USA, Malvern, PA). This included a 4 phase CT including base, arterial phase (approximately 40 seconds), portal venous phase (approximately 90 seconds), and delayed images (3 to 5 minutes) after injection of contrast. Contrast was Omnipaque 350 (GE Healthcare, Princeton, NJ) injected at rate of 3 to 5 mL/second for a total of 125 mL using a power injector. Images were acquired on a 1.5 Tesla General Electric Signa MRI Scanner system (GE Medical Systems, Milwaukee, WI), equipped with a phased array torso coil for signal reception. The imaging protocol was as follows: coronal single shot fast spin echo (SSFSE) transverse SSFSE, transverse noncontrast, T1-weighted, 2D spoiled gradient echo sequence in-phase and out-of-phase, 3D fast relaxation fast spin echo coronal T2-weighted MRCP, 2D thick slab T2-weighted MRCP, and transverse precontrast T1-weighted 3D spoiled gradient echo pulse *(LAVA)* sequence. Then, usually 20 mL of Omniscan (GE Medical Systems, Milwaukee, WI) was injected intravenously at 2 cc/sec and transverse LAVA sequences were obtained with the same parameters as above during the arterial, portal venous, and equilibrium phases. Patients referred to our institution for biopsy with outside imaging were included in the study if their images were stored, deemed adequate, and available on our Picture Archiving and Communications (PAC) system. (I-Site, Koninklijke Philips Electronics, N.V., Foster City, CA).

Twenty-nine patients were excluded from our study since their imaging studies were not available on our PACs system. Fifteen additional patients were excluded as needle aspiration yielded a fluid collection or potential abscess. Since this study addressed percutaneous fine needle aspiration cytology (FNAC) biopsies of liver masses only, six patients whose biopsies were performed under endoscopic ultrasound guidance and one percutaneous biopsy of a bile duct were excluded. 189 liver biopsies which included either FNAC for cytological diagnosis or needle core biopsy (NCB) of the liver for histological diagnosis and or both were obtained. In two cases the masses were rebiopsied and in one case, the mass was biopsied three times, and thus 185 masses were included as the data set in this study. All fine needle aspirations were performed in a similar of fashion using a 22-gauge Chiba type needle with biopsy performed either with an aspiration or non-aspiration technique. At the discretion of the operator. The majority of biopsies are performed under ultrasound guidance with needle visualization documentation in the mass.

A cytotechnologist was present in the radiology suite to collect the FNAC and NCB specimens. Two slides were prepared from each pass using the "pull-apart method". One specimen was air dried and the other was fixed in alcohol and immediately evaluated for adequacy by the cytotechnologist following staining with toluidine blue. The air-dried smears were later stained with a modified Giemsa stain in the laboratory and the toluidine blue stained slides were restrained with a Papanicolaou stain; both types of preparations were evaluated for final diagnosis. The needle from each pass was rinsed in Saccomanno fixative for cell block preparation and reviewed in conjunction with the direct smears for final adequacy determination and final diagnosis. Continued needle passes were performed until cytological technologist confirmed adequacy of the specimen. For NCB, touch prep technique was used in a similar fashion.

Furthermore, liver needle core biopsies (NCB) using an automated biopsy gun or biopsy device were performed with a number of different manufacturers automated devices. Most commonly utilized are automatic 18-gauge core biopsy needle. All NCBs were performed in a similar fashion using ultrasound or CT guidance to document needle position within the lesion. NCBs were collected into formalin, processed and sectioned in the usual fashion, and stained with hematoxylin and eosin. All percutaneous liver biopsies were performed under conscious sedation usually using midazolam hydrochloride (Versed. Hoffman-La Roche) and fentanyl citrate. Study patients were subdivided into two groups based on the clinical and radiologic impression. Group I consisted of 124 biopsies (FNAC and/or NCB) in 124 masses (from 59 men and 65 women; average age 60.3 years) with a suspected diagnosis of hepatic metastases.

In Group I, if the final cytology or histology report was "adenocarcinoma, site unspecified, this was not considered as a specific diagnosis but was considered as a malignant diagnosis. Group II consisted of 65 biopsies in 61 masses from 61 patients (34 men and 27 women; average age of 58) with a suspected diagnosis of primary liver tumor. We had 185 masses in our database. For those with rebiopsy, only the most definitive biopsy result was included. Forty-nine of sixty one (80%) of Group II patients had underlying cirrhosis which was secondary to hepatitis B or C in 38 patients, alcohol-related disease in six, NASH in two, and HCV/HIV in two and autoimmune hepatitis in one. Twelve patients in Group II had no history of hepatitis or cirrhosis. In both groups, the cytology and pathology reports were obtained from the electronic medical record. These results were separated into cases in which a specific diagnosis of a neoplasm or benign entity was made. In Group II, there were 10 reports where the final diagnosis stated, "suspicious for hepatocellular carcinoma." These were considered as specific diagnoses. When equivocal cytology and pathology results were encountered in Group II,

TABLE 1: Results.

	FNA		CB		FNA and CB	
Suspected hepatic metastasis						
Specific diagnosis	56%	(70/124)	68%	(34/50)	60%	(75/124)
*Diagnosis malignant versus benign	93%	(115/124)	96%	(48/50)	94%	(117/124)
Suspected primary neoplasms						
Specific diagnosis	70.5%	(43/61)	67.5%	(27/40)	79%	(48/61)
Total	85.4%	(158/185)	83%	(75/90)	89.1%	(165/185)

*Diagnosis of malignancy, but type not specified.

the specific reports and slides were reviewed and classified as 1 = atypical hepatocyte, 2 = HCC versus METS, 3 = HCC versus regenerating nodules, 4 = HCC versus adenoma, 5 = inadequate, 6 = abscess, and 7 = No malignancy. If core biopsy or FNAC was performed on different dates then each report was listed separately.

Slides from FNAC and NCB cases for patients in Group II with equivocal diagnoses were rereviewed by a cytopathologist (LH) with more than 20 years of experience and a pathologist (JB) with more than 25 years of experience of the FNAC (LH) and the NCB specimens (JB), respectively. They reviewed for any possible misinterpretation by the original pathologist [6]. Furthermore, cell block or core material was applied if possible for immunohistological stains for HEPPAR-1 and glypican-3 [7].

The prebiopsy CT or MRI from all available cases in Group II was re-analyzed by a single radiologist (JPM) with more than 25 years of experience. They were classified as pattern I (Focal HCC)—an arterially enhanced mass with a well defined capsule and washout of contrast on delayed imaging in a patient with chronic hepatitis. This includes modification of prior imaging criteria against a background of chronic liver disease (cirrhosis) [8–10]. This also corresponded to the liver imaging and reporting data system (LI-RADS) of definitive HCC [11]. Pattern II consisted of a diffuse irregular enhancing mass with hypervascular portal vein invasion in a patient with hepatitis and chronic liver disease. This corresponded to a LI-RADs category 5V, definitive HCC. Pattern III was considered equivocal for diagnosis based upon lack of pattern I or pattern II. None of the masses were considered definitely benign.

3. Results

Overall, a definitive diagnosis of malignancy was rendered in 165/185 cases (89.1%) based on findings from FNAC and/or NCB results and included both Group I and Group II patients (Table 1). However, when considered separately, Group I and Group II demonstrated differences in the percentage of definitive diagnoses. A diagnosis of malignancy or benign was rendered more frequently in cases where metastatic disease was suspected (94%) compared to cases where hepatocellular carcinoma was suspected (79%). In 117 of 124 (94%) in Group I had a definitive malignant versus benign diagnosis. Core biopsy also more frequently demonstrated definitive malignant versus benign diagnosis than FNA in Group I in 48 of the 50 cases (96%). Furthermore, in the 2 core biopsies in this group that were equivocal, the FNAC results were diagnostic. Therefore 50 of 50 (100%) of those masses with suspected metastatic disease had a definitive malignant versus benign diagnosis by either FNAC or NCB. In Group II, 48/61 masses (79%) had a definitive malignant versus benign diagnosis. In Group II, core biopsy improved detection of primary malignant disease in only 5 additional patients.

CT and MRI were reviewed 54/61 in Group 2 cases and classified as pattern I, pattern II, or pattern III (seven CTs were not retrievable). Pattern I of a classic HCC was seen in 27 of 54 (50%) of cases. Pattern II of an infiltrating tumor and portal vein thrombosis was seen in 8 of 54 (15%) of cases. Pattern III of an equivocal CTs or MRIs was seen in 19 of 54 (35%) of cases. In 14 of 19 equivocal CTs or MRIs cytology/pathology was helpful for giving a definitive diagnosis.

Furthermore, CT and MRI were analyzed for specific imaging features of HCC in all of the 13 equivocal cytology or pathology of primary liver masses. In 8 of these cases, the radiologic characteristics were nearly pathognomonic for HCC in the setting of cirrhosis (Figures 1 and 2) (Table 2). Six of these cases were classified as pattern I (Classic HCC) with an encapsulated enhancing mass and delayed washout in a cirrhotic liver. Two masses were classified as pattern II with an infiltrating mass and portal vein thrombosis in a cirrhotic liver. 5/13 were equivocal on CT or MRI (Table 2) (Figures 3 and 4). All classic or probable HCCs identified by CT were confirmed by follow-up resection, local progression of disease, or patients expiring with the presumed diagnosis of HCC, except for one case lost to follow-up. Of the 5 equivocal cases on CT or MRI, 1 expired from HCC, 2 had progression of disease, one had a wedge resection revealing HCC and one was an adenoma (Figures 3 and 4). Of the 13 equivocal cytology/histology results, 6 were path proven after operation. Five of these were HCC and one was a hepatic adenoma after operating resection. In 5 cases there was local progression of disease or patients expired, thus with presumed diagnosis of HCC. One is alive and 1 is lost to follow-up (Table 2). The encoded report results from FNA (and core biopsy when performed) of the 13 equivocal cases are also presented in Table 2.

Of these 13 equivocal cytology or pathology cases, six had sufficient cell block or core biopsy material to permit retrospective application of immunohistochemical (IHC) stains for HEPPAR-1 and glypican-3 (Figure 2). The results are shown in Table 3. One case was inconclusive, three were positive only for HEPPAR-1, and two were positive for

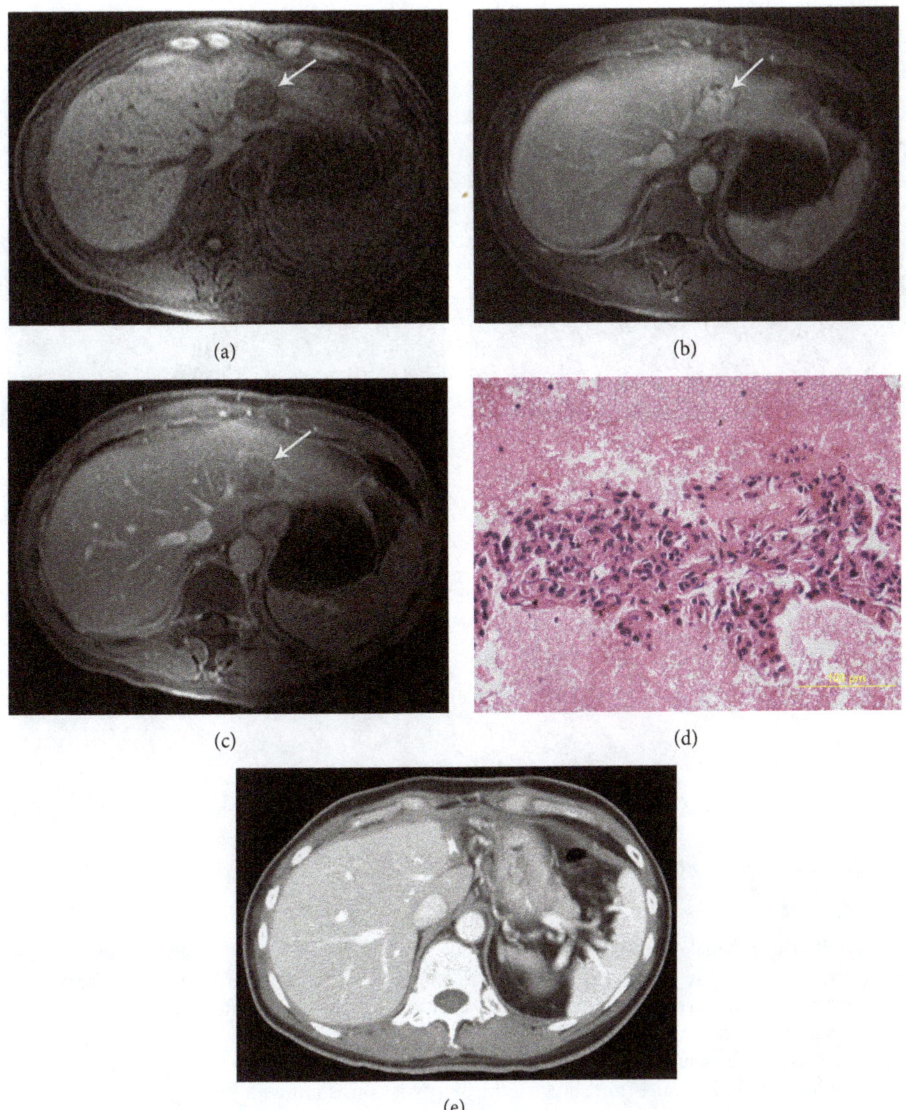

FIGURE 1: Case 5. History: 60 year-old male with cirrhosis due to hepatitis B with AFP of four. Surgically resected HCCs. Initial MRI demonstrates the following. (a) TI weighted fat suppressed LAVA base scan shows region of decreased signal intensity (arrow). (b) Post gadolinium enhanced MRI in arterial phase shows encapsulated enhancing mass in the left in the lobe of the liver (arrow). (c) After gadolinium in portal venous phase, there is a central wash-out with well-defined capsule (arrow). (d) Fine needle aspiration was deemed suspicious for well differentiated HCC but could not exclude adenoma. The cell block shows groups of hepatocytes forming a thickened trabecular pattern lined by endothelial cells. The hepatocytes have increased nuclear/cytoplasmic (N : C) ratio and occasional prominent nucleoli. (e) After resection of the mass the CT shows surgical clips. Pathology revealed well differentiated HCC.

both antibodies. If positive for both immunohistochemical stains, this is considered to be diagnostic, while if only one immunostain was positive, this was considered as equivocal [7].

4. Discussion

Percutaneous fine needle aspiration biopsy of abdominal masses guided by imaging has been performed for over 30 years [2]. With further developments, percutaneous automated biopsy needles have been used for histological retrieval of tissue from abdominal organs [1]. With improved imaging, refinements in biopsy needles, and new pathological techniques, there have been a variety of publications attesting to both high sensitivity and specificity for either fine needle aspiration biopsy or automated needle biopsy of abdominal masses. Numerous publications since the mid-1980s have demonstrated that liver FNAC has sensitivities greater than 85% and a specificity as high as 100%, with the highest sensitivity when FNAC is combined with core biopsy [3–5].

As our study demonstrates, FNAC and core biopsy have different limitations prompting equivocal diagnoses. Our findings and other reports have demonstrated that definitive diagnoses are less frequent in cases of hepatocellular

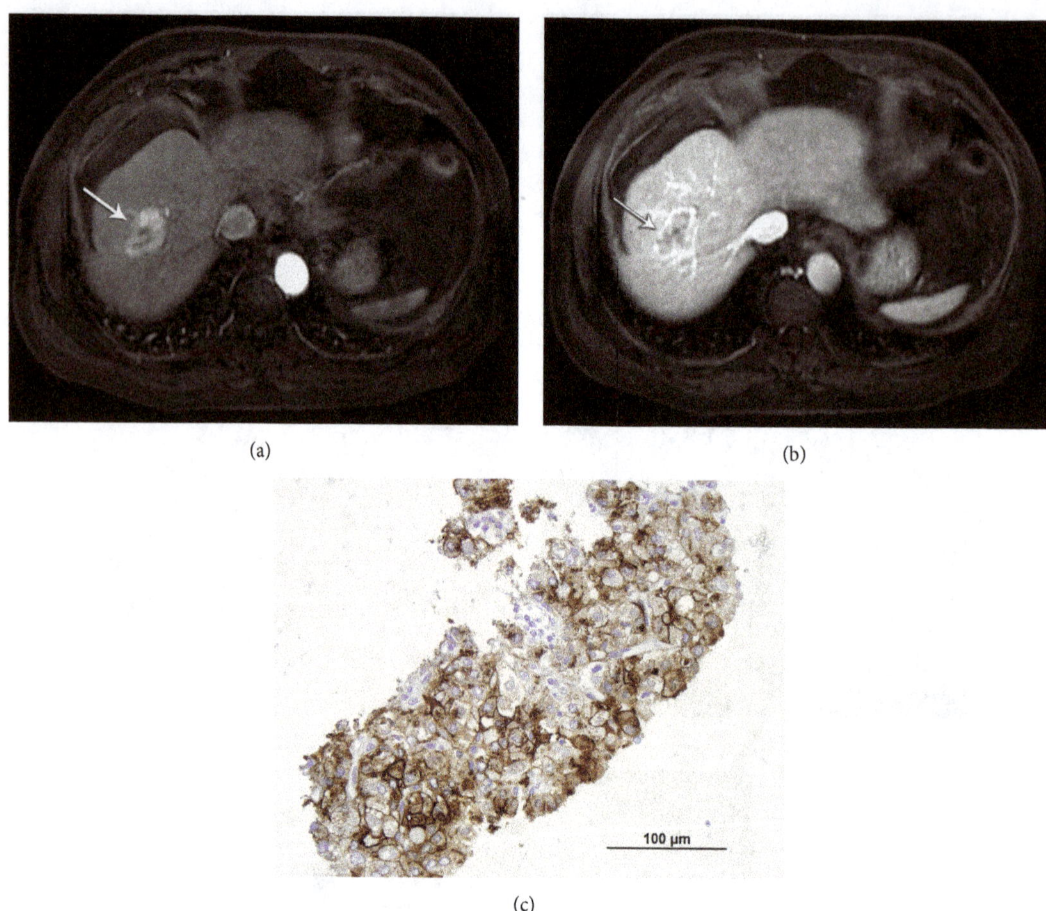

(a) (b) (c)

Figure 2: Case 11. History: 61 year-old-male with AFP of 149 with alcoholic cirrhosis and HCC after transplant. (a) Arterial phase MRI, postgadolinium LAVA sequence showing arterial enhancing lesion (arrow). (b) Post gadolinium MRI during the portal venous phase showed central washout with well defined capsule (arrow). (c) Fine needle aspiration and core were obtained. Fine needle aspiration was suspicious for well differentiated HCC but could not exclude adenoma. Deeper sections of the cell block material revealed acinar-like and branched trabecular patterns of hepatocytes as well as an altered reticulin pattern (not shown). Based on the deeper sections and the positive IHC stain results for glypican-3 (shown here) and Hep Par 1 (not shown), the biopsy is consistent with hepatocellular carcinoma, well-differentiated. Patient had RFA and then liver transplant which revealed HCC.

carcinoma than metastasis disease. This is true for other primary malignancies, including the thyroid [12, 13]. Reports by both Bru et al. and Matsushiro et al. found that FNAC diagnosis of hepatocellular carcinoma was definitive in only 62% and 61.5% respectively, even when combined with core biopsy [14, 15]. However, others have shown that combining core biopsy with FNAC can improve diagnostic accuracy. Matsushiro et al. demonstrated that adding histological exam via core biopsy improved the positive diagnosis rate to 87% of cases while cytology alone had a positivity rate of 61.5% for the diagnosis of HCC [15]. In our series, we had an overall rate of establishing a diagnosis of 89.1%. (79% for HCC and 94% for suspected metastatic disease, Table 1). So why is there such a discrepancy in establishing a diagnosis of HCC and how can diagnosis accuracy be improved?

Hepatocellular carcinoma is particularly challenging for both FNA and CB diagnosis. To better understand the challenge, we must understand that all HCCs are not the same. HCC is graded based from I to IV to reflect tumor differentiation and the presence of one or more clonelike cell population [16, 17]. Grade I HCCs can be difficult to distinguish from benign regenerative nodules and adenomas since both show minimal nuclear pleomorphism and prominent nucleoli and have abundant granular cytoplasm reflecting liver differentiation. Architectural features can be the best clues to the diagnosis and include a trabecular pattern and prominent vascular pattern which can be visible on both cytologic smear and core biopsies [18, 19]. This creates a problem for diagnosis. Grade IV HCCs are very poorly differentiated and may be difficult to distinguish from high-grade tumor of non-hepatocellular origin, since features of liver differentiation may not be present [16]. In our series, the ability to distinguish grade I HCC from regenerating nodule or adenomas was the most common reason for lack of definitive diagnosis of HCC by both cytology and histology. Hepatic adenoma was included in the differential diagnosis of

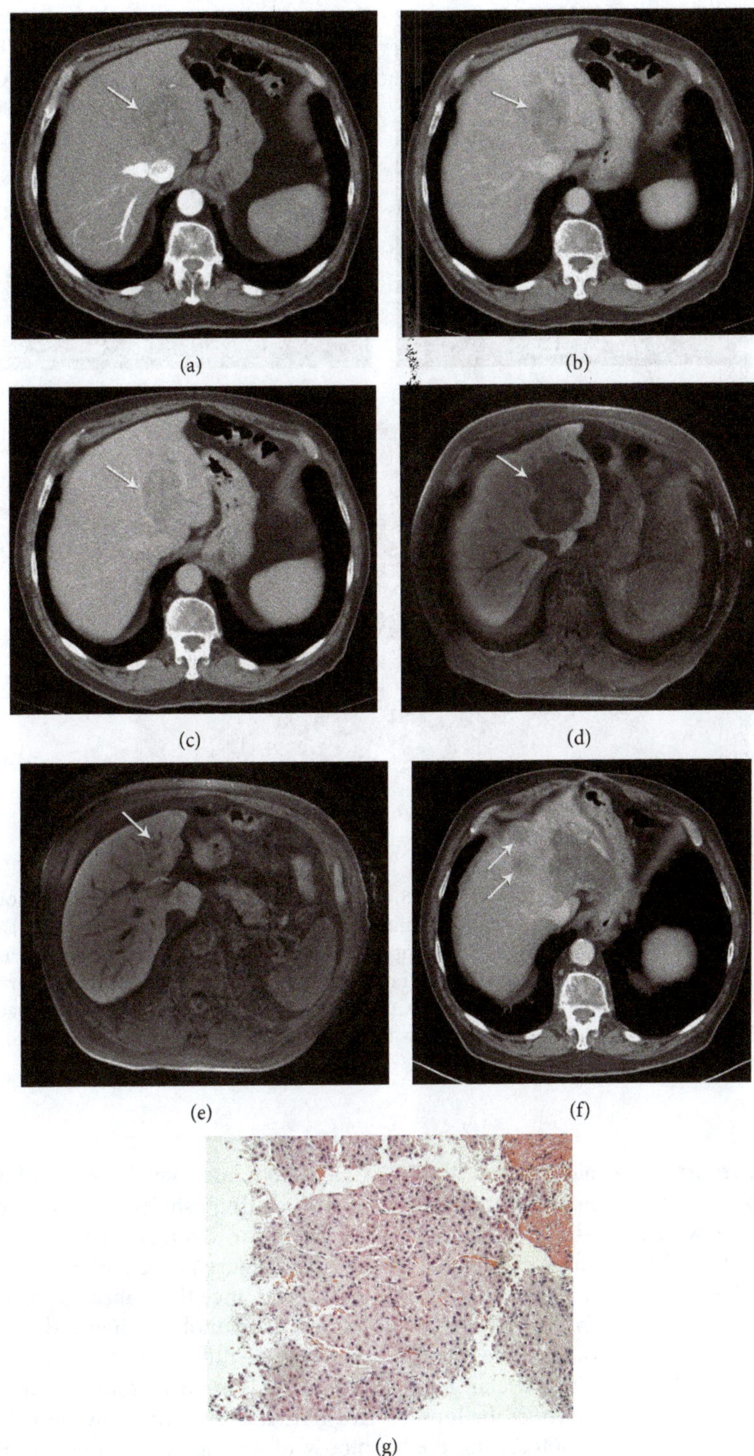

FIGURE 3: Case 8. History: 72 year-old-male with cirrhosis due to alcoholism with AFP of five. Patient had surgical wedge resection with findings consistent with HCC. (a) Initial arterial CT phase shows encapsulated mass with minimal enhancement (arrow). (b) Portal phase shows well-demarcated area of decrease density with peripheral rim (arrow). (c) Delay imaging demonstrating some washout in this lesion (arrow). This was judged as equivocal for HCC on review. At this time, five FNA's and one core sample which were thought to be nondiagnostic of HCC and were thought to be regenerating nodule versus HCC. (d) MRI with Eovist with 30 minutes delay scan demonstrating area with decrease signal intensity (arrow). (e) An addition a satellite lesion (arrow) was identified cephalad to primary lesion. Three cores were performed on the larger mass which were nondiagnostic and showed no malignancy. (f) Two year follow-up CT demonstrating mass which was locally invasive with multiple satellite lesions throughout the liver (arrows). (g) Other five FNA passes and five cores were obtained at that time which were considered to be satisfactory but nondiagnostic for malignancy. Less than 10% of the histology sample contained hepatocytes for evaluation. Some were disposed in nodules with altered reticulin (not shown). The cells have moderate N : C ratios and are not particularly atypical. Surgical wedge resection was performed which revealed HCC.

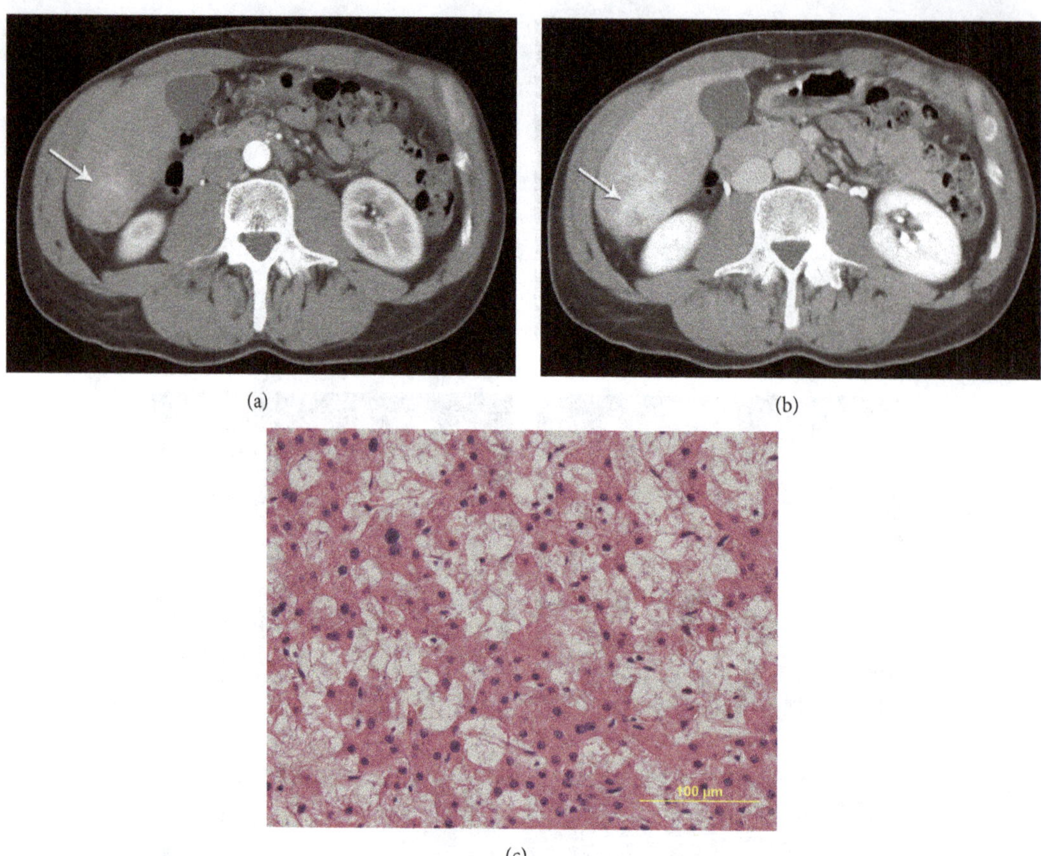

Figure 4: Case 7. History: 51 year-old-male with no cirrhosis, AFP 1.8, and no hepatitis. At surgery this was pathologically proven to represent liver adenoma. (a) Arterial phase CT demonstrating enhancing mass with lobulated margin (arrow). (b) Delay images demonstrating persisting enhancement (arrow) with focal hypodense area noted centrally. This was considered an equivocal mass on review. (c) Fine needle aspiration biopsy with three passes and three core biopsies demonstrated epithelial neoplasm and adenoma versus HCC. This was reviewed at an outside institution with the diagnosis of well-differentiated HCC. The smears are cellular and show hepatocytes with minimal atypia in sheets and small clusters. Prominent capillaries are noted within the sheets and endothelial cells are noted to be encircling clusters of hepatocytes. Post-surgery pathology revealed this to be adenoma.

the final cytology/pathology report in five masses after either FNAC or core biopsy (Table 2). Three of these patients had cirrhosis. In the other patients with cirrhosis, regenerating nodule versus HCC was mentioned in the final cytology or histology report (Table 2). This diagnostic dilemma may be occurring more frequently due to surveillance programs in patients with underlying liver disease. Not only do these patients have a background of disease with cellular features that can easily mimic malignancy such as balloon degeneration, inflammatory, infiltrate and apoptosis, but the hepatocellular carcinomas targeted for detection are more likely to be welldifferentiated, thus being particularly difficult to distinguish from the background diseased liver.

How can the problem of distinguishing a grade I HCC from a benign process be addressed? A number of immunohistochemical (IHC) markers have been put forward as possibly helpful in establishing the diagnosis of focal liver lesions. These stains are not be well known to the radiology community, but if requested, they may be useful in establishing or excluding a diagnosis of hepatocellular carcinoma. Markers such Hepatocyte Paraffin Antigen-1 (Hep Par 1), Glypican-3, CD-34, to name a few have been touted as sensitive markers to help distinguish HCC from non HCC malignancy, and are helpful to distinguish Grade 1 HCC form benign liver nodules (Figure 2). Reticulin staining has been traditionally used to enhance the trabecular architecture of primary liver lesions. Immunohistochemical staining with CD-34 may demonstrate diffuse reactivity in HCC and can also be useful [20–24]. It is important for the physicians to know that there are IHC markers that may be helpful when they obtain a biopsy of an equivocal biopsy of potential HCC. Although the best available markers may change, they currently include HepPar-1, glypican-3, and Moc-31, among others [25–27]. The European Association for the study of liver disease published recommendation in 2012 that "immunostaining for GPC3, HSP70, and glutamine synthetase and/or gene expression profiles (GPC3, LYVE1, and survivin) is recommended to differentiate high grade dysplastic nodules from early HCC. Additional staining can be considered to detect progenitor cell features (K19 and EpCAM) or assess neovascularization (CD34)" [28]. Another recent study has shown that the immunohistochemical panel of Golgi protein 73 (GP73),

TABLE 2: Features of the equivocal cases.

Case	AFP	Cirrhosis	CT	Diagnosis	FNA	Core
1	6.6	C	I (classic)	RFA-alive	1	None
2	49	B + C	III equivocal	Expired HCC	2	None
3	14.6	C + ETOH	III equivocal	Progression	1, 1	3
4	241	C	I (classic)	Path proven HCC-surgery	3	None
5	4.1	B	I (classic)	Path proven HCC-surgery	4	None
6	3.6	C	I (classic)	Path proven HCC-surgery	6	2
7	1.8	None	III equivocal	Adenoma	4	4
8	5	C	III equivocal	Path proven HCC-surgery	3, 7	7, 7, 7
9	None	ETOH	II infiltration	Died HCC	5	None
10	14,044	C	II infiltration	Hospice HCC	1, 3	7
11	149	ETOH	I (classic)	Path proven HCC-surgery. RFA transplant	4	7
12	6.4	None	III equivocal	Progression	7	4
13	19.5	C	I (classic)	Lost to follow-up	4	7

1: atypical hepatocyte; 2: HCC versus METS; 3: HCC versus regenerating nodules; 4: HCC versus adenoma; 5: inadequate; 6: abscess; 7: no malignancy. Equivocal cases including Alpha Fetoprotein (AFP) values and presence of cirrhosis including etiology for example hepatitis C (C), hepatitis B (B), or alcohol (ETOH). The review of CT results, patient follow-up and classification of results from the cytology or histology report.

TABLE 3: Results of stains applied retrospectively on equivocal biopsies.

Case	CT	Diagnosis	HepParl	Glypican3
3	III equivocal	Progression	pos	neg
5	I (classic)	Path proven HCC-surgery	Inconclusive	Inconclusive
8	I (classic)	Path proven HCC-surgery	pos	neg
10	II infiltration	Hospice HCC	pos	neg
11	I (classic)	Path proven HCC-surgery. RFA transplant	pos	pos
13	I (classic)	Lost to follow-up	pos	pos

*7 of the 13 equivocal cases did not have sufficient material for these stains.

glypican-3 (GPC 3), and CD 34, as well as reticulum stain, is highly specific in the diagnosis of HCC [29]. However, any of these staining techniques can be performed only on core biopsies (or exceptionally abundant cell blocks) and a sufficiently adequate, representative sample may not be available. In the 13 equivocal cases in our series, there was sufficient material to apply IHC markers in only six cases. Three of those six cases had CT MRI imaging pattern 1 (classic, see Table 3) of which two were positive for both markers and could, in retrospect, be considered as HCC by histopathology, using immunohistochemical markers. However, the other cases were positive for only one marker or were inconclusive (Table 3). Development of molecular tests may also eventually prove useful in distinguishing HCC from reactive disease; however, cost effectiveness will need to be considered when these are developed and implemented since molecular testing is currently very expensive.

What other things may be helpful to establish the diagnosis of HCC if there is an equivocal cytological or histological diagnosis? Rebiopsy with a larger core needle may be considered; low grade HCCs may still be difficult to distinguish from hepatocellular adenomas, as occurred in three of our cases where rebiopsy was performed (Figure 3). While there is poor diagnostic ability of serum AFP to detect HCC [30], serial increase of AFP value clinically may be helpful as a complementary method in chronic hepatitis patients under surveillance for HCC [31]. Thus increasing serum AFP in a cirrhotic patient with a new liver mass with typical features is helpful. More commonly, correlation with imaging findings in cirrhotic patients may play a key role, so that treatment may be undertaken without a definitive diagnosis. The European Association for the study of the liver has states "Noninvasive criteria can only be applied to cirrhotic patients and are based on imaging techniques obtained by 4-phase multidetector CT scan or dynamic contrast-enhanced MRI. Diagnosis should be based on the identification of the typical hallmark of HCC (hypervascular in the arterial phase with washout in the portal venous or delayed phases). While one imaging technique is required for nodules beyond 1 cm in diameter, a more conservative approach with 2 techniques is recommended in suboptimal settings" [28]. The American College of Radiology has also proposed a LI-RADS concept of referring primary liver tumors from LR 1—definitely benign to LR 5—definitely HCC. Thus LR 4 or LR 5 lesions might be considered for definitive treatment as HCC, while LR 3 lesions as intermediate probability may require the potential for biopsy for diagnosis [11]. These are the cases in which liver biopsy may be useful. In our analysis of 54 CTs or MRIs, 19 of the CTs were of pattern III with an equivocal CT diagnosis. Biopsy was definitive of HCC in 14 of 19 of these cases. However, of these 54 cases, the CT or MRI was considered to be of a pattern I or a classic appearance of HCC in 27/54 cases. In 8/54 cases, diffuse tumor with portal venous invasion was also highly suggestive of HCC. In these cases, biopsy could be considered redundant. Of interest in our equivocal biopsy, group of patients with primary liver masses, CT and MRI were very suggestive of a diagnosis in 8 of 13 masses while 5 of 13 were equivocal. Therefore, in the case with equivocal biopsy results, therapy may have to be based upon the aforementioned CT criteria and tumor behavior. Thus, eligibility inclusion criteria for diagnosis and/or treatment could include a positive biopsy with or without immunohistological stain or typical imaging features by CT or MRI in the setting of cirrhosis [11, 30, 32–34].

5. Limitations

Weakness of this paper includes the fact that this is a retrospective study and that multiple different pathologists were involved in the original interpretation and diagnosis. In addition, because this is a retrospective study, issues that may have limited specimen collection are not known, such as bleeding or technical challenges.

6. Summary

In summary, both percutaneous FNA and NCB demonstrate the ability to differentiate malignant from benign lesions in patients with suspected metastatic liver disease. However, this study confirms that the ability to provide a definitive diagnosis in HCC using FNAC with NCB or alone is more challenging. Using FNAC and NCB for suspected primary liver masses, regenerating nodules, and well-differentiated HCC frequently has overlapping cytologic features. These diagnostic challenges and their subsequent management issues may increase as surveillance of patients with liver disease becomes more commonplace. These strategies can include basing treatment on CT or MRI with specific imaging features in a cirrhotic liver with the appropriate clinical and biochemical setting. Effective management may be based upon not only definitive cytological and histological results, but also the recognition that there are special immunohistochemical stains that may prove useful in distinguishing HCC from reactive disease.

References

[1] S. H. Parker, K. D. Hopper, W. F. Yakes, M. D. Gibson, J. L. Ownbey, and T. E. Carter, "Image-directed percutaneous biopsies with a biopsy gun," *Radiology*, vol. 171, no. 3, pp. 663–669, 1989.

[2] B. Porter, W. Karp, and L. Forsberg, "Percutaneous cytodiagnosis of abdominal masses by ultrasound guided fine needle aspiration biopsy," *Acta Radiologica*, vol. 22, no. 6, pp. 663–668, 1981.

[3] P. M. Bret, J.-M. Sente, and M. Bretagnolle, "Ultrasonically guided fine-needle biopsy in focal intrahepatic lesions: six years' experience," *Canadian Association of Radiologists Journal*, vol. 37, no. 1, pp. 5–8, 1986.

[4] M. M. Pinto, N. A. Avila, C. I. Heller, and E. M. Criscuolo, "Fine needle aspiration of the liver," *Acta Cytologica*, vol. 32, no. 1, pp. 15–21, 1988.

[5] G. Sangalli, T. Livraghi, and F. Giordano, "Fine needle biopsy of hepatocellular carcinoma: improvement in diagnosis by microhistology," *Gastroenterology*, vol. 96, no. 2, part 1, pp. 524–526, 1989.

[6] B. Q. Starley, C. J. Calcagno, and S. A. Harrison, "Nonalcoholic fatty liver disease and hepatocellular carcinoma: a weighty connection," *Hepatology*, vol. 51, no. 5, pp. 1820–1832, 2010.

[7] S. Kakar, A. M. Gown, Z. D. Goodman, and L. D. Ferrell, "Best practices in diagnostic immunohistochemistry: hepatocellular carcinoma versus metastatic neoplasms," *Archives of Pathology and Laboratory Medicine*, vol. 131, no. 11, pp. 1648–1654, 2007.

[8] J. Bruix, M. Sherman, J. M. Llovet et al., "Clinical management of hepatocellular carcinoma. Conclusions of the barcelona-2000 EASL conference," *Journal of Hepatology*, vol. 35, no. 3, pp. 421–430, 2001.

[9] P. Ferenci, M. Fried, D. Labrecque et al., "World gastroenterology organisation global guideline. hepatocellular carcinoma (hcc): a global perspective," *Journal of Gastrointestinal and Liver Diseases*, vol. 19, no. 3, pp. 311–317, 2010.

[10] P. Sorrentino, L. Tarantino, S. D'Angelo et al., "Validation of an extension of the international non-invasive criteria for the diagnosis of hepatocellular carcinoma to the characterization of macroscopic portal vein thrombosis," *Journal of Gastroenterology and Hepatology*, vol. 26, no. 4, pp. 669–677, 2011.

[11] Radiology ACo, "LI-RADS concepts," http://www.acr.org/quality-safety/resources/lirads2013.

[12] E. S. Cibas and S. Z. Ali, "The Bethesda system for reporting thyroid cytopathology," *American Journal of Clinical Pathology*, vol. 132, no. 5, pp. 658–665, 2009.

[13] L. J. Layfield, J. Abrams, B. Cochand-Priollet et al., "Post-thyroid FNA testing and treatment options: a synopsis of the national cancer institute thyroid fine needle aspiration state of the science conference," *Diagnostic Cytopathology*, vol. 36, no. 6, pp. 442–448, 2008.

[14] C. Bru, A. Maroto, J. Bruix et al., "Diagnostic accuracy of fine-needle aspiration biopsy in patients with hepatocellular carcinoma," *Digestive Diseases and Sciences*, vol. 34, no. 11, pp. 1765–1769, 1989.

[15] Y. Matsushiro, M. Ebara, M. Ohto, and F. Kondo, "Usefulness of percutaneous biopsy under sonographic control and histological examination in the early diagnosis of hepatocellular carcinoma," *Japanese Journal of Gastroenterology*, vol. 90, no. 3, pp. 655–664, 1993.

[16] H. A. Edmondson and P. E. Steiner, "Primary carcinoma of the liver: a study of 100 cases among 48,900," *Cancer*, vol. 7, no. 3, pp. 462–503, 1954.

[17] T. Kanai, S. Hirohashi, and M. P. Upton, "Pathology of small hepatocellular carcinoma. A proposal for a new gross classification," *Cancer*, vol. 60, no. 4, pp. 810–819, 1987.

[18] L. G. Dodd, E. E. Mooney, L. J. Layfield, and R. C. Nelson, "Fine-needle aspiration of the liver and pancreas: a cytology primer for radiologists," *Radiology*, vol. 203, no. 1, pp. 1–9, 1997.

[19] L. Appelbaum, R. A. Kane, J. B. Kruskal, J. Romero, and J. Sosna, "Focal hepatic lesions: US-guided biopsy—lessons from review of cytologic and pathologic examination results," *Radiology*, vol. 250, no. 2, pp. 453–458, 2009.

[20] S. Bergman, F. Graeme-Cook, and M. B. Pitman, "The usefulness of the reticulin stain in the differential diagnosis of liver nodules on fine-needle aspiration biopsy cell block preparations," *Modern Pathology*, vol. 10, no. 12, pp. 1258–1264, 1997.

[21] W. B. de Boer, A. Segal, F. A. Frost et al., "Can CD34 discriminate between benign and malignant hepatocytic lesions in fine-needle aspirates and thin core biopsies?" *Cancer*, vol. 90, no. 5, pp. 273–278, 2000.

[22] N. Shafizadeh, L. D. Ferrell, and S. Kakar, "Utility and limitations of glypican-3 expression for the diagnosis of hepatocellular carcinoma at both ends of the differentiation spectrum," *Modern Pathology*, vol. 21, no. 8, pp. 1011–1018, 2008.

[23] L. Wilkens, T. Becker, B. Schlegelberger, H. H. Kreipe, and P. Flemming, "Preserved reticulin network in a case of hepatocellular carcinoma," *Histopathology*, vol. 48, no. 7, pp. 876–878, 2006.

[24] H. Hong, B. Patonay, and J. Finley, "Unusual reticulin staining pattern in well-differentiated hepatocellular carcinoma," *Diagnostic Pathology*, vol. 6, no. 1, p. 15, 2011.

[25] A. Wee, "Fine needle aspiration biopsy of hepatocellular carcinoma and hepatocellular nodular lesions: role, controversies and approach to diagnosis," *Cytopathology*, vol. 22, no. 5, pp. 287–305, 2011.

[26] E. S. Chan and M. M. Yeh, "The use of immunohistochemistry in liver tumors," *Clinics in Liver Disease*, vol. 14, no. 4, pp. 687–703, 2010.

[27] D. Jain, "Diagnosis of hepatocellular carcinoma: fine needle aspiration cytology or needle core biopsy," *Journal of Clinical Gastroenterology*, vol. 35, no. 5, supplement 2, pp. S101–S108, 2002.

[28] European Association for The Study of The L and European Organisation for R, "Treatment of C. EASL-EORTC clinical practice guidelines: management of hepatocellular carcinoma," *Journal of Hepatology*, vol. 56, no. 4, pp. 908–943, 2012.

[29] S. Yao, J. Zhang, H. Chen et al., "Diagnostic value of immunohistochemical staining of GP73, GPC3, DCP, CD34, CD31, and reticulin staining in hepatocellular carcinoma," *Journal of Histochemistry & Cytochemistry*, vol. 61, no. 9, pp. 639–648, 2013.

[30] J. Bruix and M. Sherman, "Management of hepatocellular carcinoma: an update," *Hepatology*, vol. 53, no. 3, pp. 1020–1022, 2011.

[31] S. Gupta, S. Bent, and J. Kohlwes, "Test characteristics of α-fetoprotein for detecting hepatocellular carcinoma in patients with hepatitis C: a systematic review and critical analysis," *Annals of Internal Medicine*, vol. 139, no. 1, pp. 46–50, 2003.

[32] A. S. Befeler, P. H. Hayashi, and A. M. Di Bisceglie, "Liver transplantation for hepatocellular carcinoma," *Gastroenterology*, vol. 128, no. 6, pp. 1752–1764, 2005.

[33] V. Mazzaferro, E. Regalia, R. Doci et al., "Liver transplantation for the treatment of small hepatocellular carcinomas in patients with cirrhosis," *New England Journal of Medicine*, vol. 334, no. 11, pp. 693–699, 1996.

[34] F. Y. Yao, "Liver transplantation for hepatocellular carcinoma: beyond the Milan criteria," *American Journal of Transplantation*, vol. 8, no. 10, pp. 1982–1989, 2008.

Effect of Platelet-Rich Plasma on CCl_4-Induced Chronic Liver Injury in Male Rats

Zahra Hesami,[1] Akram Jamshidzadeh,[2] Maryam Ayatollahi,[3] Bita Geramizadeh,[3] Omid Farshad,[4] and Akbar Vahdati[1]

[1] *Department of Biology, Science and Research Branch, Islamic Azad University, Fars, Iran*
[2] *Pharmaceutical Sciences Research Center, Shiraz University of Medical Sciences, Shiraz, Iran*
[3] *Transplant Research Center, Shiraz University of Medical Sciences, Shiraz, Iran*
[4] *International Branch, Shiraz University of Medical Sciences, Shiraz, Iran*

Correspondence should be addressed to Zahra Hesami; z_hesami59@yahoo.com

Academic Editor: Dirk Uhlmann

Platelet-rich plasma (PRP) has been of great concern to the scientists and doctors who are involved in wound healing and regenerative medicine which focuses on repairing and replacing damaged cells and tissues. Growth factors of platelet-rich plasma are cost-effective, available, and is more stable than recombinant human growth factors. Given these valuable properties, we decided to assess the effect of PRP on CCl_4-induced hepatotoxicity on rats. The rats received CCl_4 (1 mL/kg, i.p. 1 : 1 in olive oil) twice per week for 8 weeks. Five weeks after CCl_4 injection, the rats also received PRP (0.5 mL/kg, s.c.) two days a week for three weeks. Twenty-four hours after last CCl_4 injection, the animals bled and their livers dissected for biochemical and histopathological studies. Blood analysis was performed to evaluate enzyme activity. The results showed that PRP itself was not toxic for liver and could protect the liver from CCl_4-induced histological damages and attenuated oxidative stress by increase in glutathione content and decrease in lipid peroxidative marker of liver tissue. The results of the present study lend support to our beliefs in hepatoprotective effects of PRP.

1. Introduction

Liver is considered the key organ in the metabolism, detoxification, and secretory functions in the body, and its disorders are numerous with no effective remedies; however, the search for new medicines is still ongoing. It is a hematopoietic organ in the fetal period, and mature hepatocytes produce thrombopoietin, which can stimulate platelet production in bone marrow. However, few studies have investigated the relationship between hematic components, that is, platelets and liver regeneration [1–4].

The platelet-rich plasma (PRP) used in tissue regeneration serves as a developing area for clinicians and researchers. It is well known that platelets have a thrombotic effect. Platelets contain not only proteins needed for hemostasis but also many growth factors such as transforming growth factor (TGF), platelet-derived growth factor (PDGF), vascular endothelial growth factor (VEGF), epidermal growth factor (EGF), and insulin-like growth factor (IGF) [5].

Some study has been reported; platelets accumulate in the liver under some kinds of pathologic conditions, like ischemia/reperfusion injury [6–8], liver cirrhosis [9], cholestatic liver [10], and viral hepatitis [11].

Many in vitro studies demonstrated that platelets contain several growth factors which may theoretically contribute to the process of liver regeneration [12, 13]. However, there are few studies on the role of platelets in liver regeneration in rats that failed to identify a correlation between platelets and liver regeneration [14, 15].

Carbon tetrachloride (CCl_4) is a widely used chemical for experimental induction of fatty liver and liver fibrosis in animals [16]. Its biotransformation produces hepatotoxic metabolites, the highly reactive trichloromethyl-free radical, subsequently converted to the peroxytrichloromethyl radical

[17]. Based on the findings of different studies in this field, the present study was undertaken to investigate hepatoprotective activity of PRP on the liver injury induced by CCl_4 in experimental animal model.

2. Materials and Methods

2.1. Chemicals. CCl_4, calcium gluconate, sodium dodecyl sulfate, ethylenediaminetetraacetic acid (EDTA), 5, 5′-dithiobis-(2-nitrobenzoic acid) or DTNB, tris, thiobarbituric acid (TBA), and trichloroacetic acid were from Sigma Chemical Company, Germany. All other chemicals were of highest quality available in the market.

2.2. Preparing Platelet-Rich Plasma. Fourteen female rats (170–200 g) were selected from the Laboratory Animals Research Center in Shiraz University of Medical Sciences. The rats were maintained under controlled temperature and 12 hours light/12 hours dark conditions for one week before the start of the experiments. They were allowed to feed on standard laboratory chaw and tap water ad libitum. The research protocol complied with the guidelines for animal care of our institution.

The rats were anesthetized with ether, followed by blood collection from the rats via open chest cardiac puncture. About 100 mL of blood was collected from them after killing. The blood was then mixed with sodium citrate (3.8%) (9 parts of blood to 1 part of sodium citrate) anticoagulant solution. Then, the blood was centrifuged at 1000 rpm for 15 min at 20°C for separation of platelet rich plasma. Also, the plasma was centrifuged at 3000 rpm for 10 min at 20°C to obtain platelet pellet. The platelet concentrate dissolved in phosphate buffer saline (PBS), pooled and incubated at room temperature for 30 min on a rotating platform to eliminate platelet agglomerates. Platelets were counted using Sysmex KX-21 (Japan), resulting in a platelet number of $679 \times 10^3/\mu L$ [18]. Afterwards, autologous thrombin was prepared as per Lucarelli et al.'s method [19]. At this step, 330 μL of calcium gluconate (100 mg/mL) was added to 10 mL of plasma and 1 mL of thrombin preparation to 4 mL of platelet concentrate and incubated for 1 h at room temperature to facilitate growth factors release. The platelet secretion was centrifuged at 4000 rpm for 5 min to reduce the presence of platelet membrane fragments. The supernatant was filtered with a 0.22 μm pore filter, divided into aliquots, and frozen at −80°C for subsequent use [20]. The protein concentration in the filtrates was determined by Bradford method (150 mg/mL) [21].

2.3. Study Design. As designed, the 24 male Wistar rats (250–300 g) were randomly divided into 4 groups, each consisting of 6 animals. Group I received olive oil (0.5 mL/kg, i.p., n = 6) as normal control; group II received CCl_4 (1 mL/kg body weight as a 1 : 1 mixture with olive oil i.p., n = 6) twice per week for 8 weeks; group III received PRP (0.5 mL/kg 1 : 1 in PBS, s.c. n = 6) two days a week for three weeks; and group IV received the CCl_4 (1 mL/kg body weight as a 1 : 1 mixture with olive oil i.p.) twice per week for 8 weeks. Five weeks after CCl_4 injection, the rats received PRP (0.5 mL/kg 1 : 1 in PBS s.c. n = 6) two days a week for three weeks. Twenty-four hours after CCl_4 injection, the animals were anaesthetized by sodium thiopental injection (50 mg/kg) and their blood samples collected from the vena cava. Then, the respective sera were separated for subsequent use of different enzyme measurements. The rats were then decapitated and their livers carefully dissected and cleaned of extraneous tissues, and parts of the liver tissue were immediately transferred to 10% formalin for histopathological assessments.

2.4. Histopathological Studies. Part of the liver was removed from the animals and the tissue fixed in 10% formalin for at least 24 hours. Then, the paraffin sections were prepared (by Automatic tissue processor, Autotechnique) and cut into 5 μm thick sections by a rotary microtom. The sections then were stained with Haematoxylin-Eosin dye and studied for histopathological changes, that is, necrosis, fatty changes, ballooning degeneration, and Inflammation. Histological damage is scored as follows: 0: absent; +: mild; ++: moderate; and +++: severe.

2.5. Measurement of ALT, AST, and Albumin in Serum. Biocon standard kits and DAX-48 autoanalyzer were used to measure alanine aminotransferase (ALT), aspartate aminotransferase (AST), and albumin (ALB) activities in serum, according to Wilkinson et al.'s and Bessay et al.'s method [22, 23].

2.6. Determination of Lipid Peroxidation. The lipid peroxidation extent was assessed by measuring the amount of thiobarbituric acid-reactive substances (TBARs). In Brief, 500 mg of liver tissue gently minced in 4.5 mL of 0.25 M sucrose. The minced tissues gently homogenized and then centrifuged at 2000 rpm for 30 min. Afterwards, 0.1 mL of the supernatant was treated with a buffer containing 0.75 mL of thiobarbituric acid (0.8%, w/v), 0.75 mL of 20% acetic acid (pH = 3.5), and 0.1 mL of sodium dodecyl sulfate (8.1%, w/v). The solution was mixed up with 2 mL of distilled water and heated in a boiling water bath for 60 min. The absorbance then was measured at 532 nm by a Beckman DU-7 spectrophotometer [24].

2.7. GSH Determination. Glutathione reductase 5,50-dithio-bis-2 nitrobenzoic acid (DTNB) recycling procedure [25] was used to determine the reduced glutathione. In brief, 100 mg of liver tissues was homogenized in a buffer containing EDTA (0.2 M) to obtain 4% (w/v) whole homogenate. Then, 1.5 mL of the suspension was taken and mixed with a buffer containing 2.5 mL distilled water and 0.5 mL of 50% TCA. The mixture then was centrifuged at 3000 rpm for 15 min and 1 mL of the supernatant mixed with 1 mL of Tris buffer (0.4 M, pH = 8.9) and 0.1 mL of DTNB (0.01 M). The absorbance was measured after 5 min at 412 nm using a Beckman DU-7 spectrophotometer [26].

2.8. Statistical Analysis. The data were analyzed by student's Tukey test and one-way ANOVA, followed by Graph pad

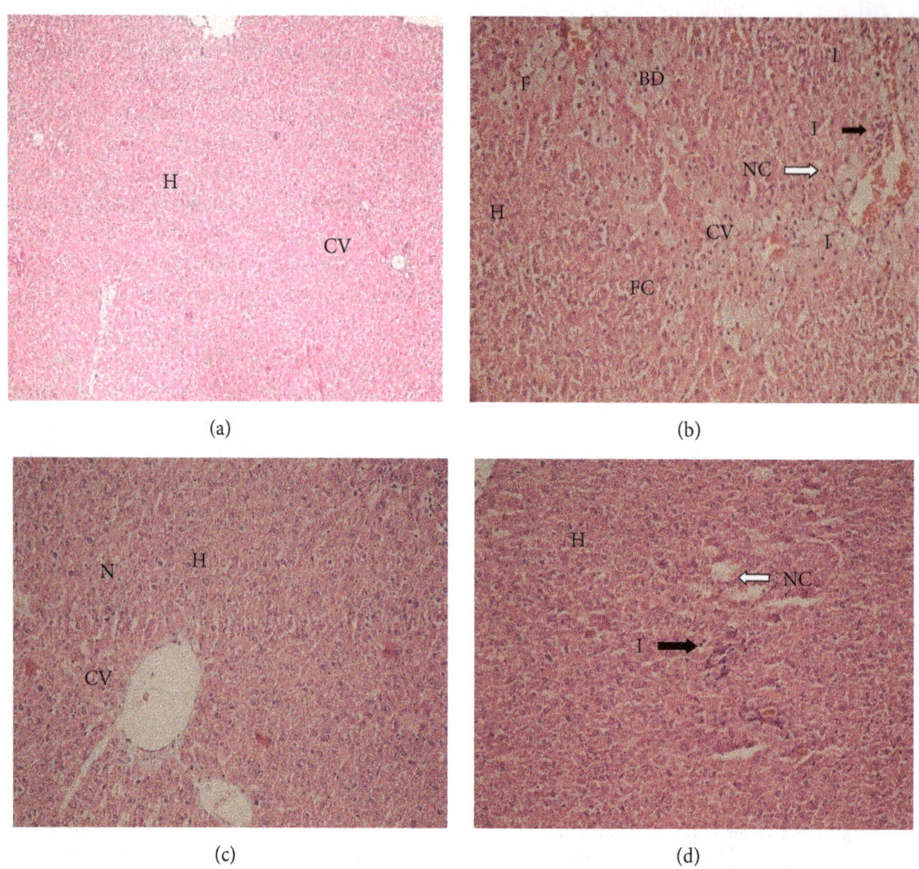

Figure 1: Effect of the platelet-rich plasma (PRP) on histopathological changes induced by CCl_4 in rats. (a) (H&E ×100) liver section of normal rats showing normal hepatocytes with prominent nucleus, cytoplasm, and central vein; (b) (H&E ×250) liver sections of CCl_4-treated (0.5 mL/kg i.p.) rats showing fatty chain, necrosis, and infiltration of inflammatory cells; (c) (H&E ×250) liver sections of the rats treated with PRP (0.5 mL/kg s.c.) showing well-brought out central vein hepatocytes with well-preserved cytoplasm and normal hepatocytes with prominent nucleus; (d) (H&E ×250) liver sections of the rats treated with CCl_4 + PRP (0.5 mL/kg + 0.5 mL/kg s.c.) showing normal architecture of hepatocytes and mild infiltration of inflammatory cells. H: hepatocyte, CV: central vein, N: nucleus, F: foamy macrophage cells, FC: fatty chain, NC: necrosis, I: infiltration of inflammatory cells, and BD: ballooning degeneration.

Table 1: Effect of the platelet-rich plasma (PRP) on histopathological liver damages induced by CCl_4 in rats.

Groups	Ballooning Degeneration	Fatty change	Hepatocyte necrosis	Inflammation	Others
Control	0	0	0	0	—
CCl_4	++	+	+++	+	Many foamy macrophages and old necrosis
PRP	0	0	0	0	—
PRP + CCl_4	0	0	+	+	—

0: absent; +: mild; ++: moderate; +++: severe.
Rats were injected (i.p.) CCL_4 with doses (0.5 mL/kg 1 : 1 in olive oil) twice per week for 8 weeks. Five weeks after CCl_4 injection, rats received PRP (0.5 mL/kg 1 : 1 in PBS, s.c.). The PRP (0.5 mL/kg 1 : 1 in PBS, s.c.) alone did not increase the levels of the enzymes. Values are mean ± SD of 6 rats per group.

Prism 5. The difference between the control and experimental groups was considered significant at $P \leq 0.05$.

3. Results

Histopathological studies revealed that CCl_4 imposed focal necrosis, fatty changes, ballooning degeneration, and infiltration of lymphocytes around the central veins (Figure 1(b); Table 1). Necrosis, which is a more severe form of injury, was markedly prevented by treatment with PRP (Figure 1(d)) and demonstrated a normal appearance, except for mild inflammation (+ in Table 1) in pericentral hepatocytes to the vein and mild necrosis (+ in Table 1). In the PRP groups that received only PRP there was no significant toxicity, which shows that PRP did not induce hepatotoxicity (Figure 1(c)).

Results of enzyme activity analysis are presented in Figure 2. Administration of CCl_4 to rats caused a significant elevation in serum ALT and AST activities after 8 weeks. Albumin (Figure 2(c)) did not show significant changes in CCl_4-treated group, compared to the control group.

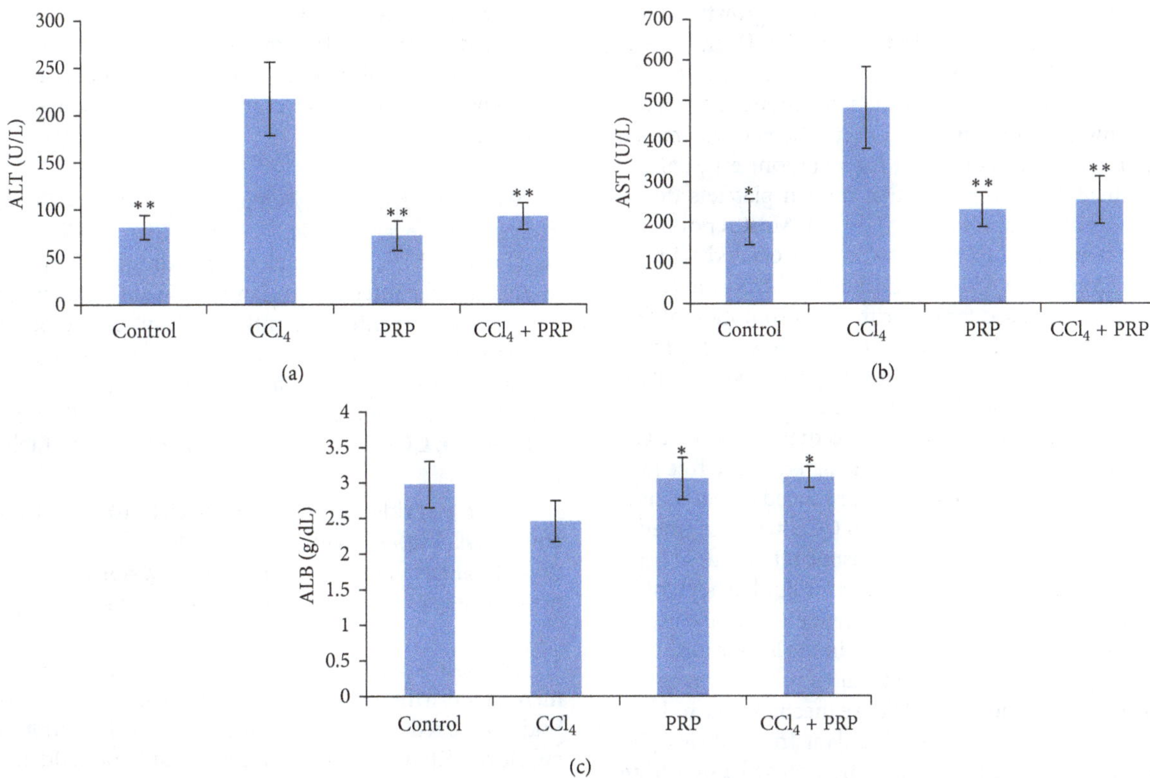

FIGURE 2: Effect of platelet rich plasma (PRP) on rat hepatic enzymes and albumin levels changed by CCl_4. (a) ALT, (b) AST, (c) albumin. Rats were injected CCL_4 with doses (0.5 mL/kg i.p. 1:1 in olive oil) twice per week for 8 weeks. Five weeks after CCl_4 injection rats received PRP (0.5 mL/kg s.c.) 2 days a week for 3 weeks. Values are mean ± SD of 6 rats per group. *Significantly different from CCl_4-treated group ($P \le 0.05$). **Significantly different from CCl_4-treated group ($P \le 0.01$).

TABLE 2: Effects of platelet-rich plasma (PRP) on GSH and TBARs levels of the liver damaged by CCl_4 in rats.

Groups	GSH (nmol/g liver)	TBARs (nmol/g liver)
Control	$0.35454 \pm 0.035^*$	$0.7 \pm 0.057^{**}$
CCL_4 (0.5 mL/kg)	0.18727 ± 0.016	4.96 ± 0.84
PRP (0.5 mL/kg)	$0.33187 \pm 0.058^*$	$0.962 \pm 0.23^{**}$
CCL_4 + PRP	$0.28774 \pm 0.034^*$	$0.981 \pm 0.035^{**}$

GSH: reduced glutathione; TBARs: thiobarbituric acid-reactive substances.
Values are mean ± SD, ($n = 6$).
$^*P \le 0.05$ mean difference, compared to CCl_4-treated rats.
$^{**}P \le 0.001$ mean difference, compared to CCl_4-treated rats.

Treatment of rats with 0.5 mg/kg i.p. of the PRP markedly prevented CCl_4-induced elevation of serum ALT and AST (Figures 2(a) and 2(b)).

As shown in Table 2, the liver's lipid peroxidation was significantly increased in the CCl_4 group when compared with the controls ($P \le 0.01$) and PRP ameliorated CCl_4-induced increases of MDA concentration ($P \le 0.01$). These findings indicate that the oxidative stress in the liver was effectively decreased when treated with PRP.

Glutathione (GSH) is measured as an index of antioxidant status of liver. There was a significant increase of GSH content in the PRP groups, compared to the group that received CCl_4 alone (Table 2).

4. Discussion

Carbon tetrachloride-induced hepatic injury is commonly used as an experimental method for the study of hepatoprotective effects of drugs or medicinal plants extracts, by in vivo and in vitro techniques [27, 28].

CCl_4 is believed to be metabolized by microsomal CYP450 in the liver to a highly reactive trichloromethyl-free radical ($^\bullet CCl3$) which can start a chain of reactive free radical formation resulting in peroxidation of lipids and damage to the proteins and components of the cells leading to cell lyses [29, 30].

Effect of platelets on liver regeneration was not addressed till the beginning of the 21st century. There are some reported studies in which platelets were shown to promote liver regeneration [27]. The following study was conducted to determine the role of platelets in liver regeneration using a thrombocytosis model in mice after 90% partial hepatectomy [28]. The entire disrupted platelets and the soluble fraction were with significant proliferative effects, whereas the membrane fraction had no significant effect. Studies indicate that the direct contact between platelets and hepatocytes could spark the release of soluble factors from the platelets such as IGF-1 and HGF; IGF-1 is contained in human platelet as the most important mediator for liver regeneration, which had a proliferative effect on them [29]. The findings in the other experiment demonstrate that exogenous platelets also enhance liver regeneration [30]. Meanwhile, growth factors, like vascular insulin-like growth factor I (IGF-I), endothelial growth factor (VEGF), and hepatocyte growth factor (HGF), contribute to hepatocyte proliferation that induced by platelet [31]. The growth factors stimulate onset of hepatocyte mitosis, which ultimately promote liver regeneration, especially in humans, since it was reported that human platelets do not contain a significant amount of HGF [32]. Most reports lend support to a decrease in platelet count associated with the severity of liver injury [33–35]. Carbon tetrachloride (CCl_4) is a chemical agent used for experimental promotion of fatty liver and liver fibrosis in animals [16]. The present study was undertaken to investigate of the hepatoprotective activity of PRP against CCl_4-induced damage in rat.

Lipid peroxidation is among the actual causes of CCl_4-induced liver injury [36, 37] and is mediated by the free radical derivatives of CCl_4. CCl_3 radicals produced in reactions by animals microsomes liver exposed to CCl_4 were assumed to attack the membrane lipid in endoplasmic reticulum of hepatocyte. When they attacked the membrane lipid in hepatocyte endoplasmic reticulum, malondialdehyde (MDA) emerged promptly [38]. The rise of MDA levels in the liver is indicative of an enhanced peroxidation that causes tissue damage and breakdown of the antioxidant defense mechanisms and thus inhibits the formation of superabundant free radicals [39]. In the present study, PRP administration caused a significant decrease in MDA levels, compared to the CCl_4-treated rat, suggesting that PRP could protect against CCl_4-induced lipid peroxidation in rats.

Unlike the toxic consequences of CCl_4 metabolism through the CYP_2E_1 pathway, the detoxification pathway involves GSH conjugation of trichloromethyl-free radicals [40]. A reduced level of GSH is crucial in the detoxification of the reactive toxic metabolites of CCl_4; liver necrosis is initiated when reserves of GSH are remarkably depleted [41]. In the present study, the hepatic content of GSH was found to be decreased significantly in CCl_4 intoxicated rats, compared to the controls. Table 2 shows that PRP treatment significantly inhibited the CCl_4-induced decrease of hepatic GSH content. When CCl_4 is administered to rats, the actions of aspartate aminotransferase (AST) and alanine aminotransferase (ALT) in rat plasma rise remarkably with necrosis and lipid accumulation of hepatocyte [42]. Both enzymes are indicators of liver injury. ALT is more sensitive to acute liver injury test, whereas AST is more sensitive to chronic injury [43]. The present study showed that PRP treatment significantly improved levels of ALT, AST, and albumin after CCl_4 administration (Figures 2(a), 2(b), and 2(c)). The most important protein synthesized by the liver is serum albumin whose main function is to regulate the colloidal osmotic pressure of blood and it reflects the extent of functioning liver cell mass. However, measuring of albumin can provide information to identify chronic injury among the experimental rats [44].

The biochemical observations are supported by the histopathological examination of rats' livers. As a result of hepatotoxicity of CCl_4, significant regenerative cellular proliferation occurs to compensate for the necrotic or damaged tissue. The Histopathological result (Figure 1) shows severe necrosis in central vein of the rats treated with CCl_4 compared to the control group that showed +++ degree (Table 1). This result is in accordance with other results [16] and shows fatty changes (+ grade in Table 1), compared to the control group.

We showed that fatty changes in PRP + CCl_4 groups decrease (0 degree, Table 1), compared to CCl_4 rat models (Figure 1(b)). The platelets are stimulated by a lot of motivation like infection, inflammation, and injury. Platelets have modulatory effects on inflammatory cell responses [45]. It seems that the histological changes in CCl_4 group, in addition to necrosis, have a foci apoptotic lesion in their livers (Figure 1(b)). The grade of necrotic foci in the liver reduced from +++ in CCl_4 to + in PRP treatment groups (Table 1).

There is evidence showing platelets to be effective in antifibrosis [46, 47], antiapoptosis [48], and liver regeneration [29]. Platelet therapy can open a new horizon to develop novel strategies for the treatments of liver diseases.

The results presented in this study indicated that the treatment of rats with the PRP 5 weeks after CCl_4-induced toxicity leads to the reduction of hepatotoxicity. The hepatoprotective effects of PRP may be due to inhibited lipid peroxidation and effective recovery of the antioxidative defense system and has a remarkable effect on signal transduction. Overall, platelet-rich plasma can be used as a complementary procedure to decrease the destructive effects of hepatotoxicants.

References

[1] S. Murata, N. Ohkohchi, R. Matsuo, O. Ikeda, A. Myronovych, and R. Hoshi, "Platelets promote liver regeneration in early period after hepatectomy in mice," *World Journal of Surgery*, vol. 31, no. 4, pp. 808–816, 2007.

[2] R. Matsuo, N. Ohkohchi, S. Murata et al., "Platelets strongly induce hepatocyte proliferation with IGF-1 and HGF in vitro," *Journal of Surgical Research*, vol. 145, no. 2, pp. 279–286, 2008.

[3] R. Hoshi, S. Murata, R. Matsuo et al., "Freeze-dried platelets promote hepatocyte proliferation in mice," *Cryobiology*, vol. 55, no. 3, pp. 255–260, 2007.

[4] M. Lesurtel, R. Graf, B. Aleil et al., "Platelet-derived serotonin mediates liver regeneration," *Science*, vol. 312, no. 5770, pp. 104–107, 2006.

[5] Y. Hiyama, I. Mahmud, and F. Karimi-Tari, "Platelet-derived growth factor and thromboxane are necessary for liver regeneration," *Cellular and Molecular Biology*, vol. 27, no. 6, pp. 593–599, 1981.

[6] A. Khandoga, P. Biberthaler, K. Messmer, and F. Krombach, "Platelet-endothelial cell interactions during hepatic ischemia-reperfusion in vivo: a systematic analysis," *Microvascular Research*, vol. 65, no. 2, pp. 71–77, 2003.

[7] A. Khandoga, M. Hanschen, J. S. Kessler, and F. Krombach, "CD4+ T cells contribute to postischemic liver injury in mice by interacting with sinusoidal endothelium and platelets," *Hepatology*, vol. 43, no. 2, pp. 306–315, 2006.

[8] S. Pak, T. Kondo, Y. Nakano et al., "Platelet adhesion in the sinusoid caused hepatic injury by neutrophils after hepatic ischemia reperfusion," *Platelets*, vol. 21, no. 4, pp. 282–288, 2010.

[9] M. M. Zaldivar, K. Pauels, P. Von Hundelshausen et al., "CXC chemokine ligand 4 (CXCl4) is a platelet-derived mediator of experimental liver fibrosis," *Hepatology*, vol. 51, no. 4, pp. 1345–1353, 2010.

[10] M. W. Laschke, S. Dold, M. D. Menger, B. Jeppsson, and H. Thorlacius, "Platelet-dependent accumulation of leukocytes in sinusoids mediates hepatocellular damage in bile duct ligation-induced cholestasis," *British Journal of Pharmacology*, vol. 153, no. 1, pp. 148–156, 2008.

[11] P. A. Lang, C. Contaldo, P. Georgiev et al., "Aggravation of viral hepatitis by platelet-derived serotonin," *Nature Medicine*, vol. 14, no. 7, pp. 756–761, 2008.

[12] K. Matsumoto and T. Nakamura, "Hepatocyte growth factor: molecular structure, roles in liver regeneration, and other biological functions," *Critical Reviews in Oncogenesis*, vol. 3, no. 1-2, pp. 27–54, 1992.

[13] A. J. Strain, J. A. McGowan, and N. L. R. Bucher, "Stimulation of DNA synthesis in primary cultures of adult rat hepatocytes by rat platelet-associated substance(s)," *In Vitro*, vol. 18, no. 2, pp. 108–116, 1982.

[14] Y. Kuwashima, K. Aoki, K. Kohyama, and T. Ishikawa, "Hepatocyte regeneration after partial hepatectomy occurs even under severely thrombocytopenic conditions in the rat," *Japanese Journal of Cancer Research*, vol. 81, no. 6-7, pp. 607–612, 1990.

[15] M. Tomikawa, M. Hashizume, H. Higashi, M. Ohta, and K. Sugimachi, "The role of the spleen, platelets, and plasma hepatocyte growth factor activity on hepatic regeneration in rats," *Journal of the American College of Surgeons*, vol. 182, no. 1, pp. 12–16, 1996.

[16] R. O. Recknagel, "Carbon tetrachloride hepatotoxicity," *Pharmacological Reviews*, vol. 19, no. 2, pp. 145–208, 1967.

[17] A. T. Williams and R. F. Burk, "Carbon tetrachloride hepatotoxicity: an example of free radical-mediated injury," *Seminars in Liver Disease*, vol. 10, no. 4, pp. 279–284, 1990.

[18] X. Xie, S. Zhao, H. Wu et al., "Platelet-rich plasma enhances autograft revascularization and reinnervation in a dog model of anterior cruciate ligament reconstruction," *Journal of Surgical Research*, vol. 183, no. 1, pp. 214–222, 2013.

[19] E. Lucarelli, A. Beccheroni, D. Donati et al., "Platelet-derived growth factors enhance proliferation of human stromal stem cells," *Biomaterials*, vol. 24, no. 18, pp. 3095–3100, 2003.

[20] S. Kazemnejad, A. Allameh, A. Gharehbaghian, M. Soleimani, N. Amirizadeh, and M. Jazayeri, "Efficient replacing of fetal bovine serum with human platelet releasate during propagation and differentiation of human bone marrow-derived mesenchymal stem cells to functional hepatocytes-like cells," *Vox Sanguinis*, vol. 95, no. 2, pp. 149–158, 2008.

[21] N. J. Kruger, "The Bradford method for protein quantitation," in *The Protein Protocols Handbook*, pp. 17–24, Springer, 2009.

[22] J. H. Wilkinson, J. H. Boutwell, and S. Winsten, "Evaluation of a new system for the kinetic measurement of serum alkaline phosphatase," *Clinical Chemistry*, vol. 15, no. 6, pp. 487–495, 1969.

[23] O. A. Bessay, O. H. Lowry, and M. J. Brock, "A method for rapid determination of alkaline phosphatase with five cubic milliliters of serum," *The Journal of Biological Chemistry*, vol. 164, pp. 321–329, 1946.

[24] I. S. Jamall and J. C. Smith, "Effects of cadmium treatment on selenium-dependent and selenium-independent glutathione peroxidase activities and lipid peroxidation in the kidney and liver of rats maintained on various levels of dietary selenium," *Archives of Toxicology*, vol. 58, no. 2, pp. 102–105, 1985.

[25] F. Tietze, "Enzymic method for quantitative determination of nanogram amounts of total and oxidized glutathione: applications to mammalian blood and other tissues," *Analytical Biochemistry*, vol. 27, no. 3, pp. 502–522, 1969.

[26] J. Sedlak and R. H. Lindsay, "Estimation of total, protein-bound, and nonprotein sulfhydryl groups in tissue with Ellman's reagent," *Analytical Biochemistry*, vol. 25, pp. 192–205, 1968.

[27] S. Murata, N. Ohkohchi, R. Matsuo, O. Ikeda, A. Myronovych, and R. Hoshi, "Platelets promote liver regeneration in early period after hepatectomy in mice," *World Journal of Surgery*, vol. 31, no. 4, pp. 808–816, 2007.

[28] A. Myronovych, S. Murata, M. Chiba et al., "Role of platelets on liver regeneration after 90% hepatectomy in mice," *Journal of Hepatology*, vol. 49, no. 3, pp. 363–372, 2008.

[29] N. Ohkohchi, S. Murata, and K. Takahashi, *Platelet and Liver Regeneration, Tissue Regeneration—from Basic Biology to Clinical Application*, 2012.

[30] R. Matsuo, Y. Nakano, and N. Ohkohchi, "Platelet administration via the portal vein promotes liver regeneration in rats after 70% hepatectomy," *Annals of Surgery*, vol. 253, no. 4, pp. 759–763, 2011.

[31] R. Matsuo, N. Ohkohchi, S. Murata et al., "Platelets strongly induce hepatocyte proliferation with IGF-1 and HGF in vitro," *Journal of Surgical Research*, vol. 145, no. 2, pp. 279–286, 2008.

[32] T. Nakamura, T. Nishizawa, M. Hagiya et al., "Molecular cloning and expression of human hepatocyte growth factor," *Nature*, vol. 342, no. 6248, pp. 440–443, 1989.

[33] S. Panzer, E. Seel, M. Brunner et al., "Platelet autoantibodies are common in hepatitis C infection, irrespective of the presence of thrombocytopenia," *European Journal of Haematology*, vol. 77, no. 6, pp. 513–517, 2006.

[34] P. Schöffski, F. Tacke, C. Trautwein et al., "Thrombopoietin serum levels are elevated in patients with hepatitis B/C infection compared to other causes of chronic liver disease," *Liver*, vol. 22, no. 2, pp. 114–120, 2002.

[35] A. Panasiuk, D. Prokopowicz, J. Zak, J. Matowicka-Karna, J. Osada, and J. Wysocka, "Activation of blood platelets in chronic hepatitis and liver cirrhosis P-selectin expression on blood platelets and secretory activity of β-thromboglobulin and platelet factor-4," *Hepato-Gastroenterology*, vol. 48, no. 39, pp. 818–822, 2001.

[36] S. Basu, "Carbon tetrachloride-induced lipid peroxidation: eicosanoid formation and their regulation by antioxidant nutrients," *Toxicology*, vol. 189, no. 1-2, pp. 113–127, 2003.

[37] M. K. Manibusan, M. Odin, and D. A. Eastmond, "Postulated carbon tetrachloride mode of action: a review," *Journal of Environmental Science and Health C*, vol. 25, no. 3, pp. 185–209, 2007.

[38] Y.-W. Hsu, C.-F. Tsai, W.-K. Chen, and F.-J. Lu, "Protective effects of seabuckthorn (Hippophae rhamnoides L.) seed oil against carbon tetrachloride-induced hepatotoxicity in mice," *Food and Chemical Toxicology*, vol. 47, no. 9, pp. 2281–2288, 2009.

[39] K. J. Lee, J. H. Choi, T. Khanal, Y. P. Hwang, Y. C. Chung, and H. G. Jeong, "Protective effect of caffeic acid phenethyl ester against carbon tetrachloride-induced hepatotoxicity in mice," *Toxicology*, vol. 248, no. 1, pp. 18–24, 2008.

[40] Y. Ou, S. Zheng, L. Lin, Q. Jiang, and X. Yang, "Protective effect of C-phycocyanin against carbon tetrachloride-induced hepatocyte damage in vitro and in vivo," *Chemico-Biological Interactions*, vol. 185, no. 2, pp. 94–100, 2010.

[41] R. O. Recknagel, E. A. Glende Jr., J. A. Dolak, and R. L. Waller, "Mechanisms of carbon tetrachloride toxicity," *Pharmacology & Therapeutics*, vol. 43, no. 1, pp. 139–154, 1989.

[42] R. Yachi, O. Igarashi, and C. Kiyose, "Protective effects of vitamin E analogs against carbon tetrachloride- induced fatty liver in rats," *Journal of Clinical Biochemistry and Nutrition*, vol. 47, no. 2, pp. 148–154, 2010.

[43] P. L. Wolf, "Biochemical diagnosis of liver disease," *Indian Journal of Clinical Biochemistry*, vol. 14, no. 1, pp. 59–90, 1999.

[44] D. Vasudevan and S. Sreekumari, "Mineral metabolism," in *Textbook of Biochemistry for Medical Students*, p. 305, Jaypee Brothers, 4th edition, 2005.

[45] M. R. Yeaman, "The role of platelets in antimicrobial host defense," *Clinical Infectious Diseases*, vol. 25, no. 5, pp. 951–970, 1997.

[46] M. Watanabe, S. Murata, I. Hashimoto et al., "Platelets contribute to the reduction of liver fibrosis in mice," *Journal of Gastroenterology and Hepatology*, vol. 24, no. 1, pp. 78–89, 2009.

[47] T. Kodama, T. Takehara, H. Hikita et al., "Thrombocytopenia exacerbates cholestasis-induced liver fibrosis in mice," *Gastroenterology*, vol. 138, no. 7, pp. 2487.e7–2498.e7, 2010.

[48] K. Hisakura, S. Murata, K. Fukunaga et al., "Platelets prevent acute liver damage after extended hepatectomy in pigs," *Journal of Hepato-Biliary-Pancreatic Sciences*, vol. 17, no. 6, pp. 855–864, 2010.

13

Histological Characterization of Biliary Intraepithelial Neoplasia with respect to Pancreatic Intraepithelial Neoplasia

Yasunori Sato,[1] Kenichi Harada,[1] Motoko Sasaki,[1] and Yasuni Nakanuma[1,2]

[1] *Department of Human Pathology, Kanazawa University Graduate School of Medicine, 13-1 Takara-machi, Kanazawa 920-8640, Japan*
[2] *Department of Pathology, Shizuoka Cancer Center, 1007 Shimonagakubo, Nagaizumi-cho, Sunto-gun, Shizuoka 411-8777, Japan*

Correspondence should be addressed to Yasuni Nakanuma; nakanuma@staff.kanazawa-u.ac.jp

Academic Editor: Masakazu Yamamoto

Biliary intraepithelial neoplasia (BilIN) is a precursor lesion of hilar/perihilar and extrahepatic cholangiocarcinoma. BilIN represents the process of multistep cholangiocarcinogenesis and is the biliary counterpart of pancreatic intraepithelial neoplasia (PanIN). This study was performed to clarify the histological characteristics of BilIN in relation to PanIN. Using paraffin-embedded tissue sections of surgically resected specimens of cholangiocarcinoma associated with BilIN and pancreatic ductal adenocarcinoma associated with PanIN, immunohistochemical staining was performed using primary antibodies against MUC1, MUC2, MUC5AC, cyclin D1, p21, p53, and S100P. For mucin staining, Alcian blue pH 2.5 was used. Most of the molecules examined here showed similar expression patterns in BilIN and PanIN, in which their expression tended to increase along with the increase in atypia of the epithelial lesions. Significant differences were observed in the increase in mucin production and the expression of S100P in PanIN-1 and the expression of p53 in PanIN-3, when compared with those in BilIN of a corresponding grade. These results suggest that cholangiocarcinoma and pancreatic ductal adenocarcinoma share, at least in part, a common carcinogenic process and further confirm that BilIN can be regarded as the biliary counterpart of PanIN.

1. Introduction

Cholangiocarcinoma that arises under conditions of chronic biliary diseases such as hepatolithiasis often undergoes the multistep carcinogenesis process [1]. Biliary intraepithelial neoplasia (BilIN) is known as a premalignant lesion of cholangiocarcinoma that represents the multistep cholangiocarcinogenesis [2]. The classification is applicable to flat atypical epithelial lesions in the intrahepatic large bile ducts and the extrahepatic bile ducts, and it is also applied to lesions in the gallbladder according to the current World Health Organization (WHO) classification for tumors of the digestive system [3].

BilIN is a concept that is proposed based on the morphological resemblance to pancreatic intraepithelial neoplasia (PanIN). Similar to PanIN, BilIN is classified into three grades according to the degree of cytological and architectural atypia: BilIN-1 (low-grade lesions), BilIN-2 (intermediate-grade lesions), and BilIN-3 (high-grade lesions, carcinoma in situ). Using the BilIN classification, there is increasing evidence that molecular and genetic alterations accumulate during the progression of BilIN to cholangiocarcinoma [4–7].

Since the biliary tract and pancreas share a common developmental process as well as morphological characteristics as duct systems, it is plausible that some biliary and pancreatic diseases show similar pathological features and biological behaviors [8]. Indeed, our recent comparative analysis showed that hilar cholangiocarcinoma and ductal adenocarcinoma of the pancreas share many clinicopathological features [9]. In addition, we showed that intraductal papillary neoplasm of the bile duct (IPNB) and intraductal papillary mucinous neoplasm (IPMN) of the pancreas, as well as mucinous cystic neoplasm (MCN) of the biliary tract and pancreas, exhibit similar immunohistochemical phenotypes, suggesting a common carcinogenic process of the tumors [10], where all these tumors were classified as premalignant lesions according to the current WHO classification.

TABLE 1: Primary antibodies used for immunohistochemical analysis.

Antigen	Clone	Company	Dilution	Antigen retrieval
MUC1	DF3	Toray Fuji Bionics (Tokyo, Japan)	1:50	MW
MUC2	Ccp58	Novocastra (Newcastle, UK)	1:100	MW
MUC5AC	CLH2	Novocastra	1:200	MW
Cytokeratin 20	Ks 20.8	DakoCytomation (Glostrup, Denmark)	1:50	MW
Cyclin D1	SP4	Nichirei (Tokyo, Japan)	Prediluted	MW*
p21	EPR3993	Abcam (Cambridge, UK)	1:100	MW
p53	DO-7	DakoCytomation	1:100	MW
S100P	EPR6143	Abcam	1:100	MW

MW: microwaving in 10 nmol/L citrate buffer (pH 6.0) for 20 minutes; MW*: microwaving in tris-ethylenediaminetetraacetic acid buffer (pH 9.0) for 20 minutes.

As far as the histological characteristics of BilIN and PanIN are concerned, previous studies have examined their features individually, and detailed data on comparative analysis of BilIN and PanIN are lacking. This study was therefore conducted to clarify the histological characteristics of BilIN with respect to PanIN.

2. Materials and Methods

2.1. Tissue Preparation. Hepatolithiatic livers associated with perihilar cholangiocarcinoma were used as a model of multistep cholangiocarcinogenesis. A total of 25 hepatolithiatic livers with cholangiocarcinoma and a total of 22 pancreatic specimens with pancreatic ductal adenocarcinoma were retrieved from the files of our laboratory and affiliated hospitals. The patients were selected during the period between 1997 and 2007. All cases were surgically resected, and all liver and pancreatic specimens were histologically accompanied by BilIN and PanIN, respectively. In all cases of cholangiocarcinoma, the main part of the tumor was located in hilar or perihilar region of the liver, and they appeared to arise from the intrahepatic large bile ducts or the right or left hepatic bile duct. Most cholangiocarcinoma cases showed macroscopic features of mass-forming type and/or intraductal growth type. Foci of BilIN were microscopically located in the intrahepatic large bile ducts and the hepatic bile ducts, and they were not observed in the septal and interlobular bile ducts. The mean age and sex distribution (male-female ratio) of the patients were 62 years and 11:14 for the liver specimens and 68 years and 12:10 for the pancreatic specimens, respectively. The samples were fixed in 10% neutral formalin and embedded in paraffin. Then, 4-μm-thick paraffin-embedded sections were prepared. One representative section from each case was used.

2.2. Histochemistry and Immunohistochemistry. Alcian blue (at pH 2.5) was used for mucin staining. Immunostaining was performed using the sections with the primary antibodies listed in Table 1. After the blocking of endogenous peroxidase, the sections were incubated in protein block solution (DakoCytomation, Glostrup, Denmark). They were then incubated overnight at 4°C with each of the primary antibodies. Their sources, optimal dilution, and antigen retrieval methods are shown in Table 1. They were treated with secondary antibodies conjugated to a peroxidase-labeled polymer using the HISTOFINE system (Nichirei, Tokyo, Japan). Color development was performed using 3,3′-diaminobenzidine tetrahydrochloride, and the sections were lightly counterstained with hematoxylin. Negative controls consisted of substitution of the primary antibodies with nonimmune serum and were consistently negative.

2.3. Histological Assessment. Semiquantitative analysis of the stained sections was performed. Staining intensity was evaluated in a high-power field for the neoplastic and nonneoplastic epithelia of the bile ducts and pancreatic ducts. From the sections of 25 liver specimens and 22 pancreatic specimens, foci of interest were selected. The number of foci examined was as follows: nonneoplastic large bile duct, 14; BilIN-1, 17; BilIN-2/3, 24, invasive carcinoma (cholangiocarcinoma), 50; nonneoplastic pancreatic duct, 13; PanIN-1, 22; PanIN-2/3, 15; invasive carcinoma (pancreatic ductal adenocarcinoma), 44.

For mucin staining with Alcian blue (pH 2.5), the signal intensity in the cytoplasm and/or on the luminal surface of the epithelial cells was evaluated using the following grading system: 1+ (mild), 2+ (moderate), and 3+ (marked). The cytoplasmic and/or luminal immunostaining of MUC1 and the cytoplasmic immunostaining of MUC2 and MUC5AC were graded as follows: 0 (negative), 1+ (mild to moderate), and 2+ (marked). For evaluation of the nuclear staining of cyclin D1, p21, p53, and S100P, the percentage of positive nuclei to the total number of nuclei of the epithelial cells was calculated, and it was graded as follows: 0 (negative), 1+ (not exceeding 10%), and 2+ (more than 10%). For p53 nuclear staining, only the proportion of intensely positive nuclei was scored.

2.4. Statistics. Statistical significance was determined using the Mann-Whitney U-test. A P value less than 0.05 was accepted as the level of statistical significance.

3. Results and Discussion

Morphological appearances such as loss of nuclear polarity, increased nucleus-to-cytoplasm ratio, nuclear hyperchromasia, and architectural atypia were basically similar between

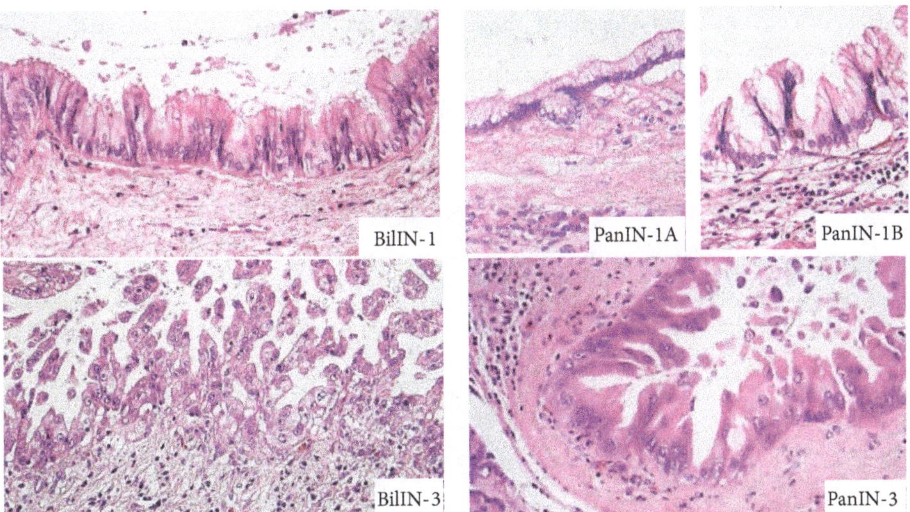

FIGURE 1: Histology of biliary intraepithelial neoplasia (BilIN) and pancreatic intraepithelial neoplasia (PanIN). Representative images of BilIN-1 and BilIN-3 and PanIN-1A, PanIN-1B, and PanIN-3 are shown. Hematoxylin and eosin staining. Original magnifications, ×400.

the corresponding grades of BilIN and PanIN, which were observed in sections stained with hematoxylin and eosin (Figure 1).

Mucin staining with Alcian blue (pH 2.5) showed that both BilIN and PanIN frequently had cytoplasmic and/or luminal surface mucin (Figure 2). According to the grade of BilIN and PanIN, PanIN-1 tended to have more abundant cytoplasmic mucin than BilIN-1, and the results of semi-quantitative analysis confirmed this tendency (Figure 3). The abundant mucin expression in PanIN-1 is consistent with the definition of PanIN-1 in which the lesion is composed of tall columnar cells with basally located nuclei and abundant supranuclear mucin [11].

The immunohistochemical expression of MUC1 was increased along with the increase in the grade of BilIN and PanIN, and no significant difference in its expression status was observed between BilIN and PanIN (Figures 2 and 3). Similarly, the expression of MUC5AC was frequently observed in all grades of both BilIN and PanIN (Figures 2 and 3). The results of the expression status of MUC1 and MUC5AC in BilIN were almost identical to those in our previous report [4].

Focal immunohistochemical expression of MUC2 was observed in several foci of BilIN, whereas MUC2 positivity was exceptional in PanIN (Figures 2 and 3). Although the expression of CK20 was typically negative in both BilIN and PanIN in this study (data not shown), BilIN is not infrequently associated with metaplastic change of intestinal type, while intestinal-type PanIN is generally not found [12, 13]. These observations may explain the focal MUC2 expression in BilIN rather than in PanIN.

The results of immunostaining of MUC1, MUC2, MUC5AC, and CK20 for BilIN and PanIN in this study are summarized in Table 2. For comparison, the results of our previous comparative analysis that examined the immunohistochemical characteristics of IPNB, IPMN of the pancreas, hepatic MCN, and pancreatic MCN [10] are also shown in Table 2. It is noteworthy that all of these premalignant lesions show similar immunoprofiles to each other between the biliary tract and pancreas, supporting the concept that BilIN, IPNB, and hepatic MCN are biliary counterparts of PanIN, IPMN, and pancreatic MCN, respectively.

As for the expression of cell cycle-related molecules, the immunohistochemical expression of cyclin D1 and p21 was absent or focal in nonneoplastic epithelium of the bile ducts and the pancreatic ducts. They were occasionally observed in BilIN-1 and PanIN-1 and more frequently in BilIN-2/3 and PanIN-2/3 (Figures 2 and 3), in which the frequency of the expression of cyclin D1 and p21 in BilIN in this study was comparable to that in our previous report [5]. Semiquantitative analysis showed that there was no significant difference in their expression status between BilIN and PanIN.

The expression of p53 was not observed in nonneoplastic epithelium of the bile ducts and the pancreatic ducts, as well as in BilIN-1/2 and PanIN-1/2. By contrast, BilIN-3 and PanIN-3 occasionally showed the expression of p53, and its frequency was significantly higher in PanIN-3 than in BilIN-3 (Figures 2 and 3). Because the process of carcinogenesis is often complicated by inflammatory changes in the biliary tract, the molecular alterations may be more complex in BilIN due to cholangitis than those seen in PanIN, where the influence of inflammation is usually insignificant in the development of pancreatic cancer. In fact, our recent study showed that the detection rate of *KRAS* mutation in BilIN was not as high as that seen in PanIN [6]. Therefore, it is predicted that factors other than genetic alterations may also affect the process of the development of BilIN and cholangiocarcinoma.

S100P is a molecule that is highly expressed by perihilar and extrahepatic cholangiocarcinoma as well as pancreatic ductal adenocarcinoma [9, 14]. In this study, the expression of S100P was frequently observed in both BilIN and PanIN of all grades (Figure 2). Semiquantitative analysis showed that its

Table 2: Immunoprofiles of premalignant lesions of the biliary tract and pancreas.

	Intraepithelial neoplasia		Intraductal papillary neoplasm		Mucinous cystic neoplasm	
	BilIN	PanIN	IPNB	IPMN	Hepatic MCN	Pancreatic MCN
MUC1	+	+	+	+	+	+
MUC2	+	−	+	+	−	−
MUC5AC	++	++	++	++	++	++
CK20	−	−	+	+	−	−

The results of comparative analysis for biliary and pancreatic neoplasms in the present study and our previous report (10) are summarized. −: likely absent; +: occasionally present; ++: usually present. BilIN: biliary intraepithelial neoplasia; CK: cytokeratin; IPMN: intraductal papillary mucinous neoplasm; IPNB: intraductal papillary neoplasm of the bile duct; MCN: mucinous cystic neoplasm; PanIN: pancreatic intraepithelial neoplasia.

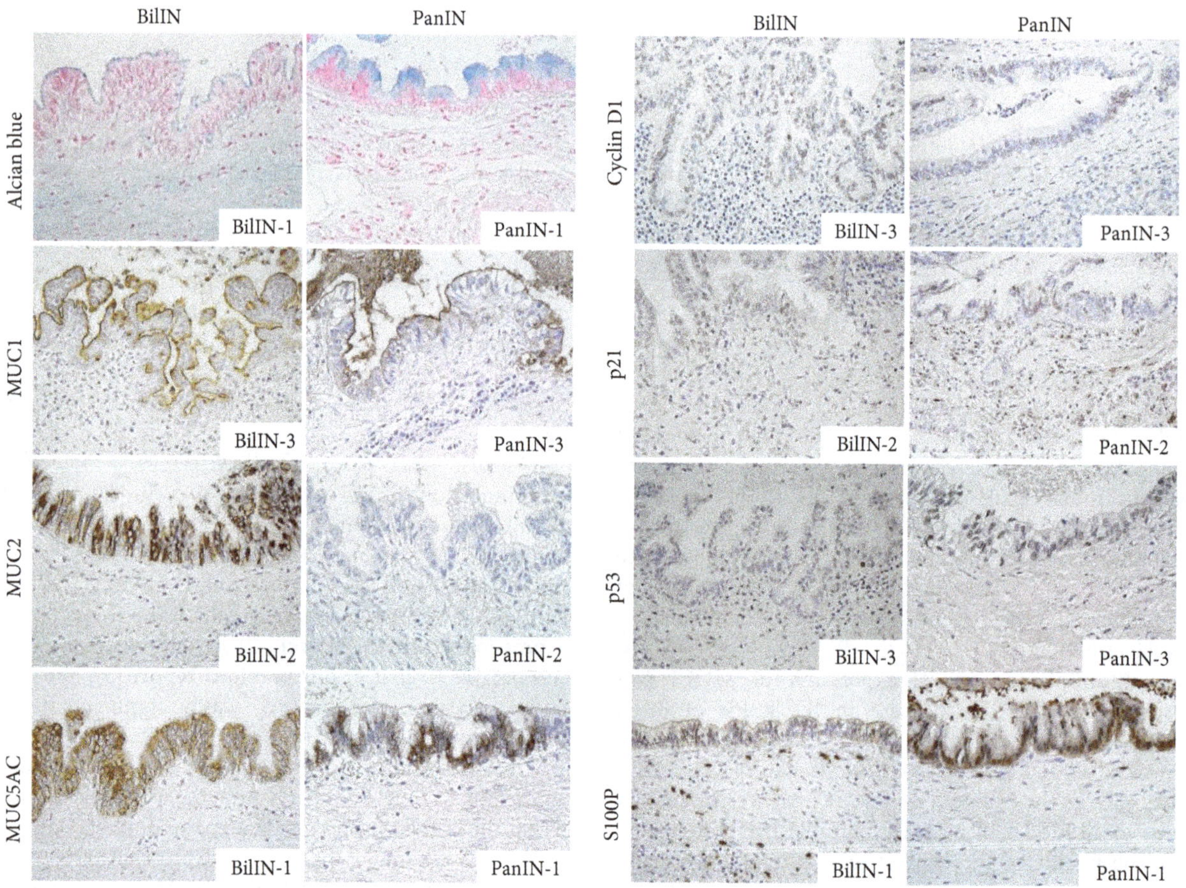

Figure 2: Representative images of histochemical and immunohistochemical staining. The results of mucin staining with Alcian blue (pH 2.5) and immunostaining of MUC1, MUC2, MUC5AC, cyclin D1, p21, p53, and S100P for biliary intraepithelial neoplasia (BilIN) and pancreatic intraepithelial neoplasia (PanIN) are shown. Original magnifications, ×400.

expression was significantly high in PanIN-1 compared with that in BilIN-1, although both BilIN-1 and PanIN-1 exhibited a high frequency of S100P expression (Figure 3).

Most of the molecules examined in this study showed similar expression patterns in BilIN and PanIN. There were significant differences in the increase in mucin production and the expression of S100P in PanIN-1 and the expression of p53 in PanIN-3, when compared with those in BilIN of corresponding grade.

The immunohistochemical expression of MUC1, cyclin D1, p21, p53, and S100P tended to be increased in invasive foci of cholangiocarcinoma and pancreatic ductal adenocarcinoma when compared to those in BilIN-2/3 and PanIN-2/3, respectively (Figure 3). These results were consistent with the concept of multistep carcinogenesis.

4. Conclusions

BilIN and PanIN showed similar histological and immunohistochemical features with several exceptions. These results suggest that cholangiocarcinoma and pancreatic ductal adenocarcinoma share, at least in part, a common carcinogenic

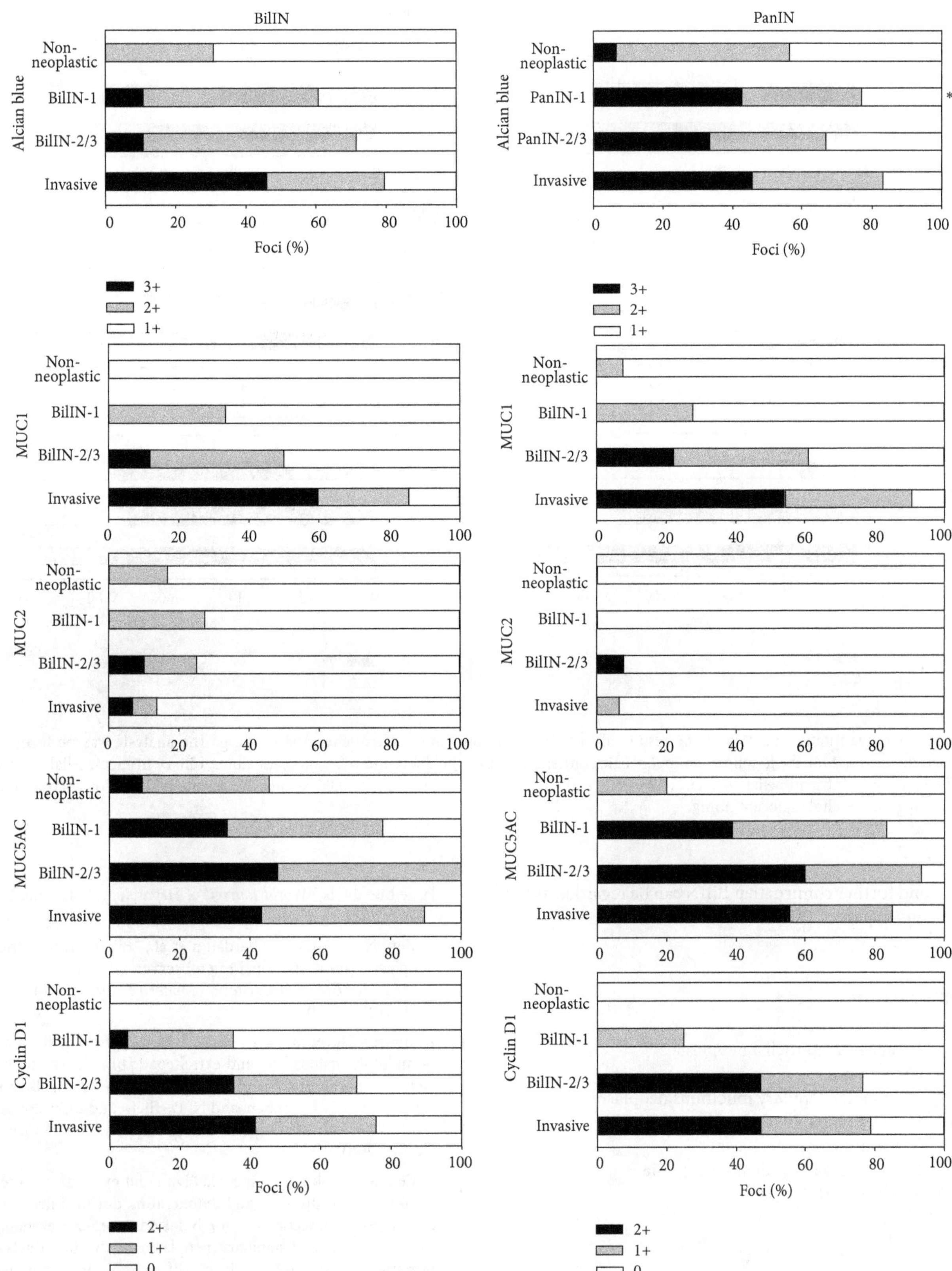

FIGURE 3: Continued.

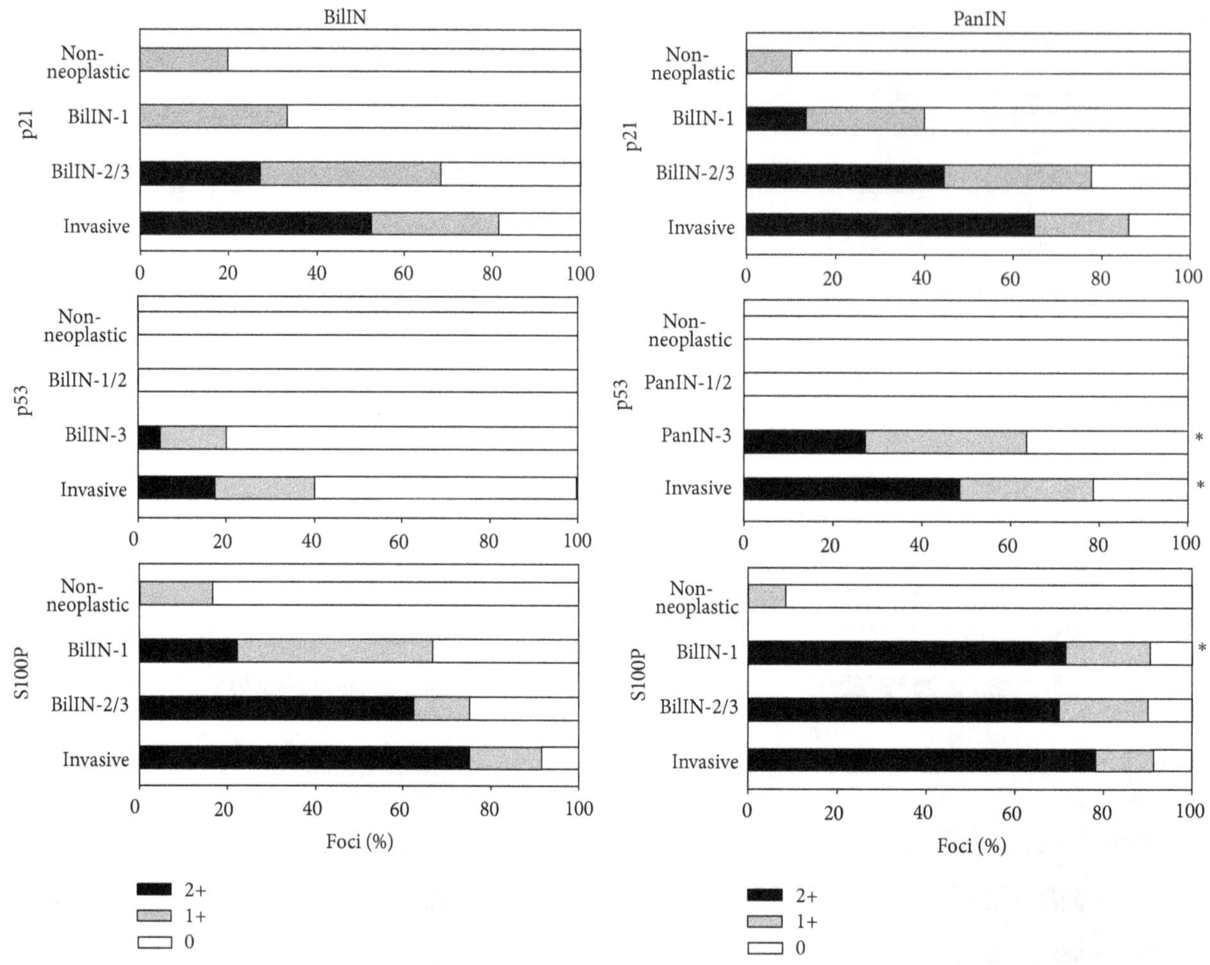

Figure 3: Semiquantitative analysis of the results of histochemical and immunohistochemical staining. The analysis was performed as described in Section 2 for the lesions of nonneoplastic epithelium of the bile ducts and the pancreatic ducts, biliary intraepithelial neoplasia (BilIN), pancreatic intraepithelial neoplasia (PanIN), and invasive carcinoma. $^{*}P < 0.05$ versus the results of BilIN of corresponding histological grade or cholangiocarcinoma.

process and further confirm that BilIN can be regarded as the biliary counterpart of PanIN.

Abbreviations

BilIN: Biliary intraepithelial neoplasia
CK: Cytokeratin
IPMN: Intraductal papillary mucinous neoplasm
IPNB: Intraductal papillary neoplasm of the bile duct
MCN: Mucinous cystic neoplasm
PanIN: Pancreatic intraepithelial neoplasia
WHO: World Health Organization.

References

[1] Y. Nakanuma, M. Sasaki, Y. Sato et al., "Multistep carcinogenesis of perihilar cholangiocarcinoma arising in the intrahepatic large bile ducts," *World Journal of Hepatology*, vol. 1, no. 1, pp. 35–42, 2009.

[2] Y. Zen, N. V. Adsay, K. Bardadin et al., "Biliary intraepithelial neoplasia: an international interobserver agreement study and proposal for diagnostic criteria," *Modern Pathology*, vol. 20, no. 6, pp. 701–709, 2007.

[3] J. Albores-Saavedra, N. V. Adsay, J. M. Crawford et al., "Carcinoma of the gallbladder and extrahepatic bile ducts," in *WHO Classification of Tumors of the Digestive System*, F. T. Bosman, F. Carneiro, R. H. Hruban, and N. D. Theise, Eds., pp. 266–273, IARC, World Health Organization of Tumors, Lyon, France, 4th edition, 2010.

[4] Y. Zen, M. Sasaki, T. Fujii et al., "Different expression patterns of mucin core proteins and cytokeratins during intrahepatic cholangiocarcinogenesis from biliary intraepithelial neoplasia and intraductal papillary neoplasm of the bile duct—an immunohistochemical study of 110 cases of hepatolithiasis," *Journal of Hepatology*, vol. 44, no. 2, pp. 350–358, 2006.

[5] Y. Nakanishi, Y. Zen, S. Kondo, T. Itoh, K. Itatsu, and Y. Nakanuma, "Expression of cell cycle-related molecules in biliary premalignant lesions: biliary intraepithelial neoplasia and

biliary intraductal papillary neoplasm," *Human Pathology*, vol. 39, no. 8, pp. 1153–1161, 2008.

[6] M. Hsu, M. Sasaki, S. Igarashi, Y. Sato, and Y. Nakanuma, "KRAS and GNAS mutations and p53 overexpression in biliary intraepithelial neoplasia and intrahepatic cholangiocarcinomas," *Cancer*, vol. 119, no. 9, pp. 1669–1674, 2013.

[7] Y. Sato, M. Sasaki, K. Harada et al., "Pathological diagnosis of flat epithelial lesions of the biliary tract with emphasis on biliary intraepithelial neoplasia," *Journal of Gastroenterology*, vol. 49, no. 1, pp. 64–72, 2014.

[8] Y. Nakanuma, K. Harada, M. Sasaki, and Y. Sato, "Proposal of a new disease concept "biliary diseases with pancreatic counterparts" Anatomical and pathological bases," *Histology and Histopathology*, vol. 29, no. 1, pp. 1–10, 2014.

[9] C. Gandou, K. Harada, Y. Sato et al., "Hilar cholangiocarcinoma and pancreatic ductal adenocarcinoma share similar histopathologies, immunophenotypes, and development-related molecules," *Human Pathology*, vol. 44, no. 5, pp. 811–821, 2013.

[10] T. Matsubara, Y. Sato, M. Sasaki et al., "Immunohistochemical characteristics and malignant progression of hepatic cystic neoplasms in comparison with pancreatic counterparts," *Human Pathology*, vol. 43, no. 12, pp. 2177–2186, 2012.

[11] R. H. Hruban, G. Klöppel, P. Boffetta et al., "Ductal adenocarcinoma of the pancreas," in *WHO Classification of Tumors of the Digestive System*, F. T. Bosman, F. Carneiro, R. H. Hruban, and N. D. Theise, Eds., pp. 281–291, IARC, World Health Organization of Tumors, Lyon, France, 4th edition, 2010.

[12] Y. Sato, K. Harada, M. Sasaki, and Y. Nakanuma, "Histological characteristics of biliary intraepithelial neoplasia-3 and intraepithelial spread of cholangiocarcinoma," *Virchows Archiv*, vol. 462, no. 4, pp. 421–427, 2013.

[13] J. Albores-Saavedra, J. Wu, T. Crook, R. H. Amirkhan, L. Jones, and R. H. Hruban, "Intestinal and oncocytic variants of pancreatic intraepithelial neoplasia. A morphological and immunohistochemical study," *Annals of Diagnostic Pathology*, vol. 9, no. 2, pp. 69–76, 2005.

[14] Y. Sato, K. Harada, M. Sasaki, and Y. Nakanuma, "Clinicopathological significance of S100 protein expression in cholangiocarcinoma," *Journal of Gastroenterology and Hepatology*, vol. 28, no. 8, pp. 1422–1429, 2013.

14

Intraductal Papillary Neoplasms of the Bile Duct

Masayuki Ohtsuka,[1] Hiroaki Shimizu,[1] Atsushi Kato,[10] Hideyuki Yoshitomi,[1] Katsunori Furukawa,[1] Toshio Tsuyuguchi,[2] Yuji Sakai,[2] Osamu Yokosuka,[2] and Masaru Miyazaki[1]

[1] *Department of General Surgery, Graduate School of Medicine, Chiba University, 1-8-1 Inohana, Chuoh-ku, Chiba 260-8670, Japan*
[2] *Department of Medicine and Clinical Oncology, Graduate School of Medicine, Chiba University, Chiba 260-8670, Japan*

Correspondence should be addressed to Masayuki Ohtsuka; otsuka-m@faculty.chiba-u.jp

Academic Editor: Valérie Paradis

Intraductal papillary neoplasm of the bile duct (IPNB) is a rare variant of bile duct tumors characterized by papillary growth within the bile duct lumen and is regarded as a biliary counterpart of intraductal papillary mucinous neoplasm of the pancreas. IPNBs display a spectrum of premalignant lesion towards invasive cholangiocarcinoma. The most common radiologic findings for IPNB are bile duct dilatation and intraductal masses. The major treatment of IPNB is surgical resection. Ultrasonography, computed tomography, magnetic resonance image, and cholangiography are usually performed to assess tumor location and extension. Cholangioscopy can confirm the histology and assess the extent of the tumor including superficial spreading along the biliary epithelium. However, pathologic diagnosis by preoperative biopsy cannot always reflect the maximum degree of atypia, because IPNBs are often composed of varying degrees of cytoarchitectural atypia. IPNBs are microscopically classified into four epithelial subtypes, such as pancreatobiliary, intestinal, gastric, and oncocytic types. Most cases of IPNB are IPN with high-grade intraepithelial neoplasia or with an associated invasive carcinoma. The histologic types of invasive lesions are either tubular adenocarcinoma or mucinous carcinoma. Although several authors have investigated molecular genetic changes during the development and progression of IPNB, these are still poorly characterized and controversial.

1. Introduction

Intraductal papillary neoplasm of the bile duct (IPNB) is a rare variant of bile duct tumors, which is characterized by papillary or villous growth within the bile duct lumen.

Formerly, attention has been drawn to biliary tumors with macroscopically visible mucin secretion, which show predominantly papillary growth within the dilated bile duct lumen and secrete a large amount of mucin. These tumors were called by various names, such as mucin-producing cholangiocarcinoma [1–4], mucin-hypersecreting bile duct tumor [5], and intraductal papillary mucinous tumor of the bile duct [6, 7], and were identified as a biliary counterpart of intraductal papillary mucinous neoplasm (IPMN) of the pancreas. On the other hand, biliary intraductal tumors without macroscopically visible mucin secretion are also known, which have a macroscopically recognizable papillary or granular structure but no clinically visible mucin secretion. Since certain morphological features of these tumors, especially intraductal papillary growth pattern, are also similar to those of IPMN of the pancreas, Zen et al. [8] proposed that they, together with tumors with macroscopically visible mucin secretion, may belong to a single tumor entity named IPNB. Now, IPNB was adopted in the 2010 World Health Organization (WHO) classification [9] as a distinct clinical and pathologic entity. In this review, we describe the concept, clinical and pathologic features, and pathogenesis of IPNB.

2. Concept of IPNB

2.1. Definition of IPNB. IPNB is defined as a biliary epithelial tumor with exophytic nature exhibiting papillary mass within the bile duct lumen and with prominent intraductal growth pattern. IPNB can develop anywhere along the biliary tree,

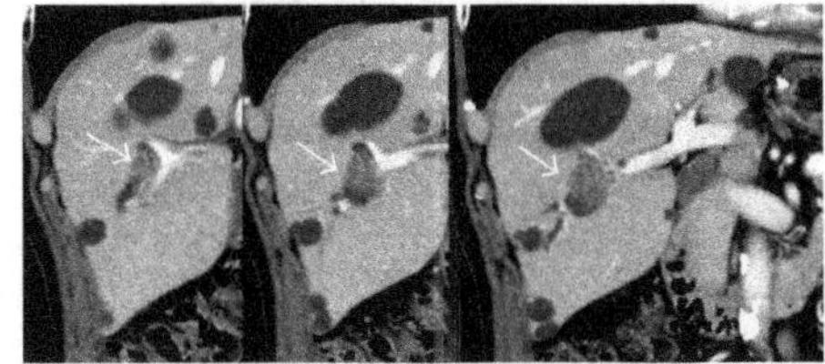

FIGURE 1: Representative images of intraductal papillary neoplasm of the bile duct on computed tomography. Localized bile duct dilatation and an intraductal mass are shown (arrows).

including both intrahepatic and extrahepatic bile ducts. Mucin hypersecretion and dilatation of the bile duct are sometimes encountered. Microscopically, IPNB is composed of papillary fronds with fine vascular cores. Neoplastic epithelial cells display a spectrum of cytoarchitectural atypia ranging from none to borderline to marked and also can be associated with invasive carcinoma. Due to these features, IPNB is regarded as a premalignant lesion towards invasive cholangiocarcinoma. In the WHO classification [9], IPNB is classified into IPN with low- or intermediate-grade intraepithelial neoplasia, IPN with high-grade intraepithelial neoplasia, and IPN with an associated invasive carcinoma. This classification is similar to that of IPMN of the pancreas, and an analogous multistep progression model is assumed in IPNB.

2.2. Diseases Included in IPNB. Before inclusion of IPNB in the WHO classification, many different terms have been used for the spectrum of this entity. These include biliary papilloma/papillomatosis, some of the intraductal growth type of cholangiocarcinoma and papillary carcinoma of the extrahepatic bile duct, and some of the biliary cystadenoma/cystadenocarcinoma. Among the intraductal growth type of intrahepatic cholangiocarcinoma and papillary carcinoma of the extrahepatic bile duct, cases with intraductal component composed of papillary fronds with fine vascular cores are exclusively included in IPNB. In the previous categories of biliary cystadenoma/cystadenocarcinoma, cystic tumors with bile duct communication and absence of ovarian-like stroma are considered as a cystic variant of IPNB [10].

3. Clinical Features

3.1. Clinical Characteristics. The prevalence of IPNB shows wide geographic variation. The highest incidence is reported in Far Eastern countries, probably because hepatolithiasis and clonorchiasis that are believed to be major risk factors of IPNB are endemic. IPNB is relatively rare and comprises 9–38% of all bile duct carcinomas [11–15]. Most patients are between 50 and 70 years of age [11–18] and show a slight male predominance in most reported series [12–14, 16–18]. Intermittent abdominal pain and acute cholangitis or jaundice are the most common clinical manifestations [11–13, 16, 18, 19], but certain frequency (5–29%) of patients have no symptoms [12, 13, 16, 18, 19]. Around 30% of patients have a previous history or concomitant existence of biliary stones, as shown in the reports from Far Eastern countries [12, 16, 20], but not from Western countries [13].

Tumor location varies by a report. Some reports showed that the majority of IPNB was located at the intrahepatic bile duct [16, 17], whereas the other showed that the most common location of IPNB was the hepatic hilum [13]. Despite these variable locations, IPNB tends to be found in the left-sided biliary ductal system, when IPNB exists in the intrahepatic bile duct, due to unknown reasons [13, 20, 21].

3.2. Radiologic Findings. The most common radiologic findings for IPNB are bile duct dilatation and intraductal masses (Figure 1). The patterns of bile duct dilatation are diffuse duct ectasia, localized duct dilatation, and cystic dilatation, which can be recognized by ultrasonography (US), computed tomography (CT), and magnetic resonance image (MRI). These modalities can also detect intraductal masses, although its sensitivity is reported to be in the range of 41.2–97% [22–24]. MRI images reveal IPNB as iso- to hypointense masses on T1-weighted image and hyperintense masses on T2-weighted image [24]. The enhancement pattern on CT scan is isodense or hyperdense during the late arterial phase and not hyperdense during the portal-venous and delayed phase, as compared with normal hepatic parenchyma [23]. Mucin, even if it exists, cannot be detected on US, CT, and MRI.

Direct cholangiography such as endoscopic retrograde cholangiography (ERC) is useful for the detection of mucobilia (Figure 2(a)) that is seen in nearly one-third of patients with IPNB, evidenced by diffuse dilatation of the bile duct with amorphous filling defect [6], and duodenoscopy shows a dilated papillary orifice with mucin (Figure 2(b)). However, the thick mucin that filled the dilated biliary tree often prevents the visualization of intraductal tumors [6, 25, 26]. In cases with IPNB without excessive mucin production, cholangiography can define the tumors as irregular filling defects.

Cholangioscopy including percutaneous transhepatic cholangioscopy (PTCS) and peroral cholangioscopy (POCS) can approach the bile duct directly, and it can confirm the histology and assess the extent of the tumor including superficial spreading along the biliary epithelium (Figure 3), which provides information to choose appropriate treatment [22], although an accurate diagnosis of the maximum degree of cytoarchitectural atypia cannot be always made by biopsy because of the existence of mixed pathologic findings in the same lesion. POCS is advantageous in the fact that it can be performed without serious complications, such as catheter dislodgement, hemobilia, and tumor seeding of the sinus tract caused by PTCS [25, 27]. In cases with IPNB with abundant mucin, however, PTCS seems to be more useful than POCS, because discrimination of the location and extent of a tumor may be difficult by POCS in some cases [27].

Intraductal ultrasonography (IDUS) is a simple method for diagnosing the location of IPNB and assessing the depth of invasion, even in the presence of thick mucin. However, IDUS image is sometimes difficult to interpret, since coexisting

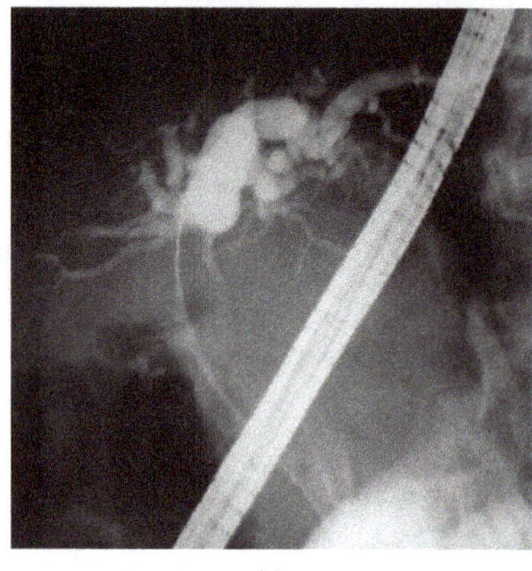

(a)

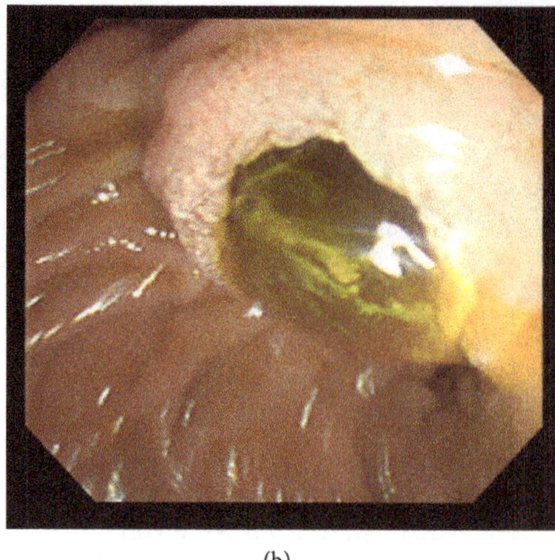

(b)

FIGURE 2: A representative case of intraductal papillary neoplasm of the bile duct with mucin hypersecretion. (a) Endoscopic retrograde cholangiogram. Diffuse dilatation of the common bile duct with amorphous filling defect is shown. (b) Duodenoscopy shows a dilated papillary orifice with mucin.

biliary sludge may have an appearance like that of elevated tumors. Furthermore, it is difficult to distinguish between inflammatory wall thickness and the superficial spreading of a tumor [25].

3.3. Treatment. Unlike patients with IPMNs of the pancreas, all patients with IPNB should be considered to treat, because papillary tumors and associated mucin often cause recurrent cholangitis and obstructive jaundice, even if these tumors are not malignant. Patients without distant metastasis are considered for surgical resection. In order to choose appropriate surgical procedure, exact preoperative assessment of tumor location and extension is important. In particular, for evaluating of the extent of superficial spreading, cholangioscopic observation and biopsy might be essential. The depth of invasion and the presence of lymph node involvement are also assessed preoperatively by CT, cholangiography, and IDUS.

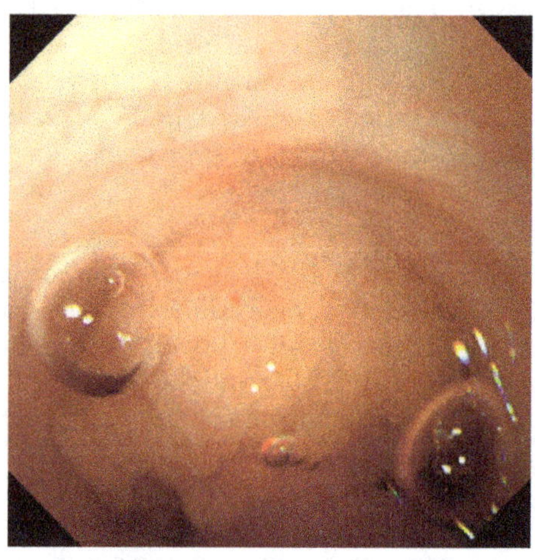

FIGURE 3: Peroral cholangioscopy reveals a papillary tumor within the lumen of the bile duct, but no obvious superficial spreading along the biliary epithelium is observed.

In principle, IPNBs should be resected in a manner similar to that employed for other types of intrahepatic cholangiocarcinomas and extrahepatic bile duct carcinomas. That is, major hepatectomy with or without extrahepatic bile duct resection or pancreaticoduodenectomy should be chosen as surgical procedure. Even though it is suspected that the tumor is premalignant, a similar strategy should be considered, because pathologic diagnosis by preoperative biopsy cannot always reflect the maximum degree of cytoarchitectural atypia. Intraoperative frozen section at the stumps of the bile duct is essential to confirm cancer-free surgical margin. Regional lymphadenectomy should also be performed.

On the other hand, in cases of IPNB with low- to high-grade intraepithelial neoplasia and limited superficial spreading and precise diagnosis which is completed preoperatively, limited resections preserving organ functions, for example, extensive hilar bile duct resection using a transhepatic approach [28, 29], can be considered as a choice among surgical procedures, although these should always be contingent on a careful intraoperative final assessment. In contrast, in cases of IPNB with extensive superficial spreading that may have positive margins or IPNB with multifocal involvement, tumor recurrence may occur with a high risk after surgical resection. In such cases, resection for the whole biliary tree by liver transplantation and pancreaticoduodenectomy can be theoretically regarded as the only curative treatment [30]. However, liver transplantation should not be performed in patients with advanced tumor invasion or with positive lymph nodes. Since accurate preoperative assessment of IPNB is usually difficult, indication of liver transplantation for patients with IPNB is very limited.

4. Pathologic Features

4.1. Macroscopic Findings. The most common macroscopic findings of IPNB are singular, or occasionally multiple, polypoid masses elevating into the lumen of the dilated bile duct and/or clinically visible granular or small papillary mucosa (Figure 4(a)). Polypoid masses occasionally extend longitudinally and fill the lumen of the bile duct, showing cast-like appearance. Multilocular, rarely unilocular, well-defined cystic mass, which contains mucinous fluid, is another manifestation of IPNB (Figure 4(b)). The internal surfaces of cystic masses are generally smooth or finely granular, and papillary mural nodules are commonly observed. Anatomic communication with the bile duct is sometimes difficult to confirm.

4.2. Microscopic Findings

4.2.1. Conventional Histology. Prominent papillary proliferation with delicate fibrovascular cores is a characteristic finding (Figure 5). Coexistence of tubulopapillary architecture can be found in IPNB, especially without mucin hypersecretion [12]. Similar to IPMNs of the pancreas, IPNBs are classified into four epithelial subtypes (Figure 5), such as pancreatobiliary, intestinal, gastric, and oncocytic types, of the intraductal component [12–14, 16, 31]. The most frequent subtype is pancreatobiliary, followed by intestinal in all IPNBs, whereas IPNBs with mucin hypersecretion are more prevalent in the intestinal subtype than those without mucin hypersecretion [12]. The pancreatobiliary or the intestinal type is commonly associated with histologic grade of more than high-grade intraepithelial neoplasia, and, therefore, most cases of IPNB are IPN with high-grade intraepithelial neoplasia or IPN with an associated invasive carcinoma. The histologic types of invasive lesions are either tubular adenocarcinoma or mucinous (colloid) carcinoma [8]. Mucinous carcinoma usually arises in association with the intestinal type of IPNB.

IPNBs, however, often exhibited marked variation in histologic grade between different regions of individual tumors, making an accurate preoperative diagnosis difficult. This feature is significantly more common in IPNBs with mucin hypersecretion than those without [12].

IPNBs manifesting cystic mass have similar morphological features to biliary mucinous cystic neoplasms. These two entities are histologically distinct. Biliary mucinous cystic neoplasms have densely cellular connective tissue resembling ovarian stroma (ovarian-like stroma) in their wall, whereas this is never seen in IPNBs [10, 32].

4.2.2. Immunohistochemical Phenotypes (Table 1). Immunohistochemical mucin core proteins are reported to be associated with epithelial subtypes in IPMN of the pancreas. Similarly, MUC1 is often detected in the pancreatobiliary type of IPNBs, but very few are expressed in the intestinal or gastric type. MUC2 is primarily expressed in the intestinal type of IPNBs compared to the pancreatobiliary or the gastric type. MUC5AC expression is common in all epithelial subtypes, including the oncocytic type. In the oncocytic type of IPNBs, MUC1 expression is focally seen [16].

Some cytokeratin is also associated with epithelial subtypes. Cytokeratin 20 is expressed in the intestinal type of IPNBs with high frequency but not in the gastric type. High expression of cytokeratin 7 is observed in the gastric type of IPNBs [33].

5. Pathogenesis

5.1. Molecular Events during Development and Progression of IPNB (Tables 2 and 3). IPNBs derive from normal epithelium of the bile duct and progress through low-, intermediate-, and high-grade intraepithelial neoplasia to invasive carcinoma. During this process, cumulative aberrations in gene expression may be associated. However, these aberrations are still poorly characterized, and it is also not well known whether progression pathways of biliary intraepithelial neoplasia (BilIN), a precursor associated with the development of nonpapillary invasive cholangiocarcinoma, and IPNB are regulated differently. Several authors have investigated molecular genetic changes during the development and progression of the IPNB lineage and compared them with those of the BilIN lineage. According to the results in these studies mentioned below, IPNB and BilIN lineages were suggested to display a lot of similarities, but some differences, in the molecular genetic changes, although there were some inconsistent data among the reports.

Cyclins D1 and p21, which are the regulators of cell cycle progression, seem to play an important role in the development and progression in both BilIN and IPNB lineages, since expressions of these molecules have been reported to increase with histologic progression from low-grade to invasive carcinoma in both IPNBs and BilINs. Itatsu et al. [34] found that the positive rate of cyclin D1 expression in the IPNB lineage (65%) was significantly higher than that in the BilIN lineage (20%), suggesting that cyclin D1 is more important to the IPNB lineage, whereas Nakanishi et al. [35] have not shown such differences. Aberrant expression of p16, another regulator of cell cycle progression, was also seen from an early phase in the development of both BilIN and IPNB lineages, although the frequency of positive cases was relatively low, and the expression reached a plateau despite histologic progression [36, 37].

C-myc, which is a transcriptional factor for modulating regulators of cell cycle progression and a target molecule of Wnt signaling pathway, is suggested to be more important in the progression of the IPNB lineage than in that of the BilIN lineage. The expression of c-myc was demonstrated to be in more than half of IPNBs [34]. Similarly, nuclear accumulation of β-catenin protein, indicating genetic alteration of Wnt signaling pathway, was found only in approximately 25% of IPNBs [34, 38], concluding that this is significantly involved in the progression of IPNBs but not BilINs. However, a recent report has shown an inconsistent conclusion, in which β-catenin protein accumulation in the nucleus is less important for the progression of IPNBs due to its infrequency (9%) [36].

v-Ki-ras2 Kirsten rat sarcoma viral oncogene homolog (KRAS) mutations are indicated to be an early event in IPNBs,

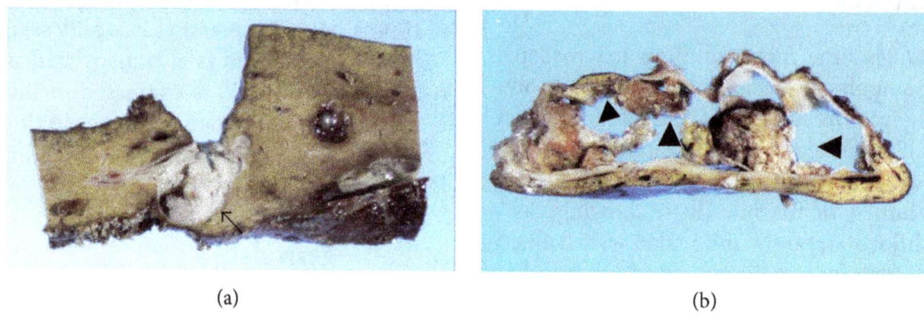

(a) (b)

FIGURE 4: Macroscopic findings of intraductal papillary neoplasm of the bile duct. (a) A polypoid mass (arrow) is elevated into the lumen of the bile duct. (b) Polypoid mural nodules (arrowheads) are observed in the well-defined cystic lesion. This lesion was communicated with the bile duct.

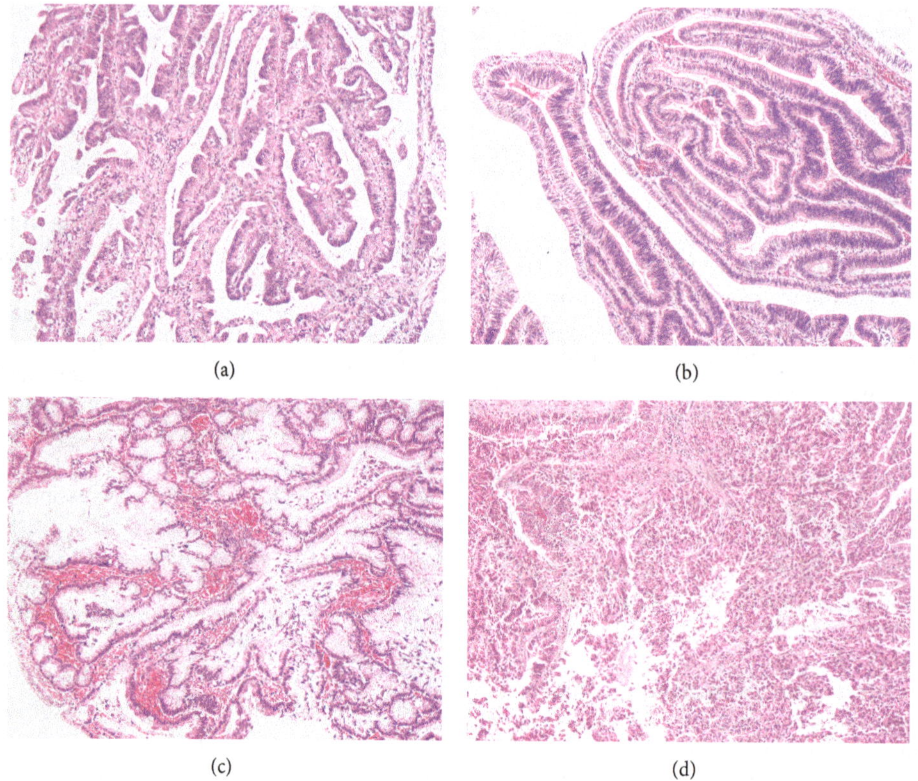

(a) (b) (c) (d)

FIGURE 5: Microscopic findings of intraductal papillary neoplasm of the bile duct. Prominent papillary proliferation with delicate fibrovascular cores is a characteristic feature. Epithelial subtypes are classified as pancreatobiliary (a), intestinal (b), gastric (c), and oncocytic (d).

TABLE 1: Immunohistochemical phenotypes in intraductal papillary neoplasms of the bile duct (IPNB) and intraductal papillary mucinous neoplasms of the pancreas (IPMN) [16, 33].

Epithelial subtypes	Mucin core proteins			Cytokeratin (CK)			
	MUC1	MUC2	MUC5AC	CK20		CK7	
				IPNB	IPMN	IPNB	IPMN
Gastric	−	−	+	0 (0/5)*	0 (0/10)	100 (5/5)	80 (8/10)
Intestinal	−	+	+	75 (3/4)	71 (12/17)	50 (2/4)	82 (14/17)
Pancreatobiliary	+	−	+	22 (2/9)	0 (0/2)	78 (7/9)	100 (2/2)
Oncocytic	− ~ +	− ~ +	+	0 (0/2)	N.D.	50 (1/2)	N.D.

*% of positive cases (positive cases/total cases examined); N.D.: not determined.

TABLE 2: Molecular events in the intraductal papillary neoplasms of the bile duct lineage and the biliary intraepithelial neoplasia lineage.

Authors	Cyclin D1		p16		c-myc		β-catenin		SMAD4/DPC4		p53			
	IPNB	BilIN	IPNB	BilIN	IPNB	BilIN	IPNB	BilIN	IPNB	BilIN	IPNB non-inv.	IPNB inv.	BilIN non-inv.	BilIN inv.
Itatsu et al. [34]	65 (17)*	20 (45)	N.D.		54 (13)	13 (45)	22 (18)	0 (45)	N.D.		N.D.			
Nakanishi et al. [35]	53 (10)	43 (11)	N.D.		N.D.		N.D.		21 (36)	27 (49)	38 (16)	36 (10)	8 (38)	82 (11)
Schlitter et al. [36]	N.D.		24 (42)	36 (22)	N.D.		9 (45)	0 (22)	7 (45)	14 (22)	60 (52)	85 (13)	N.D.	64 (22)
Sasaki et al. [37]	N.D.		29 (34)	N.D.	N.D.		N.D.		N.D.		0 (15)	30 (19)	N.D.	
Abraham et al. [38]	N.D.		N.D.		N.D.		25 (12)	N.D.	0 (12)	N.D.	0 (12)		N.D.	

*% of cases with positive staining or mutations (total cases examined); N.D.: not determined; inv.: invasive.

Table 3: KRAS and GNAS mutations in the intraductal papillary neoplasms of the bile duct lineage, the biliary intraepithelial neoplasia lineage, the intraductal papillary mucinous neoplasms of the pancreas lineage, and pancreatic ductal adenocarcinoma.

Authors	KRAS mutation				GNAS mutation			
	IPNB	BilIN	IPMN	PDAC	IPNB	BilIN	IPMN	PDAC
Furukawa et al. [39]	N.D.		47 (118)*	22 (32)	N.D.		41 (118)	0 (32)
Schlitter et al. [36]	36 (45)	14 (22)	N.D.		2 (44)	0 (22)	N.D.	
Abraham et al. [38]	29 (12)	N.D.	N.D.		N.D.	N.D.	N.D.	
Matthaei et al. [40]	18 (34)	N.D.	N.D.		4 (23)	N.D.	N.D.	
Sasaki et al. [41]	46 (26)	33 (76)	N.D.		50 (30)	0 (76)	N.D.	
Tsai et al. [42]	32 (41)	N.D.	N.D.		29 (41)	N.D.	N.D.	

*% of cases with mutations (total cases examined); N.D.: not determined.

as shown by several reports [36, 38, 40–42]. The occurrence of these mutations was more common in IPNBs (17.6 to 46.2% of cases) than in BilINs. In contrast, with regard to guanine nucleotide-binding protein, α-stimulating activity polypeptide (GNAS) codon 201 mutations, which have been exclusively detected in approximately two-thirds of IPMNs of the pancreas but not pancreatic ductal adenocarcinoma [39], there are some conflicting data among the studies. Sasaki et al. [41] showed that GNAS mutation was detected in 15 of 30 IPNBs, whereas Schlitter et al. [36] and Matthaei et al. [40] found GNAS mutation only in one of 44 IPNBs and one of 23 IPNBs, respectively. Although reasons for this discrepancy are unknown, one possible reason may be difference of phenotypes of IPNBs studied. Tsai et al. [42] recently reported that 12 of 41 IPNBs showed GNAS mutation, which was correlated with a distinct subgroup of IPNB characterized by the intestinal subtype, villous configuration, and mucin hypersecretion. These features were extremely similar to those of IPMN of the pancreas. Similarly, all IPNBs with GNAS mutation only showed high-mucin production in the study by Sasaki et al. [41], whereas GNAS mutation was detected in the intestinal subtype in both studies by Schlitter et al. [36] and Matthaei et al. [40]. Furthermore, only one IPNB with mucin hypersecretion was included in the study by Schlitter et al. [36] and only two tumors with the intestinal subtype in the study by Matthaei et al. [40].

Involvement of SMAD4/DPC4, which acts as a tumor suppressor that functions in the regulation of the TGF-β signal transduction pathway, and p53, which acts also as a tumor suppressor, during the development and progression of IPNB is still controversial. Nakanishi et al. [35] showed that loss of SMAD4/DPC4 expression was seen in both IPNB (21.4%) and BilIN (27.3%) lineages with gradually increasing frequency with progression. Schlitter et al. [36] revealed similar results despite less frequency (IPNBs, 7%; BilINs, 14%). In contrast, Abraham et al. [38] reported that immunohistochemical labeling for SMAD4/DPC4 showed intact protein expression in all the IPNBs examined. One report [35] showed that aberrant immunohistochemical expression of p53 was early on in low-grade IPNB and reached a plateau, whereas that remained low in the early phase of BilIN lineage and its expression was significantly upregulated in the cases with invasive carcinoma. However, there were reports in which aberrant expression of p53 was never seen in all IPNBs examined [38], or p53 was not aberrantly expressed in IPNBs without invasion but extensively expressed in IPNBs with invasion [37]. Another report revealed that frequency of p53 aberrant expression progressively increased from low-grade intraepithelial neoplasia to invasive carcinoma [36].

There were few studies on DNA mismatch repair functionality in IPNBs. Abraham et al. [43] showed that impaired DNA mismatch repair evidenced by microsatellite instability was seen in 8 of 17 IPNBs (high-level in 2, low-level in 1). This frequency was higher than that previously reported for extrahepatic [44] and intrahepatic cholangiocarcinoma [45], indicating that impaired DNA mismatch repair might play a role in the pathogenesis of a subset of IPNBs. However, the mechanism that causes impaired DNA mismatch repair was not clarified, and no methylation of the human Mut L homologue gene promoter was detected in IPNBs.

Mucin core proteins such as MUC1 and MUC2 are involved in the progression of both IPNB and BilIN lineages. Zen et al. [46] reported that MUC1 expression was more common in BilINs, especially in invasive lesions, than in IPNB with an associated invasive carcinoma. They supposed two progression pathways of IPNB to tubular adenocarcinoma and mucinous carcinoma, featuring the phenotypes of MUC1+/MUC2+ and MUC1−/MUC2+, respectively, which are analogous to that of IPMN of the pancreas. However, Onoe et al. [14] revealed that most IPNB with ≤50% invasive component showed MUC1+/MUC2− carcinogenetic pathway progressing to papillary/tubular adenocarcinoma, whereas a few IPNBs with ≤50% invasive progressed to mucinous carcinoma characterized by a MUC1+/MUC2+ pathway. Sasaki et al. [37] showed that the polycomb group protein enhancer of zeste homolog 2 may play a role in the regulation of MUC1 and MUC6 in IPNBs.

5.2. IPNB Originated from Peribiliary Glands. IPNB normally arises from the biliary epithelium in the extra- or intrahepatic large bile duct. However, recently, IPNBs that involved significantly the peribiliary glands and grossly showed cystic dilatation particularly aneurysmal or diverticular dilatation were reported [47–49], suggesting that some type of IPNB may arise from the peribiliary glands located within the wall or scattered in the surrounding connective tissue of the intrahepatic large bile ducts and extrahepatic bile ducts. These lesions are proposed to be IPNBs corresponding to pancreatic IPMN of the branch duct type [49, 50]. Sato et al. [51] showed that cystic and micropapillary changes of the epithelial cells of intrahepatic peribiliary glands, which were found in 9 (1%) of 938 autopsy livers, had abundant apical mucin and increased expression of MUC5AC, cyclin D1, and Ki-67. Since these characteristics were similar to those of pancreatic IPMN of the branch duct type, they insisted that cystic and micropapillary lesions of peribiliary glands may have neoplastic features and might represent a precursor of biliary epithelial neoplasms, including IPNB of "the branch duct type." Cardinale et al. [52] suggested that biliary stem/progenitor cells located in the peribiliary glands might be implicated in the carcinogenesis of mucin-producing cholangiocarcinomas. However, these are still speculative.

6. Conclusion

Originally, IPNB was proposed as a new disease entity because of striking similarities to IPMN of the pancreas, of which the disease entity and clinicopathological features are well established. Both neoplasms share intraductal papillary growth pattern, microscopic features such as papillary proliferation with delicate fibrovascular core and 4 types of epithelial subtypes, rarely occurrence of multiple lesions, and possible progression to tubular adenocarcinoma and mucinous carcinoma. However, several important differences exist between IPNB and IPMN of the pancreas. In IPNB, pancreatobiliary type is the most common and gastric type is rare. Most cases of IPNB are IPNBs with high-grade intraepithelial neoplasia or IPNBs with an associated invasive carcinoma, and IPNBs with low- or intermediate grade intraepithelial neoplasia are infrequent. Furthermore, mucin hypersecretion is usually observed in most cases with IPMN of the pancreas, whereas only one-third of IPNB cases involve mucin hypersecretion. These differences raise a question whether all IPNBs can be included in a single disease entity. In fact, our previous study [12] revealed that IPNB without mucin hypersecretion contained heterogeneous disease groups, and the majority of IPNB without mucin hypersecretion had the characteristics close to those of nonpapillary cholangiocarcinoma. Onoe et al. [14] showed that papillary cholangiocarcinoma with >50% invasive component was clinicopathologically similar to nonpapillary cholangiocarcinoma. A lot of inconsistent data with regard to the molecular events during development and progression of IPNB mentioned above may also reflect heterogeneous disease groups in the currently defined IPNB. The concept of IPNB as a biliary counterpart of IPMN of the pancreas is attractive, but the definition of this disease entity is still somewhat confused. Further study with a large number of cases is required to elucidate the essential differences between IPNBs and BilINs.

References

[1] E. Sakamoto, Y. Nimura, N. Hayakawa et al., "Clinicopathological studies of mucin-producing cholangiocarcinoma," *Journal of Hepato-Biliary-Pancreatic Surgery*, vol. 4, no. 2, pp. 157–162, 1997.

[2] M. Chen, Y. Jan, and T. Chen, "Clinical studies of mucin-producing Cholangiocellular carcinoma a study of 22 histopathology-proven cases," *Annals of Surgery*, vol. 227, no. 1, pp. 63–69, 1998.

[3] H. Shibahara, S. Tamada, M. Goto et al., "Prognostic features of mucin-producing bile duct tumors. Two histopathologic categories as counterparts of pancreatic intraductal papillary-mucinous neoplasms," *American Journal of Surgical Pathology*, vol. 28, no. 3, pp. 327–338, 2004.

[4] C. Kuo, C. Changchien, K. Wu et al., "Mucin-producing cholangiocarcinoma: clinical experience of 24 cases in 16 years," *Scandinavian Journal of Gastroenterology*, vol. 40, no. 4, pp. 455–459, 2005.

[5] H. J. Kim, M. H. Kim, S. K. Lee et al., "Mucin-hypersecreting bile duct tumor characterized by a striking homology with an intraductal papillary mucinous tumor (IPMT) of the pancreas," *Endoscopy*, vol. 32, no. 5, pp. 389–393, 2000.

[6] T. Yeh, J. Tseng, C. Chiu et al., "Cholangiographic spectrum of intraductal papillary mucinous neoplasm of the bile ducts," *Annals of Surgery*, vol. 244, no. 2, pp. 248–253, 2006.

[7] J. H. Lim, C. A. Yi, H. K. Lim, W. J. Lee, S. J. Lee, and S. H. Kim, "Radiological spectrum of intraductal papillary tumors of the bile duct," *Korean Journal of Radiology*, vol. 3, no. 1, pp. 57–63, 2002.

[8] Y. Zen, T. Fujii, K. Itatsu et al., "Biliary papillary tumors share pathological features with intraductal papillary mucinous neoplasm of the pancreas," *Hepatology*, vol. 44, no. 5, pp. 1333–1343, 2006.

[9] Y. Nakanuma, M. Curado, S. Franseschi et al., "Intrahepatic cholangiocarcinoma," in *WHO Classification of Tumours of the Digestive System*, F. Bosman, F. Carneiro, R. H. Hruban, and N. D. Theise, Eds., pp. 217–227, IARC, Lyon, France, 4th edition, 2010.

[10] Y. Zen, T. Fujii, K. Itatsu et al., "Biliary cystic tumors with bile duct communication: a cystic variant of intraductal papillary neoplasm of the bile duct," *Modern Pathology*, vol. 19, no. 9, pp. 1243–1254, 2006.

[11] J. G. Barton, D. A. Barrett, M. A. Maricevich et al., "Intraductal papillary mucinous neoplasm of the biliary tract: a real disease?" *HPB*, vol. 11, no. 8, pp. 684–691, 2009.

[12] M. Ohtsuka, F. Kimura, H. Shimizu et al., "Similarities and differences between intraductal papillary tumors of the bile duct with and without macroscopically visible mucin secretion," *American Journal of Surgical Pathology*, vol. 35, no. 4, pp. 512–521, 2011.

[13] F. G. Rocha, H. Lee, N. Katabi et al., "Intraductal papillary neoplasm of the bile duct: a biliary equivalent to intraductal papillary mucinous neoplasm of the pancreas?" *Hepatology*, vol. 56, no. 4, pp. 1352–1360, 2012.

[14] S. Onoe, Y. Shimoyama, T. Ebata et al., "Prognostic delineation of papillary cholangiocarcinoma based on the invasive proportion: a single-institution study with 184 patients," *Surgery*, vol. 155, no. 2, pp. 280–291, 2014.

[15] C. Yeh, Y. Jan, T. Yeh, T. Hwang, and M. Chen, "Hepatic resection of the intraductal papillary type of peripheral cholangiocarcinoma," *Annals of Surgical Oncology*, vol. 11, no. 6, pp. 606–611, 2004.

[16] K. M. Kim, J. K. Lee, J. U. Shin et al., "Clinicopathologic features of intraductal papillary neoplasm of the bile duct according to histologic subtype," *American Journal of Gastroenterology*, vol. 107, no. 1, pp. 118–125, 2012.

[17] G. Jung, K. M. Park, S. S. Lee et al., "Long-term clinical outcome of the surgically resected intraductal papillary neoplasm of the bile duct," *Journal of Hepatology*, vol. 57, no. 4, pp. 787–793, 2012.

[18] J. Yang, W. Wang, and L. Yan, "The clinicopathological features of intraductal papillary neoplasms of the bile duct in a Chinese population," *Digestive and Liver Disease*, vol. 44, no. 3, pp. 251–256, 2012.

[19] S. C. Choi, J. K. Lee, J. H. Jung et al., "The clinicopathological features of biliary intraductal papillary neoplasms according to the location of tumors," *Journal of Gastroenterology and Hepatology*, vol. 25, no. 4, pp. 725–730, 2010.

[20] K. Y. Paik, J. S. Heo, S. H. Choi et al., "Intraductal papillary neoplasm of the bile ducts: the clinical features and surgical outcome of 25 cases," *Journal of Surgical Oncology*, vol. 97, no. 6, pp. 508–512, 2008.

[21] K. Kubota, Y. Nakanuma, F. Kondo et al., "Clinicopathological features and prognosis of mucin-producing bile duct tumor and mucinous cystic tumor of the liver: a multi-institutional study by the Japan Biliary Association," *Journal of Hepato-Biliary-Pancreatic Sciences*, vol. 21, no. 3, pp. 176–185, 2014.

[22] S. S. Lee, M. Kim, S. K. Lee et al., "Clinicopathologic review of 58 patients with biliary papillomatosis," *Cancer*, vol. 100, no. 4, pp. 783–793, 2004.

[23] H. Ogawa, S. Itoh, T. Nagasaka, K. Suzuki, T. Ota, and S. Naganawa, "CT findings of intraductal papillary neoplasm of the bile duct: assessment with multiphase contrast-enhanced examination using multi-detector CT," *Clinical Radiology*, vol. 67, no. 3, pp. 224–231, 2012.

[24] H. J. Yoon, Y. K. Kim, K. T. Jang et al., "Intraductal papillary neoplasm of the bile ducts: description of MRI and added value of diffusion-weighted MRI," *Abdominal Imaging*, vol. 38, no. 5, pp. 1082–1090, 2013.

[25] T. Tsuyuguchi, Y. Sakai, H. Sugiyama et al., "Endoscopic diagnosis of intraductal papillary mucinous neoplasm of the bile duct," *Journal of Hepato-Biliary-Pancreatic Sciences*, vol. 17, no. 3, pp. 230–235, 2010.

[26] Y. Tsou, N. Liu, R. Wu et al., "Endoscopic retrograde cholangiography in the diagnosis and treatment of mucobilia," *Scandinavian Journal of Gastroenterology*, vol. 43, no. 9, pp. 1137–1144, 2008.

[27] Y. Sakai, T. Tsuyuguchi, T. Ishihara et al., "Usefulness of peroral cholangioscopy in preoperative diagnosis of intraductal papillary neoplasm of the bile duct," *Hepato-Gastroenterology*, vol. 57, no. 101, pp. 691–693, 2010.

[28] M. Miyazaki, F. Kimura, H. Shimizu et al., "Extensive hilar bile duct resection using a transhepatic approach for patients with hepatic hilar bile duct diseases," *American Journal of Surgery*, vol. 196, no. 1, pp. 125–129, 2008.

[29] M. Ohtsuka, F. Kimura, H. Shimizu et al., "Surgical strategy for mucin-producing bile duct tumor," *Journal of Hepato-Biliary-Pancreatic Sciences*, vol. 17, no. 3, pp. 236–240, 2010.

[30] E. Vibert, S. Dokmak, and J. Belghiti, "Surgical strategy of biliary papillomatosis in Western countries," *Journal of Hepato-Biliary-Pancreatic Sciences*, vol. 17, no. 3, pp. 241–245, 2010.

[31] Y. Ji, J. Fan, J. Zhou et al., "Intraductal papillary neoplasms of bile duct. A distinct entity like its counterpart in pancreas," *Histology and Histopathology*, vol. 23, no. 1-3, pp. 41–50, 2008.

[32] Y. Zen, F. Pedica, V. R. Patcha et al., "Mucinous cystic neoplasms of the liver: a clinicopathological study and comparison with intraductal papillary neoplasms of the bile duct," *Modern Pathology*, vol. 24, no. 8, pp. 1079–1089, 2011.

[33] J. J. Kloek, N. A. van der Gaag, D. Erdogan et al., "A comparative study of intraductal papillary neoplasia of the biliary tract and pancreas," *Human Pathology*, vol. 42, no. 6, pp. 824–832, 2011.

[34] K. Itatsu, Y. Zen, S. Ohira et al., "Immunohistochemical analysis of the progression of flat and papillary preneoplastic lesions in intrahepatic cholangiocarcinogenesis in hepatolithiasis," *Liver International*, vol. 27, no. 9, pp. 1174–1184, 2007.

[35] Y. Nakanishi, Y. Zen, S. Kondo, T. Itoh, K. Itatsu, and Y. Nakanuma, "Expression of cell cycle-related molecules in biliary premalignant lesions: biliary intraepithelial neoplasia and biliary intraductal papillary neoplasm," *Human Pathology*, vol. 39, no. 8, pp. 1153–1161, 2008.

[36] A. M. Schlitter, D. Born, M. Bettstetter et al., "Intraductal papillary neoplasms of the bile duct: stepwise progression to carcinoma involves common molecular pathways," *Modern Pathology*, vol. 27, no. 1, pp. 73–86, 2014.

[37] M. Sasaki, T. Matsubara, N. Yoneda et al., "Overexpression of enhancer of zeste homolog 2 and MUC1 may be related to malignant behaviour in intraductal papillary neoplasm of the bile duct," *Histopathology*, vol. 62, no. 3, pp. 446–457, 2013.

[38] S. C. Abraham, J. Lee, R. H. Hruban, P. Argani, E. E. Furth, and T. Wu, "Molecular and immunohistochemical analysis of intraductal papillary neoplasms of the biliary tract," *Human Pathology*, vol. 34, no. 9, pp. 902–910, 2003.

[39] T. Furukawa, Y. Kuboki, E. Tanji et al., "Whole-exome sequencing uncovers frequent GNAS mutations in intraductal papillary mucinous neoplasms of the pancreas," *Scientific Reports*, vol. 1, article no. 161, 2011.

[40] H. Matthaei, J. Wu, M. dal Molin et al., "GNAS codon 201 mutations are uncommon in intraductal papillary neoplasms of the bile duct," *HPB*, vol. 14, no. 10, pp. 677–683, 2012.

[41] M. Sasaki, T. Matsubara, T. Nitta et al., "GNAS and KRAS mutations are common inn intraductal papillary neoplasms of the bile duct," *PLOS ONE*, vol. 8, no. 12, Article ID e81706, 2013.

[42] J. H. Tsai, R. H. Yuan, Y. L. Chen et al., "GNAS is frequently mutated in a specific subgroup of intraductal papoillary neoplasms of the bile duct," *American Journal of Surgical Pathology*, vol. 37, no. 12, pp. 1862–1870, 2013.

[43] S. C. Abraham, J. Lee, J. K. Boitnott, P. Argani, E. E. Furth, and T. Wu, "Microsatellite instability in intraductal papillary neoplasms of the biliary tract," *Modern Pathology*, vol. 15, no. 12, pp. 1309–1317, 2002.

[44] T. Suto, W. Habano, T. Sugai et al., "Infrequent microsatellite instability in biliary tract cancer," *Journal of Surgical Oncology*, vol. 76, no. 2, pp. 121–126, 2001.

[45] J. Kawaki, M. Miyazaki, H. Ito et al., "Allelic loss in human intrahepatic cholangiocarcinoma: correlation between chromosome 8p22 and tumor progression," *International Journal of Cancer*, vol. 88, no. 2, pp. 228–231, 2000.

[46] Y. Zen, M. Sasaki, T. Fujii et al., "Different expression patterns of mucin core proteins and cytokeratins during intrahepatic cholangiocarcinogenesis from biliary intraepithelial neoplasia and intraductal papillary neoplasm of the bile duct—an immunohistochemical study of 110 cases of hepatolithiasis," *Journal of Hepatology*, vol. 44, no. 2, pp. 350–358, 2006.

[47] Y. Nakanishi, Y. Zen, S. Hirano et al., "Intraductal oncocytic papillary neoplasm of the bile duct: the first case of peribiliary

gland origin," *Journal of Hepato-Biliary-Pancreatic Surgery*, vol. 16, no. 6, pp. 869–873, 2009.

[48] Y. Nakanishi, Y. Nakanuma, M. Ohara et al., "Intraductal papillary neoplasm arising from peribiliary glands connecting with the inferior branch of the bile duct of the anterior segment of the liver," *Pathology International*, vol. 61, no. 12, pp. 773–777, 2011.

[49] J. H. Lim, Y. Zen, K. T. Jang, Y. K. Kim, and Y. Nakanuma, "Cyst-forming intraductal papillary neoplasm of the bile ducts: description of imaging and pathologic aspects," *American Journal of Roentgenology*, vol. 197, no. 5, pp. 1111–1120, 2011.

[50] Y. Nakanishi and Y. Sato, "Cystic and papillary neoplasm involving peribiliary glands: a biliary counterpart of branch-type intraductal papillary mucinous cystic neoplasm?" *Hepatology*, vol. 55, no. 6, pp. 2040–2041, 2012.

[51] Y. Sato, K. Harada, M. Sasaki et al., "Cystic and micropapillary epithelial changes of peribiliary glands might represent a precursor lesion of biliary epithelial neoplasms," *Virchows Archiv*, vol. 464, no. 2, pp. 157–163, 2014.

[52] V. Cardinale, Y. Wang, G. Carpino et al., "Mucin-producing cholangiocarcinoma might derive from biliary tree stem/progenitor cells located in peribiliary glands," *Hepatology*, vol. 55, no. 6, pp. 2041–2042, 2012.

15

What Are the Precursor and Early Lesions of Peripheral Intrahepatic Cholangiocarcinoma?

Yasuni Nakanuma,[1,2] Akemi Tsutsui,[1] Xiang Shan Ren,[1] Kenichi Harada,[1] Yasunori Sato,[1] and Motoko Sasaki[1]

[1] *Department of Human Pathology, Kanazawa University Graduate School of Medicine, Kanazawa 920-8640, Japan*
[2] *Department of Pathology, Shizuoka Cancer Center, Shizuoka 411-8777, Japan*

Correspondence should be addressed to Yasuni Nakanuma; nakanuma@staff.kanazawa-u.ac.jp

Academic Editor: Chawalit Pairojkul

Cholangiocarcinoma (CC) is divided into distal, perihilar, and intrahepatic CCs (ICCS), and are further subdivided into large bile duct ICC and peripheral ICC. In distal and perihilar CC and large duct ICC, biliary intraepithelial neoplasm (BilIN) and intraductal papillary neoplasm (IPN) have been proposed as precursor lesions. Peripheral ICC, bile duct adenoma (BDA), biliary adenofibroma (BAF), and von Meyenburg complexes (VMCs) are reportedly followed by development of ICCs. Herein, we surveyed these candidate precursor lesions in the background liver of 37 cases of peripheral ICC and controls (perihilar CC, 34 cases; hepatocellular carcinoma, 34 cases and combined hepatocellular cholangiocarcinoma, 25 cases). In the background liver of peripheral ICC, BDA and BAF were not found, but there were not infrequently foci of BDA-like lesions and atypical bile duct lesions involving small bile ducts (32.4% and 10.8%, resp.). VMCs were equally found in peripheral CCs and also control CCs. In conclusion, BDA, BAF, and VMCs are a possible precursor lesion of a minority of peripheral CCs, and BDA-like lesions and atypical bile duct lesions involving small bile ducts may also be related to the development of peripheral ICC. Further pathologic studies on these lesions are warranted for analysis of development of peripheral ICCs.

1. Introduction

Cholangiocarcinoma (CC) is an intractable malignant tumor with a poor prognosis. Surgical resection of CC at an early stage is crucial to improve the prognosis of CC patients [1, 2]. However, this procedure is not applicable to the majority of these patients because most CCs are diagnosed or detected at an advanced stage, and treatment options remain limited [3]. CC is generally divided into distal and perihilar CCs and intrahepatic CC (ICC) [4, 5], and their clinicopathological features, risk factors, and epidemiology are different among them [2, 6, 7].

ICC is the second most common liver primary tumor after HCC, and its incidence has increased in recent years [7–9]. ICCs themselves are known to exhibit heterogeneity in their location in the liver, histopathologies, and expression of markers [8], and this heterogeneity may reflect the heterogeneous cholangiocytes along the biliary tree [4, 6, 10, 11]. ICC can be further divided into large bile duct ICC and peripheral ICC [12]. In distal, perihilar, and intrahepatic large duct, cylindrical mucin-producing cholangiocytes are located in large bile ducts, while cuboidal non-mucin-producing cholangiocytes are located in small bile ducts and bile ductules containing bipotential hepatic progenitor cells (HPCs). Among the ICCs, peripheral ICCs, which typically present as a mass or nodular lesion, are currently considered to be derived from the cells lining small bile ducts, and large bile duct ICCs resemble perihilar CC. Many studies have recently suggested that stem or progenitor cells located in the periportal area play a role in neoplastic and nonneoplastic hepatobiliary lesions in adults [6, 13]. Liver cirrhosis, particularly that associated with HBV and HCV, has been reported as a risk factor for peripheral ICC, and hepatic

TABLE 1: Main clinicopathologic features of the cases studied.

	Peripheral ICC	Perihilar CC	HCC	cHC-CC
Number of cases	37	34	25	18
Age (years)	65 ± 1.8	61 ± 1.7	62 ± 2.1	63 ± 1.8
Sex (male/female)*	21/16	19/15	17/8	14/4
Hepatitis virus*				
HBsAg (+)	6	1	9	6
HCV (+)	7	3	13	6
HBsAg (+)/HCV (+)	0	0	0	1
HBsAg (−)/HCV (−)	24	30	3	6
Cirrhosis*	4	1	25	11
Tumor size*				
$\Phi > 3$ cm	31	20	10	8
$\Phi \leqq 3$ cm	6	11	15	9

*Number of cases. CC: cholangiocarcinoma; ICC: intrahepatic CC; HCC: hepatocellular carcinoma; cHC-CC: combined hepatocellular cholangiocarcinoma.

stem/progenitor cells located at the Canals of Hering may be involved in its carcinogenesis in such cases [2, 7, 14].

Precursor and early neoplastic lesions of CCs may provide an insight into identifying a more likely candidate for precursor lesions preceding the development of CCs. For example, two types of preneoplastic or early neoplastic lesions were recently identified for large duct ICC, perihilar and distal CCs, and gallbladder carcinomas: biliary intraepithelial neoplasm (BilIN) and intraductal papillary neoplasm (IPN) [4, 5, 15]. The former is a flat and microscopically recognizable lesion that is categorized into three grades: BilIN-1, -2, and -3, while the latter is a grossly visible papillary lesion in the dilated bile duct that is graded as low-intermediate and high. While many clinical and molecular studies have examined peripheral ICC [2, 7, 16], the precursor and premalignant lesions defined pathologically and histogenesis of peripheral CC have yet to be determined in detail.

So far, several candidate lesions, possibly followed by or associated with the development of peripheral ICC, have been proposed: bile duct adenoma, biliary adenofibroma, and von Meyenburg complexes (VMCs) [15, 17, 18]. In addition, low grade biliary epithelial malignancies such as those with ductal plate malformation- (DPM-) like features and cholangiolocellular carcinoma (bile ductular carcinoma) are known to contain the foci of classical or conventional CC [13, 18], suggesting their progression from low grade biliary epithelial malignancies to conventional CC with more malignant biological behaviors [13, 19].

Herein, we, first, reviewed the pathological features of the above-mentioned, several candidate lesions possibly followed by peripheral ICC, in the literatures. Second, we histologically surveyed such candidate lesions in the background liver of peripheral ICC in comparison with perihilar CC, HCC, and combined hepatocellular-cholangiocarcinoma (cHCC-CC) by using a total of 114 surgically resected cases. These cases were collected from the file of hepatobiliary diseases in the Department of Pathology and affiliated hospitals, and their main clinicopathological features are shown in Table 1. Finally, we discussed low grade or borderline biliary malignancies frequently followed by ordinary peripheral ICC with more aggressive behaviors.

2. Precursor and Premalignant Lesions of Peripheral ICC

New insights into the molecular and genetic mechanisms contributing to the pathogenesis of peripheral ICCs are emerging from recent epidemiological, genome-wide profiling, and laboratory-based studies [2, 7, 16]; however, their exact signaling pathways and etiology have yet to be elucidated in detail. For further elucidation and clarification of these mechanisms, a pathological entity of precursor or early neoplastic lesions in peripheral ICC cases needs to be addressed. The detailed analysis of these candidate precursors or premalignant biliary epithelial lesions may also assist in the search for the molecular and genetic studies on peripheral ICC. While the precursor lesions of peripheral ICC have not yet been identified, it appears reasonable to assume that its carcinogenesis may involve small intrahepatic bile ducts such as bile ductules, small interlobular bile ducts, or hepatic stem/progenitor cells including the canals of Hering, as indicated by the location of peripheral ICC in the liver [7, 14, 20, 21]. So far, the following lesions are known to be occasionally followed by the development of peripheral ICC in the literatures: bile duct adenoma, VMCs, and biliary adenofibroma [15, 17, 18]. While the incidence of malignant transformation may be quite low in these benign tumors, the pathological clarification and categorization of such lesions as well as more detailed molecular studies on these lesions may lead to better understanding of the carcinogenesis of peripheral ICC and may develop novel therapeutic strategies against intractable ICC.

2.1. Pathology of Candidate Precursor and Premalignant Lesions. *Bile duct adenoma* (BDA), which is also called peribiliary gland hamartoma, is regarded as a benign tumor or tumorous lesion composed of many small, uniformly sized ducts with cuboidal cells (bile ductular component)

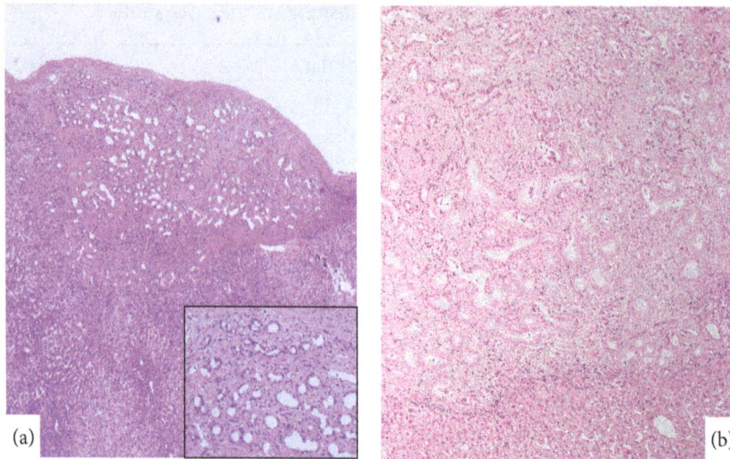

Figure 1: Bile duct adenoma. (a) Ordinary bile duct adenoma is seen under hepatic capsule, and it is composed of well-developed bile ducts of interlobular bile duct sizes (inset). HE. (b) Occasionally, bile duct adenoma with columnar epithelium and plenty cytoplasm shows compact growth. HE.

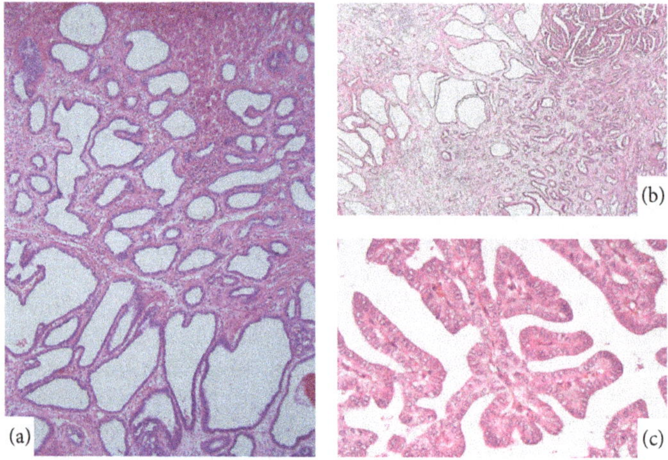

Figure 2: Biliary adenofibroma. (a) Tubular structures with fibrous stroma characterize this tumor. Focally, micropapillary features are found in the left lower corner. (b) Papillary features with complicated structures suggest an imminent malignant transformation. HE.

resembling bile ductular reactions (DRs) and variable fibrous stroma [18, 22, 23]. Allaire et al. reviewed the morphological spectrum of BDA using 152 cases [18] and found that all BDAs were asymptomatic nodules discovered incidentally during intra-abdominal surgery or at autopsy. BDAs are typically single, ranged in size from 1 to 20 mm, usually subcapsular, and well-circumscribed but nonencapsulated. BDA is known to be histologically composed of benign, noncystic ductules or interlobular bile ducts and variable degrees of inflammation and fibrosis (Figure 1(a)). Mucin is frequently detected in the cytoplasm of BDA. The immunophenotype of these ductules was shown to be similar to that of interlobular bile ducts. BDA could be distinguished from adenocarcinoma by the absence, in the former, of nuclear hyperchromasia, mitotic activity, and vascular invasion.

The biological nature of BDA has not yet been clarified in detail; however, it is generally regarded as a reactive process to a focal injury. However, interestingly, some BDAs are known to exhibit neoplastic potential followed by classical peripheral ICC [18, 22]. It seems therefore plausible that BDAs may be a heterogeneous group or have a broad morphological spectrum. Particularly, BDAs arising in chronic advanced liver diseases such as chronic viral hepatitis, those found deep in the liver parenchyma, and those with some biliary epithelial atypia and unusual features but not enough to be diagnosed as a malignancy (Figure 1(b)) may be precursor lesions for peripheral CC.

Biliary adenofibroma is characterized by a complex tubulocystic biliary epithelial tumor and abundant fibroblastic stromal components [24]. The lining epithelia of these complexes are columnar or cuboidal epithelia positive for the biliary cytokeratin marker and negative for mucin staining (Figure 2(a)) [24]. While the tumor is similar to VMCs, the large size of the lesion and absence of any typical MC characterize biliany adenofibroma. While most biliary adenofibromas are benign, one case of biliary adenofibroma with malignant transformation, recurrence, and metastasis was reported previously [17]. The patient was diagnosed with

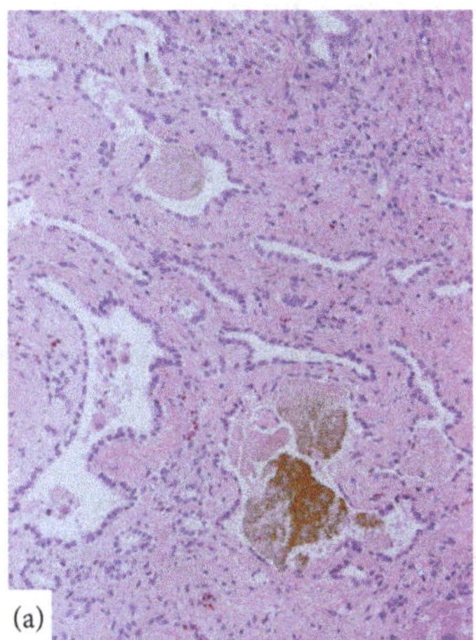

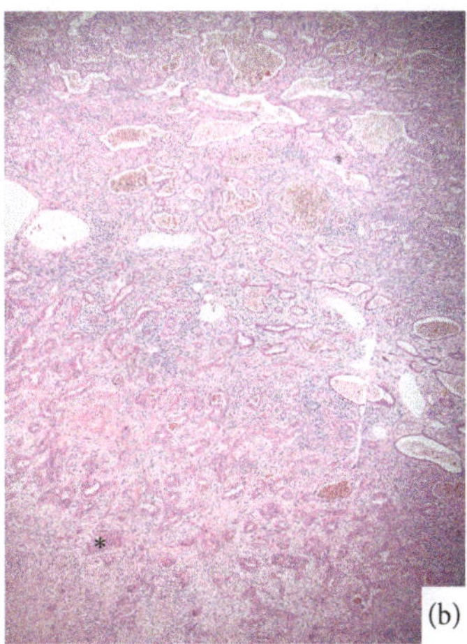

FIGURE 3: (a) Von Meyenburg complex showing a variable luminal dilatation and condensed bile. (b) Upper part shows low grade intrahepatic cholangiocarcinoma with features of von Meyenburg complex, and there are foci of ordinary cholangiocarcinoma in the low half (∗). HE.

biliary adenofibroma with malignant epithelial transformation following a pathological examination of the resected specimen. He discontinued the follow-up program for 1 year but was then admitted to the hospital with abdominal enlargement and right upper quadrant pain. A needle biopsy was performed, and a pathological examination of the biopsy specimen confirmed the recurrence of malignant biliary adenofibroma.

We recently encountered one case (69 years, female) of biliary adenofibroma with imminent malignant transformation (Tsutsui A, personal communication). The tumor (3.5 cm in a diameter) was located under the hepatic capsule in the left hepatic lobe. Most of the lesion was compatible with biliary adenofibroma, but some of it had a papillary configuration and more dysplasia (Figures 2(b) and 2(c)). A number of unusual features suggesting neoplasm were focally present, including intraluminal bile concretions and apocrine-like epithelial changes. While its expansile growth, presence of mitoses, the foci of epithelial tufting, and cellular atypia favor a neoplastic process, features indicative of overt malignancy and invasion or metastasis were not found. This case suggests that while biliary fibroadenoma is a benign tumor, it is possibly followed by the malignant transformation.

VMCs which are also called biliary microhamartoma are histopathological lesions composed of irregular small bile duct or dilated ductular structures, frequently containing concentrated bile, with a fibrous stroma, and are found at the interface of portal tracts (Figure 3(a)) [25]. While this lesion is generally considered to be a congenital or hamartomatous lesion, it is not typically found in infants and is not infrequently found in adult livers, suggesting the participation of acquired factors in the development of VMCs [26]. Several lesions are commonly found in the same liver and are occasionally multiple. Whereas VMCs are generally regarded as benign, recent case reports of CC arising from VMCs or of VMCs showing malignant transformation and also several cases of peripheral ICC, with histopathological similarities to VMCs (Figure 3(b)), arising from VMCs have been reported, raising the question of its potential role as an ICC precursor lesion [8, 27–29]. In such cases, VMCs were also found in nonneoplastic parts of the liver. For example, Xu et al. reported two cases of peripheral ICCs occurring in the liver with multiple VMCs. These cases suggested that VMCs may be a risk factor for the development of peripheral ICC, and malignant transformation has been reported in multiple VMCs [8].

In addition to the results obtained from human cases, a histological survey of hepatic parenchyma adjacent to ICC, as well as isolated regions of grossly normal livers, in an experimental animal model of ICC, which is characterized by a *K-ras* mutation and the deletion of p53, revealed several premalignant lesions [30]. Among them, some lesions, frequently found in animals with ICC, were similar to VMCs. ICCs appeared to arise directly from adjacent VMCs. The presence of these lesions in regions distal to the primary tumors suggests the multifocal initiation of VMC-like precursor lesions followed by the development of ICC. The findings of VMCs among mutant *K-ras-p53* animals provided experimental evidence for a progression model of ICC that includes VMCs.

2.2. Survey of Candidate Lesions in Our Cases. The abovementioned, three biliary lesions were surveyed in our cases (Table 1). In these cases, chronic biliary diseases such as hepatolithiasis and primary sclerosing cholangitis were not found. As shown in Table 2, biliary adenofibroma was not found in the background liver or at the rim of peripheral CCs. As for typical, subcapsular BDA, it was found in one of 25 HCC cases and one of 18 cHC-CC cases, but not in peripheral ICC. Instead, bile duct adenoma-like lesions (Figures 4(a) and 4(b)) which were a little different from BDA, itself, were found in the background liver of one-third of peripheral ICCs (32.4%). These lesions were composed of dense and localized cluster of matured interlobular bile ducts, and their overall size was rather small ranging from 1 mm to 3 mm. They were alone or several in a given liver specimen and were found in fibrous septa or enlarged portal

Table 2: Occurrence of biliary epithelial lesions related to cholangiocarcinoma.

	Peripheral ICC (n = 37)	Perihilar CC (n = 34)	HCC (n = 25)	cHC-CC (n = 18)
Biliary fibroadenoma	0 (0%)	0 (0%)	0 (0%)	0 (0%)
Bile duct adenoma	0 (0%)	0 (0%)	1 (4%)	1 (5%)
Von Meyenburg complex	9 (24.3%)	6 (17.6%)	7 (28.0%)	6 (33.3%)
Bile duct adenoma-like lesion	12 (32.4%)	4 (11.8%)	3 (12%)	6 (33.3%)
Atypical small bile duct lesion	4 (10.8%)	0 (0%)	0 (0%)	1 (5.6%)
Biliary epithelial neoplasm (BilIN) 2/3				
Perihilar bile duct	6 (16.2%)	18 (52.9%)	1 (4%)	2 (11.1%)
Peribiliary glands	4 (10.8%)	17 (50.0%)	0 (0%)	1 (5.6%)

CC: cholangiocarcinoma; ICC: intrahepatic CC; HCC: hepatocellular carcinoma; cHC-CC: combined hepatocellular cholangiocarcinoma.

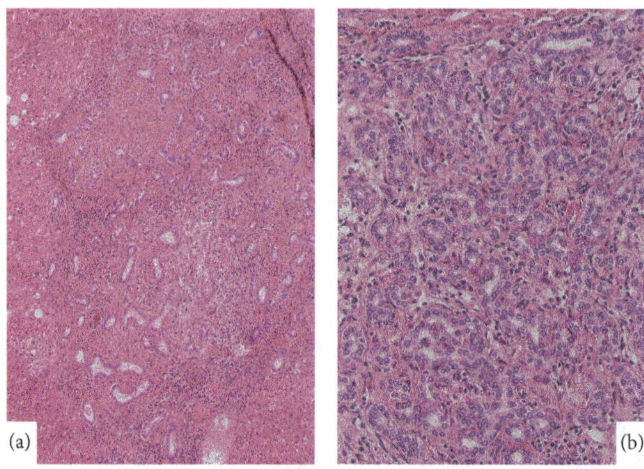

Figure 4: Bile duct adenoma-like lesion. (a) Small nodule composed of abundant interlobular bile ducts and fibrous stroma is found in the deep part of the liver. HE. (b) Small nodule of dense small interlobular bile ducts is found in the deep part of the liver. HE.

tract of the deep hepatic parenchyma. While these lesions were also found in 33.3% of cHC-CC cases, such lesions were infrequent in perihilar CC and HCC (11.8% and 12%, resp.), suggesting that this type of lesion could be related to peripheral ICC. As for VMCs, they were found focally and multiple in 24.3% of peripheral ICC cases and also other three controls (17.6% of hilar CC, 28% of HCC, and 33.3% of cHC-CC).

As a precursor or premalignant lesion of CC, BilINs are known and they are usually found in intrahepatic large bile ducts and perihilar and extrahepatic bile ducts [4, 5]. BilIN lesions were histologically classified as BilIN-1 (mild atypia), BilIN-2 (moderate atypia), and BilIN-3 (severe atypia including *in situ* carcinoma). While histological features of BilIN lesions were documented, it remains controversial whether BilIN-1 lesions contain some reactive hyperplastic changes. So, in this histological survey, only BilIN-2 and -3 lesions evaluated as neoplastic or preinvasive epithelial lesions were surveyed. In fact, it was found in this study that BilIN-2/3 lesions were found frequently in hilar bile ducts and peribiliary glands of hilar CC (52.9% and 50%, resp.) (Table 2). However, such lesions were infrequent or rare in these biliary anatomical components of biliary tree in peripheral CC, cHC-CC, and HCC. In our clinical experience, dysplastic biliary epithelial changes sharing features of BilIN are occasionally encountered in small bile ducts in peripheral CCs (Figures 5(a) and 5(b)). They showed that pleomorphic nuclei, nuclear hyperchromasia or stratification, and this size of affected bile ducts were enlarged, but not so atypical for making a diagnosis of CC or intraductal spread of carcinoma from CC. So, we surveyed such lesions in small bile ducts remote from CC itself of peripheral CC cases. It was found in this study that such small bile ducts showing atypical features were focally found in 10.8% of peripheral ICC. Interestingly, such lesions were found in 5.6% of cHCC-CC and not found in HCC and hilar CC. Further pathological and molecular studies are warranted for such small bile duct lesions which have not been reported in the literatures.

3. Progression from Low Grade Malignant or Borderline Biliary Lesions to More Aggressive ICC

Peripheral ICC is characterized by an aggressive course and early metastasis with a poor prognosis [7]. However, the histological features of ICC are known to be heterogeneous,

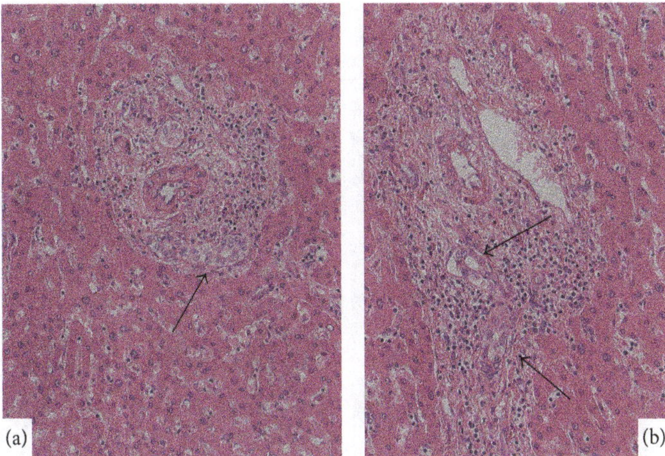

Figure 5: Atypical small bile duct lesion. (a) Small interlobular bile duct shows cellular and nuclear atypia. HE. (b) Small interlobular bile duct shows nuclear atypia and disturbed polarity. HE.

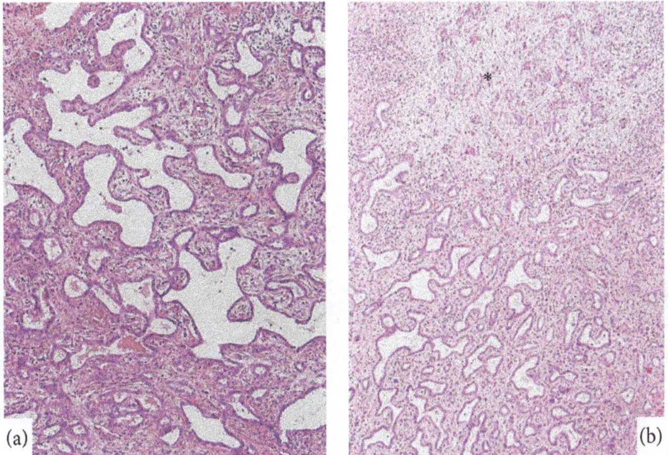

Figure 6: (a) Intrahepatic cholangiocarcinoma with features of ductal plate malformation. They appear to be blunt and lack aggressive features (low grade malignancy). (b) Within this type of cholangiocarcinoma (lower half), there are foci of ordinary cholangiocarcinoma (∗). HE.

with low grade malignancies or borderline biliary epithelial lesions with blunt histologies being reported among them [20, 30]. The foci of conventional ICCs have also been observed within these lesions and such low malignant lesions remain at the rim of ordinary peripheral ICC [18, 20], suggesting the transition of these lesions to conventional ICC with a more aggressive lesion. The following examples have been reported.

3.1. Cholangiolocellular Carcinoma (Bile Ductular Carcinoma). Cholangiolocellular carcinoma (CLC), a subtype of CC, exhibits the characteristic features of small monotonous and/or anastomosing glands. These tumors are accompanied by a variable fibrous stroma. Epithelial components are typically benign in appearance with blunt histologies showing the features of reactive bile ductules, and CLC is thought to originate from the bile ductules/canals of Hering, in which hepatic progenitor cells (HPCs) are located [13, 20]. These cells are also positive for hepatic progenitor markers, such as neural cell adhesion molecule (NCAM) in addition to CK7 and CK19.

While the majority of these tumors are mainly composed of neoplasms that appear to be benign, there are frequently foci of papillary and/or clear glandular formation with mucin production, representing CC areas. The latter lesion is commonly located in the central part of the tumor, while CLC components are typically found in the peripheral part. Transitional zones have also been reported in these tumors, suggesting that CLC is followed by ordinary peripheral ICC.

3.2. Cholangiocarcinoma with DPM Features. We recently reported an atypical form of peripheral highly differentiated adenocarcinoma (peripheral ICC) mimicking DPM features [19]. The ductal plate (DP) can be found in certain developmental stages of the fetal liver, and DPM was used for an excess of embryonic bile duct structures with a DP configuration, reflecting the lack of remodeling in the DP [31, 32]. Microscopically, the tumor was composed of many

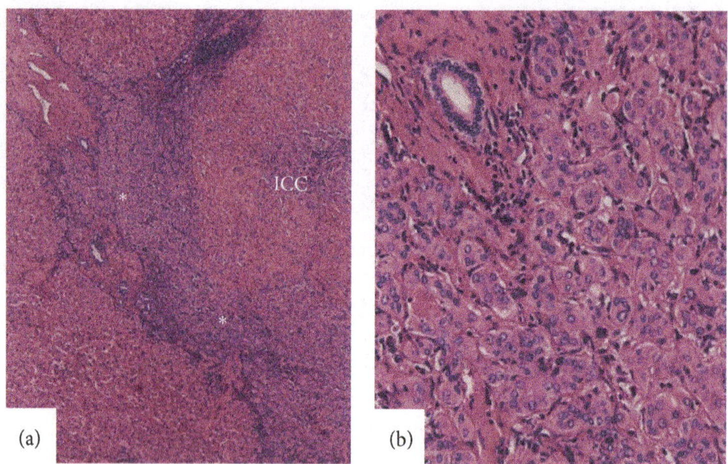

FIGURE 7: At the periphery (∗) of intrahepatic cholangiocarcinoma (ICC), there is well-differentiated lesion or bile duct adenoma-like lesion. (a) Lower magnification of ICC and (b) higher magnification of the rim (∗).

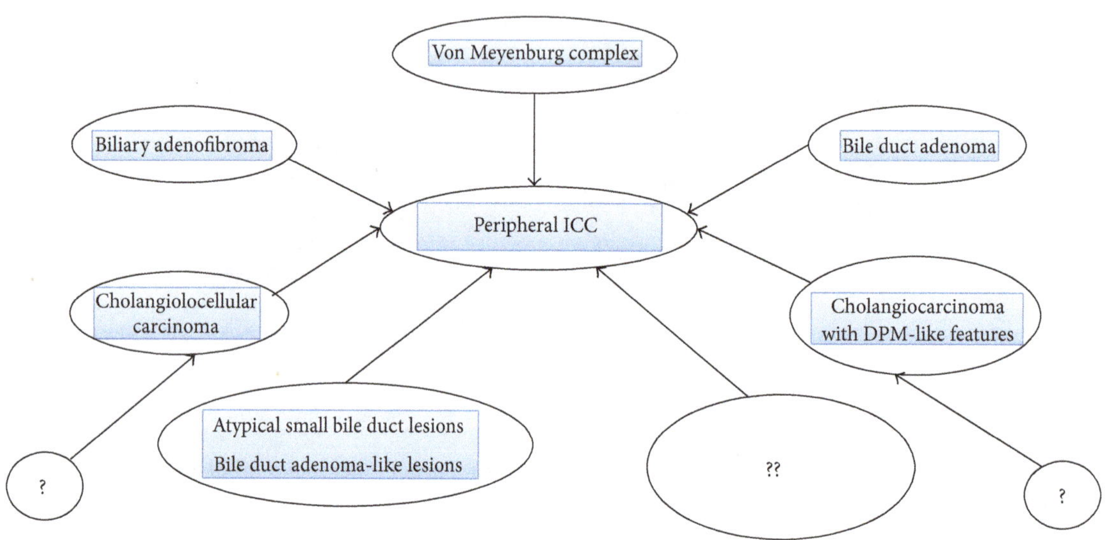

FIGURE 8: Schema of precursor lesions of peripheral intrahepatic cholangiocarcinoma (peripheral-ICC). Some of so-called benign lesions such as bile duct adenoma, von Meyenburg complex, and biliary adenofibroma are occasionally followed by the development of peripheral-ICC, and some of low grade cholangiocarcinoma (cholangiolocellular carcinoma and cholangiocarcinoma with ductal plate malformation (DPM)-like features) are also followed by ordinary peripheral-ICC. In addition, bile duct adenoma-like lesion and atypical small bile duct lesions described here could be also related to the development of peripheral ICC. Unidentified factors or lesions and may also be involved in the development of peripheral ICC.

vague, small nodular carcinomatous areas with desmoplastic reactions, and neoplastic glands had an irregularly dilated lumen lined with a single layer of cuboidal or low columnar carcinoma cells and irregular protrusions and bulges (Figure 6(a)), which resembled DPM [19]. At its border, the tumor appeared to replace nonneoplastic hepatic lobules or regenerative nodules. The central parts of the tumor were more or less hypocellular and fibrotic. The Ki-67 labeling index was less than 10% and the expression of p53 was very low. This subtype is thought to originate from bile ductules with DPM features. The foci of ordinary CC with aggressive histological features were observed in approximately half of these tumors [19], suggesting the transition of well-differentiated ICC with DPM features to more aggressive ordinary ICC (Figure 6(b)).

3.3. Rim of Low Grade or Borderline Malignancies in Conventional ICC. Peripheral ICC is typically well- to moderately differentiated tubular adenocarcinoma, while cord-like patterns are also frequently reported. While their histologies are commonly atypical enough to diagnose malignancy, highly differentiated adenocarcinoma or the appearance of borderline malignancy is occasionally observed at the peripheral rim of such ICCs, including the above-mentioned so-called benign lesions (bile duct adenoma, biliary adenofibroma, and VMCs) (Figures 7(a) and 7(b)), CLC (bile ductular carcinoma), and CC with DPM-like structures. These combinations suggest the progression of CLC or CC with DPM-like structures to more malignant or aggressive ICC. Based on the findings of our recent study [10], the foci of DPM-like features and foci of CLC were identified in approximately 10% and 30% of peripheral ICCs examined, respectively. These findings suggest that dedifferentiation may have occurred in preceding CLC or ICC with DPM-like structures and that the previous lesion remains as the peripheral rim.

In conclusion, several precursor or early neoplastic lesions of peripheral ICC reported in the literature were reviewed in the present study (Figure 8). Bile duct adenoma, biliary adenofibroma, and VMCs are reportedly associated with histologic features of malignancy or borderline lesions, and these lesions may be followed by carcinoma in a minority of peripheral ICC. Survey of unusual or atypical biliary lesions in peripheral ICC showed that bile duct adenoma-like lesions and atypical biliary lesions of small bile ducts were not infrequent in the background liver, possibly related to the development of peripheral ICC. In addition, several borderline or low grade biliary malignancies such as CLC or ICC with DPM-like structures frequently contain the foci of ordinary peripheral ICC, suggesting their transition to peripheral ICC and multistep cholangiocarcinogenesis. In hilar and extrahepatic CCs, the precursor lesions such as BilIN and IPN of bile duct are now being recognized and have been studied actively. More extensive surveys on precursor or premalignant lesions as well as more sophisticated studies based on pathologically confirmed precursor lesions in peripheral ICC as well as on those in hilar and extrahepatic CCs may lead to the earlier detection of and a better prognosis after surgical resection of peripheral ICC and hilar and extrahepatic CCs.

Authors' Contribution

Yasuni Nakanuma, Akemi Tsutsui, Xiang Shan Ren, Kenichi Harada, Yasunori Sato, and Motoko Sasaki equally contributed to this paper.

References

[1] M. Nagino, T. Ebata, Y. Yokoyama et al., "Evolution of surgical treatment for perihilar cholangiocarcinoma: a single-center 34-year review of 574 consecutive resections," *Annals of Surgery*, vol. 258, pp. 129–140, 2013.

[2] S. Rizvi and G. J. Gores, "Pathogenesis, diagnosis, and management of cholangiocarcinoma," *Gastroenterology*, vol. 145, no. 6, pp. 1215–1229, 2013.

[3] R. Higuchi, T. Ota, T. Araida, M. Kobayashi, T. Furukawa, and M. Yamamoto, "Prognostic relevance of ductal margins in operative resection of bile duct cancer," *Surgery*, vol. 148, no. 1, pp. 7–14, 2010.

[4] Y. Nakanuma, M. P. Curabo, S. Franceschi et al., "Intrahepatic cholangiocarcinoma," in *WHO Classification of Tumours of the Digestive System; World Health Organization of Tumours*, F. T. Bosman, F. Carneiro, R. H. Hruban, and N. D. Theise, Eds., pp. 217–224, IARC, Lyon, France, 4th edition, 2010.

[5] J. Albores-Saavedra, N. V. Adsay, J. M. Crawford et al., "Carcinoma of the gallbladder and extrahepatic bile ducts," in *WHO Classification of Tumours of the Digestive System; World Health Organization of Tumours*, F. T. Bosman, F. Carneiro, R. H. Hruban, and N. D. Theise, Eds., pp. 266–273, IARC, Lyon, France, 4th edition, 2010.

[6] M. Komuta, O. Govaere, V. Vandecaveye et al., "Histological diversity in cholangiocellular carcinoma reflects the different cholangiocyte phenotypes," *Hepatology*, vol. 55, pp. 1876–1888, 2012.

[7] T. Patel, "New insights into the molecular pathogenesis of intrahepatic cholangiocarcinoma," *Journal of Gastroenterology*, vol. 49, no. 2, pp. 165–172, 2014.

[8] A. M. Xu, Z. H. Xian, S. H. Zhang, and X. F. Chen, "Intrahepatic cholangiocarcinoma arising in multiple bile duct hamartomas: report of two cases and review of the literature," *European Journal of Gastroenterology and Hepatology*, vol. 21, pp. 580–584, 2009.

[9] Y. Shaib and H. B. El-Serag, "The epidemiology of cholangiocarcinoma," *Seminars in Liver Disease*, vol. 24, pp. 115–125, 2004.

[10] K. Harada, Y. Nakanuma, and H. Ikeda, "Heterogeneity in intrahepatic cholangiocarcinoma," *Hepatology Research*, 2014, in press.

[11] C. Gandou, K. Harada, Y. Sato et al., "Hilar cholangiocarcinoma and pancreatic ductal adenocarcinoma share similar histopathologies, immunophenotypes, and development-related molecules," *Human Pathology*, vol. 44, pp. 811–821, 2013.

[12] Y. Nakanuma, Y. Sato, K. Harada, M. Sasaki, J. Xu, and H. Ikeda, "Pathological classification of intrahepatic cholangiocarcinoma based on a new concept," *World Journal of Hepatology*, vol. 2, pp. 419–427, 2010.

[13] M. Komuta, B. Spee, S. V. Borght et al., "Clinicopathological study on cholangiolocellular carcinoma suggesting hepatic progenitor cell origin," *Hepatology*, vol. 47, no. 5, pp. 1544–1556, 2008.

[14] C. Sempoux, C. Fan, P. Singh et al., "Cholangiolocellular carcinoma: an innocent-looking malignant liver tumor mimicking ductular reaction," *Seminars in Liver Disease*, vol. 31, no. 1, pp. 104–110, 2011.

[15] Y. Zen, M. Sasaki, T. Fujii et al., "Different expression patterns of mucin core proteins and cytokeratins during intrahepatic cholangiocarcinogenesis from biliary intraepithelial neoplasia and intraductal papillary neoplasm of the bile duct—an immunohistochemical study of 110 cases of hepatolithiasis," *Journal of Hepatology*, vol. 44, no. 2, pp. 350–358, 2006.

[16] Y. Jiao, T. M. Pawlik, R. A. Anders et al., "Exome sequencing identifies frequent inactivating mutations in BAP1, ARID1A and PBRM1 in intrahepatic cholangiocarcinomas," *Nature Genetics*, 2013.

[17] O. Akin and M. Coskun, "Biliary adenofibroma with malignant transformation and pulmonary metastases: CT findings," *American Journal of Roentgenology*, vol. 179, no. 1, pp. 280–281, 2002.

[18] G. S. Allaire, L. Rabin, K. G. Ishak, and I. A. Sesterhenn, "Bile duct adenoma. A study of 152 cases," *American Journal of Surgical Pathology*, vol. 12, no. 9, pp. 708–715, 1988.

[19] Y. Nakanuma, Y. Sato, H. Ikeda et al., "Intrahepatic cholangiocarcinoma with predominant "ductal plate malformation" pattern: a new subtype," *American Journal of Surgical Pathology*, vol. 36, pp. 1629–1635, 2012.

[20] K. Kozaka, M. Sasaki, T. Fujii et al., "A subgroup of intrahepatic cholangiocarcinoma with an infiltrating replacement growth pattern and a resemblance to reactive proliferating bile ductules: "Bile ductular carcinoma"," *Histopathology*, vol. 51, no. 3, pp. 390–400, 2007.

[21] Y. Nakanuma, M. Hoso, T. Sanzen, and M. Sasaki, "Microstructure and development of the normal and pathologic biliary tract in humans, including blood supply," *Microscopy Research and Technique*, vol. 38, pp. 552–570, 1997.

[22] A. C. Pinho, R. B. Melo, M. Oliveira et al., "Adenoma-carcinoma sequence in intrahepatic cholangiocarcinoma," *International Journal of Surgery Case Reports*, vol. 3, pp. 131–133, 2012.

[23] K. G. Ishak, Z. D. Goodman, and J. T. Stocker, "Benign cholangiocellular tumors," in *Tumors of the Liver and Intrahepatic Bile Ducts*, J. Rosai and L.H. Sobin, Eds., Tumor Pathology 3rd series, pp. 49–70, Armed Force Institute of Pathology (AFIP), Washington, DC, USA, 2001.

[24] W. M. S. Tsui, K. T. Loo, L. T. C. Chow, and C. C. H. Tse, "Biliary adenofibroma: a heretofore unrecognized benign biliary tumor of the liver," *American Journal of Surgical Pathology*, vol. 17, no. 2, pp. 186–192, 1993.

[25] P. J. Karhunen, "Adult polycystic liver disease and biliary microhamartomas (von Meyenburg's complexes)," *Acta Pathologica Microbiologica et Immunologica Scandinavica*, vol. 94, no. 6, pp. 397–400, 1986.

[26] M. S. Redston and I. R. Wanless, "The hepatic von Meyenburg complex with hepatic and renal cysts," *Modern Pathology*, vol. 9, no. 3, pp. 233–237, 1996.

[27] J. S. Song, Y. J. Lee, K. W. Kim, J. Huh, S. J. Jang, and E. Yu, "Cholangiocarcinoma arising in von Meyenburg complexes: report of four cases," *Pathology International*, vol. 58, pp. 503–512, 2008.

[28] D. Jain, V. R. Sarode, F. W. Abdul-Karim, R. Homer, and M. E. Robert, "Evidence for the neoplastic transformation of von-Meyenburg complexes," *American Journal of Surgical Pathology*, vol. 24, pp. 1131–1139, 2000.

[29] T. Orii, N. Ohkohchi, K. Sasaki, S. Satomi, M. Watanabe, and T. Moriya, "Cholangiocarcinoma arising from preexisting biliary hamartoma of liver—report of a case," *Hepato-Gastroenterology*, vol. 50, no. 50, pp. 333–336, 2003.

[30] M. R. O'Dell, J. L. Huang, C. L. Whitney-Miller et al., "KrasG12D and p53 mutation cause primary intrahepatic cholangiocarcinoma," *Cancer Research*, vol. 72, no. 6, pp. 1557–1567, 2012.

[31] Y. Nakanuma, T. Terada, G. Ohta, M. Kurachi, and F. Matsubara, "Caroli's disease in congenital hepatic fibrosis and infantile polycystic disease," *Liver*, vol. 2, pp. 346–354, 1982.

[32] T. Sanzen, K. Harada, M. Yasoshima, Y. Kawamura, M. Ishibashi, and Y. Nakanuma, "Polycystic kidney rat is a novel animal model of Caroli's disease associated with congenital hepatic fibrosis," *American Journal of Pathology*, vol. 158, no. 5, pp. 1605–1612, 2001.

16

New Insights into the Pathogenesis of Alcohol-Induced ER Stress and Liver Diseases

Cheng Ji

USC Research Center for Liver Disease, Department of Medicine, Keck School of Medicine of USC, University of Southern California, 2011 Zonal Avenue, HMR-101, Los Angeles, CA 90089, USA

Correspondence should be addressed to Cheng Ji; chengji@usc.edu

Academic Editor: Shigeru Marubashi

Alcohol-induced liver disease increasingly contributes to human mortality worldwide. Alcohol-induced endoplasmic reticulum (ER) stress and disruption of cellular protein homeostasis have recently been established as a significant mechanism contributing to liver diseases. The alcohol-induced ER stress occurs not only in cultured hepatocytes but also *in vivo* in the livers of several species including mouse, rat, minipigs, zebrafish, and humans. Identified causes for the ER stress include acetaldehyde, oxidative stress, impaired one carbon metabolism, toxic lipid species, insulin resistance, disrupted calcium homeostasis, and aberrant epigenetic modifications. Importance of each of the causes in alcohol-induced liver injury depends on doses, duration and patterns of alcohol exposure, genetic disposition, environmental factors, cross-talks with other pathogenic pathways, and stages of liver disease. The ER stress may occur more or less all the time during alcohol consumption, which interferes with hepatic protein homeostasis, proliferation, and cell cycle progression promoting development of advanced liver diseases. Emerging evidence indicates that long-term alcohol consumption and ER stress may directly be involved in hepatocellular carcinogenesis (HCC). Dissecting ER stress signaling pathways leading to tumorigenesis will uncover potential therapeutic targets for intervention and treatment of human alcoholics with liver cancer.

1. Introduction

The endoplasmic reticulum (ER) is an essential organelle of eukaryotic cells functioning in secretory protein synthesis and processing, lipid synthesis, calcium storage/release, and detoxification of drugs. The ER ensures correct protein folding and maturation. Unfolded proteins are retained in the ER and targeted for retrotranslocation to the cytoplasm for rapid degradation. Under normal physiological conditions, there is a balance between the unfolded proteins and the ER folding machinery. Disruption of the balance results in accumulation of unfolded proteins, a condition termed ER stress [1–5]. The ER stress triggers the unfolded protein response (UPR), which attenuates protein translation, increases protein folding capacity, and promotes degradation of unfolded proteins, thus restoring ER homeostasis. However, prolonged UPR leads to an attempt to delete the cell causing injuries. Molecular chaperones such as the glucose-regulated protein 78 (GRP78/BiP) interact with three ER membrane resident stress sensors: inositol-requiring enzyme-1 (IRE1α), transcription factor-6 (ATF6), and PKR-like eukaryotic initiation factor 2α kinase (PERK), and play a vital role in maintaining the protein homeostasis inside the ER [1–5]. Many human diseases such as metabolic syndrome, neurodegenerative diseases, alcohol-induced organ disorders, and inflammatory diseases involve ER stress and impaired UPR signaling [1–7]. Increasing evidence supports ER stress as a key mechanism in alcohol-induced liver disease (ALD), a disease that affects over 140 million people worldwide. Potential molecular mechanisms underlying alcohol-induced ER stress in major organs including liver, brain, pancreas, lung, and heart have been discussed previously [8–10]. In this review, I will focus on updates and new insights into the pathogenesis of alcohol-induced ER stress and discuss an emerging role of alcohol-induced ER stress in liver tumorigenesis and hepatocellular carcinogenesis.

TABLE 1: Alcohol-induced endoplasmic reticulum stress (AERR) and injuries occur in many species.

Experimental system	Cause	Injury	Remark	Reference
Chronic intragastric infusion				
Mouse	Hyperhomocysteinemia	Necroinflammation	Mouse strain difference	[11–13]
	Methionine deficiency	Apoptosis	Rat and mouse difference	[14–18]
	Acetaldehyde adducts	Fatty liver	Synergy with obesity	[19]
Rat	High SAH	Fibrosis		[20]
	Low SAM/SAH			
	Epigenetic alterations			
Chronic oral feeding				
Micropig	Folate deficiency	Steatosis		[21]
Mouse	Chaperone deficiency	Apoptosis	Interaction of alcohol with	[22]
	Synergy with HFD/drugs	Fibrosis	anti-HIV/HCV drugs	[23]
	Excess iron	Cirrhosis	Involvement of autophagy	[24, 25]
	Oxidative stress		Oxidative stress precedes AERR	[26, 27]
Acute alcohol exposure				
Liver perfusion	Acetaldehyde, ROS	Fat accumulation	Role of alcohol metabolites in AERR	[28]
Mouse gavage	Synergy with drugs	Apoptosis		[22]
	Ca^{2+} homeostasis	Fibrosis	AERR parallels LPS-TLR4	[29, 30]
	Inflammation		Suppressed UPR	[31]
Zebrafish	CDIPT deficiency	Hepatomegaly		[32–34]
Nematode	Not known	Not characterized	No AERR without the liver	[35]
Alcohol treated cells				
Human cells	ROS	Apoptosis	Basal ER stress in HepG2	[36–38]
	Excessive homocysteine	Steatosis		
Patient liver biopsies				
Human alcoholics	Toxic lipid species	Apoptosis	Clinical relevance	[39–42]
	Oxidative stress	Steatohepatitis	Role of mitochondrial	
	Insulin resistance	Fibrosis/cirrhosis	Dysfunctions in AERR	

2. Multiple Mechanisms for Alcohol-Induced Hepatic ER Stress

Alcohol is mainly metabolized in the liver and liver cells are rich in ER, which assume synthesis of a large amount of secretory and membrane proteins. The UPR plays a pivotal role in maintaining ER homeostasis in the liver under both physiological and pathological conditions [4, 5, 9]. In the early 80s, stress-induced ER damages in the liver were observed in ultrastructural, morphological, and histological studies [43, 44]. However, little was known then about occurrence and mechanisms of alcohol-induced ER stress. A role of ER in alcohol metabolism began to be recognized as NADH from the hepatic alcohol oxidation by alcohol dehydrogenase (ADH) was also found to support microsomal alcohol oxidations [43–46]. The inducible microsomal ethanol oxidizing system (MEOS) is associated with ER proliferation and concomitant induction of cytochrome P4502E1 (CYP2E1) in rats and in humans [45, 46]. Free radical release, as a consequence of CYP2E1 activities in the ER and subsequent oxidative stress, and lipid peroxidation generally contribute to ALD. However, alcohol-induced ER stress response (AERR) that involves the UPR was not recognized until recently. Molecular evidence for an impaired UPR was first found in the mice with chronic intragastric alcohol infusion (CIAI) (Figure 1; Table 1) [11]. Alterations of some ER stress markers: GRP78, GRP94, CHOP (C/EBP homologous protein), and BAD (the Bcl-2-associated death promoter), in DNA microarrays were associated with severe steatosis, scattered apoptosis, and necroinflammation. SREBP-1c (sterol regulatory element-binding protein-1c) was found to be a strong candidate linking ER stress to alcoholic fatty liver, because SREBP-1c knockout mice were protected against triglyceride accumulation [12]. CHOP was found to be a key factor in AERR-caused cell death, as knocking out CHOP resulted in minimal alcohol-induced apoptosis in the liver [13].

Upstream of ER stress, altered methionine metabolism, and elevated homocysteine were initially proposed to be responsible for AERR because alcohol-induced hyperhomocysteinemia (HHcy) is often seen in rodents and humans [47–50] and homocysteine is known to modify proteins biochemically [8, 9, 11]. A few lines of molecular evidence support the methionine/homocysteine mechanism. First,

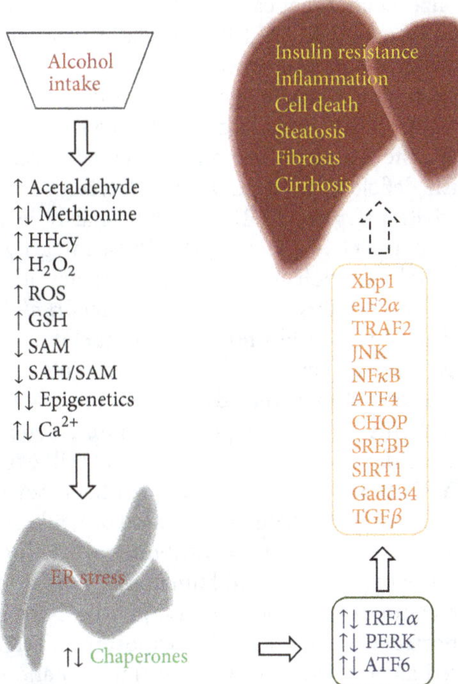

FIGURE 1: Identified molecular mechanisms for alcohol-induced endoplasmic reticulum stress and hepatic injuries. See the context for details.

betaine is a methyl donor for remethylation of homocysteine to methionine catalyzed partially by betaine-homocysteine methyltransferase (BHMT). Simultaneous betaine feeding or transgenic expression of BHMT in CIAI mice decreased the elevated homocysteine and abrogated AERR in parallel with decreased ALT and amelioration of ALD [11, 14, 15]. Second, an intragastric infusion with both high fat and alcohol induced moderate obesity and much severe ALD [16], which resulted from synergistic effects of an accentuated ER stress by the alcohol-induced HHcy in combination with mitochondrial stress, nitrosative stress, and adiponectin resistance. Third, rats with CIAI do not have a significant HHcy [17]. Consequently, the rat animals have a minimal ER stress response and are more resistant to ALD, which correlates with a significant induction of BHMT. Fourth, in a study with 14 inbred mouse strains with CIAI, profound differences in ALD were observed among the strains in spite of consistently high levels of urine alcohol [18]. ER stress related genes were induced only in strains with the most liver injury, which were closely associated with expression patterns of methionine metabolism-related genes and plasma homocysteine levels. Thus, abnormal protein modifications by excessive homocysteine as a result of aberrant one-carbon metabolism [18] and methionine deficiency [4] are likely responsible for the alcoholic ER stress and UPR in CIAI mice that lack a sufficient upregulation of BHMT.

However, other causes for the alcoholic ER stress are present in the CIAI model. For instance, in a study with CIAI rats to examine effects of selective inhibition of CYP2E1 on the development of alcoholic fatty liver [19], liver triglycerides were lower. ER stress indicated by the ER stress marker TRB3 (a mammalian homolog of *Drosophila* tribbles functions as a negative modulator of protein kinase B) was increased after ethanol and was further increased upon inhibition of CYP2E1 or overall ethanol metabolism. This suggests a contributing role of alcohol metabolites, for example, acetaldehyde, or oxidants to the alcoholic ER stress response. In another study with cystathionine β synthase (CBS) heterozygous mice treated with CIAI [20], steatohepatitis was accompanied with upregulations of hepatic ER stress components including GRP78, ATF4 (activating transcription factor 4), CHOP, and SREBP-1c and negatively correlated with S-adenosylmethionine (SAM) to S-adenosylhomocysteine (SAH) ratio. AERR was associated with a decrease in levels of suppressor chromatin marker trimethylated histone H3 lysine-9 (3meH3K9) in the promoter regions of the ER stress markers. Similarly, epigenetic mechanism for AERR might also occur in human alcoholics, as DNA hypermethylation of the promoter of HERP (homocysteine-induced ER protein) gene downregulates its mRNA expression in patients with alcohol dependence [51].

3. Diverse Models and Species with Alcohol-Induced ER Stress

AERR occurs not only in the aforementioned CIAI models but also in other chronic or acute models/systems (Table 1), which have been providing additional insights into AERR and ALD. In micropigs fed alcohol orally [21], liver steatosis and apoptosis were shown to be accompanied by increased mRNA levels of CYP2E1 and selective ER stress markers. Folate deficiency appeared to be responsible for the ER stress and injury. In mice, however, oral alcohol feeding *ad libitum* does not usually result in HHcy as remarkable as seen in the CIAI mice. Correspondingly, the degree of AERR and subsequent liver injury may depend on additional genetic and/or dietary factors. For instance, in the mice with liver specific deletion of GRP78/BiP [22], a robust ER stress response was observed at moderate oral alcohol doses (e.g., 4 g/kg), which was accompanied by much aggravated hepatosteatosis and hepatic fibrosis. Thus, compared to the homocysteine-ER stress mechanism, the liver BiP deletion represents a genetic predisposition that unmasks a distinct mechanism by which alcohol induces ER stress, one that is largely obscured by compensatory changes in normal animals or presumably in the majority of human population who have low-to-moderate drinking [8, 22]. The effect of genetic predisposition on AERR and hepatic injury is also observed in a recent study using mice with low alcohol-induced plasma homocysteine and deficient in the acid sphingomyelinase (ASMase) [23]. Strong AERR and enhanced susceptibility to lipopolysaccharides (LPS) or concanavalin-A were present in ASMase $^{-}/^{-}$ mice fed alcohol orally, indicative of a mitochondrial effect on AERR. In addition, in iron overloaded mice deficient in the hemochromatosis gene (Hfe $^{-}/^{-}$), cofeeding *ad libitum* with alcohol and a high-fat diet (HFD) led to profound steatohepatitis and fibrosis [24, 25]. XBP1 splicing, activation of IRE-1α and PERK, and increased CHOP protein expression were associated with impaired autophagy response, suggesting that preconditioning with iron overloading may modulate AERR and promote liver injury through interacting with other adaptive or compensatory mechanisms.

Alternatively, the contributing role of ER stress to ALD in oral feeding models could be secondary. This is indicated by a time-course study with a mouse model of early-stage ALD [26]. Mice with oral alcohol feeding exhibited significant hepatic steatosis and elevated plasma ALT values. At 1 to 2 weeks after alcohol feeding, oxidative stress indicated by 4-hydroxynonenal- (4-HNE-) modified proteins was increased, whereas hepatic glutathione (GSH) levels were significantly decreased as a consequence of decreased CBS activity, increased GSH utilization, and increased protein glutathionylation. Except for 4-HNE adduction to the ER disulfide isomerase (PDI), significant upregulations of other ER markers and SREBP pathways were not detected *in vivo* during the same early period of alcohol feeding [26, 27]. Although the actual blood alcohol levels were not measured in this study, which might not reach a critical point and vary widely among individual mice at a liberal access to alcohol, the results may suggest a secondary role of AERR in this early ALD model. Thus, interplay or cross-talk between AERR and other stresses might be critical in ALD. This notion is supported by a few most recent reports, which appears more evident in cell or animal models with acute alcohol exposure. First, cell death is not readily observed in acute ethanol intoxication. However, in a perfused rat liver system, downregulation of GRP78 and activation of c-Jun N-terminal kinase (JNK) and protein kinase B (PKB/Akt) were enhanced by a cotreatment of acute ethanol with a classical inhibitor of ADH, and an antioxidant addition reduced the activation of JNK and cell death [28]. High concentrations of the pharmacological ER stress-inducing agents such as tunicamycin or brefeldin A activate JNK and inhibit mitochondrial respiration and cell death in hepatocytes [52]. Mitochondrial respiration has been shown to play an adaptive role in ALD [53]. Thus, ethanol metabolites and/or impaired mitochondrial functions may complicate AERR. Second, the mice with liver specific GRP78 deletion are sensitized to a variety of acute hepatic disorders by alcohol, a high-fat diet, anti-HIV drugs, or toxins [22]. HIV protease inhibitors inhibit the ER Ca^{2+}ATPase (SERCA) and modulate calcium homeostasis in mice and primary human hepatocytes, which aggravates AERR and ALD [29]. Alcohol-induced LPS impairs UPR promoting rat liver cirrhosis [30]. Third, the interferon regulatory factor 3 (IRF3) is activated early by ER stress in mice fed alcohol either orally or intragastrically, which involves an ER adaptor, the stimulator of interferon genes (STING) [31]. Independent of inflammatory cytokines and Type-I interferons (IFNs), IRF3 exerts its pathogenic role in ALD through causing apoptosis of hepatocytes, which strongly suggests that AERR pathways and the LPS-TLR4 (toll-like receptor 4) pathways [54] are parallel or equally important in initiating ALD.

In addition to rodents, AERR has also been found in other species including human alcoholics (Table 1). Zebrafish larvae represent an alternative vertebrate model for studying AERR and ALD because their liver possesses the pathways to metabolize alcohol that can be simply added to the water, that is, acute alcohol [32]. AERR is present in alcohol-treated zebrafish, which may also interact with other pathological factors. Upon alcohol challenge, zebrafish larvae developed signs of acute ALD, including hepatomegaly and steatosis. Further, the ER stress response appeared much robust in zebrafish deficient in the CDP-diacylglycerol-inositol 3-phosphatidyltransferase (CDIPT) that primarily locates on the cytosolic aspect of the ER [33]. Thus, integrity of the ER or alcohol metabolism might be necessary for AERR [34]. In supporting this, in the species *Caenorhabditis elegans* without a liver for alcohol digestion/metabolism, little AERR has been detected [35]. The most important and clinically relevant studies regarding AERR are from human cells and patients. AERR is reported in human monocyte-derived dendritic cells (MDDC) [36], HepG2 cells expressing human CYP2E1 [37], and primary human hepatocytes [29]. Oxidative stress resulted from the function of CYP2E1 and/or interactions with other drugs contributing to AERR in the human cells. However, cultured human cell models may not reflect the complexity of the response *in vivo*. For instance, it was reported that, upon alcohol exposure, VL-17A cells metabolized alcohol which caused ER fragmentation inside the cells, but little activation of UPR target genes was detected [38]. Nevertheless, striking upregulation of multiple ER stress signaling molecules was detected in human patients with ALD (Table 1) [39–42], which is correlated with deregulated lipid metabolism, ceramide accumulation, and impaired insulin signaling, indicating that AERR is an integrated part of pathogenesis of ALD in human alcoholics.

4. Emerging Role of AERR in Liver Tumorigenesis and HCC

It has been well accepted that the UPR is a double-edged response because both adaptive survival and eliminative apoptosis can be induced by UPR components [1–6]. It is beneficial or prosurvival if it happens transiently or lasts for a short period of time, whereas it is detrimental or deadly if it is prolonged. Recent studies indicate that the UPR is associated with solid tumor development in many types of tissues or organs including the liver [55, 56]. Since the microenvironments of solid tumors are generally hypoxic, acidic, and nutrient deficient [57, 58], which individually or collectively favor activation of ER stress response, it is conceivable that the UPR is persistently present during tumorigenesis. The question is how the cancer cells evade cell death from the prolonged UPR. Emerging evidence suggests that cancerous cells could modify and perturb the ER stress-associated cell death signaling, which permits survival and growth. For instance, the master regulator UPR, GRP78, plays a dual role in tumor cells [22, 59]. It controls early tumor development through suppressive mechanisms such as the induction of cell cycle arrest or tumor dormancy upon PERK activation [60]. On the other hand, at more advanced stages of tumor progression, during which cells are exposed to more severe stressors, GRP78 suppresses caspase 7 activation and interacts with ER stress-induced protein chaperones such as clusterin to promote cell survival and further tumor development [61]. The PERK-eIF2α-ATF4 pathway is often activated by the hypoxic condition in solid tumors [62–64], which activates angiogenic genes, vascular endothelial growth factor (VEGF), type 1 collagen inducible protein, and autophagosome components such as LC3, ensuring cell survival over hypoxia-induced ER stress [65–67]. Prolonged expression and activation of ATF6 increase the Rheb-mTOR signaling pathway and also enhance tumor cell survival [68]. In addition, the IRE1α-Xbp1 pathway interacts with antiapoptotic Bcl-2 family members and the sigma-1 receptor, which is often increased in many human cell lines [69–72]. Therefore, impaired and/or prolonged UPR has a high potential to modulate cell fates and differentiations towards tumorigenesis.

Alcohol intake increasingly contributes to mortality from liver cancer in humans [73–76]. However, the mechanisms by which alcohol exerts its carcinogenic effect are largely unknown and currently there is no effective treatment. Considering that several lines of evidence indicate that polymorphic responses of major ER chaperones to alcohol and other stressors are associated with hepatocellular carcinogenesis in human populations [77–82], it is not unusual to find a role of AERR in HCC. In fact, we recently found spontaneous hepatocellular adenomas- (HCA-) like tumors in aged female mice with a liver specific BiP deletion and under constitutive ER stress [22, 59, 83]. Active ATF6, CHOP, GSK3β, and Creld2 (cysteine rich with EGF-like domains 2) were increased in the knockout, indicative of continuous ER stress response. None of p53, HNF1α, or GP130 was significantly changed compared between wild type and knockout. β-Catenin was slightly decreased. Interestingly, cyclin D was specifically reduced in the tumor portion of the knockout mice. Since most liver tumors were found in female knockouts, expression of receptors for sex hormones such as estrogen receptors, ERα and β, and androgen receptor, ARα, was examined. Three variants of ERα were detected in the liver, and their molecular sizes are 66 kD, 46 kD, and 36 kD, respectively [83]. The ERα variant 36 kD was remarkably increased in the tumor portion of the knockout liver. In contrast, there were no significant changes in the expression of ERβ, ARα, cyclin E, or cyclin G. These findings revealed thatinhibition of cyclin D and overexpression of ER variant 36 kD are associated with the tumor development in the female knockouts under constitutive ER stress [83]. Furthermore, the tumors are highly malignant in mice with additional stresses such as high-fat diet or alcohol intake [83, 84]. The pathways of ERK1/2, Stat3, and p38 were activated, which are known to promote HCC progression [85, 86].

The constitutive ER stress-induced spontaneous liver tumors that are dominant in female animals are similar to human HCA [87–90], which are of clinical relevance since about 80% of HCA cases are from women taking oral contraceptives for years [90, 91]. The pathogenesis of HCA is not completely understood due to its heterogeneity. Known potential causesfor human HCA are mutations in HNF1α, β-catenin, GP130, or chronic inflammation [87–93]. Hepatocellular protein homeostasis has rarely been noticed to be a potential mechanism for HCA development. Thus,

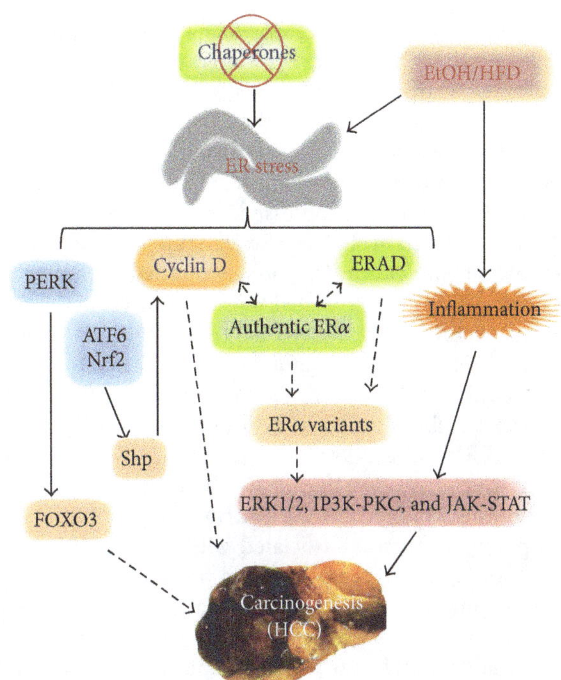

Figure 2: Proposed model depicts novel endoplasmic reticulum (ER) stress mechanisms linking alcohol (EtOH) and/or high-fat diet (HFD), cyclin D, ERAD, estrogen receptor α (ERα) variants, FOXO3, and Shp with hepatocellular carcinogenesis (HCC). Solid lines represent established pathways based on the literature; dashed lines represent emerging mechanisms under investigations. See the context for details.

the above findings on cyclin D and ERα variants may reveal a novel ER stress mechanism for HCA for several reasons (Figure 2). First, the *in vivo* inhibition of cyclin D expression upon ER stress in knockouts is consistent with an earlier study, which demonstrated that activation of the UPR in mouse NIH 3T3 fibroblasts with tunicamycin led to a decline in cyclin D and subsequent G(1) phase arrest [94–96]. Second, increased expression of cyclin D is usually associated with proliferation in other systems [97]. However, a number of studies have shown many new roles of cyclin D [98] and a surprising lack of the correlation of increased cyclin D with proliferation in tumors [99, 100]. For instance, in one subtype of human breast carcinoma, cyclin D1 protein expression was absent in the noninvasive cells [101, 102]. Similarly, a loss of cyclin D did not inhibit the proliferative response of mouse liver to mitogenic stimuli [103] and mRNA levels of cyclin D1 were downregulated in patients with HCC [104]. Most recent molecular evidence further supports this ER stress-cyclin D-tumorigenesis mechanism. Nrf2 (the nuclear factor erythroid 2-related factor 2) activities are associated with aging [105]. ER stress activates Nrf2 and ATF6, both of which regulate the orphan nuclear receptor, Shp (small heterodimer partner) which acts as a transcriptional corepressor modulating cyclin D1 and subsequent hepatic tumorigenesis [106, 107]. The ER stress sensor PERK has been shown to phosphorylate the Forkhead transcription factor 3 (FOXO3) [108] and suppressed FOXO3 exacerbates alcoholic hepatitis and insulin resistance impairing cyclin D function promoting HCC [109–111]. Thus, abnormal functions of cyclin D under ER stress conditions most likely disturb liver cell proliferation (Figure 2). Third, since the authentic ERα66 interacts with cyclin D physically [100, 101], the hepatic ERα variants may result from an unbalanced long-term molecular interaction between ERα and the suppressed cyclin D under ER stress (Figure 2). Alternatively, the ERα variants may be produced from an incomplete protein processing/maturation of ERα by an impaired ER-associated degradation (ERAD). Components of ERAD are indeed altered in the BiP knockout mouse models under constitutive UPR [22, 59, 83, 84], and there is a report indicating that an activation of the Xbp1-Hrd1 (an E3 ubiquitin ligase also called synoviolin) branch by the UPR facilitates Nrf2 ubiquitylation and degradation during liver cirrhosis [112]. Similarly, ERα could also be a target of the impaired ERAD. Fourth, considering that ERα gene polymorphism is associated with risk of HBV-related acute liver failure [113] and a switch from the authentic ERα to a predominant expression of ERα36 is associated with development and progression of HCC [114–116], the hepatic ERα variants could also play an important role in alcohol and ER stress-associated HCC. The tumorigenic signaling downstream of cyclin D and ERα variants can be activations of the ERK1/2, IP3K-PKC, or JAK-STAT pathways [117]. Overexpressed ERα36 has been associated with activation of these pathways and carcinogenesis in other systems such as breast cancer and gastric cancer [118–122]. In the liver, activations of ERK1/2 and JAK-STAT pathways were observed in the BiP knockout mice fed alcohol and high-fat diet [83, 84]. Finally, studies on hepatoma cell lines, HCC tissues, and animal models of HCC suggest a possible role of sex hormones and their receptors in HCC pathogenesis [123]. A male prevalence of HCC is often observed in young and middle aged patient populations in certain regions exposed to additional HCC risk factors [124]. However, the male prevalence of HCC tends to diminish in aged human populations [125] as well as in aged animals fed alcohol [83, 84]. Therefore, alcohol-induced ER stress and cell cycle impairment may exert specific effects on aging, hepatic expression of estrogen receptors, and subsequent tumorigenesis in females.

5. Conclusive Remarks

Alcohol-induced hepatic ER stress occurs in the liver of many species including human alcoholics, which has recently been established as an important mechanism for both acute and chronic alcohol-induced liver pathogenesis and disease development. Multiple factors commonly associated with alcohol consumption such as acetaldehyde, oxidative stress, excessive homocysteine, toxic lipid species, increased SAH, aberrant epigenetic modifications, disruption of calcium homeostasis, and insulin resistance induce ER stress response individually or collectively. However, the precise contribution of each of the factors to the ER stress induction is not clear and their importance to ALD may depend on doses, duration and patterns of alcohol exposure, presence or absence of genetic and environmental factors, cross-talks with other pathogenic pathways, and liver disease stages. The UPR, as an integrated part of liver physiology and pathology like the immune response, may occur more or less all the time during alcohol consumption, which attempts to restore ER homeostasis and protect against ALD. However, this adaptive protection is not without detrimental consequences. Prolonged UPR leads to excessive deletion of the damaged hepatocytes or cell cycle arrest, which triggers inflammatory response or interrupts normal cellular processes causing profound injuries. Emerging evidence by us and others indicates a direct involvement of long-term alcohol and constitutive ER stress in liver tumorigenesis and hepatocellular carcinogenesis. The ER stress and malfunctioning of cyclin D-caused cell cycle arrest are a well-established molecular mechanism, and the surprise overexpression of estrogen receptor α variants under constitutive UPR may result from a mal-targeting of protein processing and turnover by aberrant ERAD, which reflect complexity and depth of prolonged UPR-mediated pathogenesis. Thus, liver tumorigenesis by alcohol and ER stress may involve not only cyclin D, ERα variants, ERK1/2, PKC, and STAT pathways, but also other cell cycle targets such as IL-6, p21, p27, and CDK, other pathways such as Src/EGFR, PTEN-TGFβ, and insulin/IGF, and epigenetic regulations such as miRNAs targeting the UPR components. In addition, liver progenitor cell activation by alcohol may contribute to the malignant transformation of nonmalignant tumors developed under long-term ER stress [22, 59]. Future work should be directed to define the ER stress mechanisms leading to HCC and to develop multiple therapeutic approaches to target ER stress in human alcoholics with HCC.

Abbreviations

ADH:	Alcohol dehydrogenase
AERR:	Alcohol-induced ER stress response
ALD:	Alcohol-induced liver disease
ARα:	Androgen receptor α
ASMase:	The acid sphingomyelinase
ATF 4 or 6:	Activating transcription factor 4 or 6
BAD:	The Bcl-2-associated death promoter
BiP:	Binding immunoglobulin protein also known as 78 kDa glucose-regulated protein (GRP78)
BHMT:	Betaine-homocysteine methyltransferase
CBS:	Cystathionine β synthase
CDIPT:	CDP-diacylglycerol-inositol 3-phosphatidyltransferase
CDK:	Cyclin-dependent kinase
CHOP:	C/EBP homology protein 10
CIAI:	Chronic intragastric alcohol infusion
Creld2:	Cysteine rich with EGF-like domains 2
EGFR:	Activation of the epidermal growth factor receptor
ER:	Endoplasmic reticulum
ERα:	Estrogen receptors α
ERAD:	ER-associated degradation
ERK1/2:	Extracellular signal-regulated protein kinases 1 and 2

FOXO3: The forkhead transcription factor
HCA: Hepatocellular adenomas
HCC: Hepatocellular carcinogenesis
HERP: Homocysteine-induced ER protein
HFD: High-fat diet
HHcy: Hyperhomocysteinemia
4-HNE: 4-Hydroxynonenal
HNF1α: Hepatocyte nuclear factor 1α
Hrd1: An E3 ubiquitin ligase also called synoviolin
GADD34: Growth arrest and DNA damage-inducible protein 34
GSH: Glutathione
GP130: Glycoprotein 130
GSK3β: Glycogen synthase kinase 3β
IGF: Insulin-like growth factor
IRE1α: Inositol-requiring enzyme-1α
IRF3: The interferon regulatory factor 3
JAK: Janus kinase
JNK: c-Jun N-terminal kinases
LC3: Microtubule-associated protein 1A/1B-light chain 3
LPS: Lipopolysaccharides
Mito: Mitochondria
MDDC: Human monocyte-derived dendritic cells
MEOS: The inducible microsomal ethanol oxidizing system
mTOR: Mammalian target of rapamycin
NFκB: Nuclear factor κB
PDI: The ER disulfide isomerase
Nrf2: The nuclear factor erythroid 2-related factor 2
PGC1: PPARγ coactivator 1
PERK: PKR-like ER-localized eIF2α kinase
PKC: Protein kinase C
PTEN: Phosphatase and tensin homolog
ROS: Reactive oxygen species
SAH: S-Adenosylhomocysteine
SAM: S-Adenosylmethionine
SERCA: ER calcium transport ATPase
Shp: Small heterodimer partner
SIRT1: Silent mating type information regulation 2 homolog 1
SRC: Protooncogene tyrosine-protein kinase
SREBP: Sterol regulatory element-binding protein
STING: An ER adaptor, the stimulator of interferon genes
Stat3: Signal transducer and activator of transcription 3
TGFα: Transforming growth factor α
TLR4: Toll-like receptor 4
TRB3: A mammalian homolog of *Drosophila* tribbles functions as a negative modulator of protein kinase B (PKB)
TRAF2: TNF receptor-associated factor 2
TUDCA: Tauroursodeoxycholate
UPR: The unfolded protein response
VEGF: Vascular endothelial growth factor
XBP1: X-box binding protein 1.

Acknowledgments

This work is supported by the US National Institute of Health (NIH) Grants R01AA018612, R01AA014428, and R01AA018846. The author is grateful to the graduate students and postdoctoral fellows who contributed to the studies in his lab.

References

[1] P. Walter and D. Ron, "The unfolded protein response: from stress pathway to homeostatic regulation," *Science*, vol. 334, no. 6059, pp. 1081–1086, 2011.

[2] S. S. Cao and R. J. Kaufman, "Targeting endoplasmic reticulum stress in metabolic disease," *Expert Opinion on Therapeutic Targets*, vol. 17, no. 4, pp. 437–448, 2013.

[3] S. Fu, S. M. Watkins, and G. S. Hotamisligil, "The role of endoplasmic reticulum in hepatic lipid homeostasis and stress signaling," *Cell Metabolism*, vol. 15, no. 5, pp. 623–634, 2012.

[4] A. Henkel and R. M. Green, "The unfolded protein response in Fatty liver disease," *Seminars in Liver Disease*, vol. 33, no. 4, pp. 321–329, 2013.

[5] S. Wolff, J. S. Weissman, and A. Dillin, "Differential scales of protein quality control," *Cell*, vol. 157, no. 1, pp. 52–64, 2014.

[6] L. Ozcan and I. Tabas, "Role of endoplasmic reticulum stress in metabolic disease and other disorders," *Annual Review of Medicine*, vol. 63, pp. 317–328, 2012.

[7] M. Kitamura, "The unfolded protein response triggered by environmental factors," *Seminars in Immunopathology*, vol. 35, no. 3, pp. 259–275, 2013.

[8] C. Ji, "Dissection of endoplasmic reticulum stress signaling in alcoholic and non-alcoholic liver injury," *Journal of Gastroenterology and Hepatology*, vol. 23, no. 1, pp. S16–S24, 2008.

[9] C. Ji, "Mechanisms of alcohol-induced endoplasmic reticulum stress and organ injuries," *Biochemistry Research International*, vol. 2012, Article ID 216450, 12 pages, 2012.

[10] L. Kaphalia, N. Boroumand, J. Hyunsu, B. S. Kaphalia, and W. J. Calhoun, "Ethanol metabolism, oxidative stress, and endoplasmic reticulum stress responses in the lungs of hepatic alcohol dehydrogenase deficient deer mice after chronic ethanol feeding," *Toxicology and Applied Pharmacology*, 2014.

[11] C. Ji and N. Kaplowitz, "Betaine decreases hyperhomocysteinemia, endoplasmic reticulum stress, and liver injury in alcohol-fed mice," *Gastroenterology*, vol. 124, no. 5, pp. 1488–1499, 2003.

[12] C. Ji, C. Chan, and N. Kaplowitz, "Predominant role of sterol response element binding proteins (SREBP) lipogenic pathways in hepatic steatosis in the murine intragastric ethanol feeding model," *Journal of Hepatology*, vol. 45, no. 5, pp. 717–724, 2006.

[13] C. Ji, R. Mehrian-Shai, C. Chan, Y.-H. Hsu, and N. Kaplowitz, "Role of CHOP in hepatic apoptosis in the murine model of intragastric ethanol feeding," *Alcoholism: Clinical and Experimental Research*, vol. 29, no. 8, pp. 1496–1503, 2005.

[14] C. Ji, M. Shinohara, J. Kuhlenkamp, C. Chan, and N. Kaplowitz, "Mechanisms of protection by the betaine-homocysteine methyltransferase/ betaine system in HepG2 cells and primary

mouse hepatocytes," *Hepatology*, vol. 46, no. 5, pp. 1586–1596, 2007.

[15] C. Ji, M. Shinohara, D. Vance et al., "Effect of transgenic extrahepatic expression of betaine-homocysteine methyltransferase on alcohol or homocysteine-induced fatty liver," *Alcoholism: Clinical and Experimental Research*, vol. 32, no. 6, pp. 1049–1058, 2008.

[16] J. Xu, K. K. Y. Lai, A. Verlinsky et al., "Synergistic steatohepatitis by moderate obesity and alcohol in mice despite increased adiponectin and p-AMPK," *Journal of Hepatology*, vol. 55, no. 3, pp. 673–682, 2011.

[17] M. Shinohara, C. Ji, and N. Kaplowitz, "Differences in betaine-homocysteine methyltransferase expression, endoplasmic reticulum stress response, and liver injury between alcohol-fed mice and rats," *Hepatology*, vol. 51, no. 3, pp. 796–805, 2010.

[18] M. Tsuchiya, C. Ji, O. Kosyk et al., "Interstrain differences in liver injury and one-carbon metabolism in alcohol-fed mice," *Hepatology*, vol. 56, no. 1, pp. 130–139, 2012.

[19] M. J. Ronis, S. Korourian, M. L. Blackburn, J. Badeaux, and T. M. Badger, "The role of ethanol metabolism in development of alcoholic steatohepatitis in the rat," *Alcohol*, vol. 44, no. 2, pp. 157–169, 2010.

[20] F. Esfandiari, V. Medici, D. H. Wong et al., "Epigenetic regulation of hepatic endoplasmic reticulum stress pathways in the ethanol-fed cystathionine beta synthase-deficient mouse," *Hepatology*, vol. 51, no. 3, pp. 932–941, 2010.

[21] F. Esfandiari, J. A. Villanueva, D. H. Wong, S. W. French, and C. H. Halsted, "Chronic ethanol feeding and folate deficiency activate hepatic endoplasmic reticulum stress pathway in micropigs," *American Journal of Physiology—Gastrointestinal and Liver Physiology*, vol. 289, no. 1, pp. G54–G63, 2005.

[22] C. Ji, N. Kaplowitz, M. Y. Lau, E. Kao, L. M. Petrovic, and A. S. Lee, "Liver-specific loss of glucose-regulated protein 78 perturbs the unfolded protein response and exacerbates a spectrum of liver diseases in mice," *Hepatology*, vol. 54, no. 1, pp. 229–239, 2011.

[23] A. Fernandez, N. Matias, R. Fucho et al., "ASMase is required for chronic alcohol induced hepaticendoplasmic reticulum stress and mitochondrial cholesterol loading," *Journal of Hepatology*, vol. 59, no. 4, pp. 805–813, 2013.

[24] T. C. Tan, D. H. Crawford, L. A. Jaskowski et al., "Excess iron modulates endoplasmic reticulum stress-associated pathways in a mouse model of alcohol and high-fat diet-induced liver injury," *Laboratory Investigation*, vol. 93, no. 12, pp. 1295–1312, 2013.

[25] T. C. Tan, D. H. Crawford, L. A. Jaskowski et al., "A corn oil-based diet protects against combined ethanol and iron-induced liver injury in a mouse model of hemochromatosis," *Alcoholism: Clinical and Experimental Research*, vol. 37, no. 10, pp. 1619–1631, 2013.

[26] J. J. Galligan, R. L. Smathers, K. S. Fritz, L. E. Epperson, L. E. Hunter, and D. R. Petersen, "Protein carbonylation in a murine model for early alcoholic liver disease," *Chemical Research in Toxicology*, vol. 25, no. 5, pp. 1012–1021, 2012.

[27] J. J. Galligan, R. L. Smathers, C. T. Shearn et al., "Oxidative stress and the ER stress response in a murine model for early-stage alcoholic liver disease," *Journal of Toxicology*, vol. 2012, Article ID 207594, 12 pages, 2012.

[28] Y. Nishitani and H. Matsumoto, "Ethanol rapidly causes activation of JNK associated with ER stress under inhibition of ADH," *FEBS Letters*, vol. 580, no. 1, pp. 9–14, 2006.

[29] E. Kao, M. Shinohara, M. Feng, M. Y. Lau, and C. Ji, "Human immunodeficiency virus protease inhibitors modulate Ca(2+) homeostasis and potentiate alcoholic stress and injury in mice and primary mouse and human hepatocytes," *Hepatology*, vol. 56, no. 2, pp. 594–604, 2012.

[30] K. A. Tazi, I. Bièche, V. Paradis et al., "In vivo altered unfolded protein response and apoptosis in livers from lipopolysaccharide-challenged cirrhotic rats," *Journal of Hepatology*, vol. 46, no. 6, pp. 1075–1088, 2007.

[31] J. Petrasek, A. Iracheta-Vellve, T. Csak et al., "STING-IRF3 pathway links endoplasmic reticulum stress with hepatocyte apoptosis in early alcoholic liver disease," *Proceedings of the National Academy of Sciences of the United States of America*, vol. 110, no. 41, pp. 16544–16549, 2013.

[32] M. J. Passeri, A. Cinaroglu, C. Gao, and K. C. Sadler, "Hepatic steatosis in response to acute alcohol exposure in zebrafish requires sterol regulatory element binding protein activation," *Hepatology*, vol. 49, no. 2, pp. 443–452, 2009.

[33] P. C. Thakur, C. Stuckenholz, M. R. Rivera et al., "Lack of de novo phosphatidylinositol synthesis leads to endoplasmic reticulum stress and hepatic steatosis in cdipt-deficient zebrafish," *Hepatology*, vol. 54, no. 2, pp. 452–462, 2011.

[34] O. Tsedensodnom, A. M. Vacaru, D. L. Howarth, C. Yin, and K. C. Sadler, "Ethanol metabolism and oxidative stress are required for unfolded protein response activation and steatosis in zebrafish with alcoholic liver disease," *Disease Models & Mechanisms*, vol. 6, no. 5, pp. 1213–1226, 2013.

[35] B. Ient, R. Edwards, R. Mould, M. Hannah, L. Holden-Dye, and V. O'Connor, "HSP-4 endoplasmic reticulum (ER) stress pathway is not activated in a C. elegans model of ethanol intoxication and withdrawal," *Invertebrate Neuroscience*, vol. 12, no. 2, pp. 93–102, 2012.

[36] N. M. Boukli, Z. M. Saiyed, M. Ricaurte et al., "Implications of ER stress, the unfolded protein response, and pro- and anti-apoptotic protein fingerprints in human monocyte-derived dendritic cells treated with alcohol," *Alcoholism: Clinical and Experimental Research*, vol. 34, no. 12, pp. 2081–2088, 2010.

[37] L. Magne, E. Blanc, B. Legrand et al., "ATF4 and the integrated stress response are induced by ethanol and cytochrome P450 2E1 in human hepatocytes," *Journal of Hepatology*, vol. 54, no. 4, pp. 729–737, 2011.

[38] D. L. Howarth, A. M. Vacaru, O. Tsedensodnom et al., "Alcohol disrupts endoplasmic reticulum function and protein secretion in hepatocytes," *Alcoholism: Clinical and Experimental Research*, vol. 36, no. 1, pp. 14–23, 2012.

[39] L. Longato, K. Ripp, M. Setshedi et al., "Insulin resistance, ceramide accumulation, and endoplasmic reticulum stress in human chronic alcohol-related liver disease," *Oxidative Medicine and Cellular Longevity*, vol. 2012, Article ID 479348, 17 pages, 2012.

[40] T. Ramirez, L. Longato, M. Dostalek, M. Tong, J. R. Wands, and S. M. de la Monte, "Insulin resistance, ceramide accumulation and endoplasmic reticulum stress in experimental chronic alcohol-induced steatohepatitis," *Alcohol and Alcoholism*, vol. 48, no. 1, pp. 39–52, 2013.

[41] T. Ramirez, M. Tong, W. C. Chen, Q. G. Nguyen, J. R. Wands, and S. M. de la Monte, "Chronic alcohol-induced hepatic insulin resistance and ER stress ameliorated by PPAR-δ, agonist treatment," *Journal of Gastroenterology and Hepatology*, vol. 28, no. 1, pp. 179–187, 2013.

[42] M. Tong, L. Longato, T. Ramirez, V. Zabala, J. R. Wands, and S. M. de la Monte, "Therapeutic reversal of chronic alcohol-related steatohepatitis with the ceramide inhibitor myriocin," *International Journal of Experimental Pathology*, vol. 95, no. 1, pp. 49–63, 2014.

[43] D. L. Cinti, R. Grundin, and S. Orrenius, "The effect of ethanol on drug oxidations in vitro and the significance of ethanol-cytochrome P-450 interaction," *Biochemical Journal*, vol. 134, no. 2, pp. 367–375, 1973.

[44] C. S. Lieber, "Microsomal ethanol-oxidizing system," *Enzyme*, vol. 37, no. 1-2, pp. 45–56, 1987.

[45] C. S. Lieber, "The discovery of the microsomal ethanol oxidizing system and its physiologic and pathologic role," *Drug Metabolism Reviews*, vol. 36, no. 3-4, pp. 511–529, 2004.

[46] C. S. Lieber, "Pathogenesis and treatment of alcoholic liver disease: progress over the last 50 years," *Roczniki Akademii Medycznej w Białymstoku*, vol. 50, pp. 7–20, 2005.

[47] A. J. Barak, H. C. Beckenhauer, D. J. Tuma, and S. Badakhsh, "Effects of prolonged ethanol feeding on methionine metabolism in rat liver," *Biochemistry and Cell Biology*, vol. 65, no. 3, pp. 230–233, 1987.

[48] C. Blasco, J. Caballería, R. Deulofeu et al., "Prevalence and mechanisms of hyperhomocysteinemia in chronic alcoholics," *Alcoholism: Clinical and Experimental Research*, vol. 29, no. 6, pp. 1044–1048, 2005.

[49] B. Hultberg, M. Berglund, A. Andersson, and A. Frank, "Elevated plasma homocysteine in alcoholics," *Alcoholism: Clinical and Experimental Research*, vol. 17, no. 3, pp. 687–689, 1993.

[50] U. C. Lutz, "Alterations in homocysteine metabolism among alcohol dependent patients—clinical, pathobiochemical and genetic aspects," *Current Drug Abuse Reviews*, vol. 1, no. 1, pp. 47–55, 2008.

[51] S. Bleich, B. Lenz, M. Ziegenbein et al., "Epigenetic DNA hypermethylation of the HERP gene promoter induces down-regulation of its mRNA expression in patients with alcohol dependence," *Alcoholism: Clinical and Experimental Research*, vol. 30, no. 4, pp. 587–591, 2006.

[52] S. Win, T. A. Than, J. C. Fernandez-Checa, and N. Kaplowitz, "JNK interaction with Sab mediates ER stress induced inhibition of mitochondrial respiration and cell death," *Cell Death & Disease*, vol. 5, article e989, 2014.

[53] D. Han, M. D. Ybanez, H. S. Johnson et al., "Dynamic adaptation of liver mitochondria to chronic alcohol feeding in mice: biogenesis, remodeling, and functional alterations," *The Journal of Biological Chemistry*, vol. 287, no. 50, pp. 42165–42179, 2012.

[54] S. Inokuchi, H. Tsukamoto, E. Park, Z.-X. Liu, D. A. Brenner, and E. Seki, "Toll-like receptor 4 mediates alcohol-induced steatohepatitis through bone marrow-derived and endogenous liver cells in mice," *Alcoholism: Clinical and Experimental Research*, vol. 35, no. 8, pp. 1509–1518, 2011.

[55] Y. P. Vandewynckel, D. Laukens, A. Geerts et al., "The paradox of the unfolded protein response in cancer," *Anticancer Research*, vol. 33, no. 11, pp. 4683–4694, 2013.

[56] W. A. Wang, J. Groenendyk, and M. Michalak, "Endoplasmic reticulum stress associated responses in cancer," *Biochimica et Biophysica Acta*, 2014.

[57] J. M. Brown and A. J. Giaccia, "The unique physiology of solid tumors: opportunities (and problems) for cancer therapy," *Cancer Research*, vol. 58, no. 7, pp. 1408–1416, 1998.

[58] A. J. Giaccia, J. M. Brown, B. Wouters, N. Denko, and C. Koumenis, "Cancer therapy and tumor physiology," *Science*, vol. 279, no. 5347, pp. 12–13, 1998.

[59] A. S. Lee, "Glucose-regulated proteins in cancer: molecular mechanisms and therapeutic potential," *Nature Reviews Cancer*, vol. 14, no. 4, pp. 263–276, 2014.

[60] R. T. Weston and H. Puthalakath, "Endoplasmic reticulum stress and BCL-2 family members," *Advances in Experimental Medicine and Biology*, vol. 687, pp. 65–77, 2010.

[61] C. Wang, K. Jiang, D. Gao et al., "Clusterin protects hepatocellular carcinoma cells from endoplasmic reticulum stress induced apoptosis through GRP78," *PLoS One*, vol. 8, no. 2, article e55981, 2013.

[62] F. Martinon, "Targeting endoplasmic reticulum signaling pathways in cancer," *Acta Oncologica*, vol. 51, no. 7, pp. 822–830, 2012.

[63] C. Koumenis, "ER stress, hypoxia tolerance and tumor progression," *Current Molecular Medicine*, vol. 6, no. 1, pp. 55–69, 2006.

[64] D. R. Fels and C. Koumenis, "The PERK/eIF2alpha/ATF4 module of the UPR in hypoxia resistance and tumor growth," *Cancer Biology & Therapy*, vol. 5, no. 7, pp. 723–728, 2006.

[65] J. D. Blais, C. L. Addison, R. Edge et al., "Perk-dependent translational regulation promotes tumor cell adaptation and angiogenesis in response to hypoxic stress," *Molecular and Cellular Biology*, vol. 26, no. 24, pp. 9517–9532, 2006.

[66] T. Rzymski, M. Milani, L. Pike et al., "Regulation of autophagy by ATF4 in response to severe hypoxia," *Oncogene*, vol. 29, no. 31, pp. 4424–4435, 2010.

[67] D. Cojocari, R. N. Vellanki, B. Sit, D. Uehling, M. Koritzinsky, and B. G. Wouters, "New small molecule inhibitors of UPR activation demonstrate that PERK, but not IRE1α, signaling is essential for promoting adaptation and survival to hypoxia," *Radiotherapy & Oncology*, vol. 108, no. 3, pp. 541–547, 2013.

[68] D. M. Schewe and J. A. Aguirre-Ghiso, "ATF6α-Rheb-mTOR signaling promotes survival of dormant tumor cells in vivo," *Proceedings of the National Academy of Sciences of the United States of America*, vol. 105, no. 30, pp. 10519–10524, 2008.

[69] C. Hetz, P. Bernasconi, J. Fisher et al., "Proapoptotic BAX and BAK modulate the unfolded protein response by a direct interaction with IRE1α," *Science*, vol. 312, no. 5773, pp. 572–576, 2006.

[70] D. A. Rodriguez, S. Zamorano, F. Lisbona et al., "BH3-only proteins are part of a regulatory network that control the sustained signalling of the unfolded protein response sensor IRE1α," *EMBO Journal*, vol. 31, no. 10, pp. 2235–2437, 2012.

[71] B. J. Vilner, B. R. De Costa, and W. D. Bowen, "Cytotoxic effects of sigma ligands: sigma receptor-mediated alterations in cellular morphology and viability," *Journal of Neuroscience*, vol. 15, no. 1, part 1, pp. 117–134, 1995.

[72] T. Hayashi and T.-P. Su, "Sigma-1 Receptor Chaperones at the ER- Mitochondrion Interface Regulate Ca2+ Signaling and Cell Survival," *Cell*, vol. 131, no. 3, pp. 596–610, 2007.

[73] P. Grewal and V. A. Viswanathen, "Liver cancer and alcohol," *Clinical Liver Disease*, vol. 16, no. 4, pp. 839–850, 2012.

[74] K. R. Warren and M. M. Murray, "Alcoholic liver disease and pancreatitis: global health problems being addressed by the US National Institute on Alcohol Abuse and Alcoholism," *Journal of Gastroenterology and Hepatology*, vol. 28, supplement 1, pp. 4–6, 2013.

[75] P. D. Friedmann, "Alcohol use in adults," *The New England Journal of Medicine*, vol. 368, no. 17, pp. 1655–1656, 2013.

[76] L. Gunzerath, B. G. Hewitt, T.-K. Li, and K. R. Warren, "Alcohol research: past, present, and future," *Annals of the New York Academy of Sciences*, vol. 1216, no. 1, pp. 1–23, 2011.

[77] X. Zhu, J. Zhang, W. Fan et al., "The rs391957 variant cis-regulating oncogene GRP78 expression contributes to the risk of hepatocellular carcinoma," *Carcinogenesis*, vol. 34, no. 6, pp. 1273–1280, 2013.

[78] T. Winder, P. Bohanes, W. Zhang et al., "Grp78 promoter polymorphism rs391957 as potential predictor for clinical outcome in gastric and colorectal cancer patients," *Annals of Oncology*, vol. 22, no. 11, pp. 2431–2439, 2011.

[79] X. Zhu, L. Chen, W. Fan et al., "An intronic variant in the GRP78, a stress-associated gene, improves prediction for liver cirrhosis in persistent HBV carriers," *PLoS ONE*, vol. 6, no. 7, Article ID e21997, 2011.

[80] X. Zhu, M.-S. Chen, L.-W. Tian et al., "Single nucleotide polymorphism of rs430397 in the fifth intron of GRP78 gene and clinical relevance of primary hepatocellular carcinoma in Han Chinese: risk and prognosis," *International Journal of Cancer*, vol. 125, no. 6, pp. 1352–1357, 2009.

[81] S. Liu, K. Li, T. Li et al., "Association between promoter polymorphisms of the GRP78 gene and risk of type 2 diabetes in a Chinese han population," *DNA and Cell Biology*, vol. 32, no. 3, pp. 119–124, 2013.

[82] D. T. Merrick, "GRP78, intronic polymorphisms, and pharmacogenomics in non-small cell lung cancer," *Chest*, vol. 141, no. 6, pp. 1377–1378, 2012.

[83] M. Y. Lau, H. Han, J. Hu, and C. Ji, "Association of cyclin D and estrogen receptor α36 with hepatocellular adenomas of female mice under chronic endoplasmic reticulum stress," *Journal of Gastroenterology and Hepatology*, vol. 28, no. 3, pp. 576–583, 2013.

[84] H. Han, J. Hu, M. Y. Lau, M. Feng, L. M. Petrovic, and C. Ji, "Altered methylation and expression of ER-associated degradation factors in long-term alcohol and constitutive ER stress-induced murine hepatic tumors," *Frontiers in Genetics*, vol. 4, article 224, 2013.

[85] G. Giannelli, N. Napoli, and S. Antonaci, "Tyrosine kinase inhibitors: a potential approach to the treatment of hepatocellular carcinoma," *Current Pharmaceutical Design*, vol. 13, no. 32, pp. 3301–3304, 2007.

[86] J. Muntané, A. J. De la Rosa, F. Docobo, R. García-Carbonero, and F. J. Padillo, "Targeting tyrosine kinase receptors in hepatocellular carcinoma," *Current Cancer Drug Targets*, vol. 13, no. 3, pp. 300–312, 2013.

[87] P. Bioulac-Sage, S. Taouji, L. Possenti, and C. Balabaud, "Hepatocellular adenoma subtypes: the impact of overweight and obesity," *Liver International*, vol. 32, no. 8, pp. 1217–1221, 2012.

[88] J.-C. Nault and J. Zucman-Rossi, "Genetics of hepatobiliary carcinogenesis," *Seminars in Liver Disease*, vol. 31, no. 2, pp. 173–187, 2011.

[89] V. S. Katabathina, C. O. Menias, A. K. P. Shanbhogue, J. Jagirdar, R. M. Paspulati, and S. R. Prasad, "Genetics and imaging of hepatocellular adenomas: 2011 update," *Radiographics*, vol. 31, no. 6, pp. 1529–1543, 2011.

[90] H. Lin, J. Van Den Esschert, C. Liu, and T. M. Van Gulik, "Systematic review of hepatocellular adenoma in China and other regions," *Journal of Gastroenterology and Hepatology*, vol. 26, no. 1, pp. 28–35, 2011.

[91] H. A. Edmondson, B. Henderson, and B. Benton, "Liver cell adenomas associated with use of oral contraceptives," *The New England Journal of Medicine*, vol. 294, no. 9, pp. 470–472, 1976.

[92] P. Bioulac-Sage, G. Cubel, C. Balabaud, and J. Zucman-Rossi, "Revisiting the pathology of resected benign hepatocellular nodules using new immunohistochemical markers," *Seminars in Liver Disease*, vol. 31, no. 1, pp. 91–103, 2011.

[93] C. Guichard, G. Amaddeo, S. Imbeaud et al., "Integrated analysis of somatic mutations and focal copy-number changes identifies key genes and pathways in hepatocellular carcinoma," *Nature Genetics*, vol. 44, pp. 694–698, 2012.

[94] J. W. Brewer, L. M. Hendershot, C. J. Sherr, and J. A. Diehl, "Mammalian unfolded protein response inhibits cyclin D1 translation and cell-cycle progression," *Proceedings of the National Academy of Sciences of the United States of America*, vol. 96, no. 15, pp. 8505–8510, 1999.

[95] J. W. Brewer and J. A. Diehl, "PERK mediates cell-cycle exit during the mammalian unfolded protein response," *Proceedings of the National Academy of Sciences of the United States of America*, vol. 97, no. 23, pp. 12625–12630, 2000.

[96] R. B. Hamanaka, B. S. Bennett, S. B. Cullinan, and J. A. Diehl, "PERK and GCN2 contribute to eIF2α phosphorylation and cell cycle arrest after activation of the unfolded protein response pathway," *Molecular Biology of the Cell*, vol. 16, no. 12, pp. 5493–5501, 2005.

[97] J. K. Kim and J. A. Diehl, "Nuclear cyclin D1: an oncogenic driver in human cancer," *Journal of Cellular Physiology*, vol. 220, no. 2, pp. 292–296, 2009.

[98] R. G. Pestell, "New roles of cyclin D1," *The American Journal of Pathology*, vol. 183, no. 1, pp. 3–9, 2013.

[99] E. A. Musgrove, C. E. Caldon, J. Barraclough, A. Stone, and R. L. Sutherland, "Cyclin D as a therapeutic target in cancer," *Nature Reviews Cancer*, vol. 11, no. 8, pp. 558–572, 2011.

[100] M. Fu, C. Wang, Z. Li, T. Sakamaki, and R. G. Pestell, "Minireview: cyclin D1: normal and abnormal functions," *Endocrinology*, vol. 145, no. 12, pp. 5439–5447, 2004.

[101] T. Oyama, K. Kashiwabara, K. Yoshimoto, A. Arnold, and F. Koerner, "Frequent overexpression of the cyclin D1 oncogene in invasive lobular carcinoma of the breast," *Cancer Research*, vol. 58, no. 13, pp. 2876–2880, 1998.

[102] B. S. Shoker, C. Jarvis, M. P. A. Davies, M. Iqbal, D. R. Sibson, and J. P. Sloane, "Immunodetectable cyclin D1 is associated with oestrogen receptor but not Ki67 in normal, cancerous and precancerous breast lesions," *British Journal of Cancer*, vol. 84, no. 8, pp. 1064–1069, 2001.

[103] G. M. Ledda-Columbano, M. Pibiri, D. Concas, C. Cossu, M. Tripodi, and A. Columbano, "Loss of cyclin D1 does not inhibit the proliferative response of mouse liver to mitogenic stimuli," *Hepatology*, vol. 36, no. 5, pp. 1098–1105, 2002.

[104] J. W. Lu, Y. M. Lin, J. G. Chang et al., "Clinical implications of deregulated CDK4 and Cyclin D1 expression in patients with human hepatocellular carcinoma," *Medical Oncology*, vol. 30, no. 1, article 379, 2013.

[105] J. H. Suh, S. V. Shenvi, B. M. Dixon et al., "Decline in transcriptional activity of Nrf2 causes age-related loss of glutathione synthesis, which is reversible with lipoic acid," *Proceedings of the National Academy of Sciences of the United States of America*, vol. 101, no. 10, pp. 3381–3386, 2004.

[106] Y. Zhang and L. Wang, "Nuclear receptor small heterodimer partner in apoptosis signaling and liver cancer," *Cancers*, vol. 3, no. 1, pp. 198–212, 2011.

[107] Y. Zhang, C. H. Hagedorn, and L. Wang, "Role of nuclear receptor SHP in metabolism and cancer," *Biochimica et Biophysica Acta*, vol. 1812, no. 8, pp. 893–908, 2011.

[108] W. Zhang, V. Hietakangas, S. Wee, S. C. Lim, J. Gunaratne, and S. M. Cohen, "ER stress potentiates insulin resistance

through PERK-mediated FOXO phosphorylation," *Genes & Development*, vol. 27, no. 4, pp. 441–449, 2013.

[109] M. J. Czaja, W. X. Ding, T. M. Donohue Jr. et al., "Functions of autophagy in normal and diseased liver," *Autophagy*, vol. 9, no. 8, pp. 1131–1158, 2013.

[110] I. Tikhanovich, S. Kuravi, R. V. Campbell et al., "Regulation of FOXO3 by phosphorylation and methylation in hepatitis C virus infection and alcohol exposure," *Hepatology*, vol. 59, no. 1, pp. 58–70, 2014.

[111] J. Kopycinska, A. Kempińska-Podhorodecka, T. Haas et al., "Activation of FoxO3a/Bim axis in patients with Primary Biliary Cirrhosis," *Liver International*, vol. 33, no. 2, pp. 231–238, 2013.

[112] T. Wu, F. Zhao, B. Gao et al., "Hrdl suppresses Nrf2-mediated cellular protection during liver cirrhosis," *Genes & Development*, 2014.

[113] Z. Yan, W. Tan, Y. Dan et al., "Estrogen receptor alpha gene polymorphisms and risk of HBV-related acute liver failure in the Chinese population," *BMC Medical Genetics*, vol. 13, article 49, 2012.

[114] V. Miceli, L. Cocciadiferro, M. Fregapane et al., "Expression of wild-type and variant estrogen receptor alpha in liver carcinogenesis and tumor progression," *OMICS A Journal of Integrative Biology*, vol. 15, no. 5, pp. 313–317, 2011.

[115] S. D. Quaynor, E. W. Stradtman Jr, H. G. Kim et al., "Delayed puberty and estrogen resistance in a woman with estrogen receptor α variant," *The New England Journal of Medicine*, vol. 369, no. 2, pp. 164–171, 2013.

[116] D. J. Clegg and B. F. Palmer, "Effects of an estrogen receptor α variant," *The New England Journal of Medicine*, vol. 369, no. 17, pp. 1663–1664, 2013.

[117] A. Moeini, H. Cornellà, and A. Villanueva, "Emerging signaling pathways in hepatocellular carcinoma," *Liver Cancer*, vol. 1, no. 2, pp. 83–93, 2012.

[118] S. Vranic, Z. Gatalica, H. Deng et al., "ER-α36, a novel isoform of ER-α66, is commonly over-expressed in apocrine and adenoid cystic carcinomas of the breast," *Journal of Clinical Pathology*, vol. 64, no. 1, pp. 54–57, 2011.

[119] R. A. Chaudhri, R. Olivares-Navarrete, N. Cuenca, A. Hadadi, B. D. Boyan, and Z. Schwartz, "Membrane estrogen signaling enhances tumorigenesis and metastatic potential of breast cancer cells via estrogen receptor-α36 (ERα36)," *Journal of Biological Chemistry*, vol. 287, no. 10, pp. 7169–7181, 2012.

[120] J. Wang, J. Li, R. Fang, S. Xie, L. Wang, and C. Xu, "Expression of ERα36 in gastric cancer samples and their matched normal tissues," *Oncology Letters*, vol. 3, no. 1, pp. 172–175, 2012.

[121] X. T. Zhang, L. Ding, L. G. Kang, and Z. Y. Wang, "Involvement of ER-α36, Src, EGFR and STAT5 in the biphasic estrogen signaling of ER-negative breast cancer cells," *Oncology Reports*, vol. 27, no. 6, pp. 2057–2065, 2012.

[122] R. A. Chaudhri, R. Olivares-Navarrete, N. Cuenca, A. Hadadi, B. D. Boyan, and Z. Schwartz, "Membrane estrogen signaling enhances tumorigenesis and metastatic potential of breast cancer cells via estrogen receptor-α36 (ERα36)," *Journal of Biological Chemistry*, vol. 287, no. 10, pp. 7169–7181, 2012.

[123] M. Di Maio, B. Daniele, S. Pignata et al., "IS human hepatocellular carcinoma a hormone-responsive tumor?" *World Journal of Gastroenterology*, vol. 14, no. 11, pp. 1682–1689, 2008.

[124] M. M. Center and A. Jemal, "International trends in liver cancer incidence rates," *Cancer Epidemiology Biomarkers and Prevention*, vol. 20, no. 11, pp. 2362–2368, 2011.

[125] A. P. Venook, C. Papandreou, J. Furuse, and L. L. de Guevara, "The incidence and epidemiology of hepatocellular carcinoma: a global and regional perspective," *The Oncologist*, vol. 15, supplement 4, pp. 5–13, 2010.

17

Impact of Pretransplant HepaticEncephalopathy on Liver Posttransplantation Outcomes

Lewis W. Teperman

Division of Transplant Director, Mary Lea Johnson Richards Organ Transplantation Center, New York University Langone Medical Center, Rivergate 3, 403 E 34th Street, New York, NY 10016, USA

Correspondence should be addressed to Lewis W. Teperman; lewis.teperman@nyumc.org

Academic Editor: Matthias Bahr

Patients with cirrhosis commonly experience hepatic encephalopathy (HE), a condition associated with alterations in behavior, cognitive function, consciousness, and neuromuscular function of varying severity. HE occurring before liver transplant can have a substantial negative impact on posttransplant outcomes, and preoperative history of HE may be a predictor of posttransplant neurologic complications. Even with resolution of previous episodes of overt or minimal HE, some patients continue to experience cognitive deficits after transplant. Because HE is one of the most frequent pretransplant complications, improving patient HE status before transplant may improve outcomes. Current pharmacologic therapies for HE, whether for the treatment of minimal or overt HE or for prevention of HE relapse, are primarily directed at reducing cerebral exposure to systemic levels of gut-derived toxins (e.g., ammonia). The current mainstays of HE therapy are nonabsorbable disaccharides and antibiotics. The various impacts of adverse effects (such as diarrhea, abdominal distention, and dehydration) on patient's health and nutritional status should be taken into consideration when deciding the most appropriate HE management strategy in patients awaiting liver transplant. This paper reviews the potential consequences of pretransplant HE on posttransplant outcomes and therapeutic strategies for the pretransplant management of HE.

1. Introduction

Cirrhosis of the liver—the only cure for which is liver transplant—is associated with several serious complications, including ascites, spontaneous bacterial peritonitis, variceal bleeding, and hepatic encephalopathy (HE) [1]. Guidelines established by the American Association for the Study of Liver Diseases currently recommend referring patients with cirrhosis for liver transplant when their model for end-stage liver disease (MELD) score is ≥10 and their Child-Turcotte-Pugh (CTP) score is ≥7 or when they experience their first major complication (e.g., HE, ascites, or variceal bleeding) [2]. However, the current United Network for Organ Sharing allocation system only uses the MELD score for prioritizing adults for liver transplant [3]. The MELD scoring system evaluates a patient's short-term prognosis based on 3 common laboratory test results: serum bilirubin, international normalized ratio, and serum creatinine levels. However, this scoring system does not take into account several serious complications of cirrhosis, such as HE, when prioritizing patients for liver transplant [4]. This may have negative ramifications for patient care, as the development of HE may be associated with substantial morbidity, mortality, and cost.

HE imposes a significant burden on patients, their families, and health care resources [5, 6]. HE is characterized by alterations in behavior, cognitive abilities, consciousness, and neuromuscular function [7]. It negatively affects patient quality of life (QOL), and patients may be unable to drive, work, or adequately care for themselves because of its effects [8–11]. Patients may be less compliant with all prescribed medications, and hospitalizations related to HE may increase patient exposure to opportunistic infections and be associated with substantial costs. Furthermore, HE may be an independent predictor of mortality in patients with chronic liver disease [12]. HE occurring before liver transplant can also have a substantial negative impact on posttransplant outcomes [13–22]. This paper will review the potential consequences of pretransplant HE on posttransplant outcomes and therapeutic strategies for the pretransplant management of HE.

2. Consequences of Pretransplant HE on Posttransplant Outcomes

HE can be classified into 3 types based on the hepatic abnormality observed [7]. HE may occur in patients with acute liver failure (type A HE), in patients with portosystemic shunting but no intrinsic hepatocellular disease (type B HE), or, as in the majority of HE cases, in patients with cirrhosis and cirrhosis-related portosystemic shunting (type C HE). Because HE is a progressive neuropsychiatric condition, HE may be graded or scored based on the severity of the clinical manifestations, which may range from subtle neurologic abnormalities in mild cases to coma in severe cases. Minimal HE (sometimes referred to as covert HE), which may occur in nearly 70% of patients with cirrhosis [23], is not associated with any clinical signs of brain dysfunction [7], but patients experience cognitive abnormalities that can lead to QOL impairment [8, 24, 25]. Unlike minimal HE, overt HE can manifest as a wide spectrum of symptoms that can be observed clinically, including those related to motor and neuropsychologic functions. Overt HE has been shown to occur in nearly half of patients with cirrhosis [26] and, as with minimal HE, also has a substantial negative impact on QOL [7–10].

Although research is ongoing, the pathogenesis of HE is believed to primarily involve the exposure of the brain to elevated neurotoxin levels, particularly ammonia and other gut-derived toxins, leading to cellular morphologic changes (e.g., astrocyte swelling) and the development of a variety of neurochemical, neurotransmitter, and neuroinflammatory changes [27, 28]. Many factors that can precipitate HE (e.g., hypokalemia, infection, and gastrointestinal bleeding) serve to increase the production of ammonia or other gut-derived toxins or to reduce toxin metabolism by the liver (e.g., dehydration, anemia) [29]. Although the exact pathophysiology of HE is unclear, data are accumulating to suggest that the cascade of neuropsychiatric and neuromuscular sequelae of HE may have a longer term or more permanent negative impact on patients with chronic liver disease than originally suspected.

3. Neurologic Complications after Transplant

Neurologic complications are common following liver transplant and may include alterations in mental status, seizures, and focal motor deficits [30]. The majority (≥75%) of these complications are observed within the first month after liver transplant, suggesting a possible relationship between preoperative status and liver transplant rather than the effect of immunosuppression [13, 19, 31]. However, neurologic complications may be observed in the long term, even 1 year after transplant [19, 32]. Of the neurologic complications, encephalopathy is most commonly observed, although the reported incidence has varied widely from 12% to 84% of patients at some point postoperatively [19, 20, 31, 33–36]. A variety of factors may cause neurologic complications, including encephalopathy, infection (e.g., sepsis), perioperative complications, persistence of major portosystemic shunts, and immunosuppressant-associated toxicity. Neurologic complications have also been associated with a greater risk of patient mortality [13, 37]. Thus, encephalopathy can be seen as a neurologic complication in itself and as a potential cause of neurologic complications.

3.1. Impact of Pretransplant Overt HE on Neurologic Complications after Transplant. Preoperative history of HE is a significant predictor of posttransplant neurologic complications. In a prospective analysis of 84 patients with chronic liver disease who had undergone a liver transplant, the presence of an abnormal neurologic exam suggestive of HE before transplant was an independent risk factor for developing in-hospital central nervous system complications after transplant ($P = 0.007$) [13]. In a retrospective study of 101 patients who had undergone a liver transplant, a history of HE was strongly associated with neurologic complications after transplant (univariate odds ratio (OR), 2.6; 95% confidence interval (CI), 1.1–6.4; $P = 0.03$). Furthermore, using a multivariate analysis, HE in the immediate preoperative period was associated with posttransplant neurologic complications (adjusted OR, 10.7; 95% CI, 3.8–29.9; $P < 0.013$) [20].

Data continue to accumulate suggesting that even with resolution of prior episodes of overt HE, patients may continue to have cognitive deficits after transplant. Patients who had undergone a liver transplant, on average 17 to 19 months previously, received a battery of cognitive tests (e.g., psychometric hepatic encephalopathy score (PHES) and Repeatable Battery for the Assessment of Neuropsychological Status (RBANS; Pearson Education Inc., San Antonio, TX)) to determine if the presence of HE before liver transplant was associated with more substantial neurocognitive abnormalities within about 1.5 years after transplant [21]. Patients with a history of HE before transplant ($n = 25$) had significantly lower scores for 3 of 6 PHES domains compared with healthy individuals ($n = 20$) and for 2 of 6 PHES domains (attention domains) compared with patients without HE before transplant ($n = 14$; Figure 1) [21]. The investigators of this study did not determine the total PHES score because of a lack of available normative values. For RBANS, patients with a history of HE before transplant had significantly lower scores compared with healthy individuals in total RBANS score and 4 of the 5 RBANS subscores ($P < 0.05$). Although the total RBANS score, immediate memory, delayed memory, and attention subscores were lower for patients with HE before transplant than for patients without HE before transplant, no significant differences were observed [21].

In cross-sectional ($n = 226$) and prospective assessments ($n = 59$) of patients with cirrhosis, patients who had experienced overt HE had greater cognitive dysfunction compared with patients without overt HE [22]. Patients who had an episode of overt HE had persistent impairment in cognitive function despite normalization of mental status on lactulose therapy, and the severity of impairment increased with the number of overt HE episodes. Thus, patients who experience overt HE may have persistent and cumulative deficits in working memory, response inhibitor, and learning that are chronic, cumulative, and not readily reversible (i.e., permanent) [22]. It is possible that these deficits may remain even after liver transplantation.

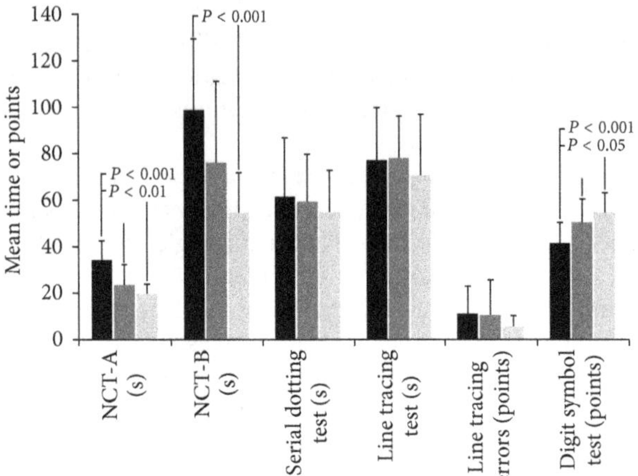

Figure 1: Psychometric HE score results for patients with a history of HE before transplant compared with patients with no history of HE before transplant and age-matched healthy individuals. HE, hepatic encephalopathy; NCT-A, number connection test A; NCT-B, number connection test B. Adapted with permission from Sotil et al., American Association for the Study of Liver Diseases [21].

Although not studied in patients who had eventually undergone a liver transplant, persistent cognitive impairment after overt HE was also supported by a study in 106 patients with cirrhosis currently without overt HE who were examined on 2 occasions within a 3-day period for the presence of mild cognitive impairment (PHES) [38]. Among 45 patients (42%) without a history of overt HE and 34 patients (32%) without a history of overt HE but with a current diagnosis of minimal HE, PHES results improved significantly from the first to the second exam ($P = 0.04$ and $P = 0.016$, resp.), suggesting a learning capacity for taking the tests involved in PHES [38]. However, there was no significant improvement in PHES results at the second exam for the 27 patients (25%) who had experienced at least 1 prior episode of overt HE, indicating a lack of learning capacity in patients with a history of overt HE [38]. Therefore, patients with a history of overt HE may have persistent cognitive impairment despite having a normal mental status and, in some cases, even in the presence of normal cognitive test results (PHES), which further supports the hypothesis that HE is not a fully reversible condition.

3.2. Impact of Pretransplant Minimal HE on Neurologic Complications after Transplant. Evidence also exists for the posttransplant persistence of cognitive dysfunction or radiologic abnormalities in patients exhibiting minimal HE before transplant [14–18]. In a small prospective study, 14 patients with minimal HE underwent liver transplant and were assessed for visuomotor function (average time of assessment, 21 months after transplant) [14]. Improvement of visuomotor and visuoconstructive skills (e.g., trail making tests, reconstruction of drawing, or picture) was observed in some patients after transplant, but worsening was observed in others. Of note, no significant improvement in posttransplant visuomotor and visuoconstructive performance was noted compared with pretreatment performance, with 50% of patients showing deterioration in performance. In addition, mean posttransplant results for the 14 patients with minimal HE were significantly lower than for 22 age-matched healthy individuals ($P = 0.04$) [14].

In another study of patients with minimal HE before transplant ($n = 23$), most assessed cognitive functions improved at 6 months after transplant, with some cognitive functions improving only 18 months after transplant (e.g., verbal short-term memory) [39].

3.3. Mechanisms by Which HE Impacts Neurologic Complications after Transplant. Data support the hypothesis that patients with a history of HE before transplant can have more pronounced cognitive dysfunction after transplant than patients without a history of HE. However, results are confounded by some studies that suggest almost complete normalization of radiologic findings after transplant, including gradual normalization of glutamine/glutamate and choline signals in a majority of patients as measured by magnetic resonance spectroscopy [40, 41]. In addition, the mechanisms by which more pronounced posttransplant cognitive impairment occurs in patients with pretransplant histories of HE are unclear, especially the lack of clearly defined variables that may play a role in short-term or long-term cognitive dysfunction. In a prospective study of 52 patients with cirrhosis who had a liver transplant (54% with minimal HE and 0% with overt HE), cognitive function significantly improved from pretransplant values for memory, attention, executive function, motor function, and visuospatial domains of the battery of tests administered ($P < 0.05$). However, 13% of patients still had global cognitive impairment 6 to 12 months after transplant [42]. In addition, after liver transplant, cognitive function in patients with cirrhosis of alcoholic etiology, diabetes mellitus, and prior HE was more severely impaired compared with patients without these factors. Posttransplant patients with alcohol-induced cirrhosis had memory decline, patients with diabetes mellitus exhibited attention impairment, and patients with histories of HE had impaired motor function (Figure 2) [42].

A multivariate analysis indicated that prior HE, diabetes mellitus, and cirrhosis of alcoholic etiology were considered risk factors for poor cognitive function that persists after transplant [42]. More research is necessary to gain a clearer understanding of the key demographics and disease characteristics that are involved to better identify patient subpopulations that are at the greatest risk for posttransplant neurologic complications.

4. Treatment of HE in the Pretransplant Setting

The development of minimal or overt HE before liver transplant may affect posttransplant outcomes, and HE is a probable risk factor for neuropsychiatric symptoms after transplantation. Therefore, although the cause of neuropsychiatric symptoms following a liver transplant is likely multifactorial,

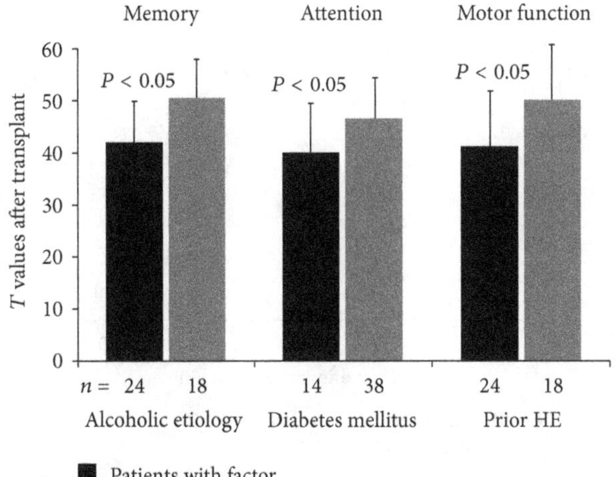

FIGURE 2: Posttransplant cognitive function (T values) in patients with or without risk factors that were determined to be associated with cognitive impairment (i.e., cirrhosis of alcoholic etiology, diabetes mellitus, and prior HE). T values were calculated using the following formula: $T = 50 + 10$ ([raw test value − mean test value]/SD of normal population). Impairment was defined as $T \leq 40$. HE, hepatic encephalopathy; SD, standard deviation. Adapted with permission from Garcia-Martinez et al., American Association for the Study of Liver Diseases [42].

improving patient HE status before transplant may improve posttransplant outcomes. Current pharmacologic therapies for HE are primarily directed at reducing the systemic levels of ammonia and other toxins produced in the gastrointestinal tract, thereby reducing cerebral exposure. Patients may be treated for minimal HE, overt HE, or the prevention of HE relapse. However, most patients with minimal HE do not currently receive treatment outside the context of clinical trials. In all of these cases, the mainstays of therapy are nonabsorbable disaccharides and antibiotics.

4.1. Nonabsorbable Disaccharides. Nonabsorbable disaccharides, such as lactulose and lactitol (not available in the United States), are metabolized in the colon by intestinal bacteria, resulting in a reduction in colonic pH. The acidic environment promotes uptake of ammonia by colonic bacteria, facilitates diffusion of ammonia from the blood into the intestine, and may reduce the survival of urease-producing bacteria. Nonabsorbable disaccharides also increase the osmotic pressure of the intestinal lumen, which induces catharsis and elimination of potential sources of gut-derived toxins from the body.

A 2004 meta-analysis of 22 randomized studies was conducted to evaluate the efficacy of nonabsorbable disaccharides compared with no treatment, placebo, or antibiotics in patients with acute, chronic, or minimal HE [43]. Nonabsorbable disaccharides appeared to improve HE (i.e., reduced the risk of no improvement) when compared with no intervention or placebo ($P = 0.002$). However, when studies of poor methodologic quality were removed from the analysis, no significant effect was observed in the few high-quality trials that had been conducted. In addition, nonabsorbable disaccharides had no significant effect on mortality compared with no treatment or placebo intervention. The authors concluded that there was insufficient evidence to support or contest the use of lactulose or lactitol for the treatment of HE [43].

A 2011 meta-analysis of 5 studies specifically evaluated nonabsorbable disaccharides for the treatment of minimal HE and concluded that compared with placebo these agents significantly improved minimal HE (i.e., reduced the risk of no improvement) ($P < 0.0001$) [44]. Another 2011 meta-analysis of 9 studies evaluating lactulose for the treatment of minimal HE confirmed that lactulose prevented the progression to overt HE, compared with either placebo or no intervention. However, no significant difference in mortality was observed [45].

Subsequent to this analysis, an open-label randomized study concluded lactulose to be effective for the primary prophylaxis of overt HE in patients with cirrhosis [46]. Twenty (19%) of 105 patients followed for 12 months developed an episode of overt HE, six (11%) in the lactulose group and 14 (28%) in the nonlactulose treated group ($P = 0.02$) [46]. However, consistent with other studies, no significant difference in mortality was observed ($P = 0.16$).

In the 2004 meta-analysis, nonabsorbable disaccharides were significantly less effective than antibiotics in improving HE (i.e., they were associated with a higher risk of no HE improvement; $P = 0.03$) and did not have a significantly different impact on mortality [43]. Patients with HE who received nonabsorbable disaccharides also had higher blood ammonia levels after treatment compared with patients who received antibiotics [43]. However, a separate meta-analysis reported similar efficacy between antibiotics and nonabsorbable disaccharides in improving HE [47].

In addition, a few studies have evaluated nonabsorbable disaccharides for the prevention of HE recurrence (i.e., secondary prophylaxis) [48–51]. In 1 randomized, and unblinded, placebo-controlled study, 140 patients with cirrhosis who had recovered from a previous HE episode were randomly assigned within 1 week of recovery to receive either lactulose 30 to 60 mL/d ($n = 70$) or placebo ($n = 70$) [49]. Thirteen patients (9%) were lost to follow-up; 61 patients in the lactulose group and 64 patients in the placebo group were followed for a median of 14 months (range, 1–20 months). Lactulose significantly reduced the percentage of patients who experienced overt HE recurrence compared with placebo (20% versus 47%, resp.; $P = 0.001$; Figure 3) [49]. However, no significant difference in the median time of HE recurrence was observed (7.5 months (range, 1–13 months) versus 6.0 months (range, 2–15 months), resp.). In addition, no significant differences between the 2 groups were reported in admissions to the liver intensive care unit for conditions other than HE or deaths during the study [49].

Adverse events (AEs) associated with nonabsorbable disaccharides are commonly gastrointestinal-related and include abdominal pain, diarrhea, flatulence, and nausea [43]. Diarrhea can also lead to secondary complications, including dehydration, hypokalemia, and hypernatremia [52]. Anorexia and vomiting have also been reported as AEs

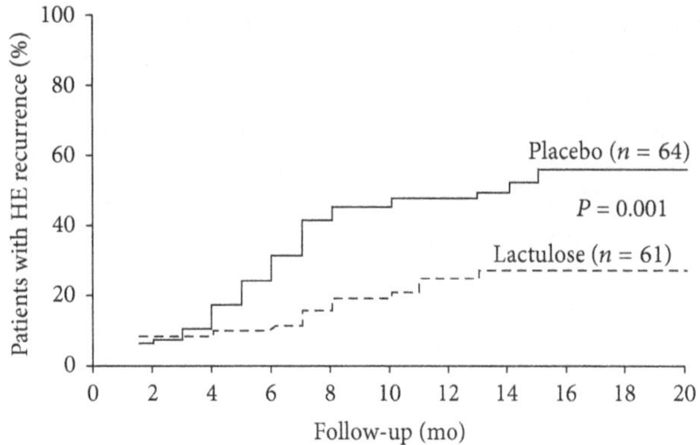

FIGURE 3: Probability of patients with cirrhosis developing HE recurrence during daily treatment with lactulose or placebo. HE, hepatic encephalopathy. Reprinted from Sharma et al., Copyright © 2009, with permission from W. B. Saunders Co. [49].

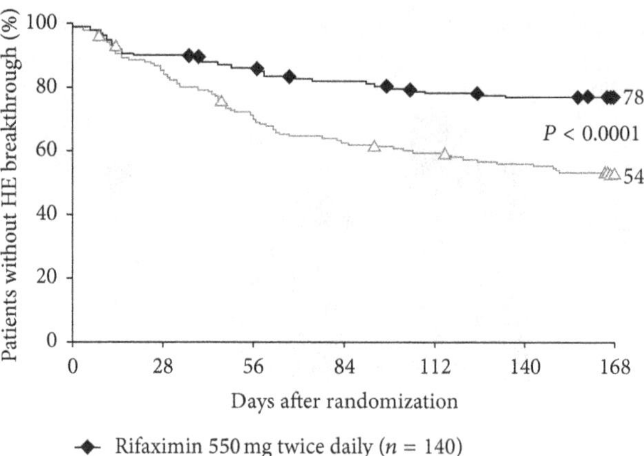

FIGURE 4: Kaplan-Meier estimate of time to first breakthrough HE episode (primary endpoint) in patients in remission for overt HE (Conn score, 0 or 1). HE breakthrough was defined as an increase in Conn score to ≥2 or, if baseline Conn = 0, a 1-unit increase each in Conn score and asterixis grade. Symbols indicate censored patients. HE, hepatic encephalopathy. Reprinted from Bass et al, Copyright © 2010, with permission from Massachusetts Medical Society [70].

occurring with use of nonabsorbable disaccharides (rate of 2% for each) [53]. One additional concern with lactulose is that administration can cause abdominal distention, which may result in technical difficulties during liver transplant [54, 55]. These gastrointestinal AEs in patients awaiting liver transplant may directly impact patient nutritional status. Nutritional status before liver transplant has also been shown to correlate with posttransplant survival [56] and is independently associated with the number of infection episodes after transplant [57]. Malnutrition, assessed by a subjective global nutritional assessment exam, was found to be an independent risk factor for the length of stay in the intensive care unit and the total number of days spent in the hospital after transplant [57]. Furthermore, alterations in specific laboratory measures (e.g., albumin, sodium, and potassium) [58–60], which may be negatively impacted by gastrointestinal AEs, have also been identified as risk factors for surgical complications in patients who received a liver transplant, and serum sodium levels are a prognostic factor for survival in patients awaiting liver transplant [61, 62]. Thus, gastrointestinal AEs may increase patient risk, particularly for patients who are prone to malnutrition because of various comorbid variables or conditions (e.g., dietary restrictions or gastroparesis) [63]. It is possible that administration of nonabsorbable disaccharides such as lactulose may exacerbate pretransplant nutritional deficits [64], thereby contributing to poor posttransplant outcomes.

4.2. Antibiotics. Antibiotics are administered to reduce systemic levels of ammonia and other gut-derived toxins by targeting gastrointestinal bacteria. Because of the risk for systemic AEs and bacterial antibiotic resistance with systemic antibiotics, nonsystemic antibiotics are preferred agents. Rifaximin is a nonsystemic gut-selective antibiotic and more than 20 studies have evaluated rifaximin for the treatment of overt HE (see review by Lawrence and Klee) [65] or minimal HE [66–68]. In 2010, rifaximin was approved by the US Food and Drug Administration for the maintenance of overt HE remission in adults [69].

In a randomized, double-blind, phase 3 trial of rifaximin for the maintenance of HE remission, patients in remission from HE were treated with rifaximin 1100 mg/d (n = 140) or placebo (n = 159) for up to 6 months [70]. Concomitant lactulose administration was permitted during the study: 91% of patients in each group received concomitant lactulose. Only 22% of patients in the rifaximin group experienced a breakthrough HE episode compared with 46% of patients in the placebo group. Furthermore, rifaximin significantly reduced the risk of HE breakthrough by 58% compared with placebo during the 6 months of treatment (hazard ratio (HR), 0.42; 95% CI, 0.28–0.64; P < 0.001; Figure 4) [70]. Data indicated that the number needed to treat (NNT) was 4 (i.e., for every 4 patients treated with rifaximin for 6 months, 1 episode of breakthrough HE would be prevented). In addition, 14% of patients in the rifaximin group reported an HE-related hospitalization compared with 23% of patients in the placebo group [70]. Rifaximin significantly (P = 0.01) reduced the risk of HE-related hospitalizations by 50% compared with placebo (HR, 0.50; 95% CI, 0.29–0.87) [70]. Data indicated that the NNT was 9 (i.e., for every 9 patients treated with rifaximin for 6 months, 1 episode of HE-related hospitalization would be prevented).

Health-related QOL in the phase 3 trial was assessed using the Chronic Liver Disease Questionnaire (CLDQ), which was administered every 4 weeks, and the time to HE breakthrough recorded [70, 71]. A significant (P = 0.0087 to 0.0436) improvement with rifaximin treatment was noted in the overall CLDQ scores and in each domain score compared with placebo treatment, and scores were significantly (P < 0.0001) lower in patients who experienced HE breakthrough compared with those who remained in remission [71].

In the phase 3 trial, rifaximin was well tolerated, with a similar incidence of AEs reported in both groups [70]. The most common AEs with rifaximin and placebo were nausea (14.3% versus 13.2%), diarrhea (10.7% versus 13.2%), fatigue (12.1% versus 11.3%), and peripheral edema (15.0% versus 8.2%). Two cases of *Clostridium difficile* infection (CDI) were reported during the double-blind portion of the trial, both in the rifaximin group. The authors noted that these 2 patients had multiple risk factors for CDI, including repeated hospitalizations during which they received multiple courses of antibiotic therapy, advanced age, and pantoprazole use. Both patients continued to receive rifaximin therapy during successful treatment for the CDI [70].

The impact of long-term rifaximin therapy on gut flora, including a risk of bacterial antibiotic resistance, is largely unknown. However, the drug appeared to have a protective effect against infections within 90 days after transplant ($P = 0.026$) in patients treated with rifaximin for HE during liver transplant candidacy and was not associated with a higher risk of multidrug-resistant bacterial infections [72].

Conventional antibiotics, neomycin and metronidazole, are also administered for the treatment of HE. However, strong clinical data supporting their efficacy in the treatment of HE are lacking. One randomized, double-blind study failed to demonstrate a benefit with neomycin ($n = 20$) compared with placebo ($n = 19$), with no significant differences observed for time to resolution of HE symptoms or for 5-day, 30-day, or 12-month mortality [73]. Two small, randomized, double-blind studies ($N = 33$ and $N = 45$) and 1 randomized, unblinded trial ($N = 173$) have suggested that neomycin and lactulose may have similar efficacy in the treatment of HE [74–76]. Two randomized studies ($N = 35$ and $N = 49$) have compared neomycin with rifaximin and suggested that they have similar efficacy in the treatment of HE, although in one of the studies, patients who received rifaximin showed improvements sooner than those who received neomycin (3 versus 5 days, resp.) [77, 78]. For metronidazole, 1 small study ($N = 18$) comparing metronidazole with neomycin suggested that both antibiotics improved mental state, reduced asterixis, and improved electroencephalogram measures [79].

However, the risk of AEs associated with neomycin and metronidazole may limit their use in patients with HE and suggest that they might not be an ideal pretransplant choice of treatment. Intestinal malabsorption and diarrhea have been observed with neomycin therapy [80] and thus could impact pretransplant nutritional status of the patients. Although neomycin is poorly absorbed, prolonged administration may result in cumulative systemic concentrations sufficient to increase the risk of serious AEs, such as ototoxicity and nephrotoxicity [80]. Because the MELD scoring system includes measures of renal dysfunction and neomycin may cause renal damage, neomycin may not be an ideal choice for patients, particularly those with high MELD scores. Metronidazole has been associated with peripheral neurotoxicity and requires dosing adjustments in patients with severe liver disease because of impaired drug clearance [80]. Metronidazole is a systemic antibiotic frequently administered for the treatment of CDI, and the potential risk of *C. difficile* resistance to metronidazole warrants judicious use of this agent [81].

Compared with nonabsorbable disaccharides, neomycin, and metronidazole, rifaximin exhibits a more favorable safety and tolerability profile [47, 65, 82]. Rifaximin has not been associated with gastrointestinal AEs such as diarrhea or nausea in clinical studies and would be unlikely to increase the risk of dehydration, weight loss, abdominal distention, malnutrition, or intestinal malabsorption in patients awaiting transplant, thereby minimizing the possible negative consequences of HE therapy on patient nutritional status.

A 2012 meta-analysis, incorporating data from 12 randomized controlled active comparator trials for the treatment of patients with HE, assessed the efficacy and psychometric outcomes of rifaximin compared with other oral therapies (including disaccharides and other antibiotics). The analysis showed that rifaximin exhibited comparable efficacy to other oral agents. However, more favorable effects were observed with rifaximin with regard to psychometric parameters and serum ammonia levels. A tolerability analysis, which included HE prevention trial data, indicated that rifaximin was also associated with fewer adverse effects [82].

5. Summary

HE is a common complication of cirrhosis that substantially affects patient morbidity and mortality. Furthermore, HE can have a detrimental impact on posttransplant outcomes, including patient survival. Data continue to emerge demonstrating the potential persistence of cognitive deficits associated with HE, even after liver transplant. Therefore, prevention of HE in patients with cirrhosis may improve pretransplant health status and thus improve posttransplant outcomes. Commonly prescribed therapies include nonabsorbable disaccharides (e.g., lactulose) and nonsystemic antibiotics (e.g., rifaximin), and their various risks and benefits should be taken into consideration when deciding the most appropriate HE management algorithm in patients awaiting liver transplant. Further studies to evaluate currently available therapies in preventing HE and improving posttransplant outcomes are warranted.

Disclosure

Lewis W. Teperman, MD, has been a member of the speakers' bureau for Salix Pharmaceuticals Inc. (Raleigh, NC).

Acknowledgments

Technical editorial and medical writing support were provided under the direction of the author by Mary Beth Moncrief, PhD, and Colette O'Sullivan, PhD, for Synchrony Medical, LLC, West Chester, PA. Funding for this support was provided by Salix Pharmaceuticals Inc., Raleigh, NC.

References

[1] G. Garcia-Tsao and J. Lim, "Management and treatment of patients with cirrhosis and portal hypertension: recommendations from the Department of Veterans Affairs Hepatitis C Resource Center Program and the National Hepatitis C Program," *American Journal of Gastroenterology*, vol. 104, no. 7, pp. 1802–1829, 2009.

[2] K. F. Murray and R. L. Carithers Jr., "AASLD practice guidelines: evaluation of the patient for liver transplantation," *Hepatology*, vol. 41, no. 6, pp. 1407–1432, 2005.

[3] Organ Procurement and Transplantation Network, "Organ distribution—allocation of livers," 2012, http://optn.transplant.hrsa.gov/PoliciesandBylaws2/policies/pdfs/policy_8.pdf.

[4] S. Saab, A. B. Ibrahim, A. Shpaner et al., "MELD fails to measure quality of life in liver transplant candidates," *Liver Transplantation*, vol. 11, no. 2, pp. 218–223, 2005.

[5] F. F. Poordad, "Review article: the burden of hepatic encephalopathy," *Alimentary Pharmacology and Therapeutics*, vol. 25, supplement 5, pp. 3–9, 2007.

[6] M. Stepanova, A. Mishra, C. Venkatesan et al., "In-hospital mortality and economic burden associated with hepatic encephalopathy in the United States from 2005 to 2009," *Clinical Gastroenterology and Hepatology*, vol. 10, no. 9, pp. 1034–1041, 2012.

[7] P. Ferenci, A. Lockwood, K. Mullen, R. Tarter, K. Weissenborn, and A. T. Blei, "Hepatic encephalopathy—definition, nomenclature, diagnosis, and quantification: final report of the Working Party at the 11th World Congresses of Gastroenterology, Vienna, 1998," *Hepatology*, vol. 35, no. 3, pp. 716–721, 2002.

[8] M. R. Arguedas, T. G. DeLawrence, and B. M. McGuire, "Influence of hepatic encephalopathy on health-related quality of life in patients with cirrhosis," *Digestive Diseases and Sciences*, vol. 48, no. 8, pp. 1622–1626, 2003.

[9] G. Kircheis, A. Knoche, N. Hilger et al., "Hepatic encephalopathy and fitness to drive," *Gastroenterology*, vol. 137, no. 5, pp. 1706–1715, 2009.

[10] J. S. Bajaj, M. Hafeezullah, Y. Zadvornova et al., "The effect of fatigue on driving skills in patients with hepatic encephalopathy," *American Journal of Gastroenterology*, vol. 104, no. 4, pp. 898–905, 2009.

[11] J. S. Bajaj, J. B. Wade, D. P. Gibson et al., "The multi-dimensional burden of cirrhosis and hepatic encephalopathy on patients and caregivers," *American Journal of Gastroenterology*, vol. 106, no. 9, pp. 1646–1653, 2011.

[12] A. Said, J. Williams, J. Holden et al., "Model for end stage liver disease score predicts mortality across a broad spectrum of liver disease," *Journal of Hepatology*, vol. 40, no. 6, pp. 897–903, 2004.

[13] A. Pujol, F. Graus, A. Rimola et al., "Predictive factors of in-hospital CNS complications following liver transplantation," *Neurology*, vol. 44, no. 7, pp. 1226–1230, 1994.

[14] S. Mechtcheriakov, I. W. Graziadei, M. Mattedi et al., "Incomplete improvement of visuo-motor deficits in patients with minimal hepatic encephalopathy after liver transplantation," *Liver Transplantation*, vol. 10, no. 1, pp. 77–83, 2004.

[15] F. Lazeyras, L. Spahr, R. DuPasquier et al., "Persistence of mild parkinsonism 4 months after liver transplantation in patients with preoperative minimal hepatic encephalopathy: a study on neuroradiological and blood manganese changes," *Transplant International*, vol. 15, no. 4, pp. 188–195, 2002.

[16] R. E. Tarter, J. Switala, A. Arria, J. Plail, and D. H. Van Thiel, "Subclinical hepatic encephalopathy. Comparison before and after orthotopic liver transplantation," *Transplantation*, vol. 50, no. 4, pp. 632–637, 1990.

[17] A. Huda, B. H. Guze, M. A. Thomas et al., "Clinical correlation of neuropsychological tests with 1H magnetic resonance spectroscopy in hepatic encephalopathy," *Psychosomatic Medicine*, vol. 60, no. 5, pp. 550–556, 1998.

[18] M. Guevara, M. E. Baccaro, B. Gómez-Ansón et al., "Cerebral magnetic resonance imaging reveals marked abnormalities of brain tissue density in patients with cirrhosis without overt hepatic encephalopathy," *Journal of Hepatology*, vol. 55, no. 3, pp. 564–573, 2011.

[19] D. J. Bronster, S. Emre, P. Boccagni, P. A. Sheiner, M. E. Schwartz, and C. M. Miller, "Central nervous system complications in liver transplant recipients—incidence, timing, and long-term follow-up," *Clinical Transplantation*, vol. 14, no. 1, pp. 1–7, 2000.

[20] R. Dhar, G. B. Young, and P. Marotta, "Perioperative neurological complications after liver transplantation are best predicted by pre-transplant hepatic encephalopathy," *Neurocritical Care*, vol. 8, no. 2, pp. 253–258, 2008.

[21] E. U. Sotil, J. Gottstein, E. Ayala, C. Randolph, and A. T. Blei, "Impact of preoperative overt hepatic encephalopathy on neurocognitive function after Liver transplantion," *Liver Transplantation*, vol. 15, no. 2, pp. 184–192, 2009.

[22] J. S. Bajaj, C. M. Schubert, D. M. Heuman et al., "Persistence of cognitive impairment after resolution of overt hepatic encephalopathy," *Gastroenterology*, vol. 138, no. 7, pp. 2332–2340, 2010.

[23] S. Prasad, R. K. Dhiman, A. Duseja, Y. K. Chawla, A. Sharma, and R. Agarwal, "Lactulose improves cognitive functions and health-related quality of life in patients with cirrhosis who have minimal hepatic encephalopathy," *Hepatology*, vol. 45, no. 3, pp. 549–559, 2007.

[24] H. Schomerus and W. Hamster, "Quality of life in cirrhotics with minimal hepatic encephalopathy," *Metabolic Brain Disease*, vol. 16, no. 1-2, pp. 37–41, 2001.

[25] M. Groeneweg, J. C. Quero, I. De Bruijn et al., "Subclinical hepatic encephalopathy impairs daily functioning," *Hepatology*, vol. 28, no. 1, pp. 45–49, 1998.

[26] M. Guevara, M. E. Baccaro, A. Torre et al., "Hyponatremia is a risk factor of hepatic encephalopathy in patients with cirrhosis: a prospective study with time-dependent analysis," *American Journal of Gastroenterology*, vol. 104, no. 6, pp. 1382–1389, 2009.

[27] M. J. McPhail, J. S. Bajaj, H. C. Thomas, and S. D. Taylor-Robinson, "Pathogenesis and diagnosis of hepatic encephalopathy," *Expert Review of Gastroenterology and Hepatology*, vol. 4, no. 3, pp. 365–378, 2010.

[28] R. F. Butterworth, "Pathophysiology of hepatic encephalopathy: a new look at ammonia," *Metabolic Brain Disease*, vol. 17, no. 4, pp. 221–227, 2002.

[29] S. M. Riordan and R. Williams, "Treatment of hepatic encephalopathy," *New England Journal of Medicine*, vol. 337, no. 7, pp. 473–479, 1997.

[30] G. Ardizzone, A. Arrigo, M. M. Schellino et al., "Neurological complications of liver cirrhosis and orthotopic liver transplant," *Transplantation Proceedings*, vol. 38, no. 3, pp. 789–792, 2006.

[31] F. H. Saner, J. Gensicke, S. W. M. O. Damink et al., "Neurologic complications in adult living donor liver transplant patients: an underestimated factor?" *Journal of Neurology*, vol. 257, no. 2, pp. 253–258, 2010.

[32] R. Moreno and M. Berenguer, "Post-liver transplantation medical complications," *Annals of Hepatology*, vol. 5, no. 2, pp. 77–85, 2006.

[33] R. Blanco, U. De Girolami, R. L. Jenkins, and U. Khettry, "Neuropathology of liver transplantation," *Clinical Neuropathology*, vol. 14, no. 2, pp. 109–117, 1995.

[34] A. J. Martinez, C. Estol, and A. A. Faris, "Neurologic complications of liver transplantation," *Neurologic Clinics*, vol. 6, no. 2, pp. 327–348, 1988.

[35] N. Ghaus, S. Bohlega, and M. Rezeig, "Neurological complications in liver transplantation," *Journal of Neurology*, vol. 248, no. 12, pp. 1042–1048, 2001.

[36] F. Saner, Y. Gu, S. Minouchehr et al., "Neurological complications after cadaveric and living donor liver transplantation," *Journal of Neurology*, vol. 253, no. 5, pp. 612–617, 2006.

[37] M. Guarino, A. Stracciari, P. Pazzaglia et al., "Neurological complications of liver transplantation," *Journal of Neurology*, vol. 243, no. 2, pp. 137–142, 1996.

[38] O. Riggio, L. Ridola, C. Pasquale et al., "Evidence of persistent cognitive impairment after resolution of overt hepatic encephalopathy," *Clinical Gastroenterology and Hepatology*, vol. 9, no. 2, pp. 181–183, 2011.

[39] K. Mattarozzi, A. Stracciari, L. Vignatelli, R. D'Alessandro, M. C. Morelli, and M. Guarino, "Minimal hepatic encephalopathy: longitudinal effects of liver transplantation," *Archives of Neurology*, vol. 61, no. 2, pp. 242–247, 2004.

[40] D. K. Atluri, M. Asgeri, and K. D. Mullen, "Reversibility of hepatic encephalopathy after liver transplantation," *Metabolic Brain Disease*, vol. 25, no. 1, pp. 111–113, 2010.

[41] T. Naegele, W. Grodd, R. Viebahn et al., "MR imaging and ^{1}H spectroscopy of brain metabolites in hepatic encephalopathy: time-course of renormalization after liver transplantation," *Radiology*, vol. 216, no. 3, pp. 683–691, 2000.

[42] R. Garcia-Martinez, A. Rovira, J. Alonso et al., "Hepatic encephalopathy is associated with posttransplant cognitive function and brain volume," *Liver Transplantation*, vol. 17, no. 1, pp. 38–46, 2011.

[43] B. Als-Nielsen, L. L. Gluud, and C. Gluud, "Non-absorbable disaccharides for hepatic encephalopathy: systematic review of randomised trials," *British Medical Journal*, vol. 328, no. 7447, pp. 1046–1050, 2004.

[44] S. Shukla, A. Shukla, S. Mehboob, and S. Guha, "Meta-analysis: the effects of gut flora modulation using prebiotics, probiotics and synbiotics on minimal hepatic encephalopathy," *Alimentary Pharmacology and Therapeutics*, vol. 33, no. 6, pp. 662–671, 2011.

[45] M. Luo, L. Li, C. Lu, and W. Cao, "Clinical efficacy and safety of lactulose for minimal hepatic encephalopathy: a meta-analysis," *European Journal of Gastroenterology and Hepatology*, vol. 23, no. 12, pp. 1250–1257, 2011.

[46] P. Sharma, B. C. Sharma, A. Agrawal et al., "Primary prophylaxis of overt hepatic encephalopathy in patients with cirrhosis: an open labeled randomized controlled trial of lactulose versus no lactulose," *Journal of Gastroenterology and Hepatology*, vol. 27, no. 8, pp. 1329–1335, 2012.

[47] Q. Jiang, X. H. Jiang, M. H. Zheng, L. Jiang, Y. Chen, and L. Wang, "Rifaximin versus nonabsorbable disaccharides in the management of hepatic encephalopathy: a meta-analysis," *European Journal of Gastroenterology and Hepatology*, vol. 20, no. 11, pp. 1064–1070, 2008.

[48] O. Riggio, G. Balducci, F. Ariosto et al., "Lactitol in prevention of recurrent episodes of hepatic encephalopathy in cirrhotic patients with portal-systemic shunt," *Digestive Diseases and Sciences*, vol. 34, no. 6, pp. 823–829, 1989.

[49] B. C. Sharma, P. Sharma, A. Agrawal, and S. K. Sarin, "Secondary prophylaxis of hepatic encephalopathy: an open-label randomized controlled trial of lactulose versus placebo," *Gastroenterology*, vol. 137, no. 3, pp. 885–891, 2009.

[50] D. Heredia, J. Teres, N. Orteu, and J. Rodes, "Lactitol vs. lactulose in the treatment of chronic recurrent portal-systemic encephalopathy," *Journal of Hepatology*, vol. 7, no. 1, pp. 106–110, 1988.

[51] A. Agrawal, B. C. Sharma, P. Sharma et al., "Secondary prophylaxis of hepatic encephalopathy in cirrhosis: an open-label, randomized controlled trial of lactulose, probiotics, and no therapy," *The American Journal of Gastroenterology*, vol. 107, no. 7, pp. 1043–1050, 2012.

[52] *Lactulose (Lactulose Solution) [Package Insert]*, Apotex Inc., Ontario, Canada, 2005.

[53] A. Watanabe, T. Sakai, S. Sato et al., "Clinical efficacy of lactulose in cirrhotic patients with and without subclinical hepatic encephalopathy," *Hepatology*, vol. 26, no. 6, pp. 1410–1414, 1997.

[54] J. Polson and W. M. Lee, "AASLD position paper: the management of acute liver failure," *Hepatology*, vol. 41, no. 5, pp. 1179–1197, 2005.

[55] L. W. Teperman and V. P. Peyregne, "Considerations on the impact of hepatic encephalopathy treatments in the pretransplant setting," *Transplantation*, vol. 89, no. 7, pp. 771–778, 2010.

[56] B. W. Shaw Jr., R. P. Wood, R. D. Gordon, S. Iwatsuki, W. P. Gillquist, and T. E. Starzl, "Influence of selected patient variables and operative blood loss on six-month survival following liver transplantation," *Seminars in Liver Disease*, vol. 5, no. 4, pp. 385–393, 1985.

[57] M. Merli, M. Giusto, F. Gentili et al., "Nutritional status: its influence on the outcome of patients undergoing liver transplantation," *Liver International*, vol. 30, no. 2, pp. 208–214, 2010.

[58] S. A. McCluskey, K. Karkouti, D. N. Wijeysundera et al., "Derivation of a risk index for the prediction of massive blood transfusion in liver transplantation," *Liver Transplantation*, vol. 12, no. 11, pp. 1584–1593, 2006.

[59] G. Fusai, P. Dhaliwal, N. Rolando et al., "Incidence and risk factors for the development of prolonged and severe intrahepatic cholestasis after liver transplantation," *Liver Transplantation*, vol. 12, no. 11, pp. 1626–1633, 2006.

[60] G. N. Ioannou, "Development and validation of a model predicting graft survival after liver transplantation," *Liver Transplantation*, vol. 12, no. 11, pp. 1594–1606, 2006.

[61] S. W. Biggins, H. J. Rodriguez, P. Bacchetti, N. M. Bass, J. P. Roberts, and N. A. Terrault, "Serum sodium predicts mortality in patients listed for liver transplantation," *Hepatology*, vol. 41, no. 1, pp. 32–39, 2005.

[62] H. Selcuk, I. Uruc, M. A. Temel et al., "Factors prognostic of survival in patients awaiting liver transplantation for end-stage liver disease," *Digestive Diseases and Sciences*, vol. 52, no. 11, pp. 3217–3223, 2007.

[63] A. J. Sanchez and J. Aranda-Michel, "Nutrition for the liver transplant patient," *Liver Transplantation*, vol. 12, no. 9, pp. 1310–1316, 2006.

[64] M. Merli, M. Caschera, C. Piat, G. Pinto, M. Diofebi, and O. Riggio, "The effect of lactulose and lactitol administration on fecal fat excretion in patients with liver cirrhosis," *Journal of Clinical Gastroenterology*, vol. 15, no. 2, pp. 125–127, 1992.

[65] K. R. Lawrence and J. A. Klee, "Rifaximin for the treatment of hepatic encephalopathy," *Pharmacotherapy*, vol. 28, no. 8, pp. 1019–1032, 2008.

[66] S. S. Sidhu, O. Goyal, B. P. Mishra, A. Sood, R. S. Chhina, and R. K. Soni, "Rifaximin improves psychometric performance and health-related quality of life in patients with minimal hepatic encephalopathy (the RIME trial)," *American Journal of Gastroenterology*, vol. 106, no. 2, pp. 307–316, 2011.

[67] J. S. Bajaj, D. M. Heuman, J. B. Wade et al., "Rifaximin improves driving simulator performance in a randomized trial of patients with minimal hepatic encephalopathy," *Gastroenterology*, vol. 140, no. 2, pp. 478–487, 2011.

[68] R. Testa, C. Eftimiadi, and G. S. Sukkar, "A non-absorbable rifamycin for treatment of hepatic encephalopathy," *Drugs under Experimental and Clinical Research*, vol. 11, no. 6, pp. 387–392, 1985.

[69] "FDA approves new use of Xifaxan for patients with liver disease," 2010, http://www.drugs.com/newdrugs/fda-approves-new-xifaxan-patients-liver-2078.html.

[70] N. M. Bass, K. D. Mullen, A. Sanyal et al., "Rifaximin treatment in hepatic encephalopathy," *New England Journal of Medicine*, vol. 362, no. 12, pp. 1071–1081, 2010.

[71] A. Sanyal, Z. M. Younossi, N. M. Bass et al., "Randomised clinical trial: rifaximin improves health-related quality of life in cirrhotic patients with hepatic encephalopathy-a double-blind placebo-controlled study," *Alimentary Pharmacology and Therapeutics*, vol. 34, no. 8, pp. 853–861, 2011.

[72] H. Y. Sun, M. Wagener, T. V. Cacciarelli, and N. Singh, "Impact of rifaximin use for hepatic encephalopathy on the risk of early post-transplant infections in liver transplant recipients," *Clinical Transplantation*, vol. 26, no. 6, pp. 849–852, 2012.

[73] E. Strauss, R. Tramote, E. P. S. Silva et al., "Double-blind randomized clinical trial comparing neomycin and placebo in the treatment of exogenous hepatic encephalopathy," *Hepato-Gastroenterology*, vol. 39, no. 6, pp. 542–545, 1992.

[74] H. O. Conn, C. M. Leevy, and Z. R. Vlahcevic, "Comparison of lactulose and neomycin in the treatment of chronic portal systemic encephalopathy. A double blind controlled trial," *Gastroenterology*, vol. 72, no. 4, pp. 573–583, 1977.

[75] C. E. Atterbury, W. C. Maddrey, and H. O. Conn, "Neomycin-sorbitol and lactulose in the treatment of acute portal-systemic encephalopathy. A controlled, double-blind clinical trial," *American Journal of Digestive Diseases*, vol. 23, no. 5, pp. 398–406, 1978.

[76] F. Orlandi, U. Freddara, and M. T. Candelaresi, "Comparison between neomycin and lactulose in 173 patients with hepatic encephalopathy. A randomized clinical study," *Digestive Diseases and Sciences*, vol. 26, no. 6, pp. 498–506, 1981.

[77] D. Festi, G. Mazzella, M. Orsini et al., "Rifaximin in the treatment of chronic hepatic encephalopathy; resultes of a multicenter study of efficacy and safety," *Current Therapeutic Research*, vol. 54, no. 5, pp. 598–609, 1993.

[78] F. Miglio, D. Valpiani, S. R. Rossellini, A. Ferrieri, and N. Canova, "Rifaximin, a non-absorbable rifamycin, for the treatment of hepatic encephalopathy. A double-blind, randomised trial," *Current Medical Research and Opinion*, vol. 13, no. 10, pp. 593–601, 1997.

[79] M. H. Morgan, A. E. Read, and D. C. E. Speller, "Treatment of hepatic encephalopathy with metronidazole," *Gut*, vol. 23, no. 1, pp. 1–7, 1982.

[80] A. T. Blei and J. Córdoba, "Hepatic encephalopathy," *American Journal of Gastroenterology*, vol. 96, no. 7, pp. 1968–1976, 2001.

[81] S. H. Cohen, D. N. Gerding, S. Johnson et al., "Clinical practice guidelines for *Clostridium difficile* infection in adults: 2010 update by the Society for Healthcare Epidemiology of America (SHEA) and the Infectious Diseases Society of America (IDSA)," *Infection Control and Hospital Epidemiology*, vol. 31, no. 5, pp. 431–455, 2010.

[82] K. M. Eltawil, M. Laryea, K. Peltekian, and M. Molinari, "Rifaximin vs conventional oral therapy for hepatic encephalopathy: a meta-analysis," *World Journal of Gastroenterology*, vol. 18, no. 8, pp. 767–777, 2012.

18

Shorter Leukocyte Telomere Length in Relation to Presumed Nonalcoholic Fatty Liver Disease in Mexican-American Men in NHANES 1999–2002

Janet M. Wojcicki,[1] David Rehkopf,[2] Elissa Epel,[3] and Philip Rosenthal[1]

[1]*Department of Pediatrics, University of California, San Francisco, CA, USA*
[2]*Department of Medicine, Stanford University, Stanford, CA, USA*
[3]*Department of Psychiatry, University of California, San Francisco, CA, USA*

Correspondence should be addressed to Janet M. Wojcicki; wojcicki@gmail.com

Academic Editor: Brijesh K. Singh

Leukocyte telomere length is shorter in response to chronic disease processes associated with inflammation such as diabetes mellitus and coronary artery disease. Data from the National Health and Nutrition Examination Survey (NHANES) from 1999 to 2002 was used to explore the relationship between leukocyte telomere length and presumed NAFLD, as indicated by elevated serum alanine aminotransferase (ALT) levels, obesity, or abdominal obesity. Logistic regression models were used to evaluate the relationship between telomere length and presumed markers of NAFLD adjusting for possible confounders. There was no relationship between elevated ALT levels, abdominal obesity, or obesity and telomere length in adjusted models in NHANES (OR 1.13, 95% CI 0.48–2.65; OR 1.17, 95% CI 0.52–2.62, resp.). Mexican-American men had shorter telomere length in relation to presumed NAFLD (OR 0.07, 95% CI 0.006–0.79) and using different indicators of NAFLD (OR 0.012, 95% CI 0.0006–0.24). Mexican origin with presumed NAFLD had shorter telomere length than men in other population groups. Longitudinal studies are necessary to evaluate the role of telomere length as a potential predictor to assess pathogenesis of NALFD in Mexicans.

1. Background

1.1. Nonalcoholic Fatty Liver Disease. Latinos are at high risk for specific complications from obesity including NAFLD [1] and insulin resistance compared with other population groups with the prevalence being higher in Latinos of Mexican and Central American origin than Latinos of Caribbean origin [2]. Furthermore, Latino males are at higher risk than Latino females [1].

1.2. Genetics and Nonalcoholic Fatty Liver Disease. Previous research has demonstrated that there is a clear genetic component (variants of the gene *PNPLA3*, I148M) to increased risk for NAFLD in Latinos of Mexican and Central American background [3]. A single nucleotide polymorphism (SNP) (rs738409) in *PNPLA*3 encodes an amino acid substitution, which results in a twofold higher liver fat accumulation among those with a GG genotype of the allele [3]. Meanwhile, however, the variant increases risk for women, not men, and Mexican and Central American origin Latinos men are at higher risk for NAFLD than women [3]. Furthermore, the addition of genetic markers to predict risk for NAFLD does not improve discriminatory ability of common clinical risk factors, suggesting the need for other biomarkers beyond genetic variants [4].

1.3. Telomere Length and Metabolic Disease. Cross-sectional data suggest that shorter telomere length could be a useful indicator of risk for metabolic disease. Studies in adults suggest that components of metabolic dysfunction including insulin resistance, abdominal obesity, and hypertension are associated with shorter telomere length [5]. Shorter telomere length also predicts development of type 2 diabetes mellitus [6] and progression of the metabolic syndrome [7].

In this study, we evaluate the role of leukocyte telomere length in presumed NAFLD in a population of US adults from two cycles of the National Health and Nutrition Examination Survey (NHANES) that tested leukocyte telomere length, with a focus on the relationship between telomere length and liver disease stratified by ethnic and racial background and gender.

2. Methods

2.1. Data Source and Sample. The National Health and Nutrition Examination Survey (NHANES) is a nationally representative survey of the noninstitutionalized US population. We used information from the questionnaire, laboratory, diet, and physical examination components for our analysis of the 1999-2000 through 2001-2002 surveys, as these included telomere measurements in a subset of the population aged 20 years and older that had blood collected for DNA purification. These years were the only two cycles of the NHANES that assessed telomere length. The total number of individuals was 3,567 in 1999-2000 and 4,260 in 2001-2002. All NHNAES participants 20 years old and over were asked to provide DNA samples. Of those who provided samples (10,291), 7,827 (76%) specifically allowed future DNA use and were tested for leukocyte telomere length [8]. The same laboratory, dietary, and physical exam measures were used in the two different cycles of NHANES. NHANES is approved by the National Center for Health Statistics (NCHS) Research Ethics Review Board, and written informed consent was obtained from participants. The Institutional Review Board at the University of California, San Francisco (Committee for Human Research (CHR)), exempted the present study from review.

2.2. Nonalcoholic Fatty Liver Disease. Our primary study outcome was the presence or absence of NAFLD. Participants were determined to have NAFLD using different indicators; if they had elevated serum alanine aminotransferase (ALT) levels (ALT $\geq$ 29 U/L) for men and $\geq$22 for women [9]. We had a secondary definition of NAFLD, which combined elevated serum ALT levels with abdominal obesity (for men > 102 centimeters and for women > 88 centimeters) [10] and a third one, which combined elevated serum ALT levels with obesity (defined using the Center for Disease Control's cut point of having a body mass index $\geq$ 30 kg/m^2). Individuals who had elevated *serum ALT* levels and abdominal obesity or overall obesity were compared with participants who had neither. Those who had one indicator of presumed nonalcoholic fatty liver disease such as elevated ALT or obesity (abdominal or high body mass index (BMI)) were excluded from analyses that focused on definitions of NAFLD that included both obesity and liver enzymes so as to have a cleaner comparison group. Participants who were known to have Hepatitis B or C, HIV, and known liver disease, were currently pregnant, and had daily consumption of alcohol or known exposure to hepatotoxic medication were excluded from all analyses. Final sample size for the dataset was 7070 after excluding those with the conditions (n = 757).

2.3. Leukocyte Telomere Length Measurements. The telomere assays were conducted in the Blackburn Laboratory at the University of California, San Francisco. The Centers for Disease Control conducted a quality control review assessment before linking the leukocyte telomere length results with NHANES public files.

Briefly, aliquots of purified DNA were provided by the National Center for Health Statistics to the Blackburn Laboratory. DNA was isolated from whole blood using the Puregene (D-50K) kit protocol (Gentra Systems, Inc., Minneapolis, Minnesota) and stored at −80°C. To measure mean leukocyte telomere length, quantitative polymerase chain reaction (PCR) assay was used to determine the relative ratio of telomere repeat copy number to single-copy reference DNA number (T/S ratio) as previously described by Cawthon (2002) [11]. The single-copy gene used as a control was human beta-globin [8]. The interassay coefficient of variability for LTL was 4%.

2.4. Control for Potential Confounders. Potential confounders included in multivariate analysis included age in years (as continuous), age squared (based on the potential for nonlinearity between age and telomere length [12, 13]), educational attainment (less than high school, high school, or more than high school), place of birth (US born or foreign born), marital status (married or unmarried), and poverty to income ratio (the ratio of household income to poverty adjusted to family size and inflation). All variables were based on self-reported status and were found to be significant predictors for leukocyte telomere length [8]. Race/ethnicity included White, Black, Mexican-American, other Hispanic, and others or mixed race. We also adjusted for cell type composition including white blood cells (SI), lymphocytes (%), monocytes (%), neutrophils (%), eosinophils (%), basophils (%), and platelets (%), following the methodology used by Rehkopf et al. (2016) [13].

2.5. Statistical Analysis. Univariate and multivariate analyses were conducted using Stata 13.0 (Stata Corp, College Station, TX). We conducted stratified analyses based on sex (male versus female) and race/ethnicity (White, Black, Mexican-American, other Hispanic, and mixed race) following the designations for these years of NHANES. We fitted an interaction term to test the hypothesis that there is significant interaction between race, specifically Mexican-American background, telomere length, and presumed NAFLD as indicated by high ALT levels. As there are significantly different patterns of incidence for NAFLD based on ethnicity and gender, we conducted stratified analysis in addition to pooled analyses adjusting for the confounders described above [14, 15]. In some cases when numbers were below 100 for stratified analyses, calculations were not conducted. Sampling weights as provided for NHANES for the examination were used to take into account the complex sampling design including clustering and stratification and were incorporated into all analyses using Stata code.

A relatively small number of individuals (<15%) were missing data for the various outcomes and covariates so we

TABLE 1: Telomere length, race, and interaction terms on suspected nonalcoholic fatty liver disease, NHANES 1999–2002. The table included interaction terms to assess the relationship between race/ethnicity and telomere length in relation to suspected nonalcoholic fatty liver disease (defined by having elevated ALT levels).

Variable	Odds ratio (OR)	*p* value	Confidence interval
Female sex	1.03	0.85	0.75–1.40
Age in years	0.98	<0.01	0.97–0.99
Telomere length	1.25	0.50	0.63–2.48
Race/ethnicity			
White (non- Hispanic)	1.00		
Black (non-Hispanic)	0.50	0.29	0.13–1.87
Mexican-American	3.96	<0.01	1.73–9.04
Other Hispanic	0.54	0.50	0.08–3.89
Other/mixed race	22.02	0.01	2.04–237.90
Interaction terms			
MexicanXtelomere	0.32	0.01	0.13–0.77
BlackXTelomere	1.36	0.70	0.38–4.87
Other Hispanic XTelomere	2.42	0.35	0.37–15.87
Other-MixedXTelomere	0.07	0.01	0.008–0.54

decided against multiple imputation. Model 1 had less than 1% of data missing, models 2 and 3 had 13% missing, and models 4 and 5 had 14% missing.

3. Results

Our initial exploratory analyses assessing the possible role of race and ethnic specific differences by telomere length in predicting presumed NALFD suggested the important role of interaction. Approximately 20–30% of the participants had the outcome in question (high ALT) with slight differences based on race/ethnicity and gender (28.1% of the population with telomere length measurements had elevated ALT levels). Specifically, Mexican ethnicity interacted with telomere length indicating shorter telomere lengths for presumed NAFLD in Mexicans (OR 0.32, 95% CI 0.13–0.77) and the other/mixed race and telomere length interaction term also indicates shorter telomere length for presumed NAFLD in this population group (OR 0.07, 95% CI 0.0008–0.54) (Table 1). Adjusting for potential confounders including demographics and cell type, the interaction term for Mexican-American ethnicity became attenuated (OR 0.46, 95% CI 0.20–1.06), although it did not become attenuated for other/mixed race individuals (OR 0.03, 95% CI 0.004–0.24) (results not shown).

3.1. Telomere Length and Elevated ALT. In unadjusted analysis, we found that longer telomere length was associated with increased risk of elevated serum ALT levels in both sexes (OR 1.87, 95% CI 1.19–2.94) with increased risk for men in particular (OR 2.95, 95% CI 1.43–6.09) and highest risk for those who self-identified as African-American males (OR 5.52, 95% CI 1.38–22.10) and other Hispanic males (OR 17.00, 95% CI 1.67–173.24) (Table 2). Non-Hispanic White males also had increased risk based on longer telomere length (OR 3.01, 95% CI 1.32–6.91). Those that defined themselves as others or mixed/race had increased risk with shorter telomere length (OR 0.14, 95% CI 0.02–0.92) (Table 2). Mexican-Americans did not have increased risk for elevated ALT with shorter or longer telomere length (OR 0.65, 95% CI 0.31–1.35).

In adjusted analyses for demographic factors, all relationships are attenuated and lose statistical significance with the exception of mixed race/other individuals. When adjusting for cell type composition, African-American men show increased risk for elevated ALT with longer telomere length (OR 4.98, 95% CI 1.03–24.13) and mixed race/other individuals continue to have increased risk with shorter telomere length (Table 2).

3.2. Telomere Length and Elevated ALT and Obesity. When elevated serum ALT levels were combined with abdominal obesity or obesity, we found that shorter telomere length was associated with presumed NAFLD in Mexican-American men (OR 0.15, 95% CI 0.03–0.64 for abdominal obesity; OR 0.012, 95% CI 0.0006–0.24 for obesity) (Table 2; models 4 and 5). Mixed race/other individuals also continued to have shorter telomere length with presumed NAFLD. Similar to the prevalence of elevated ALT, the prevalence of the outcome of high ALT and high waist or obesity was similar approximately 20–30% in the population depending on race/ethnicity (20% for high ALT and high waist and 24% for high ALT and obesity in the population as a whole).

4. Discussion

This is the first study to assess the relationship between presumed NAFLD and leukocyte telomere length in a population-based sample of mixed race and ethnicity. Telomere length was not associated with presumed NAFLD after adjustment for sociodemographic confounders in the NHANES population as a whole. However, shorter telomere length in Mexican-origin men was significantly associated

TABLE 2: Logistic regression of telomere length on elevated ALT, age 20 and older, and other indicators of suspected nonalcoholic fatty liver disease, NHANES 1999–2002.

	Model 1, unadjusted	Model 2, demographic	Model 3, demographic and cell type adjusted	Model 4, demographic, cell type, and abdominal obesity	Model 5, demographic, cell type, and obesity
All races					
All sexes	**1.87 (1.19–2.94)**** **(n = 7049)**	1.09 (0.65–1.85) (*n* = 6127)	1.14 (0.67–1.94) (*n* = 6115)	1.13 (0.48–2.65) (*n* = 2829)	1.17 (0.52–2.62) (*n* = 3373)
Male	**2.95 (1.43–6.09)**** **(n = 3621)**	1.13 (0.49–2.61) (*n* = 3195)	1.12 (0.50–2.52) (*n* = 3191)	0.98 (0.29–3.24) (*n* = 1607)	1.32 (0.42–4.17) (*n* = 1886)
Female	1.25 (0.71–2.20) (*n* = 3428)	0.91 (0.42–1.98) (*n* = 2932)	0.99 (0.44–2.22) (*n* = 2924)	1.087 (0.29–3.93) (*n* = 1222)	0.72 (0.20–2.57) (*n* = 1487)
Other Hispanic					
All sexes	**5.03 (1.05–24.13)*** **(n = 312)**	4.09 (0.54–31.18) (*n* = 269)	1.72 (0.15–19.44) (*n* = 268)	0.74 (0.08–6.94) (*n* = 128)	15.20 (0.27–860.28) (*n* = 160)
Male	**17.00 (1.67–173.24)*** **(n = 137)**	0.52 (0.008–34.10) (*n* = 126)	0.06 (0.0005–7.80) (*n* = 125)	—	—
Female	1.86 (0.27–12.75) (*n* = 175)	22.51 (0.63–807.0) (*n* = 143)	37.14 (0.65–2109.41) (*n* = 143)	—	—
African-American					
All	2.43 (0.86–6.86) (*n* = 1445)	1.86 (0.58–5.99) (*n* = 1190)	1.84 (0.64–5.18) (*n* = 1189)	2.09 (0.65–6.70) (*n* = 479)	3.23 (0.70–14.90) (*n* = 574)
Male	**5.52 (1.38–22.10)*** **(n = 696)**	3.53 (0.79–15.73) (*n* = 567)	**4.98 (1.03–24.13)*** **(n = 566)**	5.56 (0.16–192.8) (*n* = 291)	5.84 (0.29–119.55) (*n* = 315)
Female	1.34 (0.32–5.0) *n* = 749	1.46 (0.27–7.75) (*n* = 623)	1.28 (0.35–4.70) (*n* = 623)	2.25 (0.12–42.06) (*n* = 188)	2.33 (0.17–32.77) (*n* = 259)
Mexican-American					
All	0.65 (0.31–1.35) (*n* = 1201)	0.39 (0.14–1.09) (*n* = 1007)	0.41 (0.15–1.16) (*n* = 1001)	0.37 (0.09–1.52) (*n* = 537)	**0.15 (0.03–0.64)*** **(n = 594)**
Male	0.46 (0.19–1.11) (*n* = 537)	0.23 (0.05–1.04) (*n* = 471)	0.22 (0.04–1.03) (*n* = 470)	**0.07 (.006–0.79)*** **(n = 284)**	**0.012 (0.0006–0.24)**** **(n = 296)**
Female	1.10 (0.19–6.38) (*n* = 664)	1.03 (0.13–8.36) *n* = 536	1.59 (0.22–11.54) (*n* = 531)	6.00 (0.19–188.15) (*n* = 253)	0.48 (0.04–5.38) (*n* = 298)
Non-Hispanic White					
All	**1.93 (1.07–3.49)*** **(n = 3894)**	1.136 (0.62–2.07) (*n* = 3487)	1.20 (0.66–2.18) (*n* = 3483)	0.98 (0.37–2.55) (*n* = 1589)	0.99 (0.33–2.97) (*n* = 1936)
Male	**3.01 (1.32–6.91)*** **n = (2172)**	1.22 (0.50–2.96) *n* = 1959	1.31 (0.54–3.16) (*n* = 1958)	0.98 (0.265–3.82) (*n* = 934)	1.38 (0.36–5.73) (*n* = 1146)
Female	1.29 (0.56–2.97) *n* = (1722)	0.82 (0.32–2.08) *n* = 1528	0.87 (0.35–2.16) (*n* = 1525)	0.44 (0.11–1.91) (*n* = 655)	0.37 (0.07–1.90) (*n* = 790)

Table 2: Continued.

	Model 1, unadjusted	Model 2, demographic	Model 3, demographic and cell type adjusted	Model 4, demographic, cell type, and abdominal obesity	Model 5, demographic, cell type, and obesity
Others/mixed race					
All	**0.14 (0.02–0.92)*** **(n = 197)**	**0.00004 (0.000000001–0.14)**** **(n = 174)**	**1.00e – 0.06 (2.59e – 11–0.04)*** **(n = 174)**	**1.97e – 24 (1.97e – 14–0.18)** **(n = 96)**	—
Male	0.01 (0.00003–3.28) n = (79)	**0.00002 (1.62e – 09–0.18)*** **n = 72**	5.03e – 16 (8.76e – 45 – 2.90e + 13) (n = 72)	—	—
Female	0.26 (0.04–1.64) n = (118)	2.85e – 0.08 (1.61e – 17–50.50) (n = 102)	**8.46e – 08 (4.25e – 14–0.17)*** **(n = 102)**	—	—

Model 1 does not adjust for any covariates. Model 2 adjusts for the following control variables: foreign birthplace, education (less than high school, high school diploma, and more than high school), married and age (as continuous), age squared, and poverty to income ratio. Model 3 adjusts for all the variables in model 2 in addition to cell type composition, blood cells (SI), lymphocytes (%), monocytes (%), platelets (%), basophils (%), eosinophils (%), and neutrophils (%). Model 4 includes all the variables in model 3 and additionally includes abdominal obesity as an outcome (in addition to elevated ALT). Model 5 adjusts for all the variables in model 2 in addition to adding obesity as an outcome (in addition to elevated ALT). *Note.* * $p < 0.05$; ** $p < 0.01$.

with presumed NAFLD. Importantly, there were important ethnic- and gender-specific interactions between telomere length and presumed NAFLD that were uncovered through stratified analyses.

Leukocyte telomeres are particularly sensitive to oxidative stress and inflammation [16]. Mexican-origin men are known to have increased risk for NAFLD with African-American men having reduced risk compared with whites. It is possible that shorter leukocyte telomeres may precede the inflammatory cascade that results in development of fatty liver disease and Mexican-origin men are most susceptible to the inflammatory processes resulting in excess fat deposits in hepatocytes in contrast with Caucasians [17]. Other studies have found that short telomere length contributes to the inflammatory process responsible for many divergent disease conditions [18]. Leukocyte telomere shortening in Mexican-origin men may be the initial indicator regarding development of NAFLD after elevated ALTs and obesity. Indeed, a recent study found that leukocyte telomere shortening predicted onset of NAFLD in Asian patients with type 2 diabetes mellitus [19].

Mexican-origin men may be particularly sensitive to hepatic insults and inflammation associated with obesity, while other population groups, particularly African-Americans, may be more resistant to these same physiological processes.

Indeed, studies with children have shown that insulin resistance does not have the same impact on elevated serum ALT levels in African-Americans compared with Latinos [20] and that obesity explains the association between metabolic syndrome and elevated serum ALT levels in Latinos but not in other population groups [21]. Of note, longer telomere length was associated with elevated serum ALT levels in African-American men in contrast with Mexican-Americans, although this relationship disappeared after controlling for obesity.

4.1. Mixed Race/Others and Shorter Telomere Length. We also found that those NHANES participants classified as others or mixed race, most commonly of Asian, Pacific Islander, or Native American background, also had shorter telomere length in relation to presumed NAFLD. There is much less information on the prevalence of NAFLD in Asian-American and Native American populations; however, it is possible that some of the Native Americans groups may have similar genetic backgrounds with Mexican-American and hence elevated risk. The "others/mixed race" category also had a small number of individuals ($n = 197$), which limits the ability to assess specific models including those including obesity and abdominal obesity. Future studies need to sample those of mixed race and Asian, Pacific Island, and Native American race in higher numbers such that strata-specific analyses are possible.

4.2. Further Directions. Although the NHANES dataset does test fasting laboratory values for glucose and insulin, the number of samples was small as this was done in only a subset of the larger population. Future studies should assess markers of insulin resistance including HOMA levels in addition to ALT and obesity measures as well as make use of imaging studies or histology for better diagnosis of NAFLD. Lastly, studies should further investigate the differential impact of NAFLD, inflammatory process, and progression to nonalcoholic steatohepatitis (NASH) using both leukocyte and hepatocyte telomere lengths to better understand progression of disease and differential impact based on ethnicity/race and gender.

Authors' Contributions

Janet M. Wojcicki and Philip Rosenthal conceived the research hypothesis. Janet M. Wojcicki wrote the manuscript and conducted all analyses. David Rehkopf, Elissa Epel, and Philip Rosenthal helped interpret the data findings. All the authors approved the final manuscript.

References

[1] J.-J. Pan and M. B. Fallon, "Gender and racial differences in nonalcoholic fatty liver disease," *World Journal of Hepatology*, vol. 6, no. 5, pp. 274–283, 2014.

[2] E. R. Kallwitz, M. L. Daviglus, M. A. Allison et al., "Prevalence of suspected nonalcoholic fatty liver disease in hispanic/latino individuals differs by heritage," *Clinical Gastroenterology and Hepatology*, vol. 13, no. 3, pp. 569–576, 2015.

[3] S. Romeo, J. Kozlitina, C. Xing et al., "Genetic variation in PNPLA3 confers susceptibility to nonalcoholic fatty liver disease," *Nature Genetics*, vol. 40, no. 12, pp. 1461–1465, 2008.

[4] R. W. Walker, F. Sinatra, J. Hartiala et al., "Genetic and clinical markers of elevated liver fat content in overweight and obese hispanic children," *Obesity*, vol. 21, no. 12, pp. E790–E797, 2013.

[5] S. Demissie, D. Levy, E. J. Benjamin et al., "Insulin resistance, oxidative stress, hypertension, and leukocyte telomere length in men from the Framingham Heart Study," *Aging Cell*, vol. 5, no. 4, pp. 325–330, 2006.

[6] P. Willeit, J. Raschenberger, E. E. Heydon et al., "Leucocyte telomere length and risk of type 2 diabetes mellitus: new prospective cohort study and literature-based meta-analysis," *PLoS ONE*, vol. 9, no. 11, article e112483, 2014.

[7] D. Révész, Y. Milaneschi, J. E. Verhoeven, and B. W. J. H. Penninx, "Telomere length as a marker of cellular aging is associated with prevalence and progression of metabolic syndrome," *Journal of Clinical Endocrinology and Metabolism*, vol. 99, no. 12, pp. 4607–4615, 2014.

[8] B. L. Needham, N. Adlerb, S. Gregorichc et al., "Socioeconomic status, health behavior, and leukocyte telomere length in the National health and Nutrition Examination Survey, 1999–2002," *Social Science & Medicine*, vol. 85, pp. 1–8, 2013.

[9] C. E. Ruhl and J. E. Everhart, "Upper limits of normal for alanine aminotransferase activity in the United States population," *Hepatology*, vol. 55, no. 2, pp. 447–454, 2012.

[10] I. Janssen, P. T. Katzmarzyk, and R. Ross, "Waist circumference and not body mass index explains obesity-related health risk," *The American Journal of Clinical Nutrition*, vol. 79, no. 3, pp. 379–384, 2004.

[11] R. M. Cawthon, "Telomere measurement by quantitative PCR," *Nucleic Acids Research*, vol. 30, no. 10, article e47, 2002.

[12] D. H. Rehkopf, W. H. Dow, L. Rosero-Bixby, J. Lin, E. S. Epel, and E. H. Blackburn, "Longer leukocyte telomere length in Costa Rica's Nicoya Peninsula: A population-based study," *Experimental Gerontology*, vol. 48, no. 11, pp. 1266–1273, 2013.

[13] D. H. Rehkopf, B. L. Needham, J. Lin et al., "Leukocyte telomere length in relation to 17 biomarkers of cardiovascular disease risk: a cross-sectional study of US adults," *PLoS Medicine*, vol. 13, no. 11, article e1002188, 2016.

[14] M. Lazo, U. Bilal, and R. Perez-Escamilla, "Epidemiology of NAFLD and type 2 diabetes: health disparities among persons of hispanic origin," *Current Diabetes Reports*, vol. 15, no. 12, article no. 116, 2015.

[15] M. Lazo, R. Hernaez, M. S. Eberhardt et al., "Prevalence of nonalcoholic fatty liver disease in the United States: the third national health and nutrition examination survey, 1988–1994," *The American Journal of Epidemiology*, vol. 178, no. 1, pp. 38–45, 2013.

[16] C. Correia-Melo, G. Hewitt, and J. F. Passos, "Telomeres, oxidative stress and inflammatory factors: partners in cellular senescence," *Longevity & Healthspan*, vol. 3, no. 1, 2014.

[17] V. Kordinas, A. Ioannidis, and S. Chatzipanagiotou, "The telomere/telomerase system in chronic inflammatory diseases. Cause or effect?" *Genes*, vol. 7, no. 9, article 60, 2016.

[18] J. J. Carrero, P. Stenvinkel, B. Fellström et al., "Telomere attrition is associated with inflammation, low fetuin-A levels and high mortality in prevalent haemodialysis patients," *Journal of Internal Medicine*, vol. 263, no. 3, pp. 302–312, 2008.

[19] F. Ping, Z.-Y. Li, K. Lv et al., "Deoxyribonucleic acid telomere length shortening can predict the incidence of non-alcoholic fatty liver disease in patients with type 2 diabetes mellitus," *Journal of Diabetes Investigation*, vol. 8, no. 2, pp. 174–180, 2016.

[20] M. D. Deboer, R. C. Wiener, B. H. Barnes, and M. J. Gurka, "Ethnic differences in the link between insulin resistance and elevated ALT," *Pediatrics*, vol. 132, no. 3, pp. e718–e726, 2013.

[21] R. C. Graham, A. Burke, and N. Stettler, "Ethnic and sex differences in the association between metabolic syndrome and suspected nonalcoholic fatty liver disease in a nationally representative sample of US adolescents," *Journal of Pediatric Gastroenterology and Nutrition*, vol. 49, no. 4, pp. 442–449, 2009.

19

Elbasvir/Grazoprevir: A Review of the Latest Agent in the Fight against Hepatitis C

Allison M. Bell,[1] Jamie L. Wagner,[1] Katie E. Barber,[1] and Kayla R. Stover[1,2]

[1]*Department of Pharmacy Practice, University of Mississippi School of Pharmacy, Jackson, MS 39216, USA*
[2]*Department of Medicine-Infectious Diseases, University of Mississippi Medical Center, Jackson, MS 39216, USA*

Correspondence should be addressed to Allison M. Bell; abell3@umc.edu

Academic Editor: Maria Buti

Hepatitis C virus (HCV) is estimated to affect up to 150 million people worldwide. Despite worldwide prevalence, treatment modalities prior to 2011 remained suboptimal, with low virologic response rates and intolerable side effect profiles. Fortunately, the landscape of treatment for chronic hepatitis C has rapidly evolved since the introduction of HCV NS3/4 protease inhibitors in 2011. Elbasvir, a NS5A inhibitor, combined with grazoprevir, a NS3/4A protease inhibitor, is the latest FDA-approved therapy for patients with genotype 1 or 4 chronic hepatitis C, with or without compensated cirrhosis. This review will focus on the current literature and clinical evidence supporting elbasvir/grazoprevir as first-line therapy in patients with genotypes 1 and 4 chronic hepatitis C.

1. Introduction

Hepatitis C virus (HCV) is a single-stranded RNA virus that is estimated to affect 130–150 million people worldwide [1]. Although originally called simply "non-A, non-B hepatitis", HCV was soon named and identified as a predominantly parenterally transmitted member of the family of flaviviruses [2].

Since it was first isolated in 1989, advances in the understanding of the HCV life cycle have led to significant improvements in the knowledge and treatment of this disease [3, 4]. Prior to 2000, the primary management of HCV included interferon monotherapy, which boasted a sustained virologic response (SVR) of 15% after 48 weeks of therapy [5]. Shortly thereafter, combination therapy with alpha 2b interferon and ribavirin boasted an SVR of 40–50%, depending on treatment experience, after 24 weeks of therapy [5]. Although results were promising compared to monotherapy, prolonged treatment durations and severe side effects limited tolerability of these medications. With the potential for shorter required treatment durations, therapy recommendations changed to triple-drug regimens in 2011 when the first direct-acting antiviral (DAA) protease inhibitors, boceprevir and telaprevir, were approved [4, 6]. In 2014, however, treatment regimens radically changed with the development of additional, more effective DAAs [4]. These agents, including sofosbuvir, simeprevir, daclatasvir, ledipasvir, and paritaprevir/ritonavir + ombitasvir + dasabuvir, target individual portions of the viral proteins, including NS3/4A, NS5B, and NS5A [4]. With significant improvements in both efficacy and safety, these agents enable interferon-free regimens with significant hope and promise for the future of this now-curable disease [7, 8]. This paper reviews the literature available for elbasvir/grazoprevir, the newest DAA option for the treatment of HCV.

2. Elbasvir/Grazoprevir

Elbasvir/grazoprevir (Zepatier®) is a combination product with an FDA-approved indication for the treatment of chronic HCV genotypes (GTs) 1 and 4 in adults [9]. Elbasvir is an NS5A inhibitor, preventing hepatitis C viral RNA replication and virion assembly. Median EC_{50} values range from 0.2 to 3600 pmol/L, based on genotype [10]. Grazoprevir is a protease inhibitor of HCV NS3/4A that prevents cleavage of the polyprotein necessary for replication [9, 10]. Median EC_{50} values range from 0.16 to 0.8 pmol/L [10].

2.1. Resistance. Virologic failure with elbasvir/grazoprevir has been seen both *in vitro* and *in vivo*. *In vitro*, elbasvir has been associated with reduced activity in the presence of NS5A substitutions M28A/G/T, Q30D/E/H/K/R, L31M/V, H58D, and Y93C/H/N in genotype 1a, L28M, L31F, and Y93H in GT 1b, and L30S, M31V, and Y93H in GT 4 [9]. Grazoprevir has been associated with reduced activity in the presence of NS3 substitutions Y56H, R155K, A156G/T/V, and D168A/E/G/N/S/V/Y in GT 1a, F43S, Y56F, V107I, A156S/T/V, and D168A/G/V in GT 1b, and D168 A/V in GT 4 [9].

In phases 2 and 3 of clinical trials, treatment-emergent virologic failures, associated with amino acid substitutions, were identified in 37 patients with GT 1a, 8 patients with GT 1b, and 5 patients with GT 4 [9]. In GT 1a, identified NS5A substitutions included M28A/G/T, Q30H/K/R/Y, L31F/M/V, H58D, and Y93H/N/S, while NS3 substitutions included V36L/M, Y56H, V107I, R155I/K, A156G/T/V, V158A, and D168A/G/N/V/Y [9]. Prior to treatment initiation in patients with GT 1a, testing for polymorphisms associated with NS5A resistance, particularly for the resistance-associated variants 28, 30, 31, and 93, is recommended. The addition of ribavirin and extension of treatment duration to 16 weeks overcame baseline NS5A polymorphism resistance. The NS3 resistance-associated variants are less clinically relevant and do not necessarily require testing prior to initiation of therapy. Treatment-emergent NS5A-related substitutions (100% for GTs 1a and 1b) were more persistent in clinical evaluations than NS3-related substitutions (31% for GT 1a and 50% for GT 1b) at week 24 follow-up [9].

2.2. Dosing/Pharmacokinetics. Elbasvir/grazoprevir is a fixed dose tablet containing 50 mg of elbasvir and 100 mg of grazoprevir that is given once daily [9, 10]. Elbasvir/grazoprevir is given with or without ribavirin for 12–16 weeks, depending on genotype, treatment experience, and presence of baseline resistance polymorphisms [9]. No dosage adjustments are recommended in patients with renal dysfunction or mild hepatic impairment. Elbasvir/grazoprevir should not be used in patients with moderate to severe hepatic impairment (decompensated cirrhosis) [9].

After administration, peak concentrations are reached at approximately 3 hours and 2 hours for elbasvir and grazoprevir, respectively [9]. Concentrations reach steady-state within 6 days. Elbasvir and grazoprevir are highly protein bound, distributed extensively into most tissues (elbasvir) and predominantly to the liver (grazoprevir). These agents are predominately metabolized by the cytochrome P450 3A4 system, and elimination half-lives for elbasvir and grazoprevir are 24 and 31 hours, respectively, in HCV-infected patients [9].

2.3. Adverse Drug Events. In clinical trials, the most frequently reported adverse effects were headache, nausea, fatigue, decreased appetite, anemia, pyrexia, and elevations of ALT [9, 11–15]. Patients treated with elbasvir/grazoprevir should have hepatic function monitored prior to and during treatment.

2.4. Drug-Drug Interactions. Elbasvir/grazoprevir has many clinically significant drug-drug interactions [9]. It is contraindicated in patients taking organic anion transporting polypeptides 1B1/3 inhibitors (e.g., cyclosporine) due to significant increases of grazoprevir plasma concentrations when combined. Elbasvir/grazoprevir is also contraindicated with strong cytochrome P450 3A4 inducers (e.g., rifampin, phenytoin, carbamazepine, and St. John's Wort) secondary to decreased concentrations and reduced therapeutic effects of elbasvir and grazoprevir with coadministration [9]. Caution should be used with coadministration of strong cytochrome P450 3A4 inhibitors (e.g., ketoconazole and ritonavir), which may lead to increased concentrations of elbasvir and grazoprevir. Coadministration with nafcillin, bosentan, or modafinil may lead to decreases in elbasvir and grazoprevir concentrations and resultant decreases in therapeutic efficacy, so it is not recommended. Administration with tacrolimus may result in fluctuating plasma tacrolimus concentrations, which should be frequently monitored. Caution should be used with administration of elbasvir/grazoprevir with HMG-CoA reductase inhibitors (atorvastatin, rosuvastatin, fluvastatin, lovastatin, or simvastatin), and clinicians should use the lowest dose HMG-CoA reductase inhibitor possible if this combination is used (max dose: atorvastatin, 20 mg; rosuvastatin, 10 mg) [9]. See HCV-HIV Coinfection section for information about drug-drug interactions with antiretrovirals.

3. Genotypes/SVR

Since its identification, HCV has further been subcategorized into 3 different tiers: genotype, subtype, and quasispecies [16]. A total of 6 distinct genotypes have been classified. GTs 1–4 and GT 6 are further categorized, with 67 confirmed subtypes identified [17, 18]. The different genotypes are found in varying geographic regions. GT 1 is the predominate HCV genotype, estimated to comprise 46.2% of all HCV cases worldwide and approximately 70% of cases in the United States [19, 20]. HCV GT 2 is most commonly found in sub-Saharan Africa and Asia and represents approximately 13% of all HCV cases [21]. HCV GT 3 is the second most common genotype, found predominantly in Asia and representing 20–30% of HCV cases [22, 23]. GT 4 affects approximately 12–15% of patients diagnosed worldwide with HCV [23]. This genotype is most prevalent in Northern Africa and the Middle East. HCV GT 5, predominately found in South Africa, is one of the least known genotypes of all HCV strains. As a result, there is minimal treatment data for this subset of patients [24, 25]. GT 6 and its subtypes (previously categorized as GTs 7–11) are predominately found in Asian

Table 1: SVR_{12} rates of first-line therapies for the treatment of HCV genotypes 1a, 1b, and 4 [13, 28–32].

	SVR_{12} in treatment-naïve patients			
	Overall	Genotype 1a	Genotype 1b	Genotype 4
Grazoprevir-elbasvir [13]	95%	92%	99%	100%
Ledipasvir-sofosbuvir [28]	100%	NA	NA	NA
Paritaprevir-ritonavir-ombitasvir + dasabuvir [29]	91.8%	92.2%	100%	NA
Simeprevir + sofosbuvir [30, 31]	93%	NA	NA	NA
Daclatasvir + sofosbuvir [32]	100%	NA	NA	NA

NA: not applicable.

Table 2: Cost of guideline recommended therapies for HCV genotype 1a [33].

	Elbasvir-grazoprevir (Zepatier)	Simeprevir (Olysio) + sofosbuvir (Sovaldi)	Ledipasvir-sofosbuvir (Harvoni)	Ombitasvir-paritaprevir-ritonavir-dasabuvir (Viekira) + ribavirin	Daclatasvir (Daklinza) + sofosbuvir (Sovaldi)
8 weeks	NA	NA	\$63,000	NA	NA
12 weeks	\$54,600	\$150,000	\$94,500	\$84,019	\$147,000
16 weeks	\$72,800	NA	NA	NA	NA
24 weeks	NA	NA	\$189,000	\$168,038	NA

NA: not applicable.

countries [25, 26]. Excluding subtype 6a, GT 6 remains uncommon [26].

Direct-acting antivirals have become a priority in clinical development to target HCV GT 1 for multiple reasons. Not only is this the most common genotype worldwide, but it also has poor response rates to interferon-based regimens [19, 27]. Fortunately, our DAA armamentarium has dramatically increased since 2011 with the introduction of 9 new agents (12 new individual compounds). These treatment alternatives not only have much higher SVR compared to interferon-based regiments (>90% versus 10–50%) but also have shorter durations of therapy and decreased adverse effects [20]. Specifically, SVR at 12 weeks (SVR12) was observed in 95% of patients receiving immediate treatment with elbasvir/grazoprevir for the treatment of chronic HCV infections [13]. Comparisons of elbasvir/grazoprevir to other newer HCV treatment options are listed in Table 1 [13, 28–32].

4. Cost [33]

Prior to 2011, interferon-based regimens were largely utilized. The cost of peginterferon alfa-2a and alfa-2b is approximately \$9250 and \$8400, respectively, with the addition of a \$550–\$850 cost of ribavirin for a 12-week course of therapy. However, many patients received prolonged treatment with these regimens due to a lack of observed 2 $\log_{10}$ reduction in HCV RNA. As the newer HCV agents became approved, cost has become a significant concern. For a 12-week course of therapy for grazoprevir/elbasvir, the estimated cost is \$54,600. While this is substantially higher than the interferon-based treatment, other new alternative therapies are significantly higher (Table 2) [33].

5. Clinical Evidence

5.1. Treatment-Naïve Patients. The fixed dose combination tablet of elbasvir 50 mg/grazoprevir 100 mg taken orally once daily was approved by the FDA in January 2016. This combination tablet is indicated for a duration of 12 weeks in treatment-naïve patients with or without cirrhosis [9]. The 2016 AASLD/IDSA guidelines list 12 weeks of elbasvir/grazoprevir treatment as a Class 1, Level A recommendation for treatment-naïve patients with GT 1a or 1b, with or without cirrhosis [18]. In GT 1a patients who demonstrate a baseline high-fold change NS5A resistance-associated variants (RAV), treatment duration should be extended to 16 weeks and weight-based ribavirin should be added (AASLD/IDSA Class IIa, Level B recommendation). Elbasvir/grazoprevir treatment for 12 weeks is a Class IIa, Level B recommendation in the AASLD/IDSA guidelines for patients with GT 4 [18].

5.1.1. C-EDGE Treatment-Naïve [13]. The C-EDGE Treatment-Naïve study was a phase III, randomized, blinded, placebo-controlled trial designed to evaluate the safety and efficacy of elbasvir/grazoprevir in patients with chronic HCV GT 1, 4, or 6 [13]. This study included both cirrhotic and noncirrhotic treatment-naïve adults from 60 different centers around the world. Participants were entered into either an immediate or a differed treatment group. Results have only been reported for the immediate treatment group as of publication. Of the participants in the immediate treatment group (n = 316), 157 had GT 1a, 131 had GT 1b, 18 had GT 4, and 10 had GT 6. Twenty-two percent (n = 70) of participants were classified as cirrhotic. Clinical efficacy was determined by SVR12. Overall, SVR12 was achieved in 95% of participants (299/316); breakdown by GT demonstrated SVR12 of 92% for GT 1a, 99% for GT 1b, 100% for GT 4, and 80% for GT 6. The only virologic breakthrough and a majority of the virologic relapses (9 of 12) occurred in participants with GT 1a. Zeuzem et al. [13] found an association of NS5A RAVs and virologic failure when participants with GT 1a had a shift greater than 5-fold. Safety of elbasvir/grazoprevir was similar to placebo. No serious adverse events were considered to be related to elbasvir/grazoprevir. The most common adverse events were headache (17%) and fatigue (16%). Only 3 participants discontinued the study drug due to adverse events.

5.1.2. C-SCAPE [34]. The C-SCAPE trial was a phase II study designed to evaluate the efficacy and safety of grazoprevir ± elbasvir ± ribavirin in patients with GT 2, 4, 5, or 6. Participants with GT 2 received either the three-drug combination ($n = 30$) or grazoprevir + ribavirin ($n = 30$) [34]. Participants with GT 4, 5, or 6 received either the three-drug combination ($n = 10$ for GT 4, $n = 4$ for GT 5, and $n = 5$ for GT 6) or grazoprevir + elbasvir ($n = 10$ for GT 4, $n = 4$ for GT 5, and $n = 5$ for GT 6). SVR12 for participants with GT 2 was 80% (24/30) for those treated with the three-drug regimen versus 67% (20/30) for those treated with grazoprevir and ribavirin without elbasvir. SVR12 for participants with GT 4 was 100% (10/10) in the three-drug regimen group and 90% (9/10) in the grazoprevir/elbasvir without ribavirin group. For participants with GT 5, the three-drug regimen demonstrated SVR12 of 100% (4/4) while grazoprevir/elbasvir without ribavirin group demonstrated SVR of 25% (1/4). SVR12 for GT 6 participants was 80% (4/5) for both the three-drug regimen group and the grazoprevir/elbasvir without ribavirin group. The authors concluded that patients with GT 4 or 6 should be included into future phase III studies with elbasvir/grazoprevir [34].

5.1.3. C-SWIFT [35]. C-SWIFT was an open-label phase II trial to evaluate treatment duration needed with the combination of elbasvir/grazoprevir + sofosbuvir in treatment-naïve patients with HCV GT 1 or 3 [35]. Both cirrhotic and noncirrhotic patients were included. Noncirrhotic participants with GT 1 received either 4 weeks ($n = 31$) or 6 weeks ($n = 30$) of treatment. Cirrhotic participants with GT 1 received either 6 weeks ($n = 20$) or 8 weeks ($n = 21$) of treatment. Noncirrhotic participants with GT 3 received either 8 weeks ($n = 15$) or 12 weeks ($n = 14$) of treatment while cirrhotic participants received 12 weeks ($n = 12$) of treatment. Interim results have been reported. SVR at 2 weeks for all groups was 100%. SVR at 8 weeks (SVR8) was evaluated for participants with GT 1. Noncirrhotic participants who received 4 weeks of treatment demonstrated SVR8 of 37% (12/31) while those who received 6 weeks of treatment demonstrated SVR8 of 87% (26/30). Cirrhotic patients with GT 1 who received 6 weeks of treatment demonstrated SVR8 of 80% (16/20), while those who received 8 weeks of treatment showed SVR8 of 89% (17/19). Two participants in the 8-week cirrhotic group were excluded for nonvirologic discontinuation. All participants with GT 3 in the noncirrhotic group demonstrated SVR at 4 weeks (SVR4) of 100%, regardless of whether they received 8 weeks or 12 weeks of treatment. Cirrhotic participants with GT 3 demonstrated SVR4 of 90% (9/10). One patient was excluded from this group for nonvirologic discontinuation. The regimen was well tolerated. This study was completed, but final results have yet to be published [36].

5.1.4. C-SALT Part A [37]. C-SALT part A (phase II study) evaluated elbasvir/grazoprevir efficacy and safety in GT 1 patients with Child-Pugh Class B cirrhosis [37]. One aim of this study was to evaluate the pharmacokinetics of elbasvir/grazoprevir in cirrhotic patients. Cirrhotic patients received 50 mg elbasvir + 50 mg grazoprevir daily for 12 weeks. Participants in the noncirrhotic comparator group received the standard elbasvir 50 mg + grazoprevir 100 mg daily for 12 weeks. Interim results showed that all participants with cirrhosis reached undetectable HCV RNA (<15 IU/mL) by the end of treatment and at 4-week follow-up. Participants tolerated the study drug well with no significant hepatotoxicity noted. Cirrhotic patients demonstrated slightly higher plasma grazoprevir levels when compared to their noncirrhotic counterparts. This study has not yet published final results [36].

5.1.5. C-WORTHY [15]. The C-WORTHY trial examined the efficacy and safety of elbasvir/grazoprevir ± ribavirin for GT 1 patients with cirrhosis (treatment-naïve) or treatment-experienced patients with or without cirrhosis [15]. This phase II open-label study randomized treatment-naïve, well-compensated cirrhotic patients (Child-Pugh Class A) to receive elbasvir/grazoprevir ($n = 29$ for 12 weeks, $n = 31$ for 18 weeks) or elbasvir/grazoprevir + ribavirin ($n = 31$ for 12 weeks, $n = 32$ for 18 weeks). In the group of elbasvir/grazoprevir treated for 12 weeks, the SVR12 was 97% (28/29). For participants with ribavirin added and treated for 12 weeks, the SVR12 was 90% (28/31). Participants treated for 18 weeks demonstrated similar results, with SVR12 of 94% (29/31) in the elbasvir/grazoprevir arm and SVR12 of 97% (31/32) in the arm with ribavirin added. All but one of the treatment-naïve patients experiencing virologic failure had GT 1a and NS5A RAVs at virologic failure. As in other studies, the elbasvir/grazoprevir combination was well tolerated.

5.2. Treatment-Experienced Patients. The 2016 AASLD/IDSA guidelines list 12 weeks of elbasvir/grazoprevir treatment as a Class 1, Level A recommendation for treatment-experienced patients (prior exposure to peginterferon/ribavirin) with GT 1a or 1b, with or without cirrhosis [18]. In GT 1a patients who demonstrate baseline high-fold change NS5A RAVs, treatment duration should be extended to 16 weeks and weight-based ribavirin should be added (AASLD/IDSA Class I, Level B recommendation). For GT 1 patients who previously failed a NS3 protease inhibitor, elbasvir/grazoprevir plus weight-based ribavirin for 12-week duration (16 weeks if high-fold change NS5A RAV in GT 1a) is a Class IIa, Level B recommendation for patients with or without compensated cirrhosis. Elbasvir/grazoprevir treatment for 12 weeks is a Class IIa, Level B recommendation in the AASLD/IDSA guidelines for patients with GT 4 (cirrhotic and noncirrhotic) who experienced virologic relapse after treatment with peginterferon/ribavirin. Weight-based ribavirin should be added to the regimen for GT 4 patients who experienced virologic failure while on peginterferon/ribavirin, and treatment duration should be extended to 16 weeks (Class IIa, Level B) [18].

5.2.1. C-WORTHY [15]. The C-WORTHY trial examined the efficacy and safety of elbasvir/grazoprevir ± ribavirin for treatment-experienced GT 1 patients (null responders) with or without cirrhosis [15]. Treatment-naïve cirrhotic patients were also included in this study, with those results reported in the previous section. This phase II open-label study randomized patients who had previously failed peginterferon + ribavirin to receive elbasvir/grazoprevir ($n = 33$ for 12 weeks, $n = 32$ for 18 weeks) or elbasvir/grazoprevir + ribavirin ($n = 32$ for 12 weeks, $n = 33$ for 18 weeks). Cirrhotic patients represented 34–42% of the participants in the four groups. In the elbasvir/grazoprevir 12-week treatment group, the SVR12 was 91% (30/33). For participants who received elbasvir/grazoprevir + ribavirin for 12 weeks, the SVR12 was 94% (30/32). Participants treated for 18 weeks demonstrated similar results, with SVR12 of 97% (31/32) in the elbasvir/grazoprevir arm and SVR12 of 100% (33/33) in the arm with ribavirin added. All four treatment failures demonstrated NS5A RAVs at the time of virologic failure.

5.2.2. C-EDGE Treatment-Experienced [38]. The C-EDGE Treatment-Experienced phase III trial evaluated the safety and efficacy of elbasvir/grazoprevir ± ribavirin for GT 1 or GT 4 patients who previously failed peginterferon + ribavirin [38]. Both cirrhotic and noncirrhotic patients were included. Prior treatment failure included null responders and partial responders/relapses. Participants received either elbasvir/grazoprevir ($n = 105$) or elbasvir/grazoprevir + ribavirin ($n = 104$) for 12 weeks. Overall, SVR at 4 weeks (SVR4) was 95% (100/105) for the elbasvir/grazoprevir group and 98% (102/104) for the group with ribavirin added. In subgroup analysis, 95% (55/58) with GT 1a in the elbasvir/grazoprevir group achieved SVR4 while 96% (54/56) in the ribavirin added group achieved SVR4. All participants with GT 1b ($n = 38$ in elbasvir/grazoprevir, $n = 33$ in added ribavirin) achieved SVR4. Fewer participants had GT 4; 78% (7/9) in the elbasvir/grazoprevir group achieved SVR4, while 100% (15/15) in the added ribavirin group reached SVR4. Of note, one of the treatment failures was a participant who died of lymphoma during the study. Both null responders (and partial/relapse participants) responded well to elbasvir/grazoprevir (SVR4 93% [42/45] and 98% [59/60], resp.). When ribavirin was added to the regimen, null responders reached an SVR4 of 95% (42/44) and partial/relapse participants achieved an SVR4 of 100% (60/60). Participants coinfected with HIV were included in this study; all coinfected participants reached SVR4 (6/6 in elbasvir/grazoprevir, 5/5 with added ribavirin). Cirrhotic participants responded well, with SVR4 92% (34/37) in the elbasvir/grazoprevir group and SVR4 97% (35/36) in the ribavirin added group. Full study results have yet to be reported.

5.2.3. C-SALVAGE [39, 40]. The C-SALVAGE phase II study examined the use of elbasvir/grazoprevir + ribavirin for participants with GT 1 who had previously failed combination therapy of peginterferon + ribavirin + HCV NS3/4A protease inhibitor [39, 40]. Both cirrhotic and noncirrhotic participants were included. NS3 RAVs were detected in 34 participants at baseline (30 with ≤5-fold change, 4 with >5-fold change). NS5A RAVs were detected in 8 patients at baseline (3 with ≤5-fold change, 5 with >5-fold change). All participants ($n = 79$) received elbasvir 50 mg/grazoprevir 100 mg daily + weight-based ribavirin. Overall, SVR12 was 96% (76/79). This rate was maintained for an additional 12 weeks and demonstrated comparable SVR results at 24 weeks. All three virologic failures were relapses. Each of these participants had NS3 RAVs at baseline (2 with ≤5-fold change, 1 with >5-fold change). Two of the failures also had NS5A RAVs at baseline, both with >5-fold change. Both of the failures with NS5A RAVs were also cirrhotic (1 GT 1a, 1 GT 1b), while the other failure was noncirrhotic GT 1a. The authors concluded that elbasvir/grazoprevir + ribavirin for 12 weeks is a viable therapeutic option for patients who had previously failed therapy, including those with NS3 variants [39, 40].

5.3. HCV-HIV Coinfection. There are over 4 million people worldwide who are coinfected with HIV and HCV, which equates to an overall prevalence of 6.2% of all HIV-infected individuals [41]. HIV infection has demonstrated increased progression of HCV-associated liver dysfunction and has been associated with higher rates of all-cause, liver-related, and AIDS-related death [42]. Coinfected patients receiving HIV-antiretroviral therapy (ART) tend to have delayed progression to cirrhosis, especially if the HIV viral load is undetectable [43]. Concurrent treatment of HCV in these patients is common. The AASLD/IDSA guidelines recommend the use of daily elbasvir/grazoprevir in patients with HIV/HCV coinfection when the patient is not taking ART with clinically significant drug interactions (Class IIa, Level B) [18]. Elbasvir/grazoprevir was tested in coinfected patients in two trials: C-WORTHY and C-EDGE coinfection.

5.3.1. C-WORTHY Coinfection [44]. Elbasvir/grazoprevir was studied in 59 patients with HIV and HCV coinfection without cirrhosis as a substudy of the larger C-WORTHY phase 2 trial [44]. Patients with GT 1, an undetectable HIV viral load for >24 weeks, and a CD4 T-cell count >300 cells/mm^3 at screening were included. The allowed HIV ART consisted of at least 8 weeks with tenofovir or abacavir plus emtricitabine or lamivudine plus raltegravir. Patients received elbasvir/grazoprevir ± ribavirin for 12 weeks. There were 46 patients with GT 1a, of which 24 (52%) patients received ribavirin. Of the 13 patients with GT 1b, only 5 (38%) patients received ribavirin. Of the 29 patients who received ribavirin, the SVR12 rate was 97% (28/29 patients), while the SVR12 of the 30 patients who did not receive ribavirin was 87% (26/30 patients). The regimens were generally well-tolerated, with the most common adverse effects being mild-to-moderate fatigue, headache, nausea, and diarrhea.

5.3.2. C-EDGE Coinfection [12]. In this prospective single-arm clinical trial, elbasvir/grazoprevir was studied in 218 patients with treatment-naïve chronic HCV (GT 1, 4, or 6) and HIV coinfection, both with and without cirrhosis [12]. Participants could either be naïve to ART or be on stable ART with tenofovir or abacavir plus emtricitabine or lamivudine plus either raltegravir, dolutegravir, or rilpivirine for at least 8 weeks. ART-naïve patients were required to have an HIV viral load <50,000 copies/mL and a CD4 T-cell count >500 cells/μL, while patients who were stable on ART were required to have an undetectable HIV viral load. Participants received elbasvir 50 mg/grazoprevir 100 mg once daily for 12 weeks. Ninety-seven percent (211/218) of participants were on antiretroviral therapy with an undetectable HIV viral load with a median CD4 T-cell count of 568 cells/μL. Sixteen percent (35/218) of participants had compensated cirrhosis. Overall, 210/218 (96.3%) patients achieved SVR12: 139/144 (96.5%) with GT 1a, 42/44 (95.5%) with GT 1b, and 27/28 (96.4%) with GT 4. All cirrhotic patients achieved SVR12. The regimen was generally well tolerated with the most common adverse effects being fatigue (13%), headache (12%), and nausea (9%).

5.3.3. Drug-Drug Interactions [45]. HCV-HIV coinfected patients present a particular problem when selecting not only HCV regimens but also HIV regimens. Elbasvir/grazoprevir was studied in HIV patients whose ART regimens did not contain an HIV-protease inhibitor. In particular, atazanavir, darunavir, lopinavir, saquinavir, and tipranavir are protease inhibitors whose use is contraindicated with elbasvir/grazoprevir because elevated concentrations of elbasvir/grazoprevir have been observed, leading to elevated alanine aminotransferase (ALT) levels [45]. Additionally, patients in the two trials presented above were excluded if taking efavirenz, as this nonnucleoside reverse transcriptase inhibitor is contraindicated due to reductions in the concentrations of elbasvir/grazoprevir by as much as 80% [45]. Two other ART agents, cobicistat and ritonavir, although not contraindicated, should be used with caution if coadministered with elbasvir/grazoprevir [45].

5.4. Patients with Stage 4 or 5 Chronic Kidney Disease. The AASLD/IDSA guidelines recommend 12 weeks of daily elbasvir 50 mg/grazoprevir 100 mg for treatment of patients with HCV GT 1a, 1b, or 4 and severe renal impairment (creatinine clearance of <30 mL/min) (Class IIb, Level B) [18].

5.4.1. C-SURFER [11]. The phase III C-SURFER study focused on patients with HCV GT 1 with stage 4 or 5 chronic kidney disease (CKD), including patients receiving hemodialysis [11]. Safety and efficacy of elbasvir 50 mg/grazoprevir 100 mg daily for 12 weeks were evaluated. Participants were randomized to either an immediate treatment group (n = 111) or a placebo (delayed treatment) group (n = 113); eleven additional participants were included in a pharmacokinetic arm, receiving immediate treatment (n = 235 total participants). Fifty-two percent of participants had GT 1a. Seventy-six percent of participants (179/235) were on hemodialysis, 6% (14/235) had cirrhosis, and 80% (189/235) were treatment-naïve. In the immediate treatment + pharmacokinetic group, SVR12 was achieved in 94% (115/122) of participants. In a modified analysis, 6 patients were excluded for reasons other than virologic failure, resulting in a SVR12 of 99% (115/116). Adverse effects were similar between immediate treatment and placebo, with most adverse effects classified as mild to moderate in both groups. The authors concluded that elbasvir/grazoprevir for 12 weeks is an effective treatment option for GT 1 patients with stage 4 or 5 CKD [11].

5.5. Patients Who Inject IV Drugs Receiving Opioid Agonist Therapy. Injection drug use is a major risk factor for HCV infection, accounting for 50–80% of all HCV infections [46]. Study results from the trial presented below are not yet incorporated into the AASLD/IDSA guidelines but show promise for this significant population.

5.5.1. C-EDGE CO-STAR [47]. The C-EDGE CO-STAR trial evaluated the efficacy of elbasvir/grazoprevir treatment for 12 weeks in patients who inject intravenous drugs and were currently receiving opioid agonist therapy [47]. Participants with GT 1, 4, or 6 were included, with or without HIV coinfection ± cirrhosis. A total of 301 patients were randomized in 2 : 1 ratio to receive immediate or delayed treatment. Ninety-nine percent (199/201) of participants in the immediate treatment group completed 12-week treatment, with SVR4 96% (193/201). Four of these participants experienced virologic failure, detected after completion of therapy. Adverse effects were similar between the two groups. The authors concluded that preliminary data demonstrate that elbasvir/grazoprevir is safe and effective in the special population of intravenous drug users receiving opioid agonist therapy [47]. This study is currently ongoing [36] (ClinicalTrials.gov).

6. Conclusion

Elbasvir/grazoprevir has earned a spot in the current hepatitis C guidelines as a first-line option for treatment-naïve patients with GT 1a or 1b, with or without cirrhosis. It is also recommended for treatment-experienced patients with GT 1a or 1b. For patients with GT 4, elbasvir/grazoprevir is recommended for both treatment-naïve and treatment-experienced patients, with or without cirrhosis [18]. Elbasvir/grazoprevir may be used in patients with HIV coinfection or severe renal impairment. Although it does have more drug-drug interactions than other treatments, elbasvir/grazoprevir is the most cost-effective. Given the efficacy and safety data described above, elbasvir/grazoprevir should be considered a potent new weapon in the fight against chronic hepatitis C.

Competing Interests

The authors declare that they have no competing interests.

References

[1] WHO Fact Sheet, 2016, http://www.who.int/mediacentre/factsheets/fs164/en.

[2] A. J. Zuckerman, "The elusive hepatitis C virus," *British Medical Journal*, vol. 299, no. 6704, pp. 871–873, 1989.

[3] F. Douam, Q. Ding, and A. Ploss, "Recent advances in understanding hepatitis C," *F1000Research*, vol. 5, article 131, 2016.

[4] S. Zopf, A. E. Kremer, M. F. Neurath, and J. Siebler, "Advances in hepatitis C therapy: what is the current state—what come's next?" *World Journal of Hepatology*, vol. 8, no. 3, pp. 139–147, 2016.

[5] K. S. Gutfreund and V. G. Bain, "Chronic viral hepatitis C: management update," *Canadian Medical Association Journal*, vol. 162, no. 6, pp. 827–833, 2000.

[6] P. Klenerman and P. K. Gupta, "Hepatitis C virus: current concepts and future challenges," *QJM*, vol. 105, no. 1, pp. 29–32, 2012.

[7] T. Asselah, N. Boyer, D. Saadoun, M. Martinot-Peignoux, and P. Marcellin, "Direct-acting antivirals for the treatment of hepatitis C virus infection: optimizing current IFN-free treatment and future perspectives," *Liver International*, vol. 36, pp. 47–57, 2016.

[8] X. Zhang, "Direct anti-HCV agents," *Acta Pharmaceutica Sinica B*, vol. 6, no. 1, pp. 26–31, 2016.

[9] Zepatier™, *(Elbasvir and Grazoprevir) Tablets for Oral Use*, Merck & Co, Whitehouse Station, NJ, USA, 2016.

[10] G. M. Keating, "Elbasvir/Grazoprevir: first global approval," *Drugs*, vol. 76, no. 5, pp. 617–624, 2016.

[11] D. Roth, D. R. Nelson, A. Bruchfeld et al., "Grazoprevir plus elbasvir in treatment-naive and treatment-experienced patients with hepatitis C virus genotype 1 infection and stage 4-5 chronic kidney disease (the C-SURFER study): a combination phase 3 study," *The Lancet*, vol. 386, no. 10003, pp. 1537–1545, 2015.

[12] J. K. Rockstroh, M. Nelson, C. Katlama et al., "Efficacy and safety of grazoprevir (MK-5172) and elbasvir (MK-8742) in patients with hepatitis C virus and HIV co-infection (C-EDGE CO-INFECTION): a non-randomised, open-label trial," *Lancet HIV*, vol. 2, no. 8, pp. e319–e327, 2015.

[13] S. Zeuzem, R. Ghalib, K. R. Reddy et al., "Grazoprevir-elbasvir combination therapy for treatment-naive cirrhotic and noncirrhotic patients with chronic hepatitis C virus genotype 1, 4, or 6 infection: a randomized trial," *Annals of Internal Medicine*, vol. 163, no. 1, pp. 1–13, 2015.

[14] M. Lagging, A. Brown, P. S. Mantry et al., "Grazoprevir plus peginterferon and ribavirin in treatment-naive patients with hepatitis C virus genotype 1 infection: a randomized trial," *Journal of Viral Hepatitis*, vol. 23, no. 2, pp. 80–88, 2016.

[15] E. Lawitz, E. Gane, B. Pearlman et al., "Efficacy and safety of 12 weeks versus 18 weeks of treatment with grazoprevir (MK-5172) and elbasvir (MK-8742) with or without ribavirin for hepatitis C virus genotype 1 infection in previously untreated patients with cirrhosis and patients with previous null response with or without cirrhosis (C-WORTHY): a randomised, open-label phase 2 trial," *The Lancet*, vol. 385, no. 9973, pp. 1075–1086, 2015.

[16] M. Houghton, "Discovery of the hepatitis C virus," *Liver International*, vol. 29, supplement 1, pp. 82–88, 2009.

[17] D. B. Smith, J. Bukh, C. Kuiken et al., "Expanded classification of hepatitis C virus into 7 genotypes and 67 subtypes: updated criteria and genotype assignment web resource," *Hepatology*, vol. 59, no. 1, pp. 318–327, 2014.

[18] AASLD-IDSA, "Recommendations for testing, managing, and treating hepatitis C," 2016, http://www.hcvguidelines.org.

[19] J. P. Messina, I. Humphreys, A. Flaxman et al., "Global distribution and prevalence of hepatitis C virus genotypes," *Hepatology*, vol. 61, no. 1, pp. 77–87, 2015.

[20] P. Deming, M. T. Martin, J. Chan et al., "Therapeutic advances in HCV genotype 1 infection: insights from the society of infectious diseases pharmacists," *Pharmacotherapy*, vol. 36, no. 2, pp. 203–217, 2016.

[21] J. Ampuero and M. Romero-Gomez, "Hepatitis C virus current and evolving treatments for genotypes 2 and 3," *Gastroenterology Clinics of North America*, vol. 44, no. 4, pp. 845–857, 2015.

[22] E. Gower, C. Estes, S. Blach, K. Razavi-Shearer, and H. Razavi, "Global epidemiology and genotype distribution of the hepatitis C virus infection," *Journal of Hepatology*, vol. 61, supplement 1, pp. S45–S57, 2014.

[23] T. Y. Abdel-Ghaffar, M. M. Sira, and S. E. Naghi, "Hepatitis C genotype 4: the past, present and future," *World Journal of Hepatology*, vol. 7, no. 28, pp. 2792–2810, 2015.

[24] H. E. M. Smuts and J. Kannemeyer, "Genotyping of hepatitis C virus in South Africa," *Journal of Clinical Microbiology*, vol. 33, no. 6, pp. 1679–1681, 1995.

[25] M. H. Nguyen and E. B. Keeffe, "Prevalence and treatment of hepatitis C virus genotypes 4, 5, and 6," *Clinical Gastroenterology and Hepatology*, vol. 3, no. 2, pp. S97–S101, 2005.

[26] K. A. Naamani, S. A. Sinani, and M. Deschenes, "Epidemiology and treatment of hepatitis C genotypes 5 and 6," *Canadian Journal of Gastroenterology*, vol. 27, no. 1, pp. e8–e12, 2013.

[27] E. Lawitz, J. P. Lalezari, T. Hassanein et al., "Sofosbuvir in combination with peginterferon alfa-2a and ribavirin for non-cirrhotic, treatment-naive patients with genotypes 1, 2, and 3 hepatitis C infection: a randomised, double-blind, phase 2 trial," *The Lancet Infectious Diseases*, vol. 13, no. 5, pp. 401–408, 2013.

[28] M. Mizokami, O. Yokosuka, T. Takehara et al., "Ledipasvir and sofosbuvir fixed-dose combination with and without ribavirin for 12 weeks in treatment-naïve and previously treated Japanese patients with genotype 1 hepatitis C: an open-label, randomised, phase 3 trial," *The Lancet Infectious Diseases*, vol. 15, no. 6, pp. 645–653, 2015.

[29] F. Poordad, C. Hezode, R. Trinh et al., "ABT-450/r-ombitasvir and dasabuvir with ribavirin for hepatitis C with cirrhosis," *The New England Journal of Medicine*, vol. 370, no. 21, pp. 1973–1982, 2014.

[30] E. Lawitz, M. S. Sulkowski, R. Ghalib et al., "Simeprevir plus sofosbuvir, with or without ribavirin, to treat chronic infection with hepatitis C virus genotype 1 in non-responders to pegylated interferon and ribavirin and treatment-naive patients: the COSMOS randomised study," *The Lancet*, vol. 384, no. 9956, pp. 1756–1765, 2014.

[31] B. L. Pearlman, C. Ehleben, and M. Perrys, "The combination of simeprevir and sofosbuvir is more effective than that of peginterferon, ribavirin, and sofosbuvir for patients with hepatitis C-related child's class a cirrhosis," *Gastroenterology*, vol. 148, no. 4, pp. 762–770, 2015.

[32] M. S. Sulkowski, D. F. Gardiner, M. Rodriguez-Torres et al., "Daclatasvir plus sofosbuvir for previously treated or untreated chronic HCV infection," *The New England Journal of Medicine*, vol. 370, no. 3, pp. 211–221, 2014.

[33] D. H. Spach and H. N. Kim, "Medications to treat HCV," http://www.hepatitisc.uw.edu/page/treatment/drugs.

[34] A. Brown, C. Hezode, E. Zuckerman et al., "C-SCAPE: efficacy and safety of 12 weeks of grazoprevir ± elbasvir ± ribavirin in patients with HCV GT2, 4, 5, or 6 infection," in *Proceedings of the 50th Annual Meeting of the European Association for the Study of the Liver*, Abstract P0771, Vienna, Austria, April 2015.

[35] F. Poordad, E. Lawitz, J. Gutierrez et al., "C-SWIFT: grazoprevir/elbasvir + sofosbuvir in cirrhotic and noncirrhotic, treatment-naïve patients with hepatitis C virus genotype 1 infection, for durations of 4, 6, or 8 weeks and genotype 3 infection for durations of 8 or 12 weeks," in *Proceedings of the 50th Annual Meeting of the European Association for the Study of the Liver*, Abstract O006, Vienna, Austria, April 2015.

[36] ClinicalTrials.gov, http://www.clinicaltrials.gov.

[37] I. M. Jacobsen, F. Poordad, R. Firpi-Morell et al., "Efficacy and safety of grazoprevir and elbasvir in hepatitis C genotype 1-infected patients with Child-Pugh class B cirrhosis (C-SALT)," in *Proceedings of the 50th Annual Meeting of the European Association for the Study of the Liver*, Abstract O008, Vienna, Austria, April 2015.

[38] P. Kwo, E. Gane, C.-Y. Peng et al., "Efficacy and safety of grazoprevir/elbasvir ± RBV for 12 or 16 weeks in patients with HCV G1, G4, or G6 infection who previously failed peginterferon/RBV: C-EDGE treatment-experienced," in *Proceedings of the 50th Annual Meeting of the European Association for the Study of the Liver*, Abstract P0886, Vienna, Austria, April 2015.

[39] X. Forns, S. C. Gordon, E. Zuckerman et al., "Grazoprevir and elbasvir plus ribavirin for chronic HCV genotype-1 infection after failure of combination therapy containing a direct-acting antiviral agent," *Journal of Hepatology*, vol. 63, no. 3, pp. 564–572, 2015.

[40] M. Buti, S. C. Gordon, E. Zuckerman et al., "Grazoprevir, elbasvir, and ribavirin for chronic hepatitis c virus genotype 1 infection after failure of pegylated interferon and ribavirin with an earlier-generation protease inhibitor: final 24-week results from C-SALVAGE," *Clinical Infectious Diseases*, vol. 62, no. 1, pp. 32–36, 2016.

[41] L. Platt, P. Easterbrook, E. Gower et al., "Prevalence and burden of HCV co-infection in people living with HIV: a global systematic review and meta-analysis," *The Lancet Infectious Diseases*, 2016.

[42] T. Von Schoen-Angerer, J. Cohn, T. Swan, and P. Piot, "UNITAID can address HCV/HIV co-infection," *The Lancet*, vol. 381, no. 9867, p. 628, 2013.

[43] J. Y. Chen, E. R. Feeney, and R. T. Chung, "HCV and HIV co-infection: mechanisms and management," *Nature Reviews Gastroenterology and Hepatology*, vol. 11, no. 6, pp. 362–371, 2014.

[44] M. Sulkowski, C. Hezode, J. Gerstoft et al., "Efficacy and safety of 8 weeks versus 12 weeks of treatment with grazoprevir (MK-5172) and elbasvir (MK-8742) with or without ribavirin in patients with hepatitis C virus genotype 1 mono-infection and HIV/hepatitis C virus co-infection (C-WORTHY): a randomised, open-label phase 2 trial," *The Lancet*, vol. 385, no. 9973, pp. 1087–1097, 2015.

[45] *Clinical Pharmacology [database online]*, Gold Standard, Tampa, Fla, USA, 2016, http://www.clinicalpharmacology.com.

[46] B. Hajarizadeh, J. Grebely, and G. J. Dore, "Epidemiology and natural history of HCV infection," *Nature Reviews Gastroenterology and Hepatology*, vol. 10, no. 9, pp. 553–562, 2013.

[47] G. Dore, F. Altice, A. H. Litwin et al., "C-EDGE CO-STAR: efficacy of grazoprevir and elbasvir in persons who inject drugs (PWID) receiving opioid agonist therapy," in *Proceedings of the Annual Meeting of the American Association for the Study of Liver Diseases*, Abstract 40, San Francisco, Calif, USA, November 2015.

20

Therapeutic Potential of HGF-Expressing Human Umbilical Cord Mesenchymal Stem Cells in Mice with Acute Liver Failure

Yunxia Tang,[1] Qiongshu Li,[1] Fanwei Meng,[1] Xingyu Huang,[1] Chan Li,[1] Xin Zhou,[1] Xiaoping Zeng,[1] Yixin He,[1] Jia Liu,[1] Xiang Hu,[1] Ji-Fan Hu,[2,3] and Tao Li[1]

[1]*Shenzhen Beike Cell Engineering Research Institute, Yuanxing Science and Technology Building, Nanshan, Shenzhen 518057, China*
[2]*Stem Cell and Cancer Center, First Hospital, Jilin University, Changchun 130012, China*
[3]*Stanford University Medical School, Palo Alto Veterans Institute for Research, Palo Alto, CA 94304, USA*

Correspondence should be addressed to Xiang Hu; huxiang@beike.cc, Ji-Fan Hu; jifan@stanford.edu, and Tao Li; litao@beike.cc

Academic Editor: Shigeru Marubashi

Human umbilical cord-derived mesenchymal stem cells (UCMSCs) are particularly attractive cells for cellular and gene therapy in acute liver failure (ALF). However, the efficacy of this cell therapy in animal studies needs to be significantly improved before it can be translated into clinics. In this study, we investigated the therapeutic potential of UCMSCs that overexpress hepatocyte growth factor (HGF) in an acetaminophen-induced acute liver failure mouse model. We found that the HGF-UCMSC cell therapy protected animals from acute liver failure by reducing liver damage and prolonging animal survival. The therapeutic effect of HGF-UCMSCs was associated with the increment in serum glutathione (GSH) and hepatic enzymes that maintain redox homeostasis, including γ-glutamylcysteine synthetase (γ-GCS), superoxide dismutase (SOD), and catalase (CAT). Immunohistochemical staining confirmed that HGF-UCMSCs were mobilized to the injured areas of the liver. Additionally, HGF-UCMSCs modulated apoptosis by upregulating the antiapoptotic Bcl2 and downregulating proapoptotic genes, including Bax and TNFα. Taken together, these data suggest that ectopic expression of HGF in UCMSCs protects animals from acetaminophen-induced acute liver failure through antiapoptosis and antioxidation mechanisms.

1. Introduction

Acute liver failure (ALF), a severe liver damage caused by a variety of factors, is characterized by serious liver dysfunction of synthesis, detoxification, excretion, and biotransformation. Epidemiological data have shown that therapy-associated or suicide-driven overdosage of acetaminophen (APAP) is the most common etiology of ALF in developed countries [1, 2]. The mechanism of the APAP-induced ALF is related to oxidative stress in liver cells, resulting in the death of a large number of liver cells. Liver transplantation is the most commonly used therapy but has significant limitations due to organ rejection, lack of donors, and high cost [3–5].

Recently, cell-based therapies have focused on the use of mesenchymal stem cells (MSC) for liver regeneration [6], including those MSCs from human bone marrow [7, 8], umbilical cord blood [9], fetal liver [10, 11], or adipose tissue [1, 12–14]. These MSC recipes have been approved to induce host liver recovery and stimulate endogenous regeneration programs [2, 3, 12, 14, 15]. However, the efficacy of these MSC therapies in animal studies still needs to be significantly improved before they can be translated into clinics.

Hepatocyte growth factor (HGF), a potent hepatic mitogen, has multiple physiological and biochemical functions. HGF improves DNA synthesis and acts as an antioxidant factor by decreasing oxidative stress in the liver [16]. In addition, HGF also participates in regulation of various processes in the liver and has been proved to stimulate liver regeneration against liver failure [17, 18]. The HGF/c-Met signaling pathway has been implicated as a key regulator of the cellular redox homeostasis and oxidative stress. The signaling pathway protects against oxidative stress-induced cellular damage [19].

In this study, we determined whether ectopic expression of the human HGF gene would enhance the therapeutic potential of UCMSCs in APAP-induced ALF mice. We hypothesized that this unique therapeutic approach would combine the regenerative role of UCMSCs with the antioxidation activity of HGF factor. For this, we established an ALF mouse model by lethal dose of APAP and examined the therapeutic potential of the HGF-expressing UCMSCs.

2. Materials and Methods

2.1. Isolation and Flow Cytometry Phenotyping of UCMSCs. Umbilical cords were collected from delivering full-term infants in hospital after obtaining written parental consent. Isolation of UCMSC was performed as described previously [20, 21]. Briefly, Wharton's Jelly was cut into small pieces, treated with collagenase type 1 (Sigma, MO), and then cultured in DMEM containing 10% fetal calf serum (FCS) and antibiotics at 37°C in a 5% CO_2 humidified atmosphere. Cells that migrated out from the explants after 5–7 days were collected and expanded. Cells at passage 3 were used for cell transplantation. The protocol was approved by the Human Medical Ethical Review Committee from Shenzhen Beike Cell Engineering Research Institute.

The cultured UCMSCs were characterized by cytometry. Cells were trypsinized and suspended at a concentration of 1×10^6 cells/mL in phosphate-buffered saline (PBS) containing 0.1% BSA. Cells were incubated at 4°C with antibodies against MSCs markers (CD90, CD73, and CD105), hematopoietic cell markers (CD45, CD34, CD14, and CD19), and receptors for extracellular matrix (CD29, CD44) and major histocompatibility (HLA-DR) (all from BD Biosciences). After 30 minutes, cells were washed and suspended in 300 μL PBS. Flow cytometry was performed using FACSAria III cell 4 Sorter (BD Biosciences, CA). The experiment was repeated three times, and the results are representative of three independent experiments.

2.2. Cloning of Hepatocyte Growth Factor (HGF). The following PCR primers were used to amplify the human HGF cDNA: HGFNheI-F: 5′-TGCTAGCGCCACCATGTGGGTGACCAAACTCCTGCCAGC-3′ and HGFSalI-R: 5′-AGTCGACCTATGACTGTGGTACCTTATATGTTA-3′. The HGF cDNA was amplified by PCR using pSNAV2.0-hHGF plasmid as the template. PCR products were digested by NheI and SalI restriction enzymes, extracted from agarose gels, and cloned into pDC315 adenoviral vector with T4 DNA ligase.

2.3. Generation of HGF-Expressing UCMSCs. Adenoviruses were packaged and produced using the method as previously reported [22, 23]. Adenoviral packaging 293 cells (1×10^5 cells/well) were seeded in 24 well plates in Dulbecco's modified Eagle's medium (DMEM) supplemented with 10% fetal bovine serum (FBS) and incubated at 37°C with 5% CO_2 overnight. The medium was replaced with Opti-MEM (Invitrogen, CA) before transfection. The cells were transfected at 80%–90% confluence, with the backbone plasmids pBHGlox(delta) E1, 3 Cre and shuttle plasmids pDC315-HGF using Lipofectamine 2000 (Invitrogen, CA) according to the manufacturer's instructions. Six days after transfection, viral plaques appeared and were collected for the production of Ad-HGF.

Human UCMSCs were seeded in T175 flask at a concentration of 10^6 cells/flask and incubated with growth medium for 24 h. Cells were switched to Dulbecco's modified Eagle medium (DMEM) containing 5 μM HP4 without serum and infected with adenoviral carrying HGF at multiplicity of infection of 50 (MOI = 50). Four hours after viral exposure, medium was changed by normal growth medium and cells were incubated for 48 h. Infected cells were harvested 48 hours later. Flow cytometry was used to characterize the phenotype of HGF-UCMSCs that were transfected with adenoviral HGF.

2.4. Immunofluorescence Staining. Immunofluorescence was carried out to study the gene expression in infected cells and control cells. Cultured cells were fixed with freshly prepared 4% paraformaldehyde (PFA) for 10 minutes at RT and permeabilized with 0.1% Triton X-100 for 3–5 minutes on ice. After being blocked with blocking buffer (4% BSA) for 30 min at RT, cells were incubated with rabbit anti-human HGF antibody overnight at 4°C, washed with PBS, and then incubated with the secondary antibodies goat anti-rabbit antibody labeled with PE at RT for 1 h. Slides were washed with PBS. DAPI (4′,6-diamidoino-2-phenylindole, Invitrogen, CA) was used to visualize nuclei. Immunofluorescence was observed under the fluorescent microscope (Observer A1, Zeiss, Germany).

2.5. Osteogenic and Adipogenic Differentiation. Cells were seeded at 5×10^3 cells/cm^2 and were then differentiated using osteogenic and adipogenic differentiation kit (Invitrogen, CA). About 21 to 28 days later, cells were stained with the oil red O or Alizarin Red to detect the presence of neutral lipid vacuoles in differentiated adipocytes and calcium deposition in osteocytes, respectively.

2.6. Cell Transplantation into Mice with APAP-Induced Liver Injury. Male BALB/c mice (body weight 18–20 g) were purchased from the Medical Laboratory Animal Center of Guangdong Province, China. Mice were maintained under standard conditions. APAP (Aladdin, Shanghai, China) was dissolved in sterile normal saline (NS) at the concentration of 18.75 mg/mL for the lethal study. An ALF model was generated in 6–8-week-old mice by intraperitoneal administration of a single dose of 800 μL/20 g body weight sterile normal saline (NS) containing 15 μg APAP. After one hour, the mice underwent intravenous tail vein transplantation of HGF-UCMSCs (n = 10) or UCMSCs (n = 10) at a concentration of 1×10^6 cells per mouse. Control mice were receiving 800 μL/20 g body weight sterile normal saline (NS; n = 10). Mouse survival rate was calculated at different time points.

In a second experiment, APAP was prepared as the concentration of 12.5 μg/mL for a sublethal study. In this set of experiments, mice were intraperitoneally injected with 10 μg APAP to make a sublethal ALF model. After cell transplantation, livers were collected for analysis of pathological change and liver functions were assessed.

Animals were euthanized by standard CO_2 inhalation procedure at the end of the study or if they show the sign of death. All studies were performed under the guidelines and protocols approved by Institutional Animal Ethic Committee of Shenzhen Beike Cell Engineering Research Institute.

2.7. Serum Parameter and Antioxidative Enzyme Detection. Blood samples of the sublethal ALF mice were collected at 4 hours, 8 hours, and 24 hours after APAP injected. Blood samples were centrifuged at 3000x rpm, and serum was collected to determine the activities of aspartate aminotransferase (AST), alanine aminotransferase (ALT), and lactate dehydrogenase (LDH). Serum levels of AST, ALT, and LDH in mouse blood were measured with an automated biochemical analyzer (Mindray, Shenzhen, China). One week after transplantation, mice were sacrificed with CO_2. Parts of the livers were weighed and liver homogenate was made with tissue homogenate machine (IKA). Protein concentration of the liver homogenate was measured with automated biochemical analyzer. The activities of superoxide dismutase (SOD), catalase (CAT), γ-glutamylcysteine synthetase (γ-GCS), and the levels of malondialdehyde (MDA) and glutathione (GSH) in liver tissues were measured with SOD Assay Kit, γ-GCS Assay Kit, CAT Assay Kit, GSH Assay Kit, and MDA Assay Kit (Nanjing Jiancheng Bioengineering Institute, China), respectively. The activities of SOD, CAT, and γ-GCS were recorded as the relative activity by normalizing protein concentration of the homogenate. Similarly, the levels of MDA and GSH were recorded as the relative level by normalizing over the protein concentration in homogenates.

2.8. Histological and Immunohistochemical Examination. At the end of the study, livers of sublethal ALF mice were removed and weighed. About 50 mg of the liver tissue was grinded in TRIZOL and stored at −80°C for real time PCR. The remainder of each liver sample was fixed in 4% paraformaldehyde for 24 hours and processed for histological and immunohistochemical analyses. Fixed liver samples were cut into small pieces (three from each liver), dehydrated, paraffin-embedded, and cut into 5 μm thickness sections. Sections were stained with hematoxylin eosin for pathological observation. The relative necrotic areas were calculated in three fields under a microscope using the following formula: relative necrotic areas = (necrotic area/total area of image) × 100%. Immunohistochemistry stain was conducted using the method as previously described [8, 24]. Rabbit anti-human HGF monoclonal antibody (Santa Cruz Biotechnologies, CA) and rabbit anti-human CD90 monoclonal antibody (BD Biosciences, CA) were used as the primary antibodies. Goat anti-rabbit polyclonal antibody probed with DAB was used as the second antibody.

2.9. Quantitative Real-Time PCR. One week after transplantation, total RNA of sublethal ALF mice was prepared using TRIzol (Invitrogen, CA). RNA was treated by DNase I master mix and converted to cDNA by MMLV RT Mix (Invitrogen, CA). Aliquots of cDNA were tested in PCR assay using SYBR Premix Ex Tq II (Takara, Japan) in a Bio-Rad CFX96 real-time system under standard cycling conditions of 2 min at 95°C, followed by 40 cycles of PCR with 20 sec at 95°C, 30 sec at 56°C, and 30 sec at 72°C. Expression of the target genes (P65, TNFα, Bcl-2, and Bax) was calculated as the relative value by normalizing over the expression of GAPDH, using the $\Delta\Delta$Ct method [24, 25]. Data were presented as the fold change in gene expression relative to the negative control group (normal mice). Three replicates were performed for every condition and experiment, with each sample assayed in duplicate for each amplicon. The primers used for PCR included the following:

P65 F: ACAGACCCAGGAGTGTTCACAGA

P65 R: CATGGACACACCCTGGTTCAG

TNFα F: ATGAGAAGTTCCCAAATGGC

TNFα R: CTCCACTTGGTGGTTTGCTA

mBcl2-E1F: GCATCTGCACACCTGGATCCAGGAT

mBcl2-E2R: GAAATCAAACAGAGGTCGCATGCTG

mBax-E4F: ACCATCATGGGCTGGACACTGGACT

mGAPDH-F: AGGTCGGTGTGAACGGATTTG

mGAPDH-R: TGTAGACCATGTAGTTGAGGTCA

2.10. Western Blotting Analysis. The cells were lysed in radioimmunoprecipitation assay (RIPA) lysis buffer (Santa Cruz Biotechnology, CA), and the protein content was determined using Bio-Rad protein assay reagent (Bio-Rad, Hercules, CA). Equal amounts of cell lysate protein were separated by 10% SDS-PAGE and transferred to PVDF membranes (Millipore, Billerica, MA, USA). The primary antibodies against HGF, p65, and β-actin (1:1000) were derived from Santa Cruz Biotechnology, CA. After washing the membranes with Tris-buffered saline containing 0.05% Tween 20 (washing buffer), horseradish peroxidase (HRP) conjugated secondary antibody (1:1000; Santa Cruz Biotechnology, CA) was added. After further washing, color was developed using luminol reagent (Santa Cruz Biotechnology, CA), and the HRP activity of the blots was analyzed using a LAS1000 imager (Fuji film, Tokyo, Japan).

2.11. Statistical Analysis. Data were presented as the mean ± standard deviation (SD). The one-way analysis of variance (ANOVA) with the Bonferroni correction was used to analyze differences between two groups of serum parameters. Animal survival was analyzed using the Kaplan-Meier log rank method. $P < 0.05$ was considered to be statistically significant. Data were analyzed with SPSS statistical software.

3. Results

3.1. Ectopic Expression of HGF Does Not Affect the Multipotency of UCMSCs. UCMSCs were cultured from human umbilical cord tissues [20]. Adherent UCMSCs began to grow 8–12 days after the initial tissue plating. UCMSCs were infected with HGF adenovirus at a multiplicity of infection of 50. As seen in Figure 1(a), immunofluorescent staining detected the expression of HGF two days after viral transduction (right panel). The parent UCMSCs, however, did not express HGF (left panel). Western blot also validated the expression of HGF in virally transfected UCMSCs (Figure 1(b)).

We then examined the property of HGF-UCMSCs by inducing osteogenic and adipogenic differentiation. After differentiation, we did not observe significant differences between the parent UCMSCs and HGF-UCMSCs in the appearance of intracytoplasmic lipid droplets stained by oil red O (Figure 1(c), right panels) and calcium deposits stained by Alizarin Red (Figure 1(c), middle panels). These data suggest that ectopic expression of HGF does not affect the potential of adipogenic and osteogenic differentiation in UCMSCs.

We further characterized the phenotype of HGF-UCMSCs using flow cytometry 48 hours after viral infection. We found that stem cell markers CD105, CD73, CD90, CD44, and CD29 were equally expressed between the parent and the HGF-expressing UCMSCs (Figures 1(d)-1(e)). Negative markers CD45, CD34, CD14, CD19, and HLA-DR were expressed at very low level in HGF-UCMSCs. Thus, adenoviral expression of HGF does not affect the expression of mesenchymal markers, such as CD90, CD105, and CD73.

3.2. HGF-UCMSCs Protect Hepatic Injuries in ALF Mice. To evaluate the therapeutic potential in liver regeneration, HGF-UCMSCs were transplanted into mice with ALF. The ALF model was established in mice by intraperitoneal injection of APAP using a dose that is known to induce oxidative stress, hepatocyte necrosis, extensive vacuolar degeneration, and inflammatory cell infiltration in most of the zones of the parenchyma [26]. To determine the efficacy of HGF-UCMSC in ALF, we performed a titration experiment to determine the appropriate dose of cells and the timing window of cell treatment. We found that 1×10^6 UCMSC could lead to a decrease in the transaminase level. Intravenous transplantation was the most effective method to deliver HGF-UCMSCs. Thus, 1×10^6 HGF-UCMSCs were intravenously transplanted into APAP-injured mice an hour after ALF induction.

As compared with the control mice (Figure 2(a)), the sublethal APAP treated mice displayed severe internal bleeding and necrosis in the liver (Figure 2(b)). Remarkably, transplantation of HGF-UCMSCs dramatically attenuated the liver damage (Figure 2(c)). H&E staining of liver sections also confirmed the therapeutic potential of HGF-UCMSCs in attenuating the APAP-induced necrosis (Figure 2(g)). Overall, HGF-UCMSCs showed a better therapeutic potency than UCMSCs along in treating ALF (Figures 2(d), 2(h), and 2(i)).

In a separate study, animals were given a lethal dose of APAP to assess the role of HGF-UCMSCs in improving ALF survival. A single dose of 1×10^6 cells was transplanted intravenously into recipient animals. We found that transplantation of HGF-UCMSCs and UCMSCs showed a significantly increased animal survival rate compared to the NS control. ALF mice in the HGF-UCMSC group had a better survival than those in the UCMSC group (85.7% versus 78.6%), although the difference was not statistically different (Figure 2(j)).

3.3. Functional Improvement of Injured Liver by HGF-UCMSCs. The extent of liver damage in mice induced by sublethal dose of APAP was monitored by serum levels of total hepatic protein and albumin over the 24 h time course of the study. We found that total hepatic protein did not show much difference between different treatment groups (Figure 3(a)). However, serum albumin levels were 1.5-fold higher at 24 h in the mice treated with HGF-UCMSCs than that in the untreated APAP-mouse group and the group treated with UCMSCs (Figure 3(b)).

Hepatic function was also evaluated by the measurement of serum AST, ALT, and LDH. We observed that all of the enzymes were elevated in the ALF mice compared to the control but were decreased at all time points (4 h, 8 h, and 24 h) in the HGF-UCMSC treatment group ($P < 0.05$, Figures 3(c)–3(e)), compared to the untreated APAP-mouse group. Most importantly, the AST and ALT levels at 24 h and the LDH level at 4 h were significantly lower in mice treated with HGF-UCMSC than that in the group treated with UCMSCs.

3.4. Migration of HGF-UCMSCs into the Injured Hepatic Zones. To delineate mechanisms underlying the protective effect of HGF-UCMSCs in sublethal dose of APAP-induced ALF animals, we tracked the transplanted cells by immunohistochemical staining of human HGF and human CD90 positive cells in the livers of mice on day 7 after transplantation. Using anti-human HGF and anti-human CD90 antibodies, we found that HGF-UCMSCs were detected in the injured liver of mice (Figure 4). These data suggest that the transplanted UCMSCs were able to migrate to the injured area.

3.5. HGF-UCMSCs Reduce Oxidative Stress in ALF Mice. Overdosage of APAP can induce oxidant stress in hepatocytes, especially GSH exhaustion. The HGF/c-Met signaling pathway is a key regulator of the cellular redox homeostasis and oxidative stress [19]. We thus examined if the treatment of HGF-UCMSCs protected the sublethal dose of APAP-induced ALF animals through a mechanism by modifying the oxidative stress. For this, we examined the level of GSH in the liver. Hepatic GSH was slightly decreased in the APAP-injured mice at 4 h and 8 h compared to the control. Treatment of animals with UCMSCs had no significant effects on the GSH level. However, treatment of HGF-UCMSC significantly improved the GSH level at 4 h and 24 h (Figure 5(a)).

Reactive oxygen species (ROS) are scavenged by cell's antioxidant defense system including superoxide dismutase

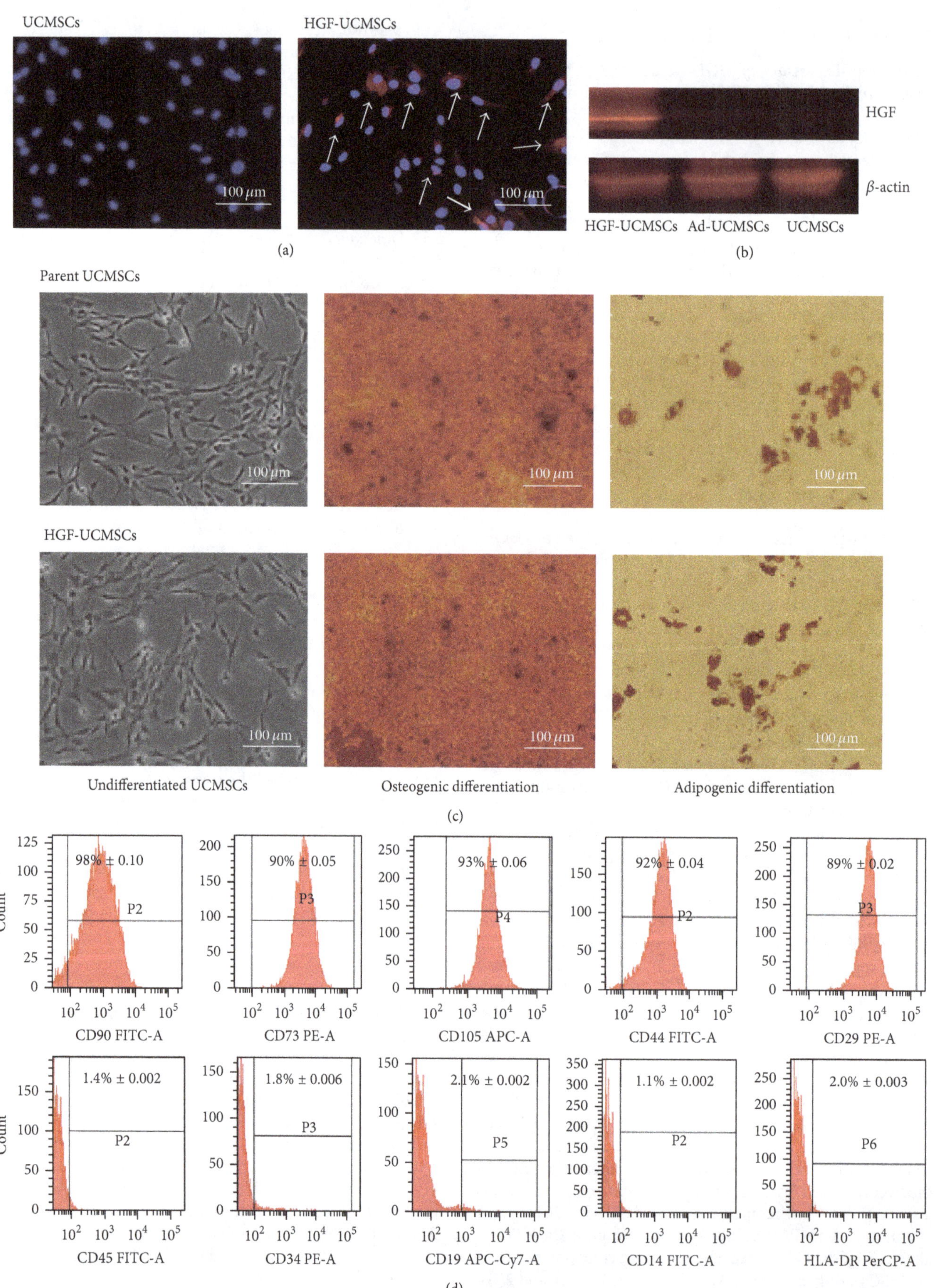

Figure 1: Continued.

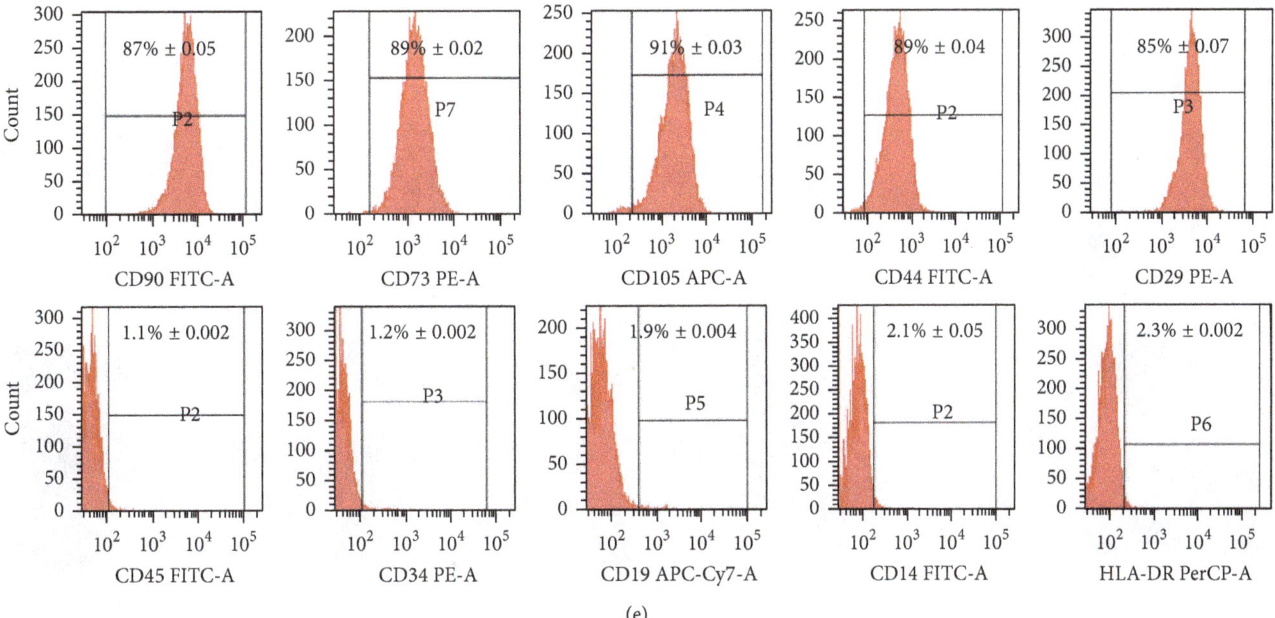

FIGURE 1: Characterization of human umbilical cord-derived mesenchymal stem cells. (a) Immunofluorescent staining of HGF protein in the liver of HGF-UCMSC treated mice. No HGF was detected in livers from the control group. Cells were HGF-positive (red) two days after HGF adenovirus infection at MOI 50. (b) Western blot of HGF in the liver of treated mice. Ad-UCMSCs: UCMSCs transfected with adenovirus carrying the control vector. (c) Differentiation of human umbilical cord-derived mesenchymal stem cells. Osteogenic differentiation was detected by calcium deposits stained by Alizarin Red. Adipogenic differentiation was detected by oil red O staining (400×). Morphology of UCMSCs and HGF-UCMSCs at day 10 of culture (40x). (d-e) Mesenchymal stem cell marker profile of the parent UCMSCs and HGF-UCMSCs. The data are representative of three independent experiments.

(SOD), catalase, and glutathione peroxidase. In this system, the SOD enzyme catalyzes the conversion of superoxide anion ($O_2^{\bullet -}$) radical into hydrogen peroxide plus molecular oxygen. Glutathione peroxidase and catalase control the balance of oxidants, including ROS, reactive nitrogen species (RNS), and sulphur containing radicals [27–29]. We thus measured these enzymes in our ALF animals. As shown in Figures 5(b)-5(c), the HGF-UCMSC therapy enhanced the activity of both enzymes in APAP-induced ALF animals at 8 h and 24 h.

γ-Glutamylcysteine synthetase (γ-GCS), a rate-limiting enzyme of GSH synthesis, determines the amount of GSH within the cell. By measuring the activity of hepatic γ-GCS in different experiment groups, we found that the HGF-UCMSC treatment increased hepatic γ-GCS activity (Figure 5(d))

Exposure to APAP caused the elevation of malondialdehyde (MDA) in the serum. We found that treatment of HGF-UCMSCs significantly suppressed the increment of serum MDA (Figure 5(e)). Notably, HGF-UCMSCs eliminated serum MDA more effectively than UCMSCs at any time points.

3.6. HGF-UCMSCs Alleviate Oxidative Stress-Induced Apoptosis. Antiapoptosis and regeneration of hepatocytes are critical for preventing the toxicity in sublethal dose of APAP-induced ALF mice. We used quantitative PCR to measure mRNA expression of genes that are associated with cell apoptosis, including Bcl-2, Bax, P65, and TNFα. We found that the HGF-UCMSC recipe upregulated the antiapoptotic Bcl-2, but downregulated the proapoptotic Bax and TNFα gene at a better efficacy than the USMSC recipe ($P < 0.01$, Figure 6(a)).

Nuclear factor-κB (NF-κB) is a pleiotropic transcription factor that regulates over 200 genes involved in cell growth, apoptosis, tumorigenesis, tumor metastasis, embryonic development, and inflammatory effects. We found that the HGF-UCMSC treatment upregulated the expression of P65 in ALF mice (Figure 6(a)). Similarly, using Western blot we found that the active nuclear P65 of NF-κB was elevated by HGF-UCMSCs (Figure 6(b)). As expected, human HGF was expressed only in the liver of mice from the HGF-UCMSC group. Together, these data suggest that the altered expression of these genes may provide a potential molecular basis for the action of HGF-UCMSCs in the ALF model.

4. Discussion

In this study, we for the first time prove the therapeutic potential of the HGF-expressing UCMSCs in mice with ALF. This approach combines the cellular therapy of mesenchymal stem cells with the role of the virally expressed HGF. While UCMSCs aid the regeneration of APAP-induced hepatic necrosis, HGF reduces tissue damage through multiple mechanisms. We demonstrate that systemically administered HGF-UCMSCs protect animals with acute liver failure by alleviating hepatic injuries and prolonging the survival.

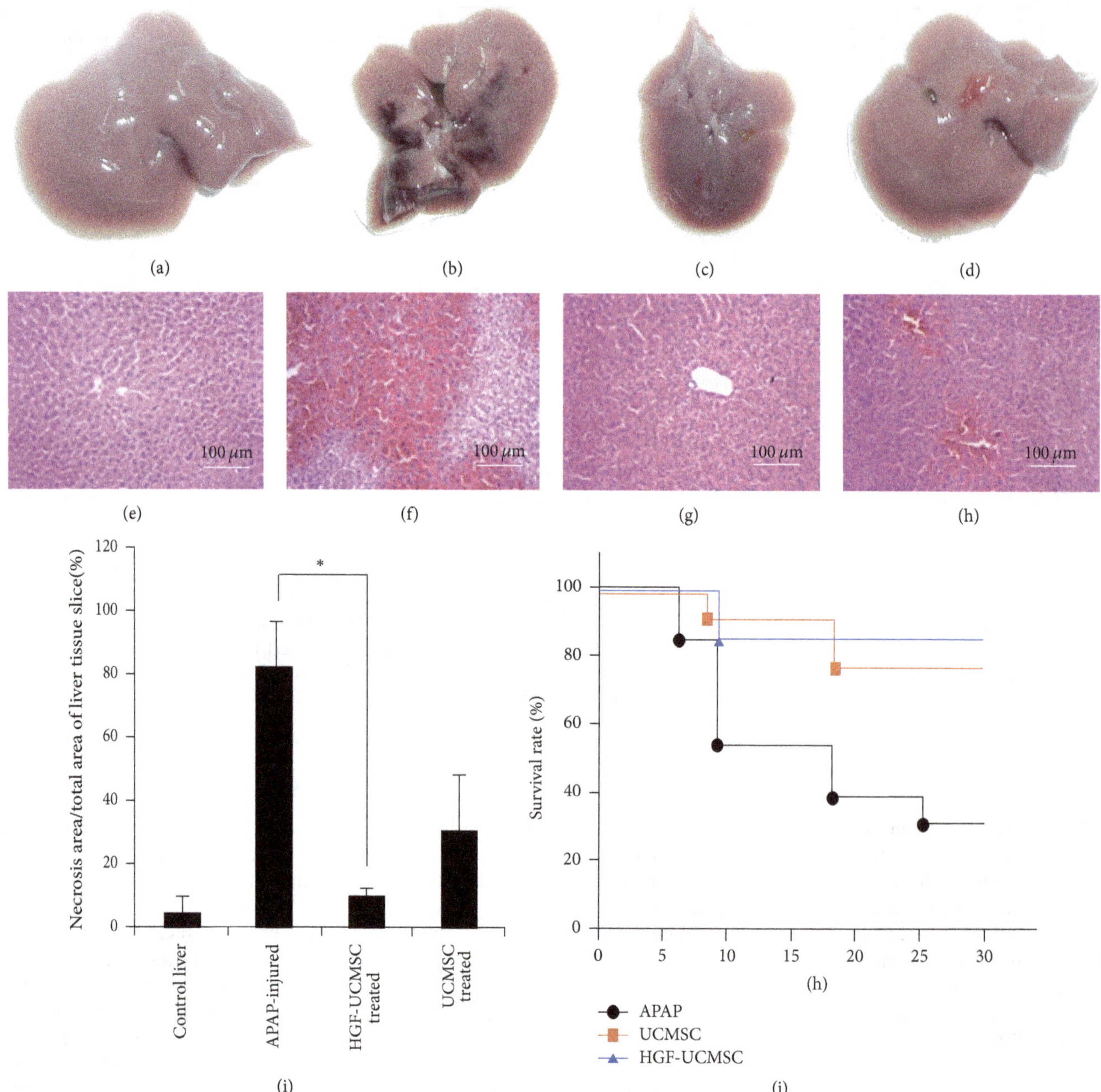

Figure 2: HGF-UCMSC treatment reduces hepatic damage in ALF mice. (a–d) Morphological analysis of the liver. (e–i) HE staining of the necrosis area in liver sections in ALF mice induced by 750 mg/kg acetaminophen. (j) Treatment with HGF-UCMSC and UCMSC significantly prolonged the survival of mice that received a lethal dose of Acetaminophen compared with nontreated animals.

Notably, overexpression of HGF via adenoviral infection has no detrimental effect on the morphology and multipotent differentiation of UCMSCs.

It is interesting to note that HGF-UCMSCs are capable of improving the survival rate of the injured mice more pronouncedly than the parental UCMSCs. We also detected a better efficacy of HGF-UCMSCs than UCMSCs in improving liver function and pathological changes. Immunohistochemical and HE staining further proved the presence of the homing HGF-UCMSCs within mouse livers, where they may act locally in the injured area to reduce liver necrosis and cell inflammatory infiltration.

HGF, also known as scatter factor, supports diverse cellular functions, including morphogenesis, motility, proliferation, and apoptosis protection [30]. HGF and its receptor c-Met activate signaling pathways that promote cell survival against apoptotic inducers. There are several reports that strongly support the antiapoptotic effects of HGF/c-Met [31–34], primarily by the induction of ant-apoptotic proteins such as Bcl-2, Bcl-XL, or Mcl-1 [35]. In this study, we also found that ALF mice that received the HGF-UCMSC treatment expressed much higher antiapoptotic Bcl2 in the liver than mice that receive the UCMSC treatment. At the same time, the therapy also downregulates the proapoptotic genes, Bax,

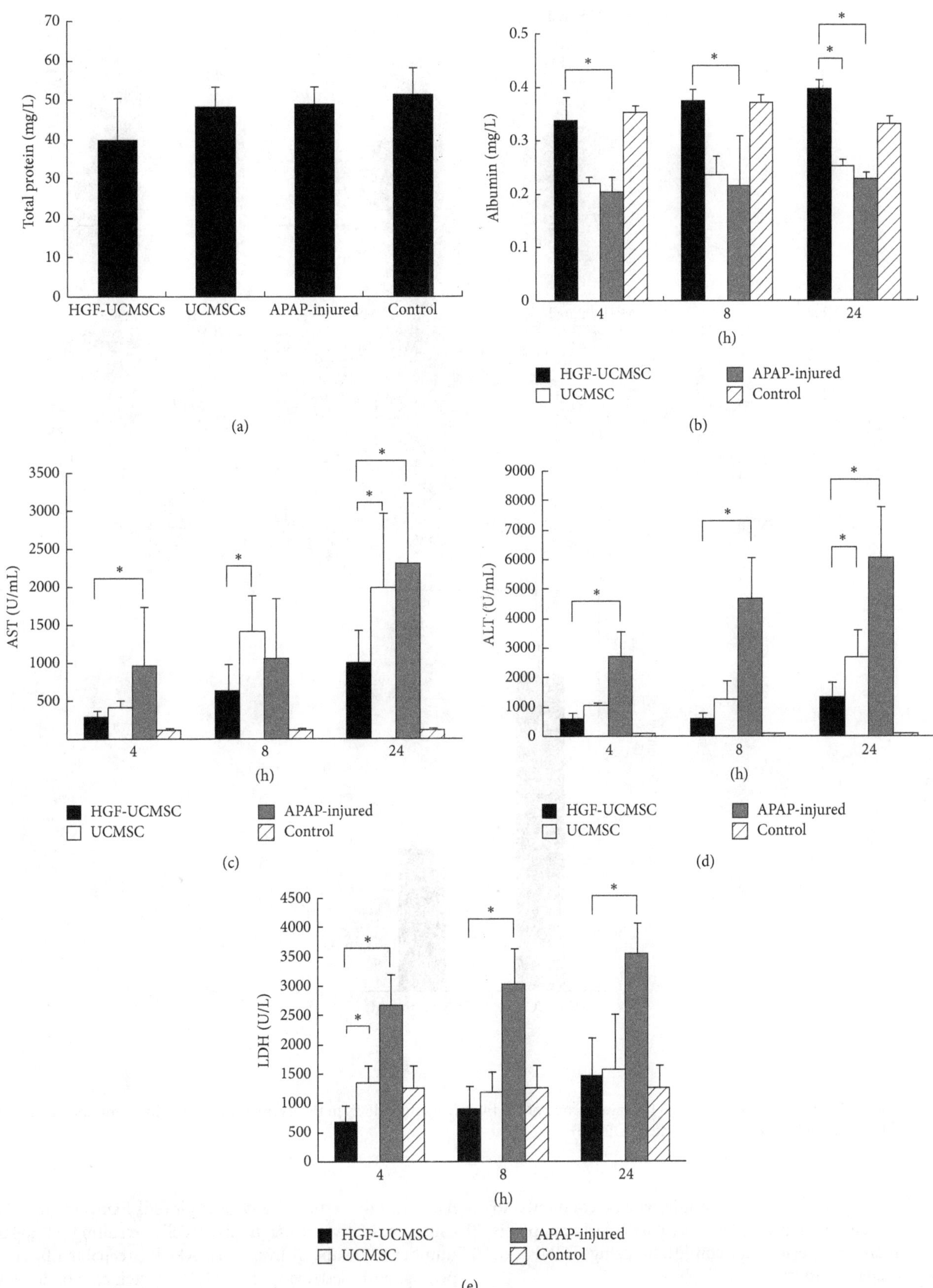

FIGURE 3: Hepatic function after transplantation of UCMSCs or HGF-UCMSCs. (a) Serum total protein in different groups at time point 24 h. (b) Serum albumin levels in different groups at different time points. (c–e) Biochemical analysis of aspartate aminotransferase (AST), alanine transaminase (ALT), and lactate dehydrogenase in serum. The data are expressed as the means ± SD of three independent experiments. $^{*}P < 0.5$ compared with the control.

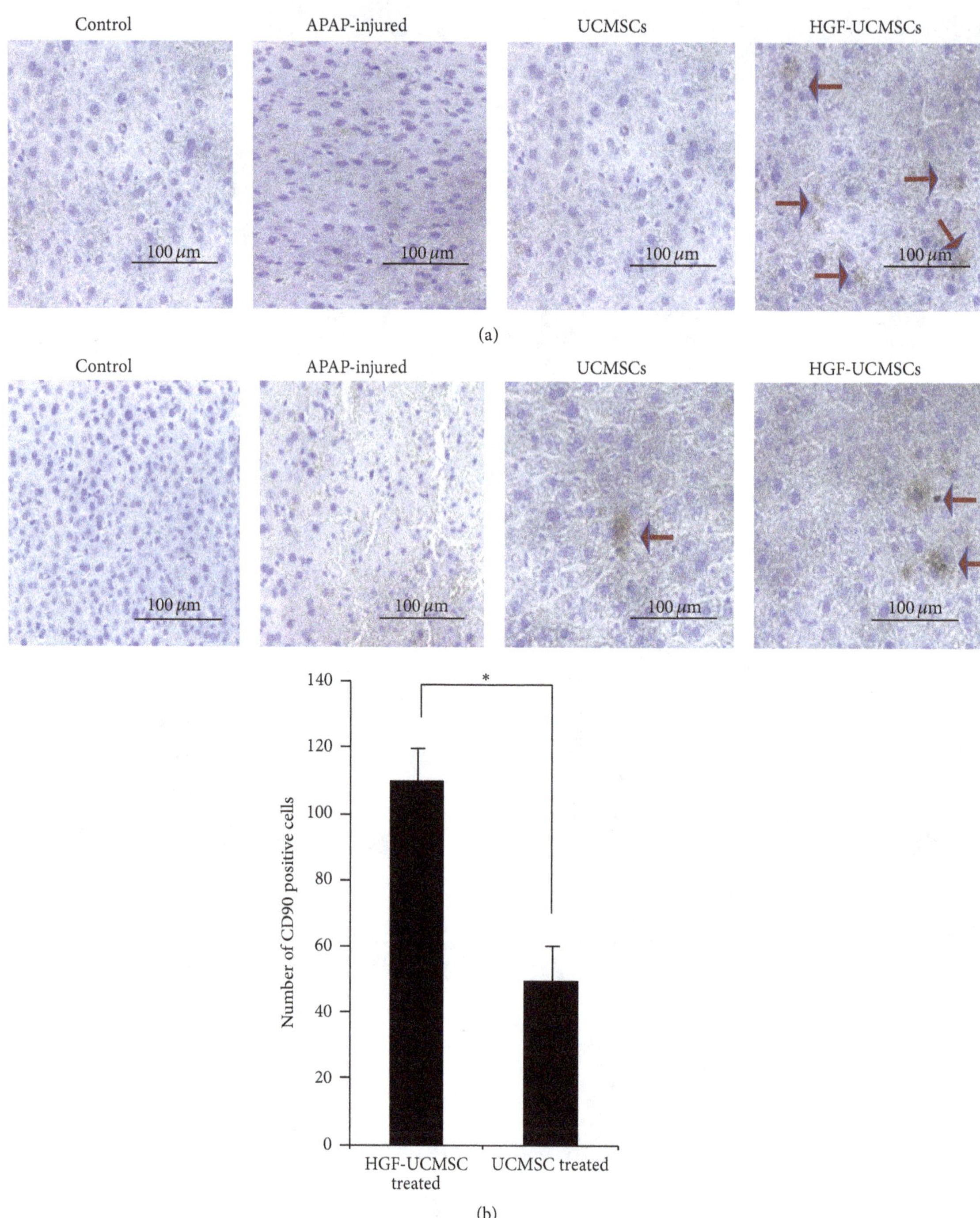

FIGURE 4: Migration of HGF-UCMSCs into the injured area of the liver. Migrated MSCs in the liver were detected by immunohistochemical staining of HGF (a) and mesenchymal marker CD90 (b).

and TNFα (Figure 6(a)). Future studies will be conducted to investigate the detailed mechanisms, particularly apoptosis under different experimental conditions using TUNEL or cleaved-caspase 3 assays.

The role of the HGF/c-Met pathway on oxidative stress protection remains poorly defined. Some published reports indicate that HGF can protect from oxidative damage [36, 37], but the effect of this growth factor on APAP-induced liver damage is practically unexplored. Exposure to APAP causes oxidative stress in liver cells, resulting in a large number of deaths of liver cells. APAP is capable of decomposing and destroying N-acetyl-L-cysteine, which is the necessary synthetic amino acid for glutathione. Cytochrome P450 within the liver cells can eliminate APAP-derived major toxic metabolite and result in the formation of N-acetyl-p-benzoquinoneimine (NAPQI). Sustained formation

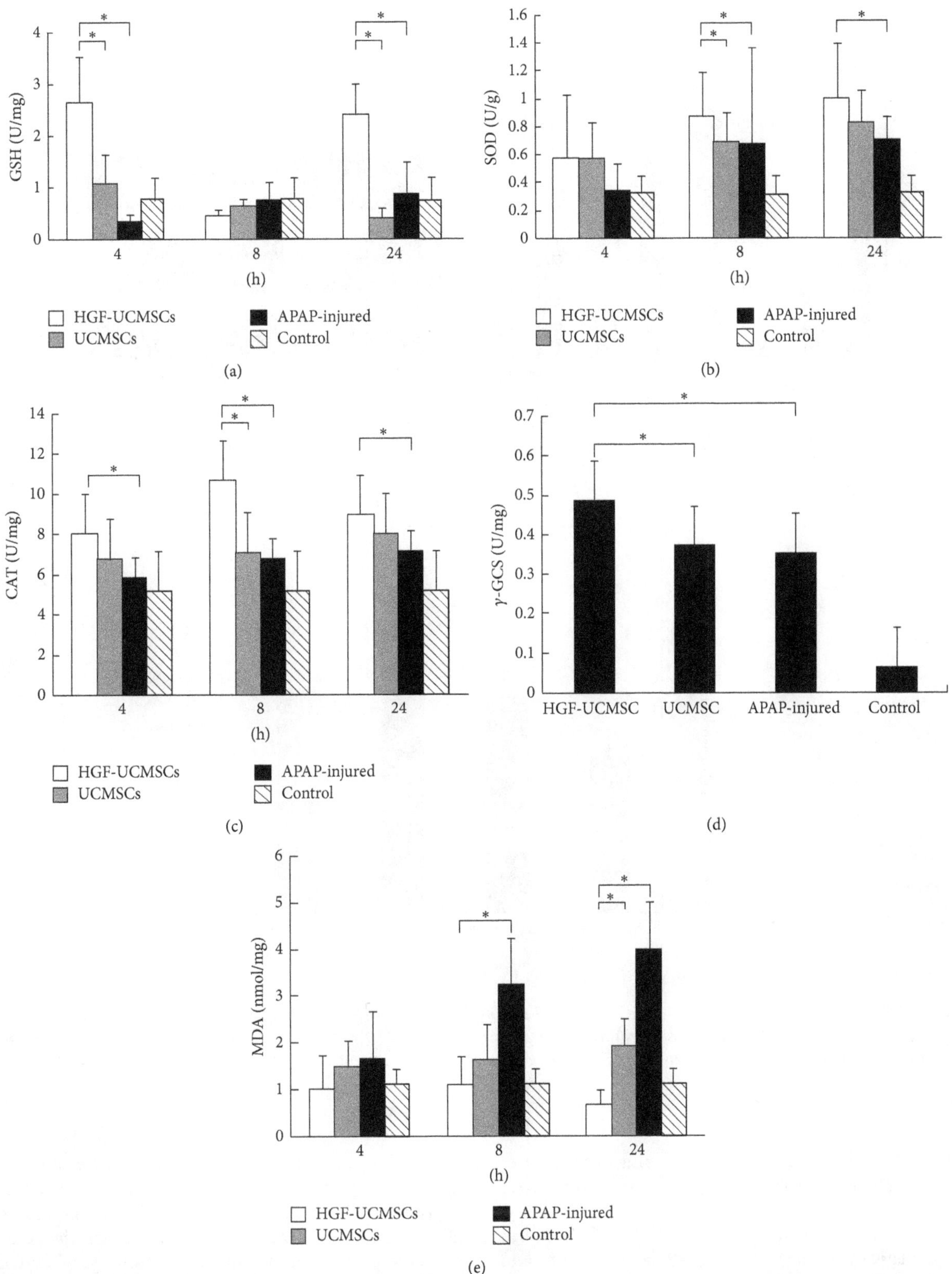

FIGURE 5: Antioxidant indexes in liver tissue of ALF mice. (a) Level of glutathione. (b) Activity of superoxide dismutase in liver tissue. (c) Activity of catalase in liver tissue. (d) Activity of γ-glutamylcysteine synthetase (γ-GCS). (e) Level of malondialdehyde (MDA). The data are expressed as the means ± SD of three independent experiments. $^{*}P < 0.5$ compared with the control.

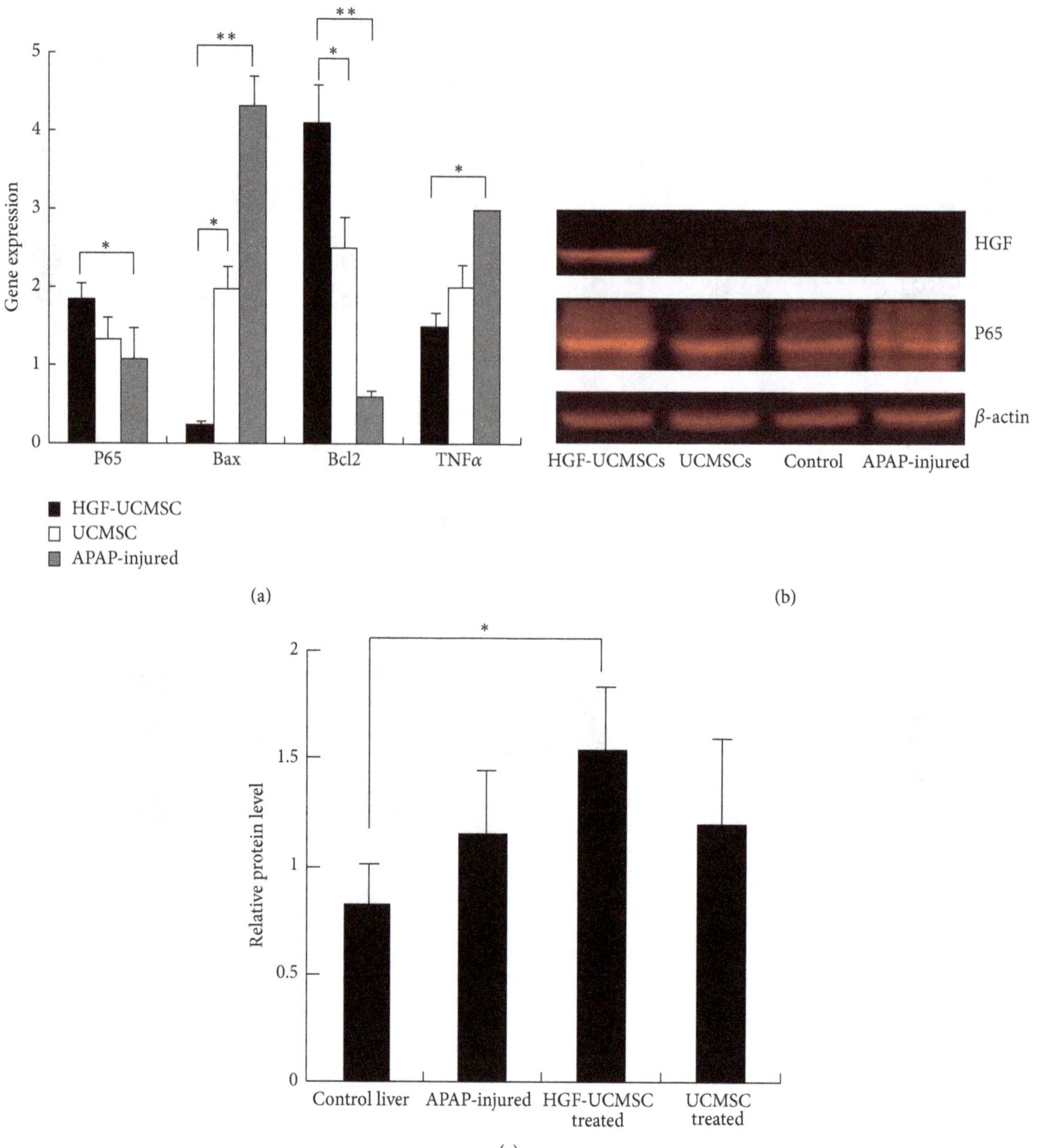

Figure 6: HGF-UCMSCs reduce apoptosis in the liver of ALF mice. (a) Quantitative PCR analysis of mRNA expression of P65, Bcl-2, Bax, and TNFα genes in the liver collected from different treatment groups. $^{*}P < 0.05$; $^{**}P < 0.01$. (b-c) Western blot of HGF and P65 in the liver of ALF mice. The data are expressed as the means ± SD of three independent experiments. $^{*}P < 0.5$ compared with the control.

of NAPQI is conjugated to glutathione and finally causes depletion of glutathione, which then leads to oxidative stress within liver cells [7].

In this study, we demonstrate that HGF-UCMSCs can reduce oxidative stress by increasing cellular glutathione and decreasing MDA content, probably through its ability to enhance the activity of three enzymes (SOD, CAT, and γ-GCS) that participate in the maintenance of cellular redox homeostasis. Taken together, our data demonstrate that the HGF-UCMSC therapy combines the unique regenerative role of UCMSCs with the antioxidative activity of human HGF.

MSCs can be directly differentiated into hepatocytic cells under appropriate culture conditions. HGF can induce the expression of liver specific genes, including alpha-fetoprotein, albumin, and cytokeratins, in MSCs through the activation of its receptor c-Met [38–40]. The Mesenchymal and Tissue Stem Cell Committee of the International Society for Cellular Therapy (ISCT) has proposed minimal criteria for human MSCs, including the potential to differentiate into osteoblasts, adipocytes, and chondroblasts *in vitro* [41]. In this preclinical study, we followed the ISCT's criteria and just examined the potential of osteogenic and adipogenic differentiation.

The role of HGF in the induction of hepatocytic lineage from UCMSCs will be investigated in future studies. Furthermore, oxidants produced in the cell, including ROS, reactive nitrogen species (RNS), and sulphur containing radicals, are controlled by both pro- and antioxidant enzymes [27, 28]. Future studies are needed to address the changes of oxidants, especially ROS, in our HGF-UCMSC treated ALF model.

In summary, the exposure to various factors, such as drugs, xenobiotics, and viruses, may cause hepatic failure. Findings from this study demonstrate the potential of HGF-expressing UCMSCs in treating ALF. This approach combines the unique regenerative role of UCMSCs with the antioxidation and antiapoptosis properties of human HGF. Our data thus highlight the clinical potential of a valuable two-pronged approach for the treatment of patients with severe liver damage.

Abbreviations

ALF: Acute liver failure
ALT: Alanine aminotransferase
AST: Aspartate aminotransferase
ELISA: Enzyme linked immunosorbent assay
FCS: Fetal calf serum
GSH: Glutathione
HGF: Hepatocyte growth factor
UCMSC: Human umbilical cord-derived mesenchymal stem cells
MDA: Malondialdehyde
MSC: Mesenchymal stem cells
NS group: Nontransplantation group
NS: Normal saline
PBS: Phosphate-buffered saline
SOD: Superoxide dismutase
CAT: Catalase
SD: Standard deviation
TNFα: Tumor necrosis factor-alpha
APAP: Acetaminophen.

Authors' Contribution

Yunxia Tang, Qiongshu Li, and Fanwei Meng equally contributed to the project.

Acknowledgments

This study was supported by Shenzhen Research Grant (GJ200807210024A, CXZZ20150430152511042) to Tao Li and Xiang Hu; Shenyang Research Grant (F13-205-9-00) to Tao Li; Guangdong Research Grant (2013B070704118); California Institute of Regenerative Medicine (CIRM) Grant (RT2-01942); Jilin International Collaboration Grant (20120720); and the National Natural Science Foundation of China Grant (81272294, 31430021) to Ji-Fan Hu.

References

[1] W. A. Bower, M. Johns, H. S. Margolis, I. T. Williams, and B. P. Bell, "Population-based surveillance for acute liver failure," *American Journal of Gastroenterology*, vol. 102, no. 11, pp. 2459–2463, 2007.

[2] W. M. Lee, R. T. Stravitz, and A. M. Larson, "Introduction to the revised American Association for the Study of Liver Diseases Position Paper on acute liver failure 2011," *Hepatology*, vol. 55, no. 3, pp. 965–967, 2012.

[3] D. van Poll, B. Parekkadan, C. H. Cho et al., "Mesenchymal stem cell-derived molecules directly modulate hepatocellular death and regeneration in vitro and in vivo," *Hepatology*, vol. 47, no. 5, pp. 1634–1643, 2008.

[4] G. K. Michalopoulos and M. C. DeFrances, "Liver regeneration," *Science*, vol. 276, no. 5309, pp. 60–65, 1997.

[5] T. Cantz, M. P. Manns, and M. Ott, "Stem cells in liver regeneration and therapy," *Cell and Tissue Research*, vol. 331, no. 1, pp. 271–282, 2008.

[6] E. Schmelzer, L. Zhang, A. Bruce et al., "Human hepatic stem cells from fetal and postnatal donors," *The Journal of Experimental Medicine*, vol. 204, no. 8, pp. 1973–1987, 2007.

[7] I. Aurich, L. P. Mueller, H. Aurich et al., "Functional integration of hepatocytes derived from human mesenchymal stem cells into mouse livers," *Gut*, vol. 56, no. 3, pp. 405–415, 2007.

[8] X.-R. Tao, W.-L. Li, J. Su et al., "Clonal mesenchymal stem cells derived from human bone marrow can differentiate into hepatocyte-like cells in injured livers of SCID mice," *Journal of Cellular Biochemistry*, vol. 108, no. 3, pp. 693–704, 2009.

[9] A. D. Sharma, T. Cantz, R. Richter et al., "Human cord blood stem cells generate human cytokeratin 18-negative hepatocyte-like cells in injured mouse liver," *The American Journal of Pathology*, vol. 167, no. 2, pp. 555–564, 2005.

[10] Y. Y. Dan, K. J. Riehle, C. Lazaro et al., "Isolation of multipotent progenitor cells from human fetal liver capable of differentiating into liver and mesenchymal lineages," *Proceedings of the National Academy of Sciences of the United States of America*, vol. 103, no. 26, pp. 9912–9917, 2006.

[11] A. A. Khan, M. V. Shaik, N. Parveen et al., "Human fetal liver-derived stem cell transplantation as supportive modality in the management of end-stage decompensated liver cirrhosis," *Cell Transplantation*, vol. 19, no. 4, pp. 409–418, 2010.

[12] A. Banas, T. Teratani, Y. Yamamoto et al., "IFATS collection: in vivo therapeutic potential of human adipose tissue mesenchymal stem cells after transplantation into mice with liver injury," *Stem Cells*, vol. 26, no. 10, pp. 2705–2712, 2008.

[13] M. J. Seo, S. Y. Suh, Y. C. Bae, and J. S. Jung, "Differentiation of human adipose stromal cells into hepatic lineage in vitro and in vivo," *Biochemical and Biophysical Research Communications*, vol. 328, no. 1, pp. 258–264, 2005.

[14] H. Aurich, M. Sgodda, P. Kaltwaßer et al., "Hepatocyte differentiation of mesenchymal stem cells from human adipose tissue in vitro promotes hepatic integration in vivo," *Gut*, vol. 58, no. 4, pp. 570–581, 2009.

[15] J. Chamberlain, T. Yamagami, E. Colletti et al., "Efficient generation of human hepatocytes by the intrahepatic delivery of clonal human mesenchymal stem cells in fetal sheep," *Hepatology*, vol. 46, no. 6, pp. 1935–1945, 2007.

[16] L. B. Ware and M. A. Matthay, "Keratinocyte and hepatocyte growth factors in the lung: roles in lung development, inflammation, and repair," *The American Journal of Physiology—Lung*

Cellular and Molecular Physiology, vol. 282, no. 5, pp. L924–L940, 2002.

[17] F. Böhm, U. A. Köhler, T. Speicher, and S. Werner, "Regulation of liver regeneration by growth factors and cytokines," *The EMBO Molecular Medicine*, vol. 2, no. 8, pp. 294–305, 2010.

[18] K. Nejak-Bowen, A. Orr, W. C. Bowen Jr., and G. K. Michalopoulos, "Conditional genetic elimination of hepatocyte growth factor in mice compromises liver regeneration after partial hepatectomy," *PLoS ONE*, vol. 8, no. 3, Article ID e59836, 2013.

[19] A. Valdés-Arzate, A. Luna, L. Bucio et al., "Hepatocyte growth factor protects hepatocytes against oxidative injury induced by ethanol metabolism," *Free Radical Biology and Medicine*, vol. 47, no. 4, pp. 424–430, 2009.

[20] P. Salehinejad, N. B. Alitheen, A. M. Ali et al., "Comparison of different methods for the isolation of mesenchymal stem cells from human umbilical cord Wharton's jelly," *In Vitro Cellular & Developmental Biology—Animal*, vol. 48, pp. 75–83, 2012.

[21] A. Reinisch and D. Strunk, "Isolation and animal serum free expansion of human umbilical cord derived mesenchymal stromal cells (MSCs) and endothelial colony forming progenitor cells (ECFCs)," *Journal of Visualized Experiments*, no. 32, Article ID e1525, 2009.

[22] J. Gan, F. Meng, X. Zhou et al., "Hematopoietic recovery of acute radiation syndrome by human superoxide dismutase-expressing umbilical cord mesenchymal stromal cells," *Cytotherapy*, vol. 17, no. 4, pp. 403–417, 2015.

[23] Z. Liu, F. Meng, C. Li et al., "Human umbilical cord mesenchymal stromal cells rescue mice from acetaminophen-induced acute liver failure," *Cytotherapy*, vol. 16, no. 9, pp. 1207–1219, 2014.

[24] H. Tabatabaeian and Z. Hojati, "Assessment of HER-2 gene overexpression in Isfahan province breast cancer patients using Real Time RT-PCR and immunohistochemistry," *Gene*, vol. 531, no. 1, pp. 39–43, 2013.

[25] T. Li, J.-F. Hu, X. Qiu et al., "CTCF regulates allelic expression of Igf2 by orchestrating a promoter-polycomb repressive complex 2 intrachromosomal loop," *Molecular and Cellular Biology*, vol. 28, no. 20, pp. 6473–6482, 2008.

[26] X. Wang, S. Ge, G. McNamara, Q.-L. Hao, G. M. Crooks, and J. A. Nolta, "Albumin-expressing hepatocyte-like cells develop in the livers of immune-deficient mice that received transplants of highly purified human hematopoietic stem cells," *Blood*, vol. 101, no. 10, pp. 4201–4208, 2003.

[27] C. Peng, X. Wang, J. Chen et al., "Biology of ageing and role of dietary antioxidants," *BioMed Research International*, vol. 2014, Article ID 831841, 13 pages, 2014.

[28] N. Sivaranjani, S. V. Rao, and G. Rajeev, "Role of reactive oxygen species and antioxidants in atopic dermatitis," *Journal of Clinical and Diagnostic Research*, vol. 7, no. 12, pp. 2683–2685, 2013.

[29] S. K. Venugopal, J. Wu, A. M. Catana et al., "Lentivirus-mediated superoxide dismutase1 gene delivery protects against oxidative stress-induced liver injury in mice," *Liver International*, vol. 27, no. 10, pp. 1311–1322, 2007.

[30] R. Zarnegar and G. K. Michalopoulos, "The many faces of hepatocyte growth factor: from hepatopoiesis to hematopoiesis," *Journal of Cell Biology*, vol. 129, no. 5, pp. 1177–1180, 1995.

[31] A. Suzuki, M. Hayashida, H. Kawano, K. Sugimoto, T. Nakano, and K. Shiraki, "Hepatocyte growth factor promotes cell survival from Fas-mediated cell death in hepatocellular carcinoma cells via Akt activation and Fas-death-inducing signaling complex suppression," *Hepatology*, vol. 32, no. 4, pp. 796–802, 2000.

[32] C.-G. Huh, V. M. Factor, A. Sánchez, K. Uchida, E. A. Conner, and S. S. Thorgeirsson, "Hepatocyte growth factor/c-met signaling pathway is required for efficient liver regeneration and repair," *Proceedings of the National Academy of Sciences of the United States of America*, vol. 101, no. 13, pp. 4477–4482, 2004.

[33] G.-H. Xiao, M. Jeffers, A. Bellacosa, Y. Mitsuuchi, G. F. Vande Woude, and J. R. Testa, "Anti-apoptotic signaling by hepatocyte growth factor/Met via the phosphatidylinositol 3-kinase/Akt and mitogen-activated protein kinase pathways," *Proceedings of the National Academy of Sciences of the United States of America*, vol. 98, no. 1, pp. 247–252, 2001.

[34] H. Schulze-Bergkamen, D. Brenner, A. Krueger et al., "Hepatocyte growth factor induces Mcl-1 in primary human hepatocytes and inhibits CD95-mediated apoptosis via Akt," *Hepatology*, vol. 39, no. 3, pp. 645–654, 2004.

[35] M. Okada, K. Sugita, T. Inukai et al., "Hepatocyte growth factor protects small airway epithelial cells from apoptosis induced by tumor necrosis factor-α or oxidative stress," *Pediatric Research*, vol. 56, no. 3, pp. 336–344, 2004.

[36] H. Li, T. Jiang, Y. Lin, Z. Zhao, and N. Zhang, "HGF protects rat mesangial cells from high-glucose-mediated oxidative stress," *American Journal of Nephrology*, vol. 26, no. 5, pp. 519–530, 2006.

[37] T. Takami, P. Kaposi-Novak, K. Uchida et al., "Loss of hepatocyte growth factor/c-Met signaling pathway accelerates early stages of *N*-nitrosodiethylamine induced hepatocarcinogenesis," *Cancer Research*, vol. 67, no. 20, pp. 9844–9851, 2007.

[38] S.-H. Oh, M. Miyazaki, H. Kouchi et al., "Hepatocyte growth factor induces differentiation of adult rat bone marrow cells into a hepatocyte lineage in vitro," *Biochemical and Biophysical Research Communications*, vol. 279, no. 2, pp. 500–504, 2000.

[39] H. C. Fiegel, M. V. Lioznov, L. Cortes-Dericks et al., "Liver-specific gene expression in cultured human hematopoietic stem cells," *STEM CELLS*, vol. 21, no. 1, pp. 98–104, 2003.

[40] S. Kakinuma, Y. Tanaka, R. Chinzei et al., "Human umbilical cord blood as a source of transplantable hepatic progenitor cells," *Stem Cells*, vol. 21, no. 2, pp. 217–227, 2003.

[41] M. Dominici, K. Le Blanc, I. Mueller et al., "Minimal criteria for defining multipotent mesenchymal stromal cells. The International Society for Cellular Therapy position statement," *Cytotherapy*, vol. 8, no. 4, pp. 315–317, 2006.

21

Hyperammonemia Is Associated with Increasing Severity of Both Liver Cirrhosis and Hepatic Encephalopathy

Abidullah Khan, Maimoona Ayub, and Wazir Mohammad Khan

KTH Peshawar, Peshawar, Pakistan

Correspondence should be addressed to Abidullah Khan; dr.abidk@yahoo.com

Academic Editor: Daisuke Morioka

Background. Hyperammonemia resulting from chronic liver disease (CLD) can potentially challenge and damage any organ system of the body, particularly the brain. However, there is still some controversy regarding the diagnostic or prognostic values of serum ammonia in patients with over hepatic encephalopathy, especially in the setting of acute-on-chronic or chronic liver failure. Moreover, the association of serum ammonia with worsening Child-Pugh grade of liver cirrhosis has not been studied. *Objective.* This study was conducted to solve the controversy regarding the association between hyperammonemia and cirrhosis, especially hepatic encephalopathy in chronically failed liver. *Material and Methods.* In this study, 171 cirrhotic patients had their serum ammonia measured and analyzed by SPSS version 16. Chi-squared test and one-way ANOVA were applied. *Results.* The study had 110 male and 61 female participants. The mean age of all the participants in years was 42.33 ± 7.60. The mean duration (years) of CLD was 10.15 ± 3.53 while the mean Child-Pugh (CP) score was 8.84 ± 3.30. Chronic viral hepatitis alone was responsible for 71.3% of the cases. Moreover, 86.5% of participants had hepatic encephalopathy (HE). The frequency of hyperammonemia was 67.3%, more frequent in males ($N = 81$, z-score = 2.4, and $P < 0.05$) than in females ($N = 34$, z-score = 2.4, and $P < 0.05$), and had a statistically significant relationship with increasing CP grade of cirrhosis ($\chi^2(2) = 27.46$, $P < 0.001$, Phi = 0.40, and $P < 0.001$). Furthermore, serum ammonia level was higher in patients with hepatic encephalopathy than in those without it; $P < 0.001$. *Conclusion.* Hyperammonemia is associated with both increasing Child-Pugh grade of liver cirrhosis and hepatic encephalopathy.

1. Introduction

Chronic liver disease (CLD) and liver cirrhosis are clinicopathologically defined disease entities. The main causes of cirrhosis of the liver, include chronic infection by viral agents (hepatitis B and C viruses), as well as metabolic toxic/drug-induced and autoimmune causes, resulting in persistent inflammation and progressive fibrosis. In fact, it is the chronic activation of the wound healing response which is the major driving force for progressive accumulation of extracellular matrix (ECM) components, eventually leading to liver cirrhosis and hepatic failure [1].

The symptoms associated with chronic liver disease depend on the level of degeneration within the liver itself. The early stages are often asymptomatic and can only be detected by specific medical tests like liver function tests and abdominal ultrasound. However, liver diseases which have progressed to a chronic stage can be recognized by mental confusion, severe jaundice, coagulopathy, and so forth [2].

Normal blood ammonia concentration is less than 35 μmol/L. Normally, blood ammonia comes from the bacterial hydrolysis of urea and other nitrogenous compounds in the intestine, the purine-nucleotide cycle and amino acid transamination in skeletal muscle, and other metabolic processes in the kidneys and liver [3, 4].

Mathews suggested an association between hyperammonemia and confusion in 1922 [5]. Similarly, further studies demonstrated a role of hyperammonemia, in the causation of hepatic coma [6, 7]. However, hyperammonemia alone is not always responsible for causing hepatic encephalopathy and, at times, patients with hepatic coma may have normal blood ammonia levels and vice versa [8–10].

The rationale of this study was to document an association between hyperammonemia and hepatic encephalopathy and to correlate serum ammonia with worsening Child-Pugh score/grade.

2. Material and Methods

This descriptive, cross-sectional study was conducted in the department of medicine of Khyber Teaching Hospital, Peshawar, Pakistan, between February and August 2016. A total of 250 patients were assessed for their suitability in the study. However, only 171 patients satisfied the inclusion and exclusion criteria and were included in the final study.

The inclusion criteria included (1) all patients with established chronic liver disease (CLD) with or without hepatic encephalopathy (CLD was diagnosed on the basis of any of the clinical features like finger clubbing, palmar erythema, spider naevi, splenomegaly, hepatomegaly or shrunken liver, or the persistent elevation for more than 6 months of the liver enzymes, namely, alanine aminotransferase (ALT), aspartate aminotransferase (AST), alkaline phosphatase (ALP), and gamma glutamyl transferase (GGT), plus a positive abdominal ultrasound for irregular liver margins, coarse liver appearance, and a dilated portal vein measuring 13–15 mm or more), (2) both genders, and (3) patients aged from 18 to 70 years.

The exclusion criteria included (1) patients already diagnosed with inherited urea cycle defect, (2) patients with chronic kidney disease, (3) hypertensive patients, (4) patients on parental nutrition or high protein diet, and (5) patients on drugs like alcohol, barbiturates, diuretics, valproate, and narcotics and smokers.

This study was approved by the hospital ethics review committee. An informed written consent was obtained from every participant. All the data was recorded on a structured questionnaire, including demographic details, duration of CLD, and serum ammonia levels. After 6 hours of overnight fasting, three mL of venous blood was drawn from every participant. Serum ammonia was determined by the same technician in the laboratory of our hospital. Those who had serum ammonia levels greater than 35 umol/L were classified as having hyperammonemia.

Data was stored and analyzed by the statistical program, SPSS Version 16. All the quantitative variables like age, blood ammonia levels, disease duration, and so forth were analyzed for mean ± standard deviation. Frequencies and percentages were calculated for qualitative variables like gender, hyperammonemia, Child-Pugh (CP) grade of liver cirrhosis, and so forth. By using Chi-square test, hyperammonemia was stratified amongst age, gender, disease severity (CP grade), grades of hepatic encephalopathy (HE grade), and so forth to see effect modification. To see any evidence of relationship of serum ammonia with both CP and HE grades, one-way ANOVA was run. P value of less than 0.05 was taken as criterion standard.

3. Results

The mean age of all the participants in years was 42.33 ± 7.60. The minimum age was 26 and the maximum was 54 years. The mean duration of chronic liver disease was 10.15 years (SD = 3.53). The study group comprised 110 (64.3%) males and 61 females (35.7%). 75% of the patients were Pakistanis (N = 128), against 25% of Afghanis (N = 43).

The most common cause of chronic liver disease was chronic viral hepatitis either chronic hepatitis B or C or both. Metabolic causes of the chronic liver disease, namely, Wilson's disease, hemochromatosis, and alpha-1 antitrypsin deficiency, and so forth, were the least encountered etiologies (Table 1). The mean Child-Pugh score was 8.84 ± 3.30 (Table 2).

TABLE 1: Details of different causes of chronic liver disease in our study group.

Etiology of CLD	Number of patients	Patients (%)
HCV	73	42.6%
HBV	41	24%
Both HCV & HBV	8	4.7%
Metabolic (Wilson's disease, etc.)	9	5.3%
Autoimmune (PBC, PSC, AIH, etc.)	11	6.4%
NAFLD	21	12.3%
Alcoholic liver disease	3	1.8%
Idiopathic etiology & others	5	2.9%

TABLE 2: Division of the patients in different groups as per Child-Pugh scoring system.

Child-Pugh grade	Number of the patients	% of the patients
A	47	27.5%
B	64	37.4%
C	60	35.1%

All the patients had splenomegaly. The splenic size was measured in centimeters on ultrasound of the abdomen (M = 16.57 and SD = 1.86%). It is worth mentioning that 32% of the patients had hematemesis which brought them to the hospital against 68% who had no such evidence. Ascites was another problem reported by most of our patients (Figure 1). Other clinical features of chronic liver disease, in our patients, included palmar erythema (45%), leuckonychia (50%), spider naevi (33%), jaundice (86%), cachexia (15%), purpura and ecchymosis (49%), fetor hepaticus (7%), and flapping tremor (43%). Liver disease related complications were commonly seen as well (Table 3). The ultrasonography findings are shown as follows (Table 4).

Amongst all the participants, 86.5% had hepatic encephalopathy (HE). West-Haven classification was used to stratify patients with HE into different groups (Table 5). The mean serum ammonia level was 45.91 ± 16.97. The minimum value of blood ammonia was 25 μmol/L against the maximum value of 99 μmol/L. 67.3% of the participants had hyperammonemia. The association of hyperammonemia with different grade of HE is given below (Table 6).

In order to see the relationship between serum ammonia and hepatic encephalopathy, one-way ANOVA was used. The assumption of homogeneity of variance was tested which

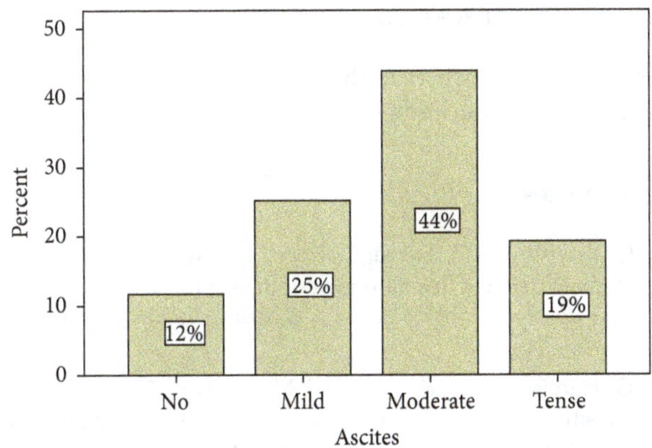

FIGURE 1: Percentage of patients with different grades of ascites on ultrasonography.

TABLE 3: Number of patients who had developed different complications of chronic liver disease.

Feature	Number (N)	Percent (%)
Hepatopulmonary syndrome (HPS)	28	16.4%
Hepatorenal syndrome (HRS)	43	25.1
Spontaneous bacterial peritonitis (SBP)	112	65.5
Esophageal varices	117	65%
Hypoglycemia	20	12%
Hepatocellular carcinoma (HCC)	24	14%

TABLE 4: Number of patients having different detectable liver abnormalities on an abdominal ultrasound.

Ultrasonography findings	Number (N)	Percent (%)
Coarse liver	171	100%
Irregular liver margins	154	90.1%
Dilated portal vein (PV)	151	88.3%

TABLE 5: Distribution of patients into different grades of hepatic encephalopathy (HE) as per West-Haven criteria.

Grade of HE	Number (N)	Percent (%)
No encephalopathy	23	13.5%
Grade 1 HE	41	34%
Grade 2 HE	38	22.2%
Grade 3 HE	40	23.4%
Grade 4 HE	29	17%

showed violation and Levene's $P < 0.05$. However, robust tests of equality of means (Welch and Brown-Forsythe) were statistically significant $P < 0.001$. The results of ANOVA showed that serum ammonia level was higher in patients with high-grade HE, that is, grades 3 and 4 ($N = 40$, M = 51.98 ±8.01, and $P < 0.001$ and $N = 29$, M = 76.28 ± 10.70, and $P < 0.001$, resp.), than in the patients with low-grade

TABLE 6: Chi-square test statistics of distribution of hyperammonemia across different grades of hepatic encephalopathy (HE).

HE Grade	Patients (%) with hyperammonemia	z-score
No HE	1.7%	−6.4
Grade 1	15.7	−3.7
Grade 2	22.6	0.2
Grade 3	34.8	5
Grade 4	25.2	4.1
χ^2 value	$\chi^2(4) = 79.58$, $P < 0.001$, Phi = 0.68, and $P < 0.001$	

HE, that is, grades 1 and 2 ($N = 41$, M = 35.17 ± 4.72, and $N = 38$. M = 37.61 ± 4.22, resp.). Patients with no evidence of HE had the lowest levels of blood ammonia ($N = 23$, M = 29.91 ± 3.32, and $P < 0.001$). Thus one-way ANOVA showed a statistically significant difference between the groups with regard to serum ammonia level; $F(4) = 229.29$, $P < 0.001$, and Eta squared = 0.85. Hence, it can be postulated, that the higher the grade of hepatic coma, the higher the blood ammonia level will be.

It must be noted that post hoc analysis via Tukey HSD revealed that patients with grades 3 and 4 of HE were significantly different from patients with either no coma or grade 1 or 2 coma; $P < 0.001$. However, there was no statistically significant difference between patients with grade 1 coma and those with grade 2; $P = 0.49$. There was little but statistically significant difference between patients with grade 1 or grade 2 coma and patients with no coma; $P < 0.02$ and $P < 0.001$, respectively.

Hyperammonemia was also stratified amongst gender using Chi-square test. The results showed that hyperammonemia was more prevalent in males ($N = 81$ and z-score = 2.4) than in females ($N = 34$ and z-score = 2.4) at a statistically significant level ($\chi^2(1) = 5.70$ and $P = 0.01$). The effect size was again significant; Phi = 0.18 and $P = 0.01$.

Finally χ^2 test was used to assess any association between hyperammonemia and the different grades of cirrhosis taking $P < 0.005$ as criterion standard. The results revealed that 46.1% of patients ($N = 53$) with Child-Pugh grade C cirrhosis had hyperammonemia at statistically significant level (z-score = 4.3 and $P < 0.05$). In contrast, 50% ($N = 28$) of the patients with grade A cirrhosis had no hyperammonemia (z-score = 4.6 and $P < 0.05$). In patients with grade B, 37.4% ($N = 43$) had hyperammonemia; however it was not statistically significant (z-score = 0.0 and $P > 0.05$). The overall Chi-square test result showed a strong evidence of relationship between hyperammonemia and increasing severity of liver cirrhosis (Child-Pugh grade); $\chi^2(2) = 27.46$ and $P < 0.001$. The effect size was statistically significant too; Phi = 0.40 and $P < 0.001$.

4. Discussion

Cirrhosis of the liver was the cause of 1.2 million deaths in 2013 in comparison with less than a million deaths in 1990 [11]. Chronic viral hepatitis is the main culprit behind liver cirrhosis. HCV alone infects more males than females in the fifth decade of life and is more common in drug abusers and blood transfusion dependent patients [12–15]. Our results are comparable to these statistics.

Hyperammonemia is associated with both hepatic encephalopathy and fetor hepaticus [16]. Similarly, Iwasa et al. did a study to clarify the relationships amongst psychometric testing results, serum ammonia (NH3) levels, electrolyte disturbance, and degree of inflammation and their correlations with the development of hepatic encephalopathy (HE). They concluded that serum ammonia level was significantly higher in patients with hepatic coma [17]. Our results are comparable with these observations.

As gut microbiota is important in producing ammonia, their eradication with certain nonabsorbable antibiotics like rifaximin is the mainstay of treatment of hepatic coma. Studies suggest that the beneficial effects of both lactulose and rifaximin could be due to a change in the microbial metabolic function, leading to bacterial survival disadvantage as well as an improvement in dysbiosis via direct eradication [18, 19]. This data is supported further by our study, as most of the patients showed dramatic response to treatment with rifaximin and lactulose.

It is notable that 15% of the patients in our study group were cachectic. This is in contrast with other studies where muscle wasting was seen in as much as 40–50% of the cirrhotic patients. This needs to be treated with regular exercises and nutritional support [20, 21]. As ammonia inhalation has been shown to cause vasodilation, it can be assumed that the arteriovenous shunting in hepatopulmonary syndrome or even the causation of esophageal varices is partly contributed by hyperammonemia [22, 23]. Our study results support these finding, as more than two-thirds of the patients in our study group had both hyperammonemia and accompanying esophageal varices.

Currently, hyperammonemia in cirrhotic patients is treated with laxatives (lactulose), antibiotics like rifaximin, and/or neomycin and the administration of branched chain amino acids (BCAAs) and so forth. However, in an experimental study by Kosenko et al., the erythrocytes obtained from mice were loaded with the enzyme glutamine synthetase, called ammocytes and infused into hyperammonemic mice. The results were exceptional, as up to 50% reduction in ammonia levels of hyperammonemic mice was seen. The researchers observed that ammocytes were able to maintain their integrity, normal energy metabolism, and the inserted glutamine synthetase activity [24].

The results of our studies were according to expectations of the authors, but we recommend further studies, including bigger sample sizes, to clarify the true link between ammonia and hepatic encephalopathy and severity of cirrhosis.

5. Conclusion

It can be concluded that both chronic hepatitis B and chronic hepatitis C are the leading causes of liver cirrhosis in our region. Furthermore, ammonia in cirrhosis is positively related with both hepatic encephalopathy and Child-Pugh grade.

Competing Interests

The authors declare that there is no conflict of interests regarding the publication of this manuscript.

References

[1] C. Paternostro, E. David, E. Novo, and M. Parola, "Hypoxia, angiogenesis and liver fibrogenesis in the progression of chronic liver diseases," *World Journal of Gastroenterology*, vol. 16, no. 3, pp. 281–288, 2010.

[2] G. Garcia-Tsao, J. K. Lim, and Members of Veterans Affairs Hepatitis C Resource Center Program, "Management and treatment of patients with cirrhosis and portal hypertension: recommendations from the Department of Veterans Affairs Hepatitis C Resource Center Program and the National Hepatitis C Program," *The American Journal of Gastroenterology*, vol. 104, no. 7, pp. 1802–1829, 2009.

[3] E. Crisan, J. Chawla, and J. S. Huff, *Hyperammonemia*, Medscape, 2014.

[4] M. O. Qureshi, N. Khokhar, and F. Shafqat, "Ammonia levels and the severity of hepatic encephalopathy," *Journal of the College of Physicians and Surgeons Pakistan*, vol. 24, no. 3, pp. 160–163, 2014.

[5] S. Matthews, "Ammonia, a causative factor in meat poisoning in Eck fistula dogs," *American Physiological Society*, vol. 59, pp. 459–460, 1922.

[6] E. Phear, S. Sherlock, and W. H. J. Summerskill, "Blood ammonium levels in liver disease and hepatic coma," *The Lancet*, vol. 265, no. 6869, pp. 836–840, 1955.

[7] D. L. Shawcross, S. S. Shabbir, N. J. Taylor, and R. D. Hughes, "Ammonia and the neutrophil in the pathogenesis of hepatic encephalopathy in cirrhosis," *Hepatology*, vol. 51, no. 3, pp. 1062–1069, 2010.

[8] L. Noiret, S. Baigent, and R. Jalan, "Arterial ammonia levels in cirrhosis are determined by systemic and hepatic hemodynamics, and by organ function: a quantitative modelling study," *Liver International*, vol. 34, no. 6, pp. e45–e55, 2014.

[9] O. Riggio, G. Mannaioni, L. Ridola et al., "Peripheral and splanchnic indole and oxindole levels in cirrhotic patients: a study on the pathophysiology of hepatic encephalopathy," *American Journal of Gastroenterology*, vol. 105, no. 6, pp. 1374–1381, 2010.

[10] J. O. Clemmesen, A. L. Gerbes, V. Gülberg et al., "Hepatic blood flow and splanchnic oxygen consumption in patients with liver failure. Effect of high-volume plasmapheresis," *Hepatology*, vol. 29, no. 2, pp. 347–355, 1999.

[11] GBD, Mortality and Causes of Death, and Collaborators, "Global, regional, and national age-sex specific all-cause and cause-specific mortality for 240 causes of death, 1990–2013: a systematic analysis for the Global Burden of Disease Study 2013," *The Lancet*, vol. 385, no. 9963, pp. 117–171, 2013.

[12] M. A. Maan, H. Fatma, and J. Muhammad, "Epidemiology of hepatitis C viral infection in Faisalabad, Pakistan: a retrospective study (2010–2012)," *African Health Sciences*, vol. 14, no. 4, pp. 810–815, 2014.

[13] Y. Waheed, T. Shafi, S. Z. Safi, and I. Qadri, "Hepatitis C virus in Pakistan: a systematic review of prevalence, genotypes and risk factors," *World Journal of Gastroenterology*, vol. 15, no. 45, pp. 5647–5653, 2009.

[14] L. Ur Rehman, I. Ullah, I. Ali et al., "Active hepatitis C infection and HCV genotypes prevalent among the IDUs of Khyber Pakhtunkhwa," *Virology Journal*, vol. 8, article 327, 2011.

[15] S. Attaullah, S. Khan, and I. Ali, "Hepatitis C virus genotypes in Pakistan: a systemic review," *Virology Journal*, vol. 8, article 433, 2011.

[16] C. Shimamoto, I. Hirata, and K.-I. Katsu, "Breath and blood ammonia in liver cirrhosis," *Hepato-Gastroenterology*, vol. 47, no. 32, pp. 443–445, 2000.

[17] M. Iwasa, R. Sugimoto, R. Mifuji-Moroka et al., "Factors contributing to the development of overt encephalopathy in liver cirrhosis patients," *Metabolic Brain Disease*, vol. 31, no. 5, pp. 1151–1156, 2016.

[18] R. Rai, V. A. Saraswat, and R. K. Dhiman, "Gut microbiota: its role in hepatic encephalopathy," *Journal of Clinical and Experimental Hepatology*, vol. 5, supplement 1, pp. S29–S36, 2015.

[19] J. S. Bajaj, "The role of microbiota in hepatic encephalopathy," *Gut Microbes*, vol. 5, no. 3, pp. 397–403, 2014.

[20] M. Kalafateli, C. Konstantakis, K. Thomopoulos, and C. Triantos, "Impact of muscle wasting on survival in patients with liver cirrhosis," *World Journal of Gastroenterology*, vol. 21, no. 24, pp. 7357–7361, 2015.

[21] G. Davuluri, D. Krokowski, B. J. Guan et al., "Metabolic adaptation of skeletal muscle to hyperammonemia drives the beneficial effects of L-leucine in cirrhosis," *Journal of Hepatology*, vol. 65, no. 5, pp. 929–937, 2016.

[22] C. Chen, K. B. Bain, J. A. Iuppa, R. D. Yusen, D. E. Byers, and G. A. Patterson, "Hyperammonemia syndrome after lung transplantation: a single center experience," *Transplantation*, vol. 100, no. 3, pp. 678–684, 2016.

[23] K. Oi, T. Okado, H. Togo, S. Iimori, N. Yui, and E. Sohara, "Two cases of hemodialysis-associated Chronic Portal-Systemic Shunt Encephalopathy (CPSE) with opposite changes in the blood ammonia concentrations during hemodialysis: a case report and literature review," *Internal Medicine Journal*, vol. 54, no. 11, pp. 1375–1380, 2015.

[24] E. A. Kosenko, N. I. Venediktova, A. A. Kudryavtsev et al., "Encapsulation of glutamine synthetase in mouse erythrocytes: a new procedure for ammonia detoxification," *Biochemistry and Cell Biology*, vol. 86, no. 6, pp. 469–476, 2008.

A Population-Based Cross-Sectional Study of the Association between Liver Enzymes and Lipid Levels

Subrata Deb[1] **Prasanth Puthanveetil,**[2] **and Prashant Sakharkar**[2]

[1]*Department of Pharmaceutical Sciences, College of Pharmacy, Larkin University, Miami, FL 33169, USA*
[2]*Roosevelt University College of Pharmacy, Schaumburg, IL 60173, USA*

Correspondence should be addressed to Prashant Sakharkar; psakharkar@roosevelt.edu

Academic Editor: Simon Bramhall

Background. To examine the association between low-density lipoprotein (LDL) and high-density lipoprotein (HDL) levels and liver enzyme functions. *Methods.* The National Health and Nutrition Examination Survey (NHANES) data from 1999 to 2012 was used to examine the association between liver enzymes and lipid levels amongst adults in the United States. *Results.* Sixteen percent adults had ALT > 40 U/L, 11% had AST > 40 U/L, and 96% had ALP > 120 U/L. Age, gender, and race/ethnicity showed significant association with LDL, HDL, and triglycerides levels. LDL greater than borderline high was associated with little over two times higher odds of elevated ALT (OR: 2.33, 95% CI: 2.17, 2.53, $p \leq 0.001$) and AST (OR: 2.79, 95% CI: 2.55, 3.06, $p \leq 0.001$). High HDL was associated with 50% higher odds for elevated ALT (OR: 1.51, 95% CI: 1.39, 1.64, $p \leq 0.001$) and over two-and-half fold elevated AST (OR: 2.77, 95% CI: 2.47, 3.11, $p \leq 0.001$). LDL-C, HDL-C, and triglycerides were found to be good predictor of elevated ALT, AST, and ALP levels. Similarly, old age and female gender were significant predictor of elevated ALT and AST ($p \leq 0.001$). *Conclusions.* Underlying hepatic pathophysiology from dyslipidemia deserves further exploration due to its potential effects on hepatic drug metabolism/detoxification.

1. Introduction

Elevated lipid induced complications are significantly higher in North America and worldwide. Higher lipid levels are known to cause complications without sparing any organs including central nervous system, cardiovascular and endocrine systems, and even hepatic and renal systems [1]. Even though all the organ systems are affected by elevated lipid levels, liver is considered to be the generator and balancer of lipoprotein particles in the body including low-density lipoprotein (LDL), very low-density lipoprotein (VLDL), and high-density lipoprotein (HDL) [1]. An increase in the cholesterol levels considered to be detrimental, specifically LDL and VLDL, has always been a predictor for cardiovascular disease [1].

Approximately 30% of Americans are living with fatty liver disease, an epidemic that is rising in geometric proportions because of the calorie rich diet, lack of physical activity, and diabetes [2]. Genetically and nongenetically induced lipid disorders can lead to accumulation of excess fat bodies in the liver. This excess lipid thus brings about a change in liver anatomy, physiology, metabolism, and even survival of individual hepatocytes ultimately resulting in fibrosis and damage of hepatic tissue [2]. One of the major consequences resulting from such events could be tremendous oxidative stress that is generated because of the excess lipid accumulation in hepatocytes leading to their inflammation and cell death [2].

Even though there are published studies that have investigated the effect of lipids on cardiovascular system [3], there are limited studies which have looked into the impact of lipids on liver function. The goal of the present study was to examine the association between LDL and HDL levels and liver enzyme functions in the population of United States (US). We have utilized National Health and Nutrition Examination Survey (NHANES) of noninstitutional civilian population of the US to accumulate data for this particular study. The prominent aminotransferases such as alanine amino transferases (ALT) and aspartate aminotransferases (AST) are considered as markers of hepatic stress or injury

[4]. ALT is predominantly a hepatic residing enzyme but also found in muscle tissues and kidneys. ALT levels tend to increase in population suffering from viral attack on hepatic tissues, metal overloads, and metabolic stress, whereas AST is a rate limiting enzyme involved in transamination reaction which exists in cytosolic and mitochondrial compartments [4]. Like ALT, AST is also found in liver, muscle tissues, and kidneys, with their levels tending to increase in case of high alcohol consumption, chemical, and lipid induced hepatotoxicity [4]. In our study, we have also included the alkaline phosphatase levels (ALP), which have enhanced expression in lipid induced hepatic inflammatory diseases [4]. This work provides us evidence about the connection between high lipids and liver function in the absence of any confounding factors like metabolic syndrome and diabetes.

2. Materials and Methods

2.1. Study Population. We analyzed the sample of adults 20 years and older who participated in NHANES, an ongoing population-based statistical survey to estimate the health status of the noninstitutionalized civilian US population, based on interview, examination, and laboratory information from representative samples of US households. In-person interviews were conducted in sampled households, and subjects were invited to participate in medical examinations. Participants were selected using a stratified multistage probability design with oversampling of certain age and ethnic groups. We extracted data on individuals with age equal or above 20 years old, who participated in NHANES from 1999 through 2012 into a combined dataset (NHANES 1999–2012) to increase sample size for greater estimator reliability (NHANES Analytic Guidelines) [5]. Of 71,916 total participants who completed a home interview, 68,705 (96%) were screened. We excluded individuals with hepatitis B surface antibody ($n = 6179$), hepatitis B surface antigen, hepatitis D antibody and hepatitis C confirmed antibody combined ($n = 653$), and hepatitis A antibody and hepatitis B core antibody ($n = 17649$). We also excluded participants with missing AST and ALT levels ($n = 2532$). Participants ($n = 7249$) had missing data on one or more covariates, leaving final adjusted sample of 34,443 participants for analyses.

2.2. Covariates. Covariates included age, gender and ethnicity, blood pressure, cardiovascular disease, alcohol use, and use of lipid-lowering drugs. Age, race, and ethnicity were self-reported by the participants.

2.3. Study Definitions. Hyperlipidemia was defined in accordance with "National Cholesterol Education Program-Adult Treatment Panel" (NCEP-ATP III) guidelines [6]. Individuals were considered hyperlipidemic, if they had LDL 130 mg/dl or higher; HDL 40 mg/dl or lower in male; and 50 mg/dl or lower in female. Body mass index, a measure of obesity defined as weight in kilograms divided by height in meters squared, was categorized according to clinical guidelines set by the National Institute of Health [7].

2.4. Statistical Analysis. The statistical analyses for this study were performed using STATA, version 14 (STATA Corp, College Station, Texas) a statistical software package that takes into account sample weighting and the complex, multistage probability sample design of NHANES [8]. Demographic characteristics were compared by age, gender, race/ethnicity, education, lipid, and glycemic markers using the Chi-square test. Sampling weights were applied to take into account selection probabilities, oversampling, nonresponse, and differences between the sample and the US adolescent male population. We examined the association between lipid levels and ALT or AST. A multivariate logistic regression model was constructed to evaluate the associations of lipid levels with abnormal ALT or AST. There is no universal agreement about the cut-off values for ALT and AST in published literature. In this study, we defined abnormal ALT and AST as values greater than 40 U/L for total sample population. We also used gender based cut-off value of ALT (>40 U/L for male and >31 U/L for female) and AST (>37 U/L for male and >31 U/L for female) to explore if this change in cut-off value produces any difference in associations [9]. These cut-off values were chosen as it represents common institutional reference values and commonly used in the clinical practice. Similar cut-offs have been used in both adolescent and adult epidemiological studies. Regression model was adjusted for age, gender, and ethnicity. For interpretability, we treated lipid values as categories using clinical cut-off values: LDL ≥ 130 mg/dl; HDL ≤ 40 in male and ≤50 in female; triglyceride ≥ 150 mg/dl. Taylor series linearization was used for variance estimation. A p value of ≤0.05 or ≤0.001 was considered statistically significant.

3. Results

3.1. Study Participants. Table 1 presents the demographic and the baseline characteristics of individuals with low, medium, or high LDL, HDL, or triglyceride. A total of 34,443 adults (20 years and above) were included in this study. Sample mean age was 46 ± 0.22 yrs. and 62% individuals were 40 years of age and older, 52% were female, 70% were non-Hispanic White, and 57% had some college or graduate level education.

In overall sample, 27% adults had LDL levels > 130 mg/dl (borderline high) and 19% participants had HDL levels < 40 mg/dl (low). However, based on NCEP-ATP recommendation for female, 40% female had HDL levels less than 50 mg/dl. Twenty-six percent had triglycerides levels greater than 150 mg/dl (borderline high) according to NCEP-ATP III guidelines. Sixteen percent adults had ALT > 40 U/L, 11% had AST > 40 U/L, and 96% had ALP > 120 U/L in overall sample (Table 1).

The mean LDL, HDL, and triglyceride levels were 117.3 mg/dl, 45.8 mg/dl in male and 56.1 mg/dl in female, and 126.9 mg/dl, respectively, all within the normal range, with the exception of HDL being little high. Adults had mean body mass index (BMI) of 28.2 and mean waist circumference of 97.5 cm, well within the normal range with the cut-off values of 30 for BMI, 102 cm for men, and 88 cm for women for waist circumference (Table 2). Mean LDL, HDL, and triglycerides in overall sample among adults who had ALT and AST

Table 1: Demographic characteristics and lipid and liver enzyme laboratory data.

	N (%)
Age (yrs.)	
20–29	6256 (19)
30–39	5907 (19)
40–49	5754 (21)
50–59	4817 (17)
≥60	11709 (24)
Gender	
Male	16538 (48)
Female	17905 (52)
Ethnicity	
Mexican American	6518 (7.9)
Other Hispanics	2473 (5.3)
Non-Hispanic White	16275 (70)
Non-Hispanic black	7107 (11)
Other	2070 (5.8)
Education	
<High school	8530 (18.5)
High school	7050 (24)
Some college degree	8264 (30)
Graduate degree and above	6163 (27)
Participant with BMI ≥ 30	7504 (34.8)
Participants with Hypertension	2883 (12.0)
Told by Doctor of having high cholesterol	3417 (10.6)
On lipid lowering drugs	1123 (7.8)
Five or more alcohol drinks/day	2065 (15.0)
LDL (mg/dl)	
Optimal (<100)	8514 (41.6)
Near optimal/above optimal (100–129)	6338 (30.9)
Borderline high (130–159)	3725 (18.2)
High (160–189)	1373 (6.7)
Very high (≥190)	502 (2.3)
HDL (mg/dl)	
<40	6164 (19)
≥40	28279 (81)
Triglyceride (mg/dl)	
Normal (<150)	15846 (74.1)
Borderline high (150–199)	2620 (12.3)
High (200–499)	2693 (12.6)
Very high (≥500)	214 (1.0)
Total Cholesterol (mg/dl)	
Desirable (<200)	17220 (51)
Borderline high (200–239)	9878 (29)
High (≥240)	7345 (20)
ALT (U/L)	
≤40	28828 (84)
>40	5615 (16)
AST (U/L)	
≤40	30200 (89)
>40	4243 (11)
ALP (U/L)	
≤120	1047 (3.6)
>120	33396 (96)

Table 2: Mean values of lipid biomarkers and liver enzymes among participants.

	Mean (95% CI)
LDL (mg/dl)	117.3 (116.5, 118.2)
HDL (mg/dl)	50.8 (50.1, 51.5)
HDL (mg/dl) Male	45.8 (45.1, 46.5)
HDL (mg/dl) Female	56.1 (55.1, 57.1)
Triglyceride (mg/dl)	126.9 (124.9, 128.9)
Total cholesterol (mg/dl)	202.1 (199.6, 204.6)
ALT (U/L)	25.4 (25.0, 25.8)
ALT (U/L) Male	29.9 (29.5, 30.4)
ALT (U/L) Female	21.5 (21.0, 21.9)
AST (U/L)	25.2 (24.8, 25.5)
AST (U/L) Male	27.2 (26.9, 27.5)
AST (U/L) Female	23.3 (23.0, 23.5)
ALP (U/L)	68.9 (68.2, 69.7)
Waist circumference (cm)	97.5 (97.1, 98.0)
BMI	28.2 (28.0, 28.3)
SBP (mmHg)	119.5 (119.0, 119.9)
DBP (mmHg)	71.2 (70.9, 71.6)

ALT: alanine transaminase; AST: aspartate aminotransferase; ALP: alkaline phosphatase; SBP: systolic blood pressure; and DBP: diastolic blood pressure.

> 40 U/L was 130 mg/dl and 128.3; 52 mg/dl; 45.4 mg/dl, 50.6 mg/dl; and 157.3 mg/dl and 143.9 mg/dl, respectively, again within the normal limit with the exception of HDL, which was little high (Table 3).

3.2. Association of LDL, HDL, and Triglycerides with Abnormal Liver Enzymes. We examined the association of demographic characteristics with LDL, HDL, and triglyceride levels using the Chi-square test. Age, gender, and race/ethnicity showed significant association with LDL, HDL, and triglycerides levels. Post hoc analyses showed that >40 years of age and non-Hispanic white and black ethnicity were significantly associated with high LDL and borderline high triglycerides. Age of sixty years and above was also significantly associated with high triglycerides. Female gender was significantly associated with high HDL (>40 mg/dl) and high triglyceride levels (200–499 mg/dl), respectively. Non-Hispanic black ethnicity was significantly associated with borderline high LDL, Mexican American, and non-Hispanic black ethnicity with low HDL and high triglycerides (200–499 mg/dl). Obesity and presence of cardiovascular disease (CVD) were significantly associated with high HDL, whereas being on lipid-lowering drugs demonstrated significant association with low LDL levels. Blood pressure found

Table 3: Mean lipid biomarkers and liver enzymes.

	ALT (U/L) [Mean (SE)]			AST (U/L) [Mean (SE)]		
	<40	>40	p-value	<40	>40	p-value
Overall Sample						
LDL (mg/ml)	122.3 (0.9)	130.8 (3.1)	**≤0.001*** **	123.0 (0.9)	128.3 (3.9)	**≤0.001*** **
HDL (mg/dl)	52.0 (0.4)	45.4 (1.0)	**≤0.001*** **	51.4 (0.4)	50.6 (2.0)	**≤0.001*** **
Triglyceride (mg/dl)	129.5 (1.8)	157.3 (6.8)	**≤0.001*** **	131.8 (1.8)	143.9 (9.7)	0.499
	<40	>40	p-value	<37	>37	p-value
Male						
LDL (mg/ml)	117.3 (0.6)	124.6 (1.5)	**≤0.001*** **	118.1 (0.5)	121.4 (1.8)	**≤0.05***
HDL (mg/dl)	46.3 (0.4)	43.3 (0.7)	**≤0.001*** **	45.6 (0.4)	48.2 (0.9)	**≤0.05***
Triglyceride (mg/dl)	147.2 (2.6)	191.2 (6.9)	**≤0.001*** **	151.8 (2.5)	177.9 (9.9)	**≤0.001*** **
	<31	>31	p-value	<31	>31	p-value
Female						
LDL (mg/ml)	116.7 (0.5)	120.9 (1.9)	**≤0.001*** **	116.7 (0.5)	121.2 (1.9)	**≤0.05***
HDL (mg/dl)	56.5 (0.5)	53.0 (1.2)	**≤0.001*** **	56.0 (0.4)	56.7 (1.6)	0.630
Triglyceride (mg/dl)	123.9 (1.3)	160.9 (7.5)	**≤0.001*** **	125.1 (1.3)	154.7 (8.5)	**≤0.001*** **

SE = standard error (SE); significant at $^{*}p \leq 0.05$ and $^{***}p \leq 0.001$.

Table 4: Association of lipid markers and liver enzymes (overall sample).

	ALT (U/L) (N, %)		p-value	AST (U/L) (N, %)		p-value
	<40	>40		<40	>40	
LDL (mg/dl)						
<100	4471 (33.3)	420 (27.6)		4595 (32.7)	296 (33.6)[a]	
100–129	4454 (33.2)	483 (31.8)		4654 (33.1)	283 (32.2)	
130–159	2969 (22.1)	378 (24.9)	**≤0.001*** **	3167 (22.5)	180 (20.5)	**≤0.05***
160–189	1125 (8.3)	162 (10.7)		1209 (8.6)	78 (8.9)	
≥190	401 (2.9)	75 (4.9)[a]		433 (3.0)	43 (4.9)[a]	
HDL (mg/dl)						
<40	5417 (17)	747 (2.3)	**≤0.001*** **	5827 (18)	337 (0.94)	**≤0.001*** **
≥40	23411 (68)	4868 (14)		24373 (71)	3906 (10)	
Triglyceride (mg/dl)						
<150	9834 (70.0)	901 (54.9)		10156 (68.9)	579 (61.2)	
150–199	1976 (14.1)	290 (17.6)	**≤0.001*** **	2137 (14.5)	129 (13.6)	**≤0.001*** **
200–499	2074 (14.8)	392 (23.9)[a]		2261 (15.4)	205 (21.6)[a]	
≥500	146 (1.0)	57 (3.5)[a]		170 (1.2)	33 (3.5)[a]	

Significant at $^{*}p \leq 0.05$ and $^{***}p \leq 0.001$. [a]Differed significantly from others on post hoc analyses.

significantly associated with triglyceride levels; however, LDL and HDL did not show any significant association with blood pressure status (Supplemental Tables 1(a) and 1(b)). Similarly, drinking five or more alcoholic drinks per day was found to be significantly associated with ALT and AST but showed no association with lipid markers (data not shown).

We also examined the association of LDL, HDL, and triglycerides with liver enzymes. LDL, HDL, and triglycerides were found significantly associated with liver enzymes ALT and AST (Table 4). Post hoc analysis showed low LDL significantly associated with normal ALT and AST levels, whereas, high HDL and triglycerides were associated with elevated ALT and AST. BMI of <30 and blood pressure of 130/90 were found significantly associated with normal ALT and AST in overall sample and in male and female based on gender based cut-off values with the exception of association between blood pressure and ALT in female. Taking lipid-lowering drugs and CVD found associated with normal AST; however, no such association was observed based on gender (Supplemental Table 1(c)).

We calculated the odds ratio of abnormal ALT (ALT > 40 IU/L), AST (AST > 40 IU/L) using cut-off value of borderline high LDL, low HDL, and borderline high triglycerides. LDL greater than borderline high was associated with over two times higher odds of elevated ALT (OR: 2.33, 95% CI: 2.17, 2.53, $p \leq 0.001$) and AST (OR: 2.79, 95% CI: 2.55, 3.06, $p \leq 0.001$). High HDL was associated with 50% higher odds for elevated ALT (OR: 1.51, 95% CI: 1.39, 1.64, $p \leq 0.001$) and over two-and-half fold elevated AST (OR: 2.77, 95% CI: 2.47, 3.11, $p \leq 0.001$). Triglyceride levels above borderline high were

Table 5: Odds of elevated liver enzymes with lipid biomarkers.

	ALT		AST	
	OR (95% CI)	*p* value	OR (95% CI)	*p* value
LDL (mg/dL)	2.33 (2.17–2.53)	**≤0.001*****	2.79 (2.55–3.06)	**≤0.001*****
HDL (mg/dL)	1.51 (1.39–1.64)	**≤0.001*****	2.77 (2.47–3.11)	**≤0.001*****
Triglyceride (mg/dL)	2.71 (2.51–2.93)	**≤0.001*****	3.21 (2.93–3.52)	**≤0.001*****
Male				
LDL (mg/dL)	1.39 (1.18–1.63)	**≤0.001*****	1.07 (0.865–1.31)	0.551
HDL (mg/dL)	1.34 (1.17–1.55)	**≤0.001*****	1.19 (0.99–1.44)	0.055
Triglyceride (mg/dL)	1.83 (1.59–2.09)	**≤0.001*****	1.12 (0.93–1.33)	0.209
Female				
LDL (mg/dL)	0.97 (0.88–1.06)	0.480	0.98 (0.87–1.11)	0.790
HDL (mg/dL)	0.64 (0.49–0.83)	**≤0.001*****	0.86 (0.61–1.20)	0.360
Triglyceride (mg/dL)	1.36 (1.03–1.81)	**≤0.05***	0.96 (0.69–1.34)	0.080

OR = odds ratio; CI = confidence interval; significant at * $p < 0.05$ and *** $p < 0.001$.

Table 6: Predictors of AST and ALT level on regression (adjusted model).

	ALT		AST	
	OR (95% CI)	*p* value	OR (95% CI)	*p* value
Age	0.87 (0.85, 0.89)	**≤0.001*****	0.94 (0.91, 0.97)	**≤0.001*****
Gender	0.49 (0.46, 0.53)	**≤0.001*****	0.75 (0.69, 0.82)	**≤0.001*****
Ethnicity	0.93 (0.89, 0.97)	**≤0.001*****	1.03 (0.98, 1.08)	0.134
LDL (mg/dl)	1.07 (1.01, 1.13)	**≤0.001*****	1.08 (1.01, 1.16)	0.057
HDL (mg/dl)	1.59 (1.42, 1.78)	**≤0.001*****	2.85 (2.38, 3.42)	**≤0.001*****
Triglyceride (mg/dl)	1.29 (1.21, 1.37)	**≤0.001*****	1.43 (1.32–1.55)	**≤0.001*****

OR = odds ratio; CI = confidence interval; significant at * $p < 0.05$ and *** $p < 0.001$.

associated with more than two-and-half times higher odds of abnormal ALT (OR: 2.71, 95% CI: 2.51, 2.93, $p \le 0.001$) and little over three times higher odds of elevated AST (OR: 3.21, 95% CI: 2.93, 3.52, $p \le 0.001$) compared to normal LDL, HDL, and triglyceride levels (Table 5).

We modeled the odds of abnormal ALT and AST using LDL, HDL, triglyceride, and other covariates simultaneously and calculated the odds ratio of abnormal ALT (ALT > 40 U/L), AST (AST > 40 U/L) using logistic regression model (Table 6). After adjustment, high LDL was associated with 7% and 8% higher odds of elevated ALT and AST, respectively, and high HDL was associated with 59% higher odds for abnormal ALT and close to threefold higher odds for abnormal AST (OR: 1.59; 95% CI: 1.01, 1.13, $p \le 0.001$ and OR: 2.85; 95% CI: 1.01, 1.16, $p \le 0.001$, respectively). Whereas, high triglyceride levels were associated with 29% higher odds of higher ALT and 43% higher odds of elevated AST (OR: 1.29; 95% CI: 1.21, 1.37, $p \le 0.001$ and OR: 1.43; 95% CI: 1.32, 1.55, $p \le 0.001$, respectively). Age was also significantly associated with lower odds of having elevated ALT (OR: 0.87; 95% CI: 0.85, 0.89, $p \le 0.001$) and AST (OR: 0.94; 95% CI: 0.91, 0.97, $p \le 0.001$) and female with lower ALT (OR: 0.49; 95% CI: 0.46, 0.53, $p \le 0.001$) and AST (OR: 0.75; 95% CI: 0.69, 0.82, $p \le 0.001$) suggesting that increase in age and female gender lowers the odds of elevated ALT and AST and seems to be protective.

3.3. Association of LDL, HDL, and Triglycerides with Abnormal Liver Enzymes Using Gender Based Cut-Off Values. Twenty percent male and 11% female had elevated ALT, and 9% male and 10% female had elevated AST according to the gender based cut-off values (data not shown). Mean ALT in male and female was 29.9 U/L and 21.5 U/L, respectively. Similarly, mean AST in male was 27.2 U/L and in female 23.3 U/L (Table 2).

Mean LDL, HDL, and triglycerides among male who had ALT > 40 U/L and AST > 37 was 124.6 mg/dl and 121.4 mg/dl; 43.3 mg/dl and 48.2 mg/dl; and 191.2 mg/dl and 177 9 mg/dl, respectively. In case of female, these values were 120.9 mg/dl and 121.2 mg/dl; 53 mg/dl and 56.7 mg/dl; and 160.9 mg/dl and 154.7 mg/dl, respectively, little higher for HDL and triglycerides. These differences in LDL, HDL, and triglycerides with ALT and AST were significant in both genders with the exception of HDL and AST in female ($p \le 0.001$) (Table 3). LDL, HDL, and triglyceride levels were found significantly associated with gender-specific ALT and AST cut-off values. Post hoc analysis showed that very high LDL, HDL, and borderline high triglycerides were significantly associated with elevated ALT in male, whereas low HDL and borderline high triglycerides associated with elevated ALT in female. Similarly, borderline high triglycerides were associated with elevated AST in both genders ($p \le 0.05$) (data not shown).

LDL greater than borderline high was associated with 39% higher odds (OR: 1.39; 95% CI: 1.18, 1.6, $p \le 0.001$); high

HDL was associated with 34% higher odds (OR: 1.34; 95% CI: 1.17, 1.55, $p \leq 0.001$) of ALT in male. Triglyceride above borderline was associated with 83% higher odds (OR: 1.83; 95% CI: 1.59, 2.09, $p \leq 0.001$) and 36% higher odds (OR: 1.36; 95% CI: 1.03, 1.81, $p \leq 0.05$) of ALT in female, respectively (Table 5). On regression analysis, after adjustment, high LDL was associated with 38% higher odds (OR: 1.38; 95% CI: 1.18, 1.62, $p \leq 0.001$) and triglycerides with 87% higher odds (OR: 1.87; 95% CI: 1.63, 2.14, $p \leq 0.001$) of ALT. Similarly, high HDL was associated with 38% and 21% of higher odds of elevated ALT (OR: 1.38; 95% CI: 1.20, 1.59, $p \leq 0.001$) and AST (OR: 1.21; 95% CI: 1.01, 1.47, $p \leq 0.001$) in male. Race/ethnicity and HDL were significant predictor of elevated ALT and AST and age of elevated AST in both genders. Similarly, LDL and triglyceride levels were significant predictors of ALT in male ($p \leq 0.001$) (data not shown).

4. Discussion

In the present study, we have expanded the data to include population of 34,443 individuals with age ranging from 20 years and above who are free of hepatitis A, B, C, and D. Also, we have included participants from 1999 to 2012, which is a wider time range than any of the previous studies performed using NHANES. This study helps in drawing the link between high lipid profile and its injurious effect on liver function as measured by AST, ALT, and ALP levels. The mean age of the study population was 46 years old with 62% ranging over 40 years old and 57% of the participants included had a college or graduate level education. Participants of age 60 years and above (2.6%) had normal ALT compared to other age groups; however, no single group found significantly different for AST levels. Similarly, less number of female compared to male (6% versus 9.8%) had elevated ALT and (5.2% versus 5.9%) had elevated AST on Chi-square analyses (data not shown). On the other hand, overall increase in age and female gender appears to be protective to liver health as indicated by the results of regression analysis.

The mean lipid profile and BMI in our study show an interesting pattern, because the mean LDL, HDL, and triglycerides, along with waist circumference and BMI, were all in the upper part of the borderline, with HDL mean value being relatively higher which is 50.8 mg/dl predicted to offer protection. Individuals on lipid-lowering drugs or with BMI < 30 are more likely to have normal liver function than the others with elevated lipid levels. Frequent and excessive consumption of alcoholic drinks can lead to increased AST/ALT functions but potentially without any interference with the lipid levels. Typically, a healthy liver in a subject who is involved with a more sedentary work and life style will metabolize and maintain a normal systemic lipid level in the body, by increasing hepatic reverse cholesterol transport and also uptake of VLDL and LDL by increasing the LDL receptor expression and concentration on the hepatic surface [10]. This LDL receptor mediated increased uptake of lipid remnants which try to maintain a normal lipid profile in the body, but at the same time the accumulated remnants get stored in liver which could initiate metabolic alterations and induce fibrosis and cell death of the hepatic tissue, also resulting in a dysfunctional hepatic system [11]. Relentless assault by lipids on liver while it performs regular hepatic functions adds more workload on liver and thereby alters its physiology. One of the most important factors to observe is that the accumulated lipid remnants could promote inflammation of hepatic tissue with generation of free radicals inside [11]. These free radicals could then be playing a major role in inducing fibrosis or cell death of the hepatic tissue. The damaged liver cell can release more transaminases outside and can become more permeable due to thinning from the excess stretch caused by accumulated lipid remnants or due to induction of porous and fibrous hepatic tissue by the lipid metabolites.

Our results suggest that in general there are no gender-specific differences in the systemic LDL and HDL-cholesterol levels; however, the LDL levels were slightly higher in females than males, albeit without any statistical significance. The non-Hispanic whites had a higher limit of both borderline and higher levels of LDL compared to Mexican Americans and Hispanics who had the lowest. In addition, non-Hispanic white had higher HDL levels, which reflect the finding of previous studies, where higher lipid level including HDL-cholesterol was accompanied by an increase in hepatic transaminase expression [12]. Increasing age was associated with enhanced triglyceride levels; gender was significantly associated with elevated triglycerides and ethnicity showing a significant trend in the triglyceride increases. Non-Hispanic white population shows elevated triglyceride levels along with LDL and HDL, further indication of diet pattern of specific ethnicities.

There is a significant rise in hepatic AST and ALT enzymes in proportion to raised LDL, HDL, and triglyceride levels. These findings further strengthen the claims and give a projection about the connection between the etiology and epidemiology of lipid induced hepatic dysfunction. There are substantial scientific evidence that shows how lipids can affect liver function in preclinical and also in clinical setting [13, 14]. The antioxidant capacity of human liver could be compromised with increasing lipid levels, resulting in more inflammation and reactive oxygen species in the body especially liver [11, 13]. This could result in many of the liver functions including reverse cholesterol transport, the innate ability by which liver try to keep the levels of bad cholesterol-LDL in check. Also the reactive oxygen species could hinder hepatic ability to uptake remnants through LDL receptor, scavenger receptors like SR-1, and its own ability to pack the remnant cholesterol to fully fledged lipoprotein bodies which the system can actually utilize. No significant association was observed for different lipid levels (optimal to very high) with gender on Chi-square analysis; however, gender was found to be a good predictor of the hepatic function as determined by high AST and ALT levels in male compared to female on regression analysis.

One of the previous studies by Jiang et al. [12] showed that low LDL and high HDL-cholesterol levels, which is considered beneficial, showed a negative correlation between liver function as measured by elevated levels of transaminase enzyme. Authors in this study excluded subjects who had viral hepatitis and positive HCV status and also those on lipid-lowering medications along with those subjects whose

ALT or AST data was not available. As authors stated, there were some major confounding factors which could have altered both lipid profiles and liver function as seen from the clinical and laboratory data of those participated individuals [12]. Some of the other studies that have used the NHANES data also showed a correlation between hepatic enzyme levels and metabolic dysfunction. A study by Kim et al. [15] showed an interesting phenomenon that even a small rise in AST and ALT showed characteristic features of metabolic syndrome like effects. Samadi et al. [16] in their study showed that there is a strong correlation between waist circumference, a mark of obesity to liver enzymes, AST, ALT, ALP, and gamma glutamyl transpeptidase (GGT) and also noted a significant correlation that this connection between hepatic enzymes and waist circumference only existed in Hispanic females and not in non-Hispanic black males and females.

Another interesting study by Tsai et al. [17] showed a good correlation between obesity, alcohol consumption, and liver enzyme functions using NHANES data for a 3-year period (2005–08) from more than 8300 adults with ages > 20 years as sample size found that obese females who are excess drinkers tend to have an increased AST, ALT, and GGT levels compared to nonobese and nondrinker females. Recently, Unalp-Arida and Ruhl [18] have reported NHANES data (1988–1994) with twenty-three years of mortality follow-up and suggested a strong link between hepatic disease-induced mortality and enzyme function. A patient population of 14,527 who were not tested positive for viral hepatitis B and C were chosen; also this population was not independently associated with mortalities due to other complications like cancer, diabetes, and cardiovascular disease. Individuals having hepatic steatosis with elevated ALT, AST, and GGT enzymes tend to show an elevated level of mortality due to liver disease. One important point to emphasize in our study is that gender is the only independent determinant of liver function independent of the age, ethnic background, or lipid levels in these individuals. It is important to look into the details of protective effect of female hormones, which are active during the premenopausal state and could play a role in both regulating lipid levels and exhibiting hepatoprotective function. In women who are in the postmenopausal state, this hepatic protective function of estrogen could be lost which could result in elevated AST and ALT levels.

Liver plays a vital role in the biotransformation, detoxification, and excretion of diverse lipophilic agents including medications, dietary substances, and environmental toxicants. In addition to detoxification, the drug metabolizing enzymes also play an important role in converting the prodrugs to their active form. Cytochrome P450 (CYP) and uridine diphosphate (UDP) glucuronosyltransferases (UGT) superfamily metabolizing enzymes primarily execute their functions in liver [19]. Expression and activities of hepatic CYP and UGT enzymes are closely regulated by several physiological and external factors including circulating and tissue lipid levels [20]. Thus, individuals with higher lipid levels are likely to be susceptible to altered metabolism profile. A fatty liver with inefficient functioning could lead to decrease in its ability to detoxify drugs and toxins or activate the prodrugs. This will eventually aggravate systemic oxidative stress and result in vital organ damage and elevating the morbidity and mortality in subjects suffering from nonalcoholic fatty liver disease (NAFLD) [21]. A detailed mechanistic understanding of hyperlipidemia on CYP and UGT levels would facilitate our understanding of therapeutic outcome following hyperlipidemia-related NAFLD.

Our study has some limitations. First, we used ALT and AST as a surrogate marker, which is an indirect assessment of liver dysfunction or liver diseases. Second, the proportions of people with LDL, triglycerides, high ALT, and AST were comparatively small. Therefore, despite the large dataset, the power can be limited in these categories, especially when the sample size is reduced for sensitivity analysis. Third, only a single measurement of ALT and AST levels was available for each individual in the NHANES data. Though a small number of participants had CVD, were on lipid-lowering drugs, and reported drinking more than 5 alcoholic drinks per day, perhaps they may have influenced our results. Similarly, missing data and presence of reported/unreported confounding factors such as smoking, cancer/malignancy, diabetes, and presence of liver conditions among participants are the other factors that may have contributed to our results limiting its generalizability.

5. Conclusions

Both high LDL and HDL were associated with significantly higher odds of elevated liver enzymes in the general US adult population. Age, gender, and race/ethnicity have significant association with LDL, HDL, and triglycerides levels. Our findings raise concerns about potentially unrecognized hepatic dysfunction among people with high LDL or HDL and the underlying hepatic pathophysiology can impact hepatic detoxification of drugs or environmental toxicants.

Abbreviations

LDL: Low-density lipoprotein
HDL: High-density lipoprotein
NHANES: National Health and Nutrition Examination Survey
CDC: Center for Disease Control and Prevention
ALT: Alanine amino transferases
AST: Aspartate aminotransferases
ALP: Alkaline phosphatase levels
BMI: Body mass index
VLDL: Very low-density lipoprotein
GGT: Gamma glutamyl transpeptidase
CYP: Cytochrome P450
UGT: Uridine diphosphate (UDP) glucuronosyltransferases
NAFLD: Nonalcoholic fatty liver disease.

References

[1] L. Badimon and G. Vilahur, "LDL-cholesterol versus HDL-cholesterol in the atherosclerotic plaque: inflammatory resolution versus thrombotic chaos," *Annals of the New York Academy of Sciences*, vol. 1254, no. 1, pp. 18–32, 2012.

[2] M. Ahmed, "Non-alcoholic fatty liver disease in 2015," *World Journal of Hepatology*, vol. 7, no. 11, pp. 1450–1459, 2015.

[3] R. H. Nelson, "Hyperlipidemia as a Risk Factor for Cardiovascular Disease," *Primary Care—Clinics in Office Practice*, vol. 40, no. 1, pp. 195–211, 2013.

[4] E. G. Giannini, R. Testa, and V. Savarino, "Liver enzyme alteration: a guide for clinicians," *Canadian Medical Association Journal*, vol. 172, no. 3, pp. 367–379, 2005.

[5] National Health and Nutrition Examination Survey (NHANES), National Center for Health Statistics. Hyattsville, MD; Center for Disease Control and Prevention, U.S. Department of Health and Human Services. https://wwwn.cdc.gov/nchs/nhanes/analyticguidelines.aspx, 2017.

[6] Adult Treatment Panel III (ATP III) Guidelines At-A-Glance Quick Desk Reference, National Cholesterol Education Program (NCEP), https://www.nhlbi.nih.gov/files/docs/guidelines/atglance.pdf, 2017.

[7] The Practical Guide Identification, Evaluation, and Treatment of Overweight and Obesity in Adults, NHLBI Obesity Education Initiative, National Institute of Health, https://www.nhlbi.nih.gov/files/docs/guidelines/prctgd_c.pdf, 2017.

[8] STATA 14; StataCorp, Stata Statistical Software: Release 13, College Station, TX: StataCorp LP. 2013.

[9] G. Aragon and Z. M. Younossi, "When and how to evaluate mildly elevated liver enzymes in apparently healthy patients," *Cleveland Clinic Journal of Medicine*, vol. 77, no. 3, pp. 195–204, 2010.

[10] W. Annema and U. J. F. Tietge, "Regulation of reverse cholesterol transport - A comprehensive appraisal of available animal studies," *Journal of Nutrition and Metabolism*, vol. 9, article no. 25, 2012.

[11] J. Arauz, E. Ramos-Tovar, and P. Muriel, "Redox state and methods to evaluate oxidative stress in liver damage: from bench to bedside," *Annals of Hepatology*, vol. 15, no. 2, pp. 160–173, 2016.

[12] Z. G. Jiang, K. Mukamal, E. Tapper, S. C. Robson, and Y. Tsugawa, "Low LDL-C and high HDL-C levels are associated with elevated serum transaminases amongst adults in the United States: A cross-sectional study," *PLoS ONE*, vol. 9, no. 1, Article ID e85366, 2014.

[13] M. Bertolotti, A. Lonardo, C. Mussi et al., "Nonalcoholic fatty liver disease and aging: epidemiology to management," *World Journal of Gastroenterology*, vol. 20, no. 39, pp. 14185–14204, 2014.

[14] C.-Y. Liu, C.-W. Chang, H.-C. Lee et al., "Metabolic damage presents differently in young and early-aged C57BL/6 mice fed a high-fat diet," *International Journal of Gerontology*, vol. 10, no. 2, pp. 105–111, 2016.

[15] H. C. Kim, K. S. Choi, Y. H. Jang, H. W. Shin, and D. J. Kim, "Normal serum aminotransferase levels and the metabolic syndrome: Korean National Health and Nutrition Examination Surveys," *Yonsei Medical Journal*, vol. 47, no. 4, pp. 542–550, 2006.

[16] N. Samadi, G. S. Cembrowski, and J. Chan, "Effect of waist circumference on reference intervals of liver-related enzyme tests in apparently healthy adult Mexican Americans, black and white Americans," *Clinical Biochemistry*, vol. 40, no. 3-4, pp. 206–212, 2007.

[17] J. Tsai, E. S. Ford, G. Zhao, C. Li, K. J. Greenlund, and J. B. Croft, "Co-occurrence of obesity and patterns of alcohol use associated with elevated serum hepatic enzymes in US adults," *Journal of Behavioral Medicine*, vol. 35, no. 2, pp. 200–210, 2012.

[18] A. Unalp-Arida and C. E. Ruhl, "Noninvasive fatty liver markers predict liver disease mortality in the U.S. population," *Hepatology*, vol. 63, no. 4, pp. 1170–1183, 2016.

[19] S. Deb, M. Pandey, H. Adomat, and E. S. Guns, "Cytochrome P450 3A-Mediated Microsomal Biotransformation of 1 ,25-Dihydroxyvitamin D3 in Mouse and Human Liver: Drug-Related Induction and Inhibition of Catabolism," *Drug Metabolism and Disposition*, vol. 40, no. 5, pp. 907–918, 2012.

[20] M. Hafner, T. Rezen, and D. Rozman, "Regulation of hepatic cytochromes P450 by lipids and cholesterol," *Current Drug Metabolism*, vol. 12, no. 2, pp. 173–185, 2011.

[21] S. Tangvarasittichai, "Oxidative stress, insulin resistance, dyslipidemia and type 2 diabetes mellitus," *World Journal of Diabetes*, vol. 6, no. 3, pp. 456–480, 2015.

23

A Combination of Leucine, Metformin, and Sildenafil Treats Nonalcoholic Fatty Liver Disease and Steatohepatitis in Mice

Antje Bruckbauer,[1] Jheelam Banerjee,[1] Lizhi Fu,[2] Fenfen Li,[2] Qiang Cao,[2] Xin Cui,[2] Rui Wu,[2] Hang Shi,[2] Bingzhong Xue,[2] and Michael B. Zemel[1]

[1]*NuSirt Biopharma Inc., 11020 Solway School Rd, Knoxville, TN 37931, USA*
[2]*Center for Obesity Reversal, Department of Biology, Georgia State University, 33 Gilmer Street SE, Atlanta, GA 30302, USA*

Correspondence should be addressed to Antje Bruckbauer; abruckbauer@nusirt.com

Academic Editor: Heather Francis

Sirt1, AMPK, and eNOS modulate hepatic energy metabolism and inflammation and are key players in the development of NASH. L-leucine, an allosteric Sirt1 activator, synergizes with low doses of metformin or sildenafil on the AMPK-eNOS-Sirt1 pathway to reverse mild NAFLD in preclinical mouse models. Here we tested a possible multicomponent synergy to yield greater therapeutic efficacy in NAFLD/NASH. Liver cells and macrophages or an atherogenic diet induced NASH mouse model was treated with two-way and three-way combinations. The three-way combination Sild-Met-Leu increased hepatic fatty acid oxidation and reduced lipogenic gene expression and inflammatory marker *in vitro*. In mice, Sild-Met-Leu reduced the diet induced increases of ALT, TGFβ, PAI-1, IL1β, and TNFα, hepatic collagen expression, and nearly completely reversed hepatocyte ballooning and triglyceride accumulation, while all two-way combinations had only modest effects. Therefore, these data provide preclinical evidence for therapeutic efficacy of Sild-Met-Leu in the treatment of NAFLD and NASH.

1. Introduction

Nonalcoholic steatohepatitis (NASH), the progressive form of nonalcoholic fatty liver disease (NAFLD), is characterized by the presence of >5% macrovesicular steatosis, inflammation, and liver cell ballooning [1]. Its prevalence is increasing concomitantly with prevalence of obesity and diabetes, thus representing a serious public health issue [2, 3]. About 30 to 40% of NASH progresses to fibrosis or to cirrhosis, resulting in a high risk for cardiovascular and liver-related morbidity and mortality [3]. However, treatment is presently limited to lifestyle intervention, as approved treatment options are lacking and represent a significant unmet need.

Sirt1 enzyme and AMPK are important regulators of energy metabolism and modulate hepatic glucose and lipid metabolism. In addition, Sirt1 regulates multiple inflammatory pathways such as NF-κB and TNFα [2]. Thus they play an important role in the pathophysiology of NAFLD and NASH [2, 4, 5]. Liver-specific deletion of Sirt1 results in hepatic steatosis and inflammation in mice [6], while treatment with Sirt1 activators or Sirt1 overexpression ameliorates fatty liver and reduces lipogenic gene expression [5, 7].

We have previously demonstrated that leucine acts as a direct Sirt1 activator by lowering the activation energy for NAD$^+$ and enables coactivation with other AMPK/Sirt1 activators thereby reducing the necessary concentration for each individual compound [8, 9]. Synergy with leucine was also demonstrated with metformin (met), the first-line treatment drug for diabetes, at which effects are also mediated by merging on the AMPK/Sirt1 pathway [10, 11]. Accordingly, treatment with a Met-Leu combination resulted in reduction of lipid accumulation *in vitro* and reversal of hepatic steatosis *in vivo* in a HFD-induced NAFLD mouse model [12].The endothelial nitric oxide synthase, nitric oxide and cyclic guanosine monophosphate (eNOS-NO-cGMP) signaling pathway has also been shown to affect the progression of NAFLD to NASH. High-fat diet feeding reduced eNOS-NO signaling in the liver of NAFLD models of mice and rats. This was precedent to the onset of hepatic inflammation and insulin resistance and was prevented by daily administration of sildenafil [13, 14].

The primary action of sildenafil is the inhibition of phosphodiesterase 5 (PDE5) which hydrolyses cGMP and thus terminates cGMP signaling. In addition, sildenafil activates eNOS resulting in increased NO/cGMP signaling with consecutive activation of the cGMP-dependent protein kinases (PKGs) to induce vasodilatory, anti-inflammatory, and antiproliferative effects [15–18].

This pathway also interacts with the sirtuin pathway, as it stimulates Sirtl, while Sirtl appears to deacetylate and activate eNOS and thereby elevate NO levels; thus sildenafil's effects may be partly mediated by Sirtl activation [17, 19–21]. Moreover, leucine synergizes with PDE5 inhibitors to exert amplifying downstream effects of AMPK and Sirtl activation on glucose and fat metabolism as well as reversal of hepatic steatosis and inflammation *in vitro* and *in vivo* [22]. Accordingly, the aim of this study was to evaluate the effects of a three-way interaction between leucine, metformin, and sildenafil on AMPK/Sirtl/eNOS pathway and the protective effects on hepatocyte metabolism in a NASH mouse model.

2. Methods

2.1. Cell Culture. Human hepatoma HepG2 cells (ATCC, Manassas, VA, USA) were grown in Dulbecco's modified Eagle's medium (DMEM, 5.5 mM glucose) containing 10% fetal bovine serum (FBS) and antibiotics (1% penicillin-streptomycin) at 37°C in 5% CO_2 in air. Mouse AML-12 liver cells (ATCC, Manassas, VA, USA) were grown and maintained in 1:1 mixture of DMEM and Ham's F12 medium with 0.005 mg/mL insulin, 0.005 mg/mL transferrin, 5 ng/mL selenium, 40 ng·mL dexamethasone, 10% FBS, and antibiotics (1% penicillin-streptomycin) at 37°C in 5% CO_2 in air. Mouse RAW 264.7 macrophages (ATCC, Manassas, VA, USA) were grown and maintained in DMEM containing 10% fetal bovine serum (FBS) and antibiotics (1% penicillin-streptomycin) at 37°C in 5% CO_2 in air. Media were replaced with fresh medium every 2 to 3 days. Cells were split at a 1:4 ratio at 70 to 80% confluence.

Lipid accumulation in HepG2 cells was induced by incubation in 25 mM glucose DMEM media for 48 hours. Lipid accumulation and inflammatory response in AML-12 cells and RAW 264.7 macrophages were induced by stimulation with 500 μM free fatty acids (FFA, palmitic-oleic acid mixture 1:2) and lipopolysaccharide (LPS, 1 ng/mL) for 24 hours.

Treatment (metformin 0.1 mM, leucine 0.5 mM, and sildenafil 1 nM) was added for further 24 to 48 hours.

2.2. Coculture. Mouse AML-12 liver cells and RAW 264.7 macrophages were seeded together in a ratio 4:1. Next day lipid accumulation and inflammatory response were induced by stimulation with 500 μM free fatty acids (palmitic-oleic acid mixture 1:2) and LPS (1 ng/mL) for 24 hours. The cells were then treated as indicated for 24 hours.

2.3. MCPl and TNFα Measurement in Media. AML-12 and/or RAW 264.7 macrophages were seeded and treated as described above. At the end of the treatment, the media were harvested. Monocyte chemotactic protein- (MCP-) 1 and tumor necrosis factor- (TNF-) α secretion was measured with the MCP1 Mouse Elisa kit and TNF-alpha Mouse Elisa kit (Abcam, Cambridge, MA, USA), respectively, according to manufacturer's instructions.

2.4. Western Blot. The Sirtl, phospho-AMPK (Thr172), AMPK, FAS, SCD1, PPAR-α, and PPARδ, SREBP1, and TNF-α antibodies were obtained from Cell Signaling (Danvers, MA). Protein levels of cell extracts were measured by bicinchoninic acid assay (BCA) kit (Thermo Fisher Scientific Inc., Waltham, MA). For Western blot, 10–50 μg protein was resolved on 4–15% gradient polyacrylamide gels (criterion precast gel, Bio-Rad Laboratories, Hercules, CA), transferred to PVDF or nitrocellulose membranes, incubated in blocking buffer (5% nonfat dry milk in TBS), and then incubated with primary antibody (1:1000 dilution), washed, and incubated with horseradish peroxidase- or fluorescence-conjugated secondary antibody (1:10000 dilution). Visualization was conducted using Li-COR Odyssey Fc Imaging system (Li-COR Biosciences, Lincoln, NB) and band intensity was assessed using Quantity One (Bio-Rad Laboratories, Hercules, CA), with correction for background and loading controls.

2.5. Fatty Acid Oxidation. Cellular oxygen consumption was measured using a Seahorse Bioscience XF24 analyzer (Seahorse Bioscience, Billerica, MA) in 24-well plates at 37°C. HepG2 cells were seeded at 40,000 cells per well. Lipid accumulation was induced by 48 h incubation with 25 mM glucose. Cells were treated for 24 hours with the indicated treatments, washed twice with nonbuffered carbonate-free pH 7.4 low glucose (2.5 mM) DMEM containing carnitine (0.5 mM), equilibrated with 550 μL of the same media in a non-CO_2 incubator for 30 minutes, and then inserted into the instrument for 15 minutes of further equilibration. O_2 consumption was measured in three successive baseline measurements at eight-minute intervals prior to injection of palmitate (200 μM final concentration). Post-palmitate-injection measurements were taken over a 3-hour period with cycles consisting of 10 min break and three successive measurements of O_2 consumption. The area under the curve was calculated.

2.6. Animals and Diets. Six- to eight-week-old male C57BL/6J mice were purchased from Jackson Laboratories. First NASH was induced in all animals (except low-fat diet control animals (LF)) via feeding of a high-fat atherogenic diet (HC: 60% of calories from fat, 1.25% cholesterol, and 0.5% cholate) for 6 weeks. After this induction period, the HC animals were randomized into one of the following groups with 10 animals/group and kept on their experimental diet for additional 6 weeks (12 weeks total): high-fat atherogenic diet (HC); HC + sildenafil (25 mg/kg diet, calculated as human equivalent dose of 1 mg/day) (HC + Sil); HC + leucine (24 g/kg diet) + sildenafil (HC + Leu + Sil); HC + leucine + metformin (0.25 g/kg diet, calculated as a human equivalent dose of 250 mg/day (HC + Leu + Met)); HC + metformin + sildenafil (HC + Met + Sil); HC + leucine + metformin + sildenafil (HC + Leu + Met + Sil). The LF animals were continued on their diet for an additional 6 weeks.

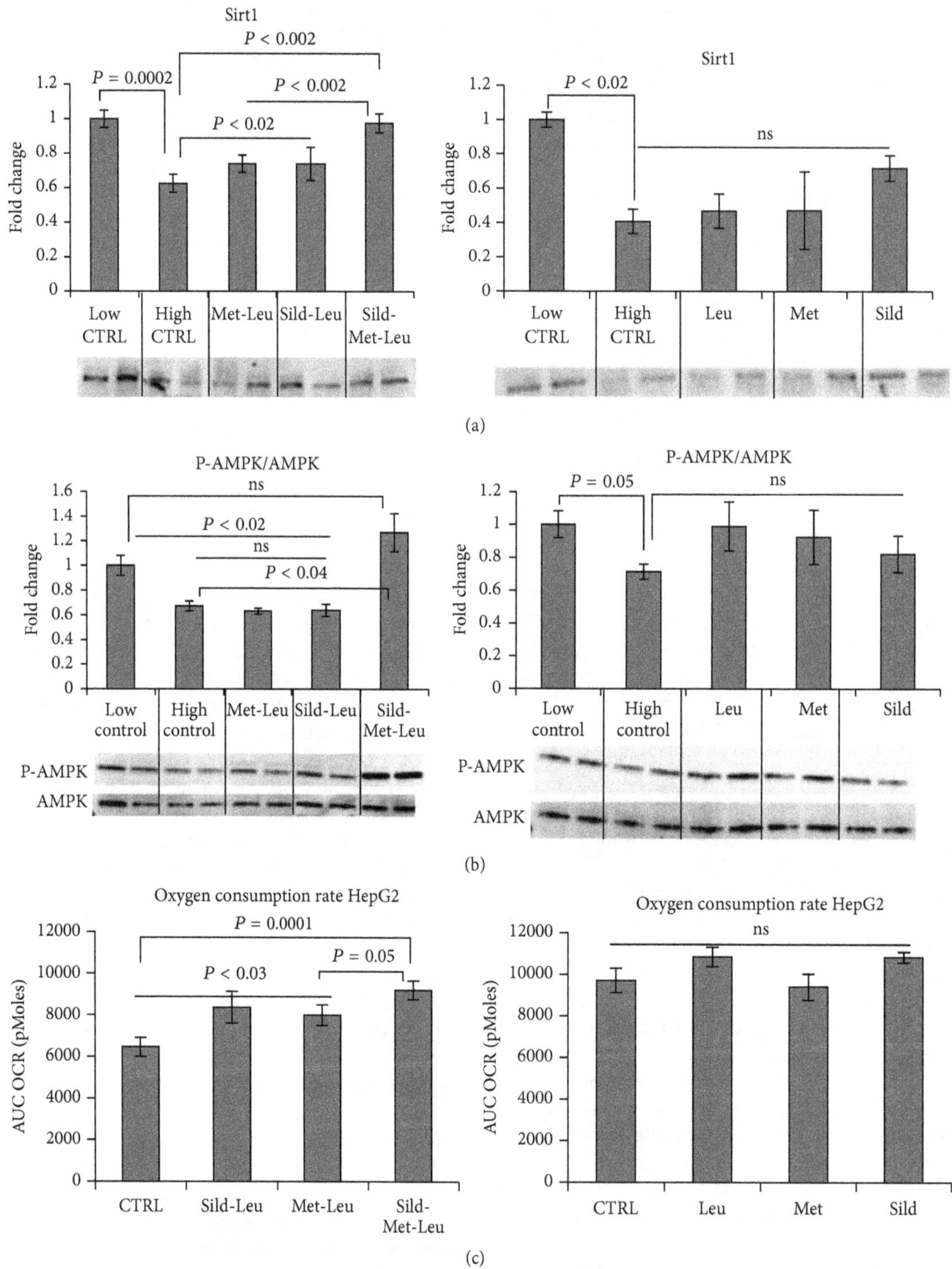

FIGURE 1: Sild-Met-Leu treatment in hepatocytes increases AMPK and Sirt1 activation and stimulates fatty acid oxidation. HepG2 cells were treated with sildenafil (Sild, 1 nM), metformin (Met, 0.1 mM), and leucine (Leu, 0.5 mM) as indicated for 24 hours after induction of lipid accumulation and compared to nontreated cells (control or CTRL high) after lipid accumulation and without lipid accumulation (CTRL low). (a) Sirt1 and (b) AMPK and phospho-AMPK protein expression was measured via Western blotting. Representative blots are shown. Data from repeated experiments are analyzed and presented as mean ± SEM (n = 2 to 8). (c) Oxygen consumption rate (OCR) after 200 μM palmitate injection was measured and the area under the curve (AUC) was calculated. Data are represented as mean ± SEM (n = 5).

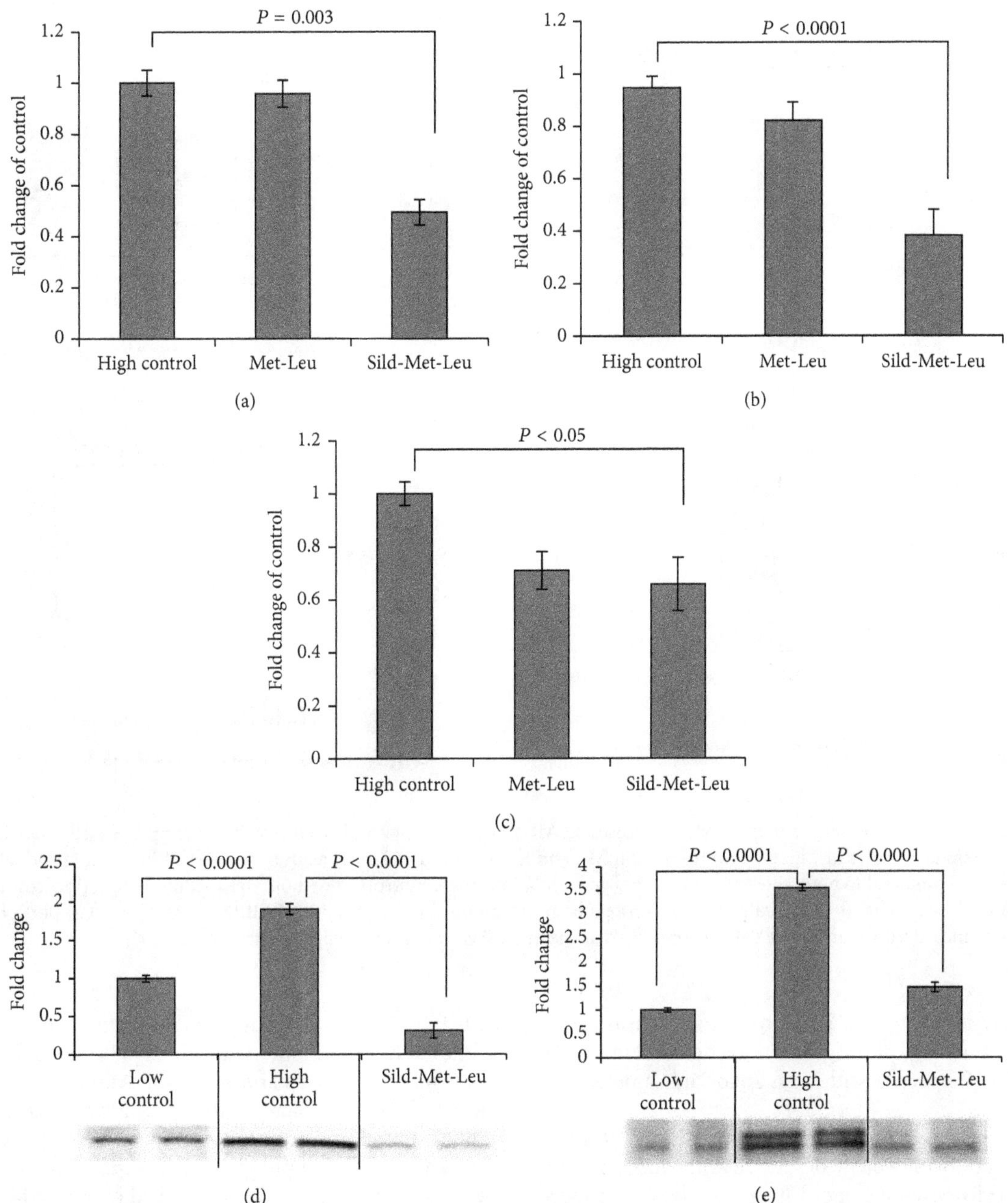

FIGURE 2: Sild-Met-Leu treatment in hepatocytes decreases lipogenic gene expression. HepG2 cells were treated with sildenafil (Sild, 1 nM), metformin (Met, 0.1 mM), and leucine (Leu, 0.5 mM) as indicated for 24 hours after induction of lipid accumulation and compared to nontreated cells after lipid accumulation (high control) or without lipid accumulation (low control). (a) Fatty acid synthase (FAS), (b) stearoyl-coenzyme A desaturase 1 (SCD1), and (c) acetyl-coenzyme A carboxylase 1 alpha (ACC 1 alpha) gene expression were measured. Data are presented as mean ± SEM ($n = 8$ to 12). ((d) and (e)) Protein expression of FAS and SCD1: quantitative data, presented as mean ± SEM, and representative blots are shown ($n = 4$).

Animals were housed in polypropylene cages at a room temperature of 22°C and a 12 h light/dark cycle. The animals had free access to water and their experimental food throughout the experiment. Body weight was measured every week. At the end of the treatment period (6 weeks) all animals were humanely euthanized with CO_2 inhalation. Blood was collected via trunk bleed and tissues were collected for further experiments as described below.

This study and all animal procedures were performed under the auspices of Institutional Animal Care and Use Committee-Approved protocol of the Georgia State University and in accordance with PHS policy and recommendations of the Guide.

2.7. Liver Histology. Liver tissues were fixed in 10% neutral formalin, embedded in paraffin, and cut into 5 μm sections.

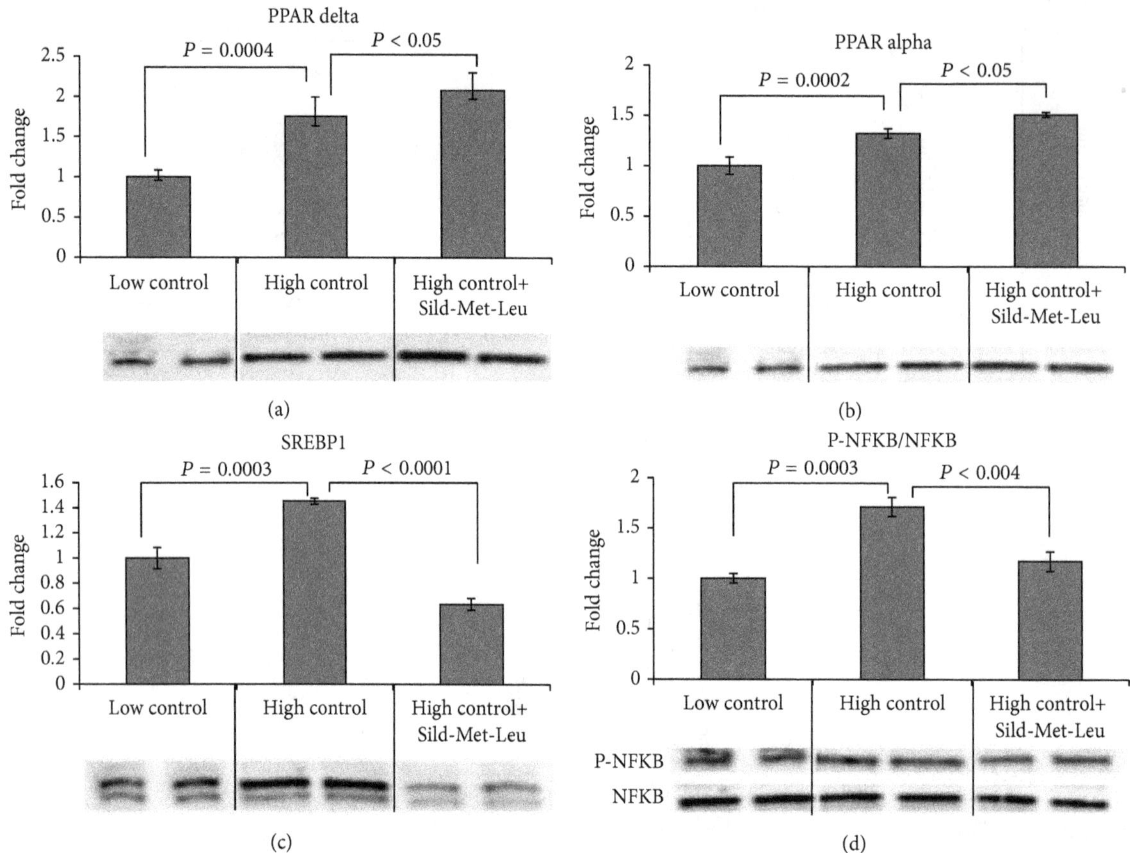

FIGURE 3: Sild-Met-Leu treatment in hepatocytes increases PPAR alpha and delta and decreases SREBP1 and NF-κB. HepG2 cells were treated with sildenafil (Sild, 1 nM), metformin (Met, 0.1 mM), and leucine (Leu, 0.5 mM) as indicated for 24 hours after induction of lipid accumulation and compared to nontreated cells after lipid accumulation (high control) or without lipid accumulation (low control). Protein expression of (a) PPAR delta, (b) PPAR alpha, (c) sterol regulatory element-binding protein (SREBP) 1, and (d) ratio of phosphorylated to total NF-κB was measured. Quantitative data are presented as mean ± SEM ($n = 4$) and representative blots are shown.

Sections were processed for hematoxylin and eosin (H&E) staining and histological images were recorded using Nikon Eclipse E800 Microscopy with Zeiss AxioCam camera.

2.8. Liver Triglyceride Measurements. Liver lipid extraction was conducted as previously described with minor modifications [23]. Briefly, ~100 mg of liver was thawed, minced, and weighted in glass tube. Lipids were extracted in 2 : 1 $CHCl_3$/methanol at room temperature overnight. The lipid portion was then dried down under N_2 and redissolved in a measured volume of 2 : 1 $CHCl_3$/methanol. Diluted H2SO4 was added to the sample, which was then vortexed and centrifuged to split the phases. The aqueous upper phase was aspirated and discarded, and an aliquot of the bottom phase was dried down and dissolved in 2% Triton X-100. The triglyceride content was then measured using TG kit/L-Type TG M (Wako Chemicals, USA) and normalized to liver weight.

2.9. ALT Measurement. Serum ALT levels were measured in fed mice after 4 weeks of diet treatment using a mouse ALT ELISA kit from BioVision.

2.10. Liver CD68 and Collagen Staining. Liver tissues were fixed in 10% neutral formalin, embedded in paraffin, and cut into 5 μm sections. For inflammation immunostaining, slides were immunoblotted with CD68 (Bio-Rad MCA 1957) as primary antibody and Biotin-SP-AffiniPure Mouse Anti-Rat IgG as secondary antibody. This was followed by the application of the immunoperoxidase technique with a Vector kit. Areas of staining were quantified with ImageJ and expressed as percentages of the field area. For fibrosis Picro Sirius Red staining, liver slides were dewaxed and hydrated, Weigert's hematoxylin stained for 8 minutes, and Picro-Sirius Red (Picro Sirius Red Stain Kit, Abcam, Cat # ab150681) stained for one hour. Acidified water wash was applied. Slides were dehydrated in three changes of 100% ethanol and cleared in xylene and mounted in a resinous medium. All of the histological images were recorded using Nikon Eclipse E800 Microscopy with Zeiss AxioCam camera. Areas of staining were quantified with ImageJ and expressed as percentages of the field area.

2.11. Gene Expression

2.11.1. In Vitro Data. Cells were grown in a 96-well plate. Cell Lysis, reverse transcription, and RT-PCR were performed using the TaqMan® Gene Expression Cells-to C_T™ Kit (Life Technologies, Cat # 4399002) according to manufacturer's instructions. Gene expression was assessed by RT-PCR using

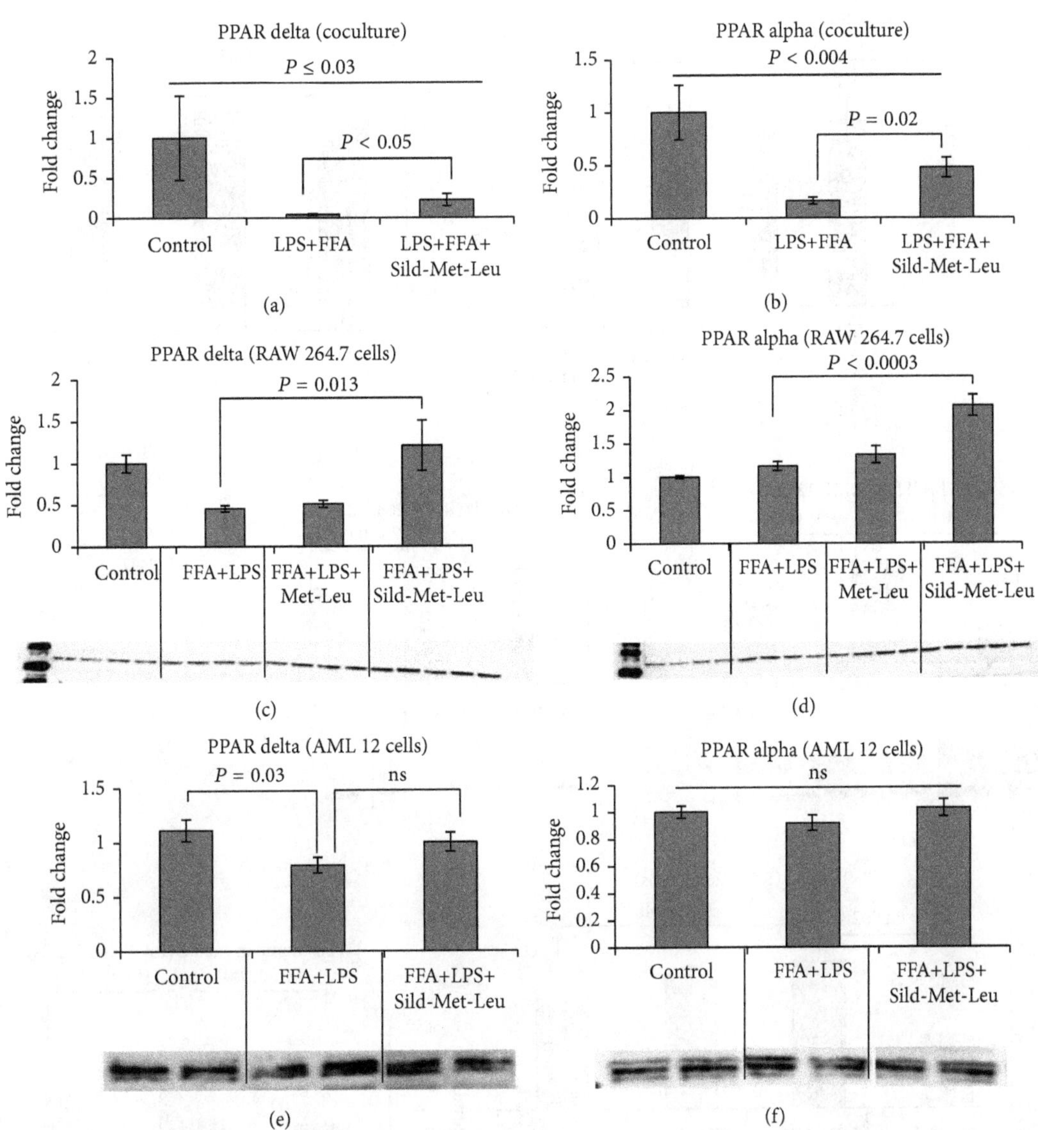

FIGURE 4: Sild-Met-Leu treatment increases PPAR alpha and delta in mouse hepatocyte-macrophage coculture. Mouse hepatocytes and macrophages, grown individually or in coculture, were treated with sildenafil (1 nM), metformin (0.1 mM), and leucine (0.5 mM) as indicated for 24 hours after induction with free fatty acids (FFA) and LPS. Nontreated cells with induction with FFA and LPS (FFA + LPS) or without (control) were included for comparison. ((a) and (b)) Gene expression of PPAR alpha and delta in hepatocyte-macrophage coculture. Data are represented as mean ± SEM of fold change of control ($n = 6$ to 8). ((c) to (f)) Protein expression of PPAR alpha and delta in RAW 264.7 macrophages and in in AML 12 hepatocytes. Quantitative data are presented as mean ± SEM ($n = 4$ to 5), and representative blots are shown.

StepOnePlus™ PCR system (Thermo Fisher Scientific) and TaqMan Gene expression assays for AMPK (Life Technologies, Cat # Mm01264789) and Sirt1 (Life Technologies, Cat # Mm01168521).

2.11.2. In Vivo Data. Total RNA from liver was extracted using the Tri-Reagent kit (Molecular Research Center, Cincinnati, OH) and gene expression was assessed by quantitative reverse transcription- (RT-) PCR (ABI Universal PCR Master Mix, Applied Biosystems, Foster City, CA) using a Stratagene Mx3000p thermocycler (Stratagene, La Jolla, CA). Cyclophilin was used to normalize the gene expression data. The primer and probe sets used in the assays were purchased from Applied Biosystems/Life Technologies (Grand Island, NY).

2.12. Statistical Analysis. All data are expressed as mean ± SEM. Data were analyzed by one-way ANOVA, and significantly different group means ($P < 0.05$) were separated by the least significant difference test using GraphPad Prism version 6 (GraphPad Software, La Jolla, California, USA, www.graphpad.com).

3. Results

Based on our previous results *in vitro* and *in vivo* showing interacting effects of leucine with either low dose metformin

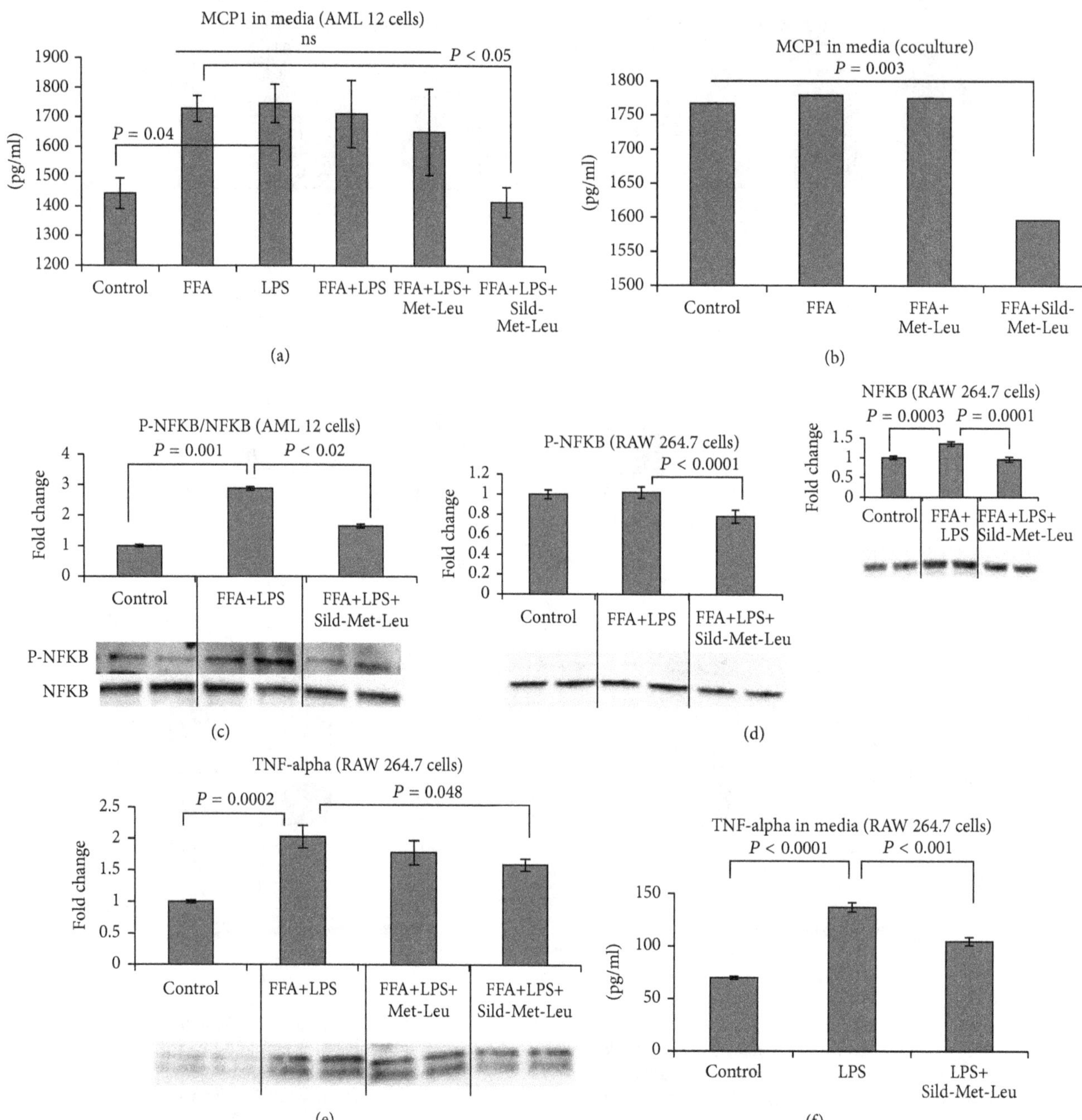

FIGURE 5: Sild-Met-Leu treatment decreases inflammatory marker in hepatocytes and macrophages. Mouse hepatocytes (AML cells) and macrophages (RAW 264.7 cells), grown individually or in coculture, were treated with sildenafil (1 nM), metformin (0.1 mM), and leucine (0.5 mM) as indicated for 24 hours after induction with free fatty acids (FFA) and/or LPS. Nontreated cells (control) were included for comparison. ((a) and (b)) Monocyte chemotactic protein- (MCP-) 1 secretion in media of AML cells and of hepatocyte-macrophage coculture. Data are presented as mean ± SEM ($n = 4$ to 10). ((c) to (e)) Protein expression of phosphorylated and total NF-κB and TNF-alpha in AML 12 hepatocytes and RAW 264.7 macrophages. Quantitative data are presented as mean ± SEM ($n = 4$), and representative blots are shown. (f) Macrophage tumor necrosis factor- (TNF-) alpha secretion was measured in the media. Data are presented as mean ± SEM ($n = 5$).

or with PDE5 inhibitors (icariin, sildenafil) on hepatic lipid metabolism, we tested in this study the three-way interaction of leucine, metformin, and sildenafil. As expected, incubation of HepG2 cells with high glucose (25 mM) medium for 48 hours caused significant downregulation of the AMPK/Sirt signaling. This was completely reversed by the three-way combination Sild-Met-Leu while the two-way combinations Met-Leu and Sild-Leu exerted a significant smaller effect (Figures 1(a) and 1(b)). The individual components had no effects. Accordingly, the palmitate-induced oxygen consumption rate in HepG2 cells, measured as a downstream effect of Sirtl/AMPK activation, was significantly increased by the three-way combination. This effect was greater than that exerted by the two-way combinations or by the individual

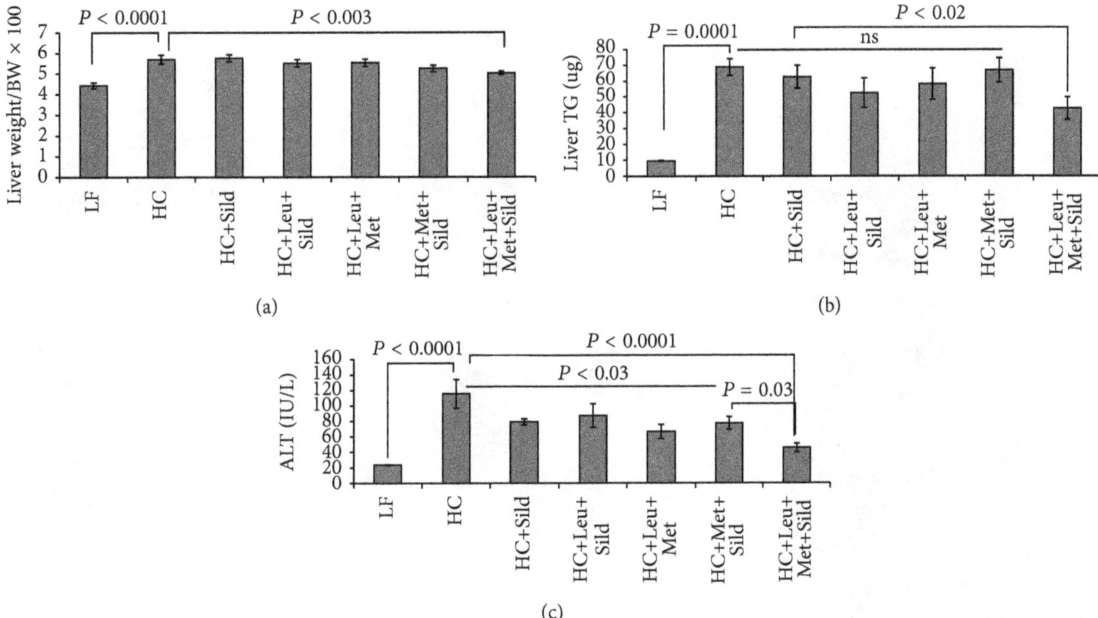

Figure 6: Sild-Met-Leu effects on liver weight, liver triglycerides, and ALT in mice. Mice were fed a low-fat (LF) diet or high-fat atherogenic (HC) diet for 6 weeks and then randomized to the indicated treatment groups for an additional 6 weeks. (a) Liver weight (expressed as ratio to total body weight), (b) liver triglycerides, and (c) alanine aminotransferase (ALT) were determined at the end of the study. Data are expressed as mean ± SEM (n = 5 to 8). Sild: sildenafil, Met: metformin, Leu: leucine.

compounds, which had no effect (Figure 1(c)). In addition, gene and protein expressions of lipogenic enzymes (FAS, SCD1 and ACC alpha), which were 2- to 3-fold upregulated after incubation with high glucose medium, were significantly suppressed by Sild-Met-Leu (Figure 2). In addition, the high glucose induced increase of SREBP1, a key transcription factor for lipid synthesis, was reversed by Sild-Met-Leu (Figure 3(c)). In contrast, PPAR alpha and delta, transcription factors regulating fatty acid oxidation, were augmented by Sild-Met-Leu (Figures 3(a) and 3(b)). Moreover, Sild-Met-Leu treatment reduced significantly the ratio of phospho-NF-κB to NF-κB, indicating a reduced inflammatory response (Figure 3(d)).

Next we tested whether these effects could be repeated using a different induction scheme and a different hepatocyte cell line. Induction of lipid accumulation with FFA and LPS had similar effects on Sirt1 and AMPK signaling in HepG2 cells as treatment with high glucose (data not shown). Also, treatment with Sild-Met-Leu increased Sirt1 protein expression in mouse AML-12 hepatocytes and reduced lipogenic protein expression of SREBP1, SCD1, and FAS similar to our observations in HepG2 cells (data not shown). These treatment effects were not caused by significant changes in cell viability (data not shown).

Since the activation of macrophages plays an important role in the pathogenesis of NASH, we used mouse hepatocytes (AML 12 cells) and mouse macrophages (RAW 264.7 cells) as an *in vitro* model of NASH. To induce lipid accumulation and an inflammatory response, cells were grown individually or in coculture and stimulated with free fatty acids (oleic/palmitic acid mixture) and/or LPS. Stimulation with LPS and FFA reduced both PPAR alpha and delta in coculture (Figures 4(a) and 4(b)) and treatment with Sild-Met-Leu reversed this effect. Sild-Met-Leu also increased PPAR alpha and delta in macrophages (Figures 4(c) and 4(d)), while there was only a trend (27% increase) for PPAR delta and no effect on PPAR alpha (Figures 4(e) and 4(f)) in AML 12 cells. Secretion of the inflammatory mediator MCP-1 was increased after stimulation of cells with FFA only, LPS only, or the combination FFA and LPS. Sild-Met-Leu completely reversed this effect in AML 12 cells and AML/RAW coculture (Figures 5(a) and 5(b)). Sild-Met-Leu also reduced the ratio of phospho-NF-κB/total NF-κB in AML 12 cells to normal control levels. However, the ratio was not changed in RAW macrophages, since Sild-Met-Leu reduced both, total and phospho-NF-κB (Figures 5(c) and 5(d)). In addition, FFA and LPS induced TNF α secretion and protein expression was significantly decreased by Sild-Met-Leu in RAW macrophages (Figures 5(e) and 5(f)).

Based on the *in vitro* data, we assessed the *in vivo* effects of Sild-Met-Leu in comparison with Met-Leu, Met-Sild and Sild-Leu in a NASH mouse model. Feeding of a high-fat atherogenic diet (HC) increased liver weight, liver triglycerides, and ALT levels (sixfold), indicating significant hepatocellular injury, while treatment with the Sild-Met-Leu combination significantly blunted these effects. Although the two-way combinations and sildenafil by itself had some effect on ALT levels, the three-way combination exerted a significantly greater effect in comparison with all other groups (Figure 6). Histology staining confirmed a pronounced increase in lipid droplets and ballooned hepatocytes induced by HC diet compared with low-fat diet control. While the two-way combinations attenuated these effects, the triple combination Sild-Met-Leu substantially reversed the

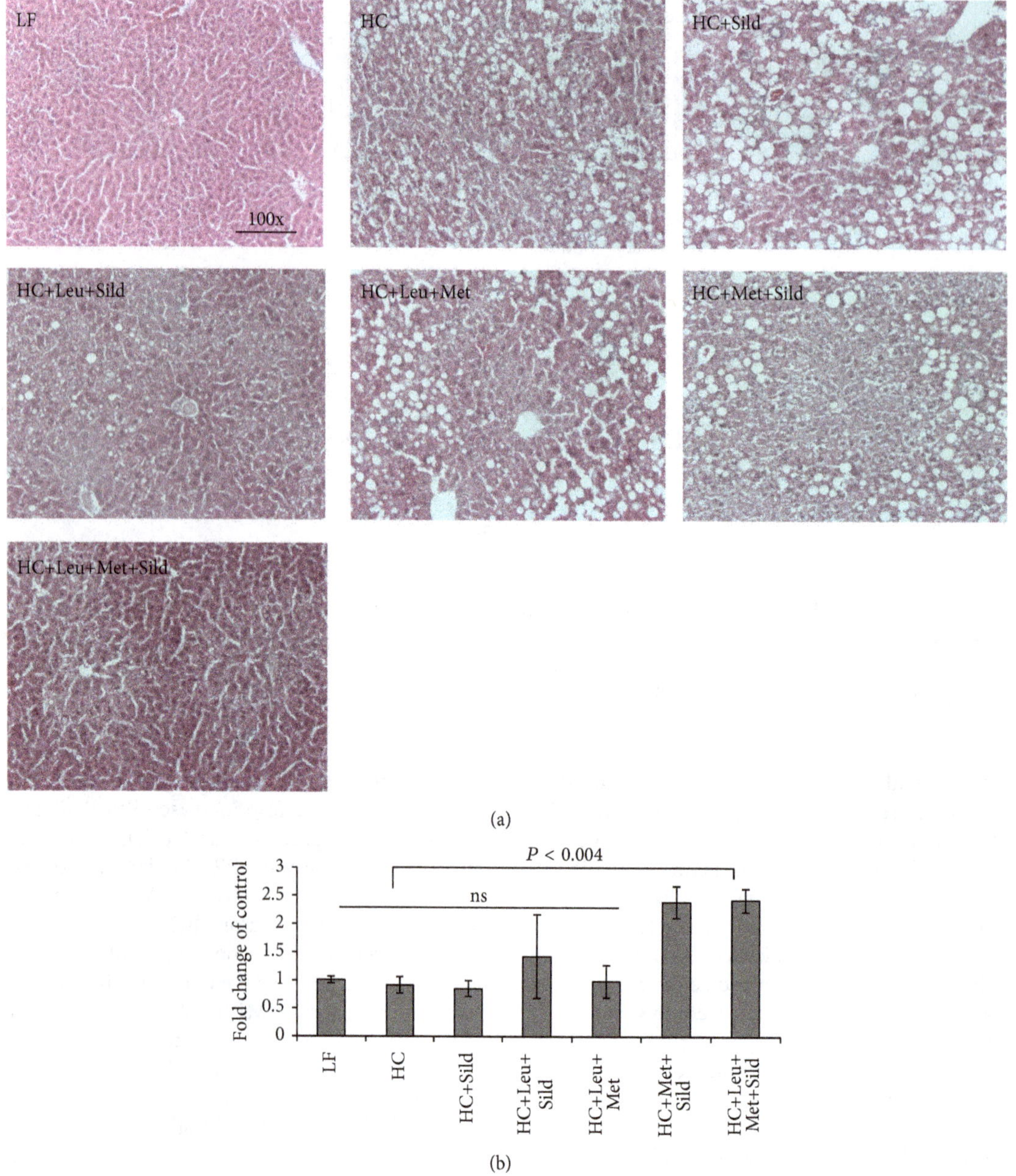

FIGURE 7: Sild-Met-Leu effects on liver histology in mice. Mice were fed a low-fat (LF) diet or high-fat atherogenic (HC) diet for 6 weeks and then randomized to the indicated treatment groups for an additional 6 weeks. (a) Liver sections were stained with hematoxylin and eosin (H&E) at the end of the study. Representative images for each group are shown. (b) PPAR alpha gene expression in liver extracts was measured and expressed as mean ± SEM of fold change of control ($n = 6$). Sild: sildenafil, Met: metformin, Leu: leucine.

steatohepatitis (Figure 7(a)). Moreover, both Met-Leu and Sild-Met-Leu increased PPAR alpha expression in the liver twofold (Figure 7(b)), consistent with activation of hepatic fatty acid oxidation. To assess the level of inflammation in the liver, sections of liver were stained with CD68. The HC diet caused a sixfold increase of CD68 staining in the liver sections, representing a substantial increase in Kupffer cell activation (Figure 8). All two-way combinations significantly attenuated this effect, while only the three-way combination fully reversed it to levels not significantly different from low-fat fed animals (Figure 8). Consistent with this, inflammatory markers such as IL1 beta, TNF-alpha, MCP-1, and PAI-1 were reduced to normal levels by Sild-Met-Leu, but not by the two-way combinations (Figure 9). Next, we assessed fibrosis in liver sections via Sirius Red staining. The increase in fibrotic changes induced by the HC diet was substantially reversed by Sild-Met-Leu and to a lesser degree by the two-way combinations (Figure 10). In accordance with this, gene expressions of the fibrotic markers Col1a1, Col1a2, Col4a1, and TGF-beta were decreased to normal levels by Sild-Met-Leu but only partly reduced by Met-Leu and Sild-Met (Figure 11).

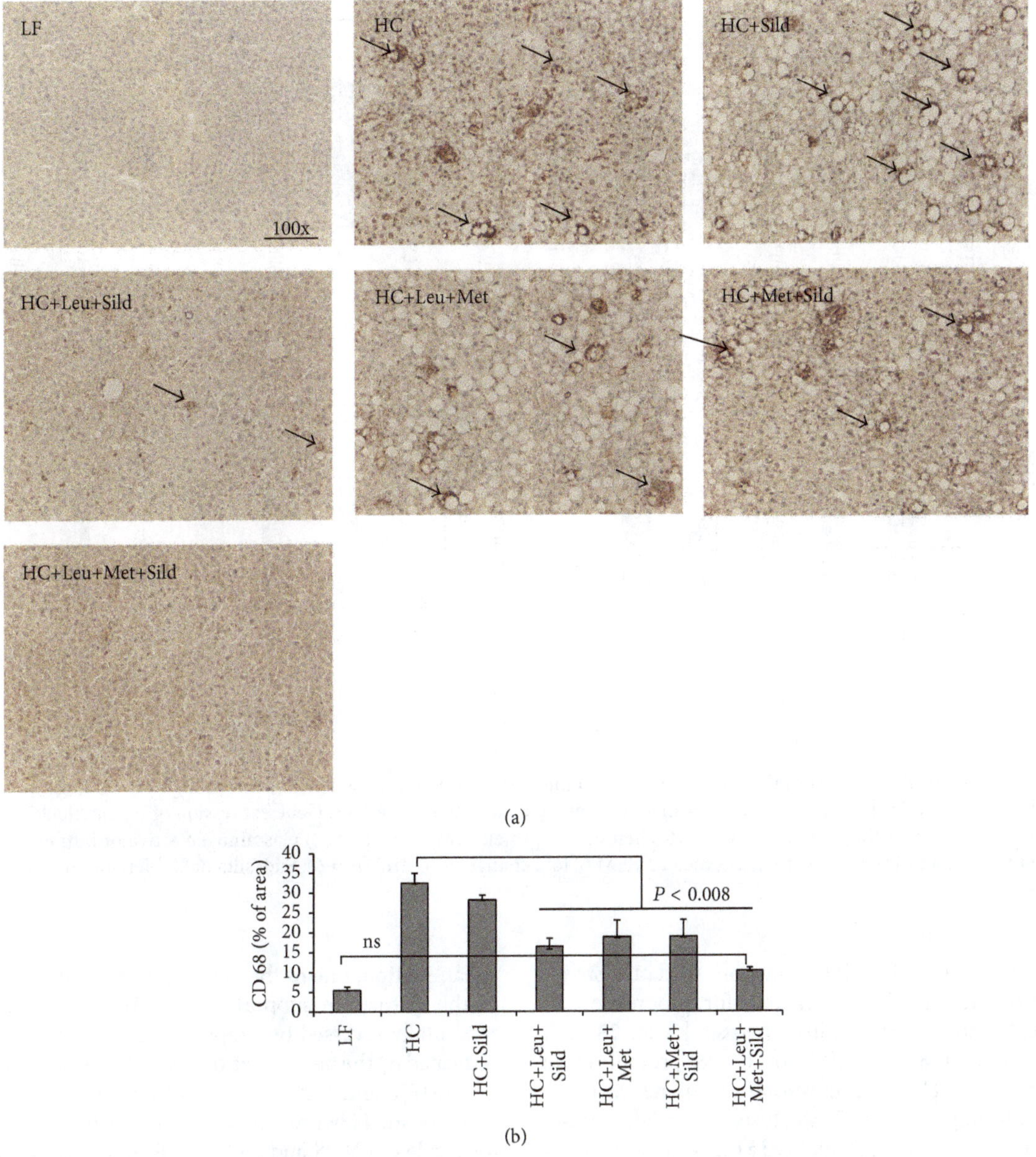

FIGURE 8: Sild-Met-Leu effects on liver Kupffer cell activation in mice. Mice were fed a low-fat (LF) diet or high-fat atherogenic (HC) diet for 6 weeks and then randomized to the indicated treatment groups for an additional 6 weeks. (a) Liver sections were stained with anti-CD68 antibody at the end of the study ($n = 2$). Representative images for each group are shown. (b) Quantitation of CD68 staining, calculated as % of the examined area. Data are expressed as mean ± SEM ($n = 2$). Sild: sildenafil, Met: metformin, Leu: leucine.

4. Discussion

Our data indicate that the triple combination of leucine, metformin, and sildenafil substantially regresses hepatic steatosis, inflammation, and fibrosis and exerts greater effects than the two-way combination, suggesting that this combination may provide a new therapeutic approach to treat NASH.

The pathophysiology of the development of NASH is thought to be a "multihit process," where multiple environmental, dietary, and genetic factors interact with others [24]. The accumulation of excess lipids in the liver is considered the first step and the prerequisite for subsequent events, which causes progression from simple steatosis to the severe form of NASH in about 30% of patients with NAFLD. Among the other factors contributing to the progression of NASH, inflammation plays an important role [25]. Chronic injury to hepatocytes or hepatocyte death due to excess free fatty acid influx leads to activation of resident macrophages (Kupffer cells) as well as other infiltrating monocytes and macrophages to release proinflammatory cytokines, including TNF-α, IL-1 beta, and IL-6, and profibrogenic factors such as TGF-β which in turn results in activation of hepatic stellate cells and fibrosis progression [26, 27].

The three-way combination Leu-Met-Sild targets the AMPK-Sirt1-eNOS network, as depicted in Figure 12. AMPK, Sirt1, and eNOS are key regulators of hepatic energy and

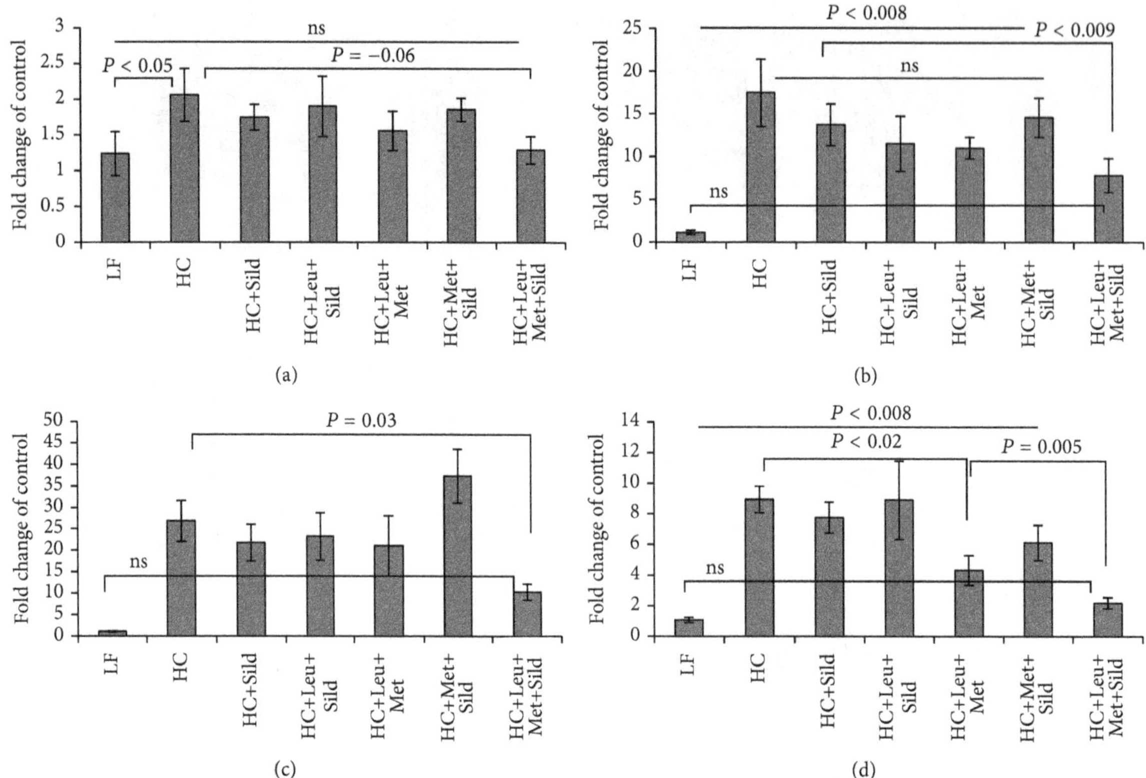

Figure 9: Sild-Met-Leu effects on liver inflammatory marker in mice. Mice were fed a low-fat (LF) diet or high-fat atherogenic (HC) diet for 6 weeks and then randomized to the indicated treatment groups for an additional 6 weeks. Gene expression of (a) interleukin- (IL-) 1 beta, (b) tumor necrosis factor- (TNF-) alpha, (c) monocyte chemotactic protein- (MCP-) 1, and (d) plasminogen activator inhibitor- (PAI-) 1 was measured in liver extracts. Data are expressed as mean ± SEM of fold change of control ($n = 6$). Sild: sildenafil, Met: metformin, Leu: leucine.

lipid metabolism, as well as inflammation, oxidative stress, and cell proliferation, the key factors for progression of simple NAFLD to NASH and liver fibrosis [2, 14, 28, 29]. Downregulation of Sirt, AMPK, or eNOS promotes the progression of NASH, while activation of this network has been shown to improve hepatic steatosis and inflammation. For example, eNOS-knockout mice fed a high-fat diet showed more extensive hepatic lipid accumulation and inflammation than wild-type mice [30] and resveratrol treatment, a known Sirt1 and AMPK activator, prevented and reversed lipid accumulation, oxidative stress, and inflammation *in vitro* and *in vivo* [31, 32]. We found the triple combination Sild-Met-Leu to upregulate AMPK and Sirt1 and to increase palmitate-stimulated oxygen consumption and decrease the expression of lipogenic genes such as FAS, ACC, and SCD1 in HepG2 cells. Moreover, treatment with Sild-Met-Leu lowered liver triglycerides and reversed the HFD-induced steatosis in mice, the prerequisite condition for developing NASH. In addition, we show a reduction of inflammatory markers *in vitro* and *in vivo* as well as a normalization of the CD68 staining in liver samples, a marker expressed by monocytes and macrophages. This was also repeated for F4/80 marker in a follow-up mouse study (data not shown), in which F4/80 was reduced by 40% by Sild-Met-Leu feeding to levels not statistically different from the control low-fat fed animals. Therefore, the triple combination also significantly improves inflammation, one of the key factors for driving progression of the disease. In support of this, the HC-induced fibrosis was totally reversed by supplementation with Sild-Met-Leu, indicated by the percentage of Sirius Red positive area in liver.

AMPK and Sirt1 are well-known regulators of hepatic metabolism. However, there is an increasing body of evidence for a role of eNOS and NO/cGMP signaling in the development of hepatic steatosis, inflammation, and progression to fibrosis [14, 30]. The liver is a highly vascularized tissue and eNOS-derived NO from sinusoidal endothelial cells (SEC) regulate vascular resistance, proliferation, and migration, as well as exerting paracrine effects on adjacent stellate cells. As the first cells exposed to portal vein components and bacterially derived lipopolysaccharides (LPS) from the gut, SECs can undergo dramatic phenotype changes and can induce inflammation and stellate cell activation [33]. eNOS is constitutively expressed in SEC and NO plays a crucial role in maintaining physiological phenotypes of SECs and stellate cells [14, 34]. NAFLD is associated with decreased eNOS activation [35]. Moreover, endothelial dysfunction and reduced NO production have been found to precede inflammation and fibrosis in a NAFLD rat model [13]. In contrast, activation of eNOS as well as increased NO production ameliorates the progression of NASH-related hepatic fibrosis [36, 37]. We previously demonstrated the amplifying effects of the Met-Leu combination on AMPK signaling and

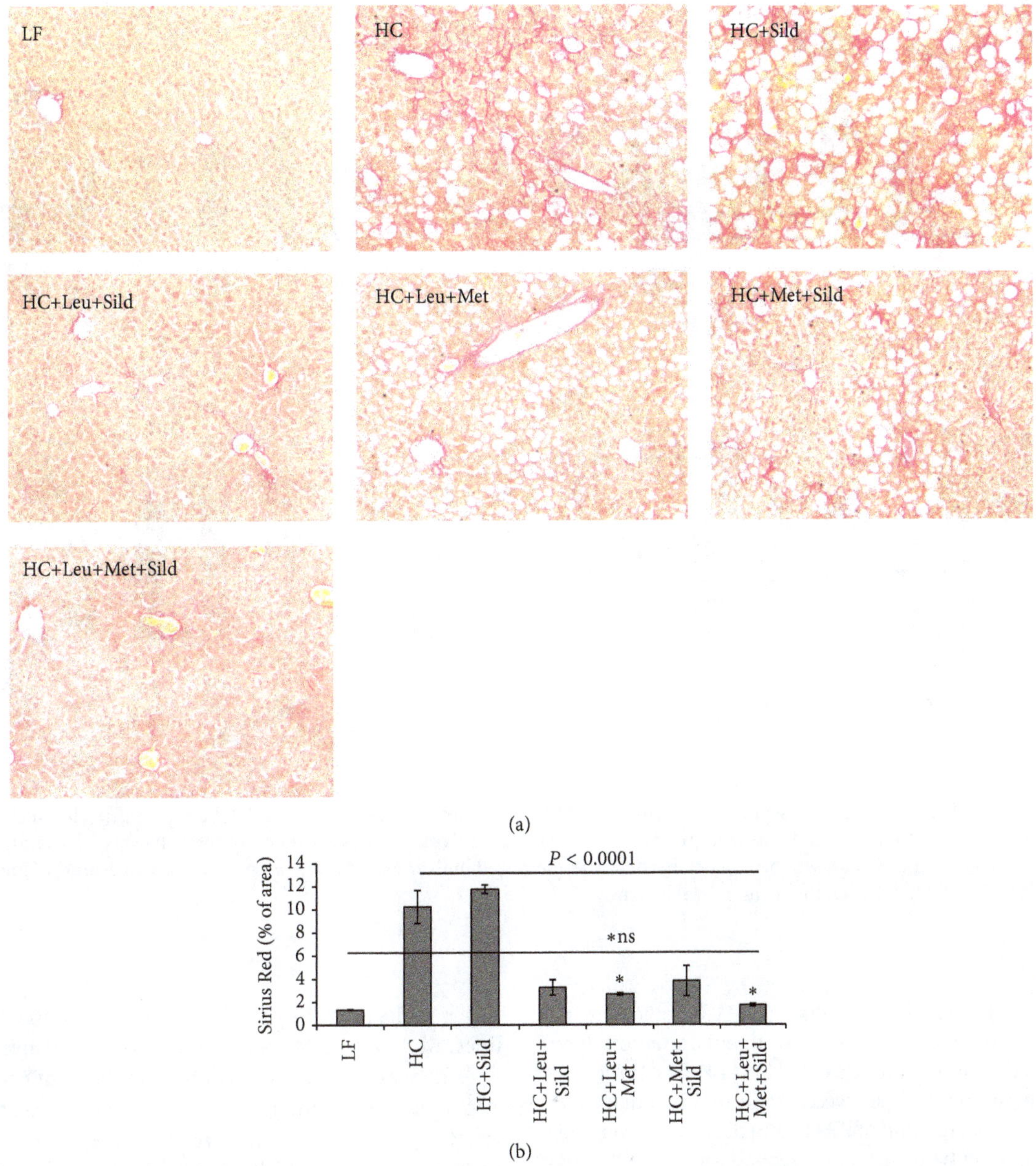

FIGURE 10: Met-Leu effects on hepatic fibrosis in mice. Mice were fed a low-fat (LF) diet or high-fat atherogenic (HC) diet for 6 weeks and then randomized to the indicated treatment groups for an additional 6 weeks. (a) Liver sections were stained with Picro Sirius Red for collagen at the end of the study ($n = 3$). Representative images for each group are shown. (b) Quantitation of Picro Sirius Red staining, calculated as % of the examined area. Data are expressed as mean ± SEM ($n = 3$). Sild: sildenafil, Met: metformin, and Leu: leucine. * indicates groups which are not significantly different from LF.

reduction of hepatic steatosis in DIO-mice [12]. Similarly, leucine with PDE5 inhibitors (sildenafil, icariin) increased fat metabolism and reduced hepatic lipid accumulation in DIO-mice which was associated with increased NO production in addition to AMPK/Sirt1 activation, indicating that the actions of the PDE5 inhibitors converge on this pathway [8, 22]. In this study, we demonstrate that the Sild-Met-Leu combination exerts greater effects on inflammatory and fibrogenic parameters than the Met-Leu or the Sild-Leu combination, suggesting that the stimulation of eNOS/NO/cGMP pathway may contribute to additional effects on the AMPK/Sirt1 signaling.

The peroxisome proliferator-activated receptors- (PPAR-) alpha and delta are transcription factors finely regulating energetic fluxes and metabolic pathways [38]. PPAR-α is highly expressed in liver and regulates the rates of fatty acid catabolism and lipogenesis in response to nutritional demands. PPAR-α deficient mice develop more severe hepatic steatosis, inflammation, and NASH when fed a HFD compared to wild-type mice [39, 40], while administration of the PPAR-α agonists reverses hepatic steatosis and fibrosis [41, 42]. PPAR-δ is constitutively expressed and regulates β-oxidation in muscle. In the liver, it controls hepatic glucose and lipoprotein metabolism and exerts anti-inflammatory

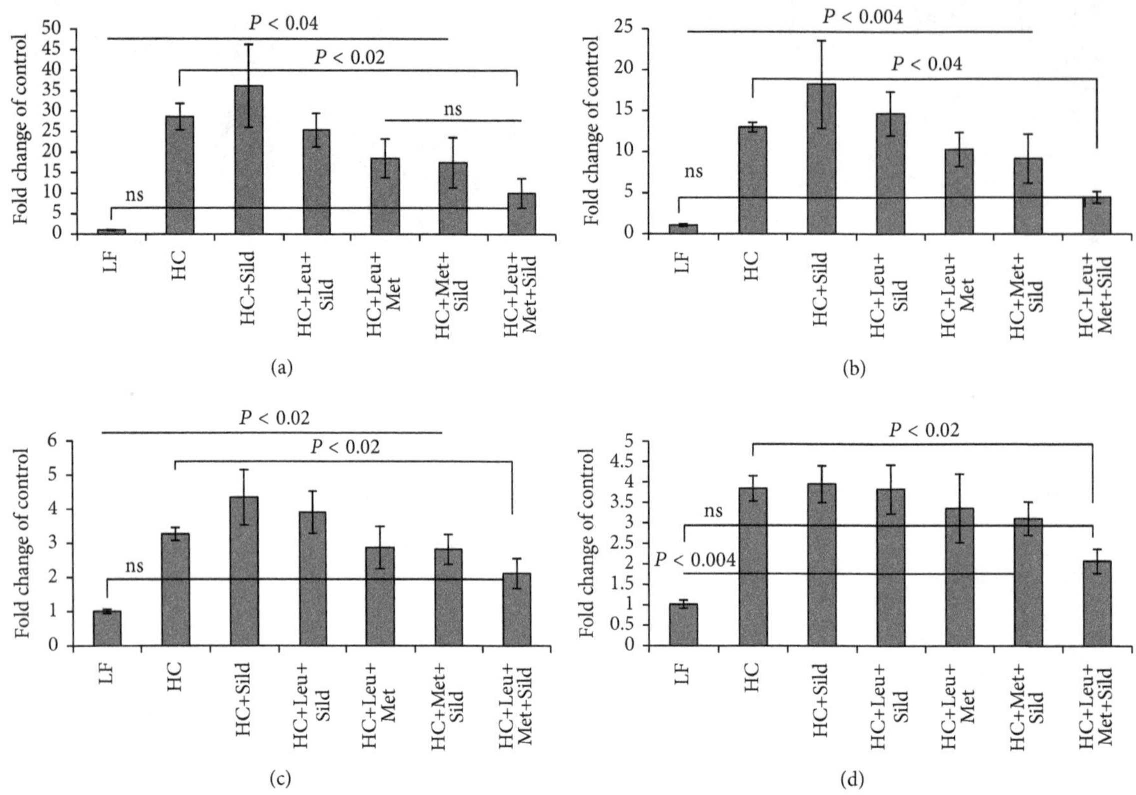

FIGURE 11: Sild-Met-Leu effects on fibrosis marker in mice. Mice were fed a low-fat (LF) diet or high-fat atherogenic (HC) diet for 6 weeks and then randomized to the indicated treatment groups for an additional 6 weeks. Gene expression of the collagens (a) Col1a1, (b) Col1a2, (c) Col4a1, and (d) transforming growth factor- (TGF-) beta was measured in liver extracts and expressed as mean ± SEM of fold change of control ($n = 6$). Sild: sildenafil, Met: metformin, Leu: leucine.

effects [38, 43]. Beneficial effects of PPAR-δ agonists on improvement of hepatic steatosis and inflammation have been reported in mouse models of NASH [44]. The three-way combination in this study showed significant upregulation of PPAR-α and -δ *in vitro* and of PPAR-α in the mouse liver. This may be an indirect treatment effect secondary to AMPK/Sirt1 stimulation, since AMPK and Sirt1 interact with PPAR-α and -δ [6, 45, 46].

We recently demonstrated the efficacy of the Met-Leu combination and a combination of leucine with the PDE5 inhibitor icariin in reducing hepatic lipid accumulation and inflammation in a HFD-induced NAFLD mouse model [12, 22]. In this study, we used a high-fat atherogenic diet (60% fat, 1.25% cholesterol, and 0.5% cholate) to induce a more severe form of NASH, as this diet induces hepatic insulin resistance, progressive steatosis, inflammation, and fibrosis over 6 to 24 weeks, mimicking the human disease pathology [47]. The animals used in this study developed a significant steatosis with ~7-fold increase in liver triglycerides, hepatic inflammation, and fibrosis within the 12 weeks of study, which is comparable to other studies using this form of diet to induce NASH [48–50].

There are some limitations to this study. We used different forms of induction for the lipid accumulation in HepG2 (high glucose) and AML cells (high concentration of FFA), which limits the ability to compare results between these cell lines. Moreover, AML and RAW cells were stimulated with FFA, LPS, or a combination of both in different experiments, although we show in Figure 3(a) that there was a comparable effect. Finally, not all *in vitro* parameters were measured *in vivo* due to limited tissue availability and since we had demonstrated AMPK/Sirt1 activation already previously for the two-way combinations in mice studies [12, 22].

In summary, we demonstrate the beneficial effects of the three-way combination Sild-Met-Leu on the reversal of hepatic steatosis, inflammation, and fibrosis in a NASH mouse model and that all the three components are necessary for maximal effect. These effects are mediated by targeting the AMPK/Sirt1/eNOS network from multiple sites, each contributing a modest effect to the overall outcome, as summarized in Figure 12. This approach allows a substantial dose reduction of each individual compound to a concentration, which has little or no independent effect on the measured outcomes. Therefore, the risk of associated adverse effects of the individual compounds will be diminished. Based on the pivotal role of the AMPK/Sirt1/eNOS network in hepatic metabolism and the promising results of this animal study, the Sild-Met-Leu combination provides a new therapeutic approach to treat NAFLD and NASH.

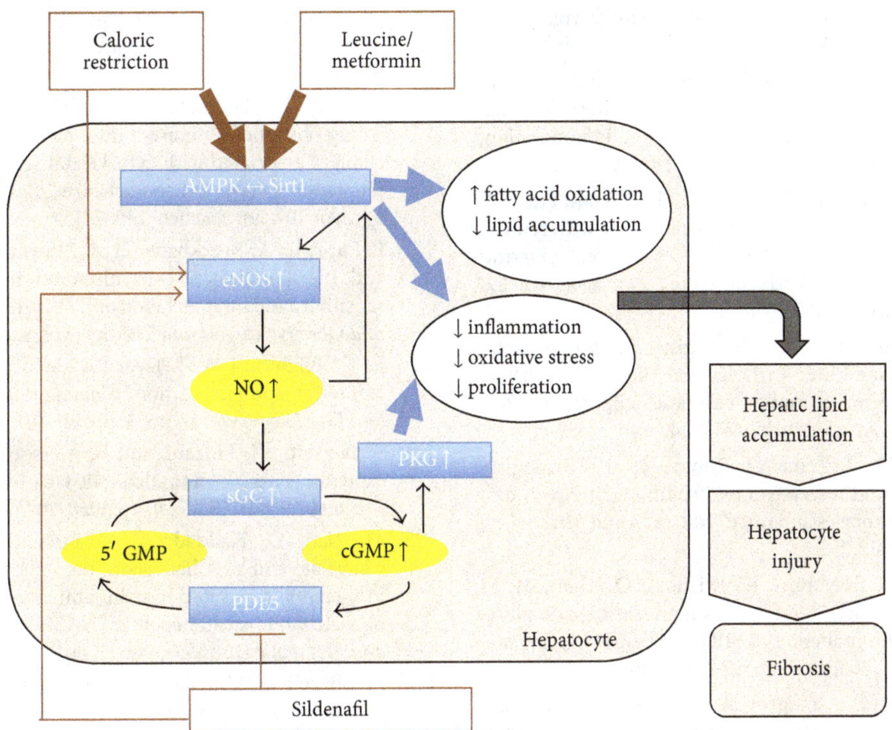

FIGURE 12: Proposed model of the interaction of leucine, metformin, and sildenafil on the AMPK/Sirtl/eNOS network. AMPK, Sirtl, and eNOS are nutrient sensors responsive to caloric restriction, regulating energy metabolism in an interacting network. In addition, they prevent inflammation and reduce oxidative stress and proliferation, the key factors for the progression of NAFLD to NASH. Leucine and metformin synergistically activate the AMPK/Sirtl pathway while sildenafil contributes to further stimulation through activation of eNOS. Moreover, sildenafil's inhibition of PDE5 results in concomitant activation of the cGMP-dependent protein kinases (PKGs). These integrated effects result in reduction of hepatic lipid accumulation, hepatic inflammation and injury, and subsequently reduction of fibrosis.

Abbreviations

eNOS: Endothelial nitric oxide synthase
NO: Nitric oxide
5′GMP: 5′Guanosine monophosphate
cGMP: Cyclic guanosine monophosphate
sGC: Soluble guanylate cyclase
PKGs: cGMP-dependent protein kinases
PDE5: Phosphodiesterase 5.

Disclosure

The funders had no role in data collection and analysis but were involved in study design, decision to publish, and preparation of the manuscript.

Competing Interests

Antje Bruckbauer, Jheelam Banerjee, and Michael B. Zemel are employees and stockholders of NuSirt Biopharma Inc. Antje Bruckbauer and Michael B. Zemel also have patents related to the reported work. All other authors have declared that no competing interests exist.

Acknowledgments

Financial support was provided by NuSirt Biopharma Inc. (http://nusirt.com). Bingzhong Xue and Hang Shi received funds from NuSirt Biopharma to conduct the animal study.

References

[1] A. J. Sanyal, E. M. Brunt, D. E. Kleiner et al., "Endpoints and clinical trial design for nonalcoholic steatohepatitis," *Hepatology*, vol. 54, no. 1, pp. 344–353, 2011.

[2] Y. Colak, O. Ozturk, E. Senates et al., "SIRT1 as a potential therapeutic target for treatment of nonalcoholic fatty liver disease," *Medical Science Monitor*, vol. 17, no. 5, pp. HY5–HY9, 2011.

[3] P. Dietrich and C. Hellerbrand, "Non-alcoholic fatty liver disease, obesity and the metabolic syndrome," *Best Practice & Research: Clinical Gastroenterology*, vol. 28, no. 4, pp. 637–653, 2014.

[4] Q. Lv, Q. Zhen, L. Liu et al., "AMP-kinase pathway is involved in tumor necrosis factor alpha-induced lipid accumulation in human hepatoma cells," *Life Sciences*, vol. 131, pp. 23–29, 2015.

[5] X. Hou, S. Xu, K. A. Maitland-Toolan et al., "SIRT1 regulates hepatocyte lipid metabolism through activating AMP-activated

protein kinase," *The Journal of Biological Chemistry*, vol. 283, no. 29, pp. 20015–20026, 2008.

[6] A. Purushotham, T. T. Schug, Q. Xu, S. Surapureddi, X. Guo, and X. Li, "Hepatocyte-specific deletion of SIRT1 alters fatty acid metabolism and results in hepatic steatosis and inflammation," *Cell Metabolism*, vol. 9, no. 4, pp. 327–338, 2009.

[7] Y. Yamazaki, I. Usui, Y. Kanatani et al., "Treatment with SRT1720, a SIRT1 activator, ameliorates fatty liver with reduced expression of lipogenic enzymes in MSG mice," *American Journal of Physiology—Endocrinology and Metabolism*, vol. 297, no. 5, pp. E1179–E1186, 2009.

[8] A. Bruckbauer and M. B. Zemel, "Synergistic effects of polyphenols and methylxanthines with leucine on AMPK/Sirtuin-mediated metabolism in muscle cells and adipocytes," *PLoS ONE*, vol. 9, no. 2, Article ID e89166, 2014.

[9] A. Bruckbauer, M. B. Zemel, T. Thorpe et al., "Synergistic effects of leucine and resveratrol on insulin sensitivity and fat metabolism in adipocytes and mice," *Nutrition and Metabolism*, vol. 9, article 77, 2012.

[10] P. W. Caton, N. K. Nayuni, J. Kieswich, N. Q. Khan, M. M. Yaqoob, and R. Corder, "Metformin suppresses hepatic gluconeogenesis through induction of SIRT1 and GCN5," *Journal of Endocrinology*, vol. 205, no. 1, pp. 97–106, 2010.

[11] W. Xu, Y.-Y. Deng, L. Yang et al., "Metformin ameliorates the proinflammatory state in patients with carotid artery atherosclerosis through sirtuin 1 induction," *Translational Research*, vol. 166, no. 5, pp. 451–458, 2015.

[12] L. Fu, A. Bruckbauer, F. Li et al., "Interaction between metformin and leucine in reducing hyperlipidemia and hepatic lipid accumulation in diet-induced obese mice," *Metabolism: Clinical and Experimental*, vol. 64, no. 11, pp. 1426–1434, 2015.

[13] M. Pasarín, V. La Mura, J. Gracia-Sancho et al., "Sinusoidal endothelial dysfunction precedes inflammation and fibrosis in a model of NAFLD," *PLoS ONE*, vol. 7, article e32785, 2012.

[14] S. Tateya, N. O. Rizzo, P. Handa et al., "Endothelial NO/cGMP/VASP signaling attenuates kupffer cell activation and hepatic insulin resistance induced by high-fat feeding," *Diabetes*, vol. 60, no. 11, pp. 2792–2801, 2011.

[15] U. Förstermann and W. C. Sessa, "Nitric oxide synthases: regulation and function," *European Heart Journal*, vol. 33, no. 7, pp. 829–837, 2012.

[16] S. G. Chrysant and G. S. Chrysant, "The pleiotropic effects of phosphodiesterase 5 inhibitors on function and safety in patients with cardiovascular disease and hypertension," *Journal of Clinical Hypertension*, vol. 14, no. 9, pp. 644–649, 2012.

[17] A. Das, D. Durrant, F. N. Salloum, L. Xi, and R. C. Kukreja, "PDE5 inhibitors as therapeutics for heart disease, diabetes and cancer," *Pharmacology and Therapeutics*, vol. 147, pp. 12–21, 2015.

[18] B. Musicki, T. J. Bivalacqua, H. C. Champion, and A. L. Burnett, "Sildenafil promotes eNOS activation and inhibits NADPH oxidase in the transgenic sickle cell mouse penis," *Journal of Sexual Medicine*, vol. 11, no. 2, pp. 424–430, 2014.

[19] I. Mattagajasingh, C.-S. Kim, A. Naqvi et al., "SIRT1 promotes endothelium-dependent vascular relaxation by activating endothelial nitric oxide synthase," *Proceedings of the National Academy of Sciences of the United States of America*, vol. 104, no. 37, pp. 14855–14860, 2007.

[20] S. Koka, H. S. Aluri, L. Xi, E. J. Lesnefsky, and R. C. Kukreja, "Chronic inhibition of phosphodiesterase 5 with tadalafil attenuates mitochondrial dysfunction in type 2 diabetic hearts: potential role of NO/SIRT1/PGC-1α signaling," *American Journal of Physiology—Heart and Circulatory Physiology*, vol. 306, no. 11, pp. H1558–H1568, 2014.

[21] S. Koka, L. Xi, and R. C. Kukreja, "Chronic treatment with long acting phosphodiesterase-5 inhibitor tadalafil alters proteomic changes associated with cytoskeletal rearrangement and redox regulation in Type 2 diabetic hearts," *Basic Research in Cardiology*, vol. 107, no. 2, article 249, 2012.

[22] L. Fu, F. Li, A. Bruckbauer et al., "Interaction between leucine and phosphodiesterase 5 inhibition in modulating insulin sensitivity and lipid metabolism," *Diabetes, Metabolic Syndrome and Obesity: Targets and Therapy*, vol. 8, pp. 227–239, 2015.

[23] E. G. Bligh and W. J. Dyer, "A rapid method of total lipid extraction and purification," *Canadian Journal of Biochemistry and Physiology*, vol. 37, no. 8, pp. 911–917, 1959.

[24] E. Buzzetti, M. Pinzani, and E. A. Tsochatzis, "The multiple-hit pathogenesis of non-alcoholic fatty liver disease (NAFLD)," *Metabolism*, vol. 65, no. 8, pp. 1038–1048, 2016.

[25] M. Nati, D. Haddad, A. L. Birkenfeld, C. A. Koch, T. Chavakis, and A. Chatzigeorgiou, "The role of immune cells in metabolism-related liver inflammation and development of non-alcoholic steatohepatitis (NASH)," *Reviews in Endocrine and Metabolic Disorders*, vol. 17, no. 1, pp. 29–39, 2016.

[26] M. Sharma, S. Mitnala, R. K. Vishnubhotla, R. Mukherjee, D. N. Reddy, and P. N. Rao, "The riddle of nonalcoholic fatty liver disease: progression from nonalcoholic fatty liver to non-alcoholic steatohepatitis," *Journal of Clinical and Experimental Hepatology*, vol. 5, no. 2, pp. 147–158, 2015.

[27] C. Trautwein, S. L. Friedman, D. Schuppan, and M. Pinzani, "Hepatic fibrosis: concept to treatment," *Journal of Hepatology*, vol. 62, no. 1, pp. S15–S24, 2015.

[28] Z. Yang, B. B. Kahn, H. Shi, and B.-Z. Xue, "Macrophage α1 AMP-activated protein kinase (α1AMPK) antagonizes fatty acid-induced inflammation through SIRT1," *The Journal of Biological Chemistry*, vol. 285, no. 25, pp. 19051–19059, 2010.

[29] J. Xie, X. Zhang, and L. Zhang, "Negative regulation of inflammation by SIRT1," *Pharmacological Research*, vol. 67, no. 1, pp. 60–67, 2013.

[30] Y. Nozaki, K. Fujita, K. Wada et al., "Deficiency of eNOS exacerbates early-stage NAFLD pathogenesis by changing the fat distribution," *BMC Gastroenterology*, vol. 15, article 177, 2015.

[31] G. Ji, Y. Wang, Y. Deng, X. Li, and Z. Jiang, "Resveratrol ameliorates hepatic steatosis and inflammation in methionine/choline-deficient diet-induced steatohepatitis through regulating autophagy," *Lipids in Health and Disease*, vol. 14, article 134, 2015.

[32] S. Heebøll, K. L. Thomsen, S. B. Pedersen, H. Vilstrup, J. George, and H. Grønbæk, "Effects of resveratrol in experimental and clinical non-alcoholic fatty liver disease," *World Journal of Hepatology*, vol. 6, no. 4, pp. 188–198, 2014.

[33] T. Greuter and V. H. Shah, "Hepatic sinusoids in liver injury, inflammation, and fibrosis: new pathophysiological insights," *Journal of Gastroenterology*, vol. 51, no. 6, pp. 511–519, 2016.

[34] G. Xie, X. Wang, L. Wang et al., "Role of differentiation of liver sinusoidal endothelial cells in progression and regression of hepatic fibrosis in rats," *Gastroenterology*, vol. 142, no. 4, pp. 918–927, 2012.

[35] R. D. Sheldon, M. H. Laughlin, R. S. Rector, J. Padilla, and N. T. Jenkins, "Reduced hepatic eNOS phosphorylation is associated with NAFLD and type 2 diabetes progression and is prevented by daily exercise in hyperphagic OLETF rats," *Journal of Applied Physiology*, vol. 116, no. 9, pp. 1156–1164, 2014.

[36] W. Wang, C. Zhao, J. Zhou, Z. Zhen, Y. Wang, and C. Shen, "Simvastatin ameliorates liver fibrosis via mediating nitric oxide synthase in rats with non-alcoholic steatohepatitis-related liver fibrosis," *PLoS ONE*, vol. 8, no. 10, Article ID e76538, pp. 1–11, 2013.

[37] Z. Dong, L. Su, S. Esmaili et al., "Adiponectin attenuates liver fibrosis by inducing nitric oxide production of hepatic stellate cells," *Journal of Molecular Medicine*, vol. 93, no. 12, pp. 1327–1339, 2015.

[38] S. Ballestri, F. Nascimbeni, D. Romagnoli, E. Baldelli, and A. Lonardo, "The role of nuclear receptors in the pathophysiology, natural course, and drug treatment of NAFLD in humans," *Advances in Therapy*, vol. 33, no. 3, pp. 291–319, 2016.

[39] A. Montagner, A. Polizzi, E. Fouché et al., "Liver PPARa is crucial for whole-body fatty acid homeostasis and is protective against NAFLD," *Gut*, vol. 65, pp. 1202–1214, 2016.

[40] E. Ip, G. C. Farrell, G. Robertson, P. Hall, R. Kirsch, and I. Leclercq, "Central role of PPARα-dependent hepatic lipid turnover in dietary steatohepatitis in mice," *Hepatology*, vol. 38, no. 1, pp. 123–132, 2003.

[41] S. Barbosa-Da-Silva, V. Souza-Mello, D. C. Magliano, T. D. S. Marinho, M. B. Aguila, and C. A. Mandarim-De-Lacerda, "Singular effects of PPAR agonists on nonalcoholic fatty liver disease of diet-induced obese mice," *Life Sciences*, vol. 127, pp. 73–81, 2015.

[42] E. Ip, G. Farrell, P. Hall, G. Robertson, and I. Leclercq, "Administration of the potent PPARα agonist, Wy-14,643, reverses nutritional fibrosis and steatohepatitis in mice," *Hepatology*, vol. 39, no. 5, pp. 1286–1296, 2004.

[43] S. Liu, B. Hatano, M. Zhao et al., "Role of peroxisome proliferator-activated receptor δ/β in hepatic metabolic regulation," *Journal of Biological Chemistry*, vol. 286, no. 2, pp. 1237–1247, 2011.

[44] H. J. Lee, J. E. Yeon, E. J. Ko et al., "Peroxisome proliferator-activated receptor-delta agonist ameliorated inflammasome activation in nonalcoholic fatty liver disease," *World Journal of Gastroenterology*, vol. 21, no. 45, pp. 12787–12799, 2015.

[45] L. Serrano-Marco, M. R. Chacón, E. Maymó-Masip et al., "TNF-α inhibits PPARβ/δ activity and SIRT1 expression through NF-κB in human adipocytes," *Biochimica et Biophysica Acta—Molecular and Cell Biology of Lipids*, vol. 1821, no. 9, pp. 1177–1185, 2012.

[46] V. A. Narkar, M. Downes, R. T. Yu et al., "AMPK and PPARδ agonists are exercise mimetics," *Cell*, vol. 134, no. 3, pp. 405–415, 2008.

[47] S. H. Ibrahim, P. Hirsova, H. Malhi, and G. J. Gores, "Animal models of nonalcoholic steatohepatitis: eat, delete, and inflame," *Digestive Diseases and Sciences*, vol. 61, no. 5, pp. 1325–1336, 2016.

[48] M. Ichimura, M. Kawase, M. Masuzumi et al., "High-fat and high-cholesterol diet rapidly induces non-alcoholic steatohepatitis with advanced fibrosis in Sprague-Dawley rats," *Hepatology Research*, vol. 45, no. 4, pp. 458–469, 2015.

[49] K. Mukai, T. Miyagi, K. Nishio et al., "S100A8 production in CXCR2-expressing CD11b+Gr-1high cells aggravates hepatitis in mice fed a high-fat and high-cholesterol diet," *Journal of Immunology*, vol. 196, no. 1, pp. 395–406, 2016.

[50] N. Matsuzawa, T. Takamura, S. Kurita et al., "Lipid-induced oxidative stress causes steatohepatitis in mice fed an atherogenic diet," *Hepatology*, vol. 46, no. 5, pp. 1392–1403, 2007.

24

Predictive Factors for a Long Hospital Stay in Patients Undergoing Laparoscopic Cholecystectomy

Wasana Ko-iam,[1,2] Trichak Sandhu,[2] Sahattaya Paiboonworachat,[3] Paisal Pongchairerks,[4] Anon Chotirosniramit,[2] Narain Chotirosniramit,[2] Kamtone Chandacham,[2] Tidarat Jirapongcharoenlap,[2] and Sunhawit Junrungsee[2]

[1]*Clinical Epidemiology, Faculty of Medicine, Chiang Mai University, Chiang Mai, Thailand*
[2]*Department of Surgery, Faculty of Medicine, Chiang Mai University, Chiang Mai, Thailand*
[3]*Department of Anesthesiology, Faculty of Medicine, Chiang Mai University, Chiang Mai, Thailand*
[4]*Department of Surgery, Bumrungrad International Hospital, Bangkok, Thailand*

Correspondence should be addressed to Sunhawit Junrungsee; sunhawit.j@gmail.com

Academic Editor: Dirk Uhlmann

Background. Although the advantages of laparoscopic cholecystectomy (LC) over open cholecystectomy are immediately obvious and appreciated, several patients need a postoperative hospital stay of more than 24 hours. Thus, the predictive factors for this longer stay need to be investigated. The aim of this study was to identify the causes of a long hospital stay after LC. *Methods*. This is a retrospective cohort study with 500 successful elective LC patients being included in the analysis. Short hospital stay was defined as being discharged within 24 hours after the operation, whereas long hospital stay was defined as the need for a stay of more than 24 hours after the operation. *Results*. Using multivariable analysis, ten independent predictive factors were identified for a long hospital stay. These included patients with cirrhosis, patients with a history of previous acute cholecystitis, cholangitis, or pancreatitis, patients on anticoagulation with warfarin, patients with standard-pressure pneumoperitoneum, patients who had been given metoclopramide as an intraoperative antiemetic drug, patients who had been using abdominal drain, patients who had numeric rating scale for pain > 3, patients with an oral analgesia requirement > 2 doses, complications, and private ward admission. *Conclusions*. LC difficulties were important predictive factors for a long hospital stay, as well as medication and operative factors.

1. Introduction

Laparoscopic cholecystectomy (LC) is one of the most common minimally invasive elective surgeries. The advantages of LC over open cholecystectomy (OC) have been immediately appreciated. These include an earlier return of bowel function, less postoperative pain, improved cosmesis, a shorter length of hospital stay, an earlier return to full activity, and decreased overall cost [1–4]. Nevertheless, there are several patients who have had a postoperative hospital stay of more than 24 hours, due to conversion to open surgery or complications. Thus, the factors predicting this should be investigated to inform the at-risk patients. The aim of this study was to identify the causes of long hospital stay after LC. From these results, a guideline for patient selection for further ambulatory surgery might be offered in the future.

2. Patients and Methods

The present study was approved by the ethics committee of the Faculty of Medicine, Chiang Mai University. In this retrospective cohort study, 500 patients who underwent elective LC at Chiang Mai University Hospital between July 2010 and June 2014 were recruited. All 500 successful LC procedures were included in the analysis. The medical records of the patients were reviewed systematically. They were divided into two groups: long hospital stay (LS group) and short hospital stay (SS group). A short hospital stay was defined as returning home within 24 hours of the operation, whereas a long hospital stay was defined as a stay of more than 24 hours after the operation. Variables were documented from medical records for comparison between the two groups. A total of 34 variables were identified for comparison. These included 20 patient variables: age, gender, American Society of Anesthesiologists (ASA) risk classification, comorbidities (including diabetes mellitus, hypertension, dyslipidemia, cirrhosis, cardiovascular disease, chronic kidney disease, thalassemia, and other factors such as asthma, COPD, and thyroid diseases), body mass index, previous upper intra-abdominal surgery, indications of surgery, and patients on anticoagulation with warfarin; eight operative variables: surgeons' status, type of procedure, use of preemptive analgesia, intraoperative antiemetic drugs, intraoperative cholangiogram, operative time, operative findings of thickened gallbladder wall, presence of adhesions, incidental perforation of gallbladder, and use of abdominal drain; and six postoperative variables: postoperative nausea or vomiting (PONV), numeric rating scale (NRS) pain score, parenteral analgesia requirement, oral analgesia requirement, complications, and type of ward admission.

2.1. Anesthetic Technique. Balanced general anesthesia with endotracheal intubation was performed in all patients. Intravenous induction was performed using thiopental (5 mg/kg body weight), and intravenous fentanyl (1 μg/kg body weight) was given as an analgesic.

2.2. Surgical Technique. The American technique (surgeon standing on the side) was used in all patients. Then, standard LC was performed by the set of surgeons.

2.3. Postoperative Treatment. At the end of the surgery, each patient received one kind of intravenous antiemetic drug including the combination of dexamethasone 8 mg and metoclopramide 10 mg [5], ondansetron 8 mg [6], or metoclopramide 10 mg alone. The score of PONV in each patient was recorded with the number 0 or 1 (0 = no nausea or vomiting, 1 = nausea or vomiting). In case of nausea and vomiting, intravenous metoclopramide 10 mg was given as a rescue drug.

A numeric rating scale (NRS) (0–10) was used to assess the postoperative pain score. Morphine 0.05 mg/kg was administered intravenously by a staff nurse as a rescue analgesic as the patient required (if NRS ≥ 6). After 2 hours postoperatively, if NRS was 3–5, pain was controlled by oral paracetamol with codeine (15 mg) 1-2 tablets and then repeated every 4–6 hours in case of minor pain.

In addition, some patients received preemptive analgesia with etoricoxib 120 mg orally two hours before surgery at the ward.

2.4. Statistical Analysis. Statistical comparison of these 34 variables was performed using Fisher's exact test for categorical variables, t-test for normally distributed continuous variables, and Mann–Whitney U test for non-normally distributed continuous variables. The pre- and postoperative factors identified as significant were included in a multivariable analysis by log risk regression to identify the predictive factors for a long hospital stay. A p value of 0.05 was considered as being statistically significant. STATA version 11.0 was used for data analysis.

TABLE 1: Reasons for long hospital stay in long stay group.

Reasons for long hospital stay	LS group ($N = 89$)
Observation of postoperative fever	19
Surgery related causes	
Postoperative pain	34
Delayed oral diet	1
Retained abdominal drain	4
Postoperative complications	
Bowel injury	2
Septicemia	1
Postoperative nausea or vomiting	10
Medical causes	13
Patient preference	5

3. Results

Of the 500 laparoscopic cholecystectomies, 411 (82.20%) could be discharged within 24 hours after operation, while 89 (17.80%) had a longer hospital stay. The postoperative stay was 1 day and 2 days (range: 2–19) in the SS group and LS group, respectively ($p < 0.001$). Reasons for long hospital stay included observation of postoperative fever ($n = 19$), surgery related causes ($n = 42$; postoperative pain = 34, delayed oral diet = 1, retained abdominal drain = 4, and postoperative complications = 3), PONV ($n = 10$), medical causes ($n = 13$), and patient preference ($n = 5$). Postoperative complications included bowel injury ($n = 2$) and septicemia ($n = 1$). The patients who stayed due to observation of postoperative fever were discharged uneventfully (Table 1).

The patient factors that were significantly associated with a long hospital stay included ASA risk classification ($p < 0.001$), history of cirrhosis ($p = 0.039$), and being on anticoagulation with warfarin ($p < 0.001$) (Table 2). In addition, several operative and postoperative factors were also associated with a long hospital stay including types of intraoperative antiemetic drug ($p = 0.021$), intraoperative cholangiogram ($p = 0.037$), operative time ($p = 0.010$), incidental perforation of the gallbladder ($p = 0.005$), use of an abdominal drain ($p < 0.001$), PONV ($p = 0.008$), postoperative pain ($p < 0.001$), parenteral analgesia requirement ($p = 0.001$), oral analgesia requirement ($p < 0.001$), and complications ($p = 0.005$) (Tables 3 and 4).

Sixteen potential factors were identified in the comparison between the SS and LS groups in the univariable analysis (Table 5). The factors that increased the risk of a long hospital stay included patients with an ASA class 3, a history of previous acute cholecystitis, cholangitis, or pancreatitis, a history of cirrhosis, being on long-term anticoagulation with warfarin, having standard-pressure pneumoperitoneum (14 mmHg), having been given metoclopramide as an intraoperative antiemetic drug, having an intraoperative cholangiogram, having an operative time of more than 60 minutes, having an incidental perforation of the gallbladder, using an abdominal drain, PONV, an NRS pain score more than 3, a

TABLE 2: Patients' variables.

Patients' variables, *n* (%)	LS group (*n* = 89)	SS group (*n* = 411)	*p* value
Age (years), mean ± SD	55.44 ± 11.75	53.55 ± 13.10	
≤60 years	61 (16.85)	301 (83.15)	0.363
>60 years	28 (20.29)	110 (79.71)	
Gender			
Male	25 (15.06)	141 (84.94)	0.321
Female	64 (19.16)	270 (80.84)	
ASA risk classification			
ASA class 1	29 (18.13)	131 (81.88)	<0.001
ASA class 2	47 (15.02)	266 (84.98)	
ASA class 3	13 (48.15)	14 (51.85)	
Comorbidities			
Diabetes mellitus	12 (18.18)	54 (81.82)	1.000
Hypertension	35 (19.13)	148 (80.87)	0.547
Dyslipidemia	16 (16.84)	79 (83.16)	0.882
Cirrhosis	8 (36.36)	14 (63.64)	0.039
Cardiovascular disease	8 (30.77)	18 (69.23)	0.108
Chronic kidney disease	5 (29.41)	12 (70.59)	0.202
Thalassemia	2 (8.70)	21 (91.30)	0.400
Others (asthma, COPD, thyroid diseases, etc.)	33 (18.86)	142 (81.14)	0.713
BMI (kg/m^2), mean ± SD	24.21 ± 4.16	24.63 ± 12.39	
Normal weight (18.5–24.9)	51 (16.56)	257 (83.44)	0.639
Overweight (25–29.9)	30 (19.11)	127 (80.89)	
Obese (30–39.9)	8 (24.24)	25 (75.76)	
Morbidly obese (≥40)	0	2 (100.00)	
Previous upper intra-abdominal surgery			
Yes	11 (19.30)	46 (80.70)	0.716
No	78 (17.61)	365 (82.39)	
Indication for surgery			
Symptomatic gallstones	84 (18.06)	381 (81.94)	0.818
Gallstones with previous ERCP	21 (21.88)	75 (78.13)	0.239
Gallstones with previous cholangitis or pancreatitis	12 (22.64)	41 (77.36)	0.343
Gallstones with previous acute cholecystitis	21 (25.93)	60 (74.07)	0.055
Gallbladder polyp	4 (15.38)	22 (84.62)	1.000
Acute cholecystitis	0	1 (100.00)	1.000
On long-term anticoagulation with warfarin			
Yes	7 (77.78)	2 (22.22)	<0.001
No	82 (16.70)	409 (83.30)	

SS: short stay; LS: long stay; ASA: American Society of Anesthesiologists; BMI: body mass index; ERCP: endoscopic retrograde cholangiopancreatography.

parenteral analgesia requirement of more than 2 doses, an oral analgesia requirement of more than 2 doses, complications, and private ward admission.

The multivariable analysis showed that 10 independent predictive factors indicated a long hospital stay (Table 6): patients with a history of cirrhosis, patients with a history of previous acute cholecystitis, cholangitis, or pancreatitis, patients on long-term anticoagulation with warfarin, patients with standard-pressure pneumoperitoneum (14 mmHg), patients who had been given metoclopramide as an intraoperative antiemetic drug, using an abdominal drain, having an NRS pain score of more than 3, having an oral analgesia requirement of more than 2 doses, complications, and private ward admission.

TABLE 3: Operative variables.

Operative variables, n (%)	LS group (n = 89)	SS group (n = 411)	p value
Surgeons' status			
Surgical attending	36 (16.22)	186 (83.78)	0.480
Resident	53 (19.06)	225 (80.94)	
Type of procedure			
Low-pressure pneumoperitoneum (7 mmHg)	39 (15.42)	214 (84.58)	0.163
Standard-pressure pneumoperitoneum (14 mmHg)	50 (20.42)	197 (79.76)	
Use of preemptive analgesia			
Yes	11 (11.96)	81 (88.84)	0.131
No	78 (19.12)	330 (80.88)	
Intraoperative antiemetic drug			
Combination of dexamethasone and metoclopramide	3 (6.00)	47 (94.00)	0.021
Ondansetron	73 (18.25)	327 (81.75)	
Metoclopramide	13 (26.00)	37 (74.00)	
Intraoperative cholangiogram			
Yes	4 (50.00)	4 (50.00)	0.037
No	85 (17.28)	407 (82.72)	
Operative time (min), mean ± SD	79.25 ± 33.11	65.24 ± 22.12	
≤60 min	33 (13.31)	215 (86.69)	0.010
>60 min	56 (22.22)	196 (77.78)	
Operative findings			
Thickened gallbladder wall	16 (25.00)	48 (75.00)	0.116
Presence of adhesions	11 (25.58)	32 (74.42)	0.208
Incidental perforation of gallbladder	25 (28.74)	62 (71.26)	0.005
Use of abdominal drain			
Yes	5 (100.00)	0	<0.001
No	84 (16.97)	411 (83.03)	

SILC: single incision laparoscopic cholecystectomy.

4. Discussion and Conclusions

Improvement in LC and anesthetic techniques, together with increased familiarity with the procedure, has led to progressively shorter hospital stays [7]. However, two studies have reported that LC patients fulfilling the following criteria had a significant association with longer hospital stays: patients aged more than 60 years, patients with ASA class 3, patients with complicated gallstones, patients with increased operative time, patients with intraoperative findings of thickened gallbladder wall, and patients with adhesions and perforations of the gallbladder [8, 9].

Our results showed that the independent predictive factors for a long hospital stay were a history of cirrhosis, a history of previous acute cholecystitis, cholangitis, or pancreatitis, being on long-term anticoagulation with warfarin, having standard-pressure pneumoperitoneum (14 mmHg), having been given metoclopramide as an intraoperative antiemetic drug, using an abdominal drain, having an NRS pain score of more than 3, having an oral analgesia requirement of more than 2 doses, complications, and private ward admission.

It is widely accepted that patients with liver cirrhosis are at higher risk of developing complications to surgical procedures, and the condition will result in a longer hospital stay of between 3 and 6.9 days (average 2.8 days) [10]. There are some technical difficulties with performing LC in patients with cirrhosis [11]. The cirrhotic liver parenchyma is stiff due to fibrous transformation and could interfere with the frequently standard maneuver in LC where retraction of the gallbladder fundus is performed to expose the triangle of Calot [12]. It has therefore been suggested that laparoscopic procedures in patients with liver cirrhosis are performed with a lower intra-abdominal pressure [10].

Previous acute cholecystitis, cholangitis, and pancreatitis all contributed to the longer hospital stay. These conditions are associated with inflammation of the right upper quadrant abdomen and cause the distortion of anatomy such as biliary fibrosis. These make the surgery difficult and result in prolonged operative time.

TABLE 4: Postoperative variables.

Postoperative variables, n (%)	LS group (n = 89)	SS group (n = 411)	p value
Postoperative nausea or vomiting			
Yes	35 (25.55)	102 (74.45)	0.008
No	54 (14.88)	309 (85.12)	
NRS pain score, mean ± SD	4.62 ± 1.30	3.29 ± 1.22	
≤3	19 (6.74)	263 (93.26)	<0.001
>3	70 (32.11)	148 (67.89)	
Parenteral analgesia requirement (dose), median (range)	1 (0–5)	1 (0–4)	
≤2 doses	56 (14.66)	326 (85.34)	0.001
>2 doses	33 (27.97)	85 (72.03)	
Oral analgesia requirement (dose), median (range)	3 (0–10)	1 (0–3)	
≤2 doses	22 (6.73)	305 (93.27)	<0.001
>2 doses	67 (38.73)	106 (61.27)	
Complications			
Yes	3 (100.00)	0	0.005
No	86 (17.30)	411 (82.70)	
Type of ward admission			
Private ward	70 (19.94)	281 (80.06)	0.056
General ward	19 (12.75)	130 (87.25)	

NRS: numeric rating scale.

Despite being minimally surgically invasive, laparoscopic surgery has yet to be proven safe in patients receiving anticoagulants. In the present study, warfarin was discontinued preoperatively in all cases. Heparin anticoagulation was individualized according to each patient's risk of thrombosis [13]. LC was completed in each patient without resulting hemorrhagic complications, but a longer hospital stay was required for the continuation of postoperative anticoagulation treatment.

Postoperative pain is an important practical problem in LC. A postoperative pain score of more than 3 was one of the predictive factors of a longer hospital stay. Oral analgesia consumption, which reflected the degree of postoperative pain, especially an oral analgesia requirement of more than 2 doses, was another predictive factor of a longer hospital stay. 78.65% (70/89) of patients in the long hospital stay group had a longer hospital stay due to a postoperative pain score of more than 3. Satisfactory pain control involved a multimodality of treatment, which included low-pressure pneumoperitoneum (7 mmHg) [14, 15], preemptive analgesia [15, 16], intraoperative local anaesthesia infiltration, and postoperative analgesia.

Several studies have shown that low-pressure pneumoperitoneum is feasible and safe and results in reduced postoperative pain compared with standard-pressure pneumoperitoneum [14, 15, 17, 18]. Our results confirmed the potential benefits of the reduced length of hospital stay when the procedure of low-pressure pneumoperitoneum was used, whereas standard-pressure pneumoperitoneum resulted in a longer hospital stay.

Although PONV was not an independent risk factor for delayed hospital stays, it was a significant risk factor in the univariable analysis in our study. Since PONV was not actively assessed after the operation, its incidence depended a great deal on complaints by the patients. Thus, inadequate documentation with underestimation of the incidence of PONV would be expected in this retrospective analysis. PONV is known to be a frequent and distressing source of discomfort during the postoperative period, especially after laparoscopic procedures, with an incidence rate as high as 70%. The use of proper antiemetic drugs during the operation might also reduce the incidence of PONV [5, 19, 20].

Based on the evidence, ondansetron is more effective than metoclopramide in preventing PONV after LC [6, 21]. Furthermore, the administration of dexamethasone combined with metoclopramide had significant effects in the prophylaxis of nausea and vomiting after LC and also shortened the hospital stay [5]. Our results from the present study confirmed that the potential effect of the combination of dexamethasone with metoclopramide is better than of ondansetron and metoclopramide for preventing PONV and shortening the hospital stay after LC.

The use of abdominal drain significantly increased the hospital stay after LC. At least 48 hours were needed before removing the drain. In addition, the complications in the present study that occur during surgery (bowel injury and bile duct injury) or after surgery (septicemia) also take several days for treatment and postoperative administration of antibiotics.

TABLE 5: Potential factors from the univariable analysis.

Factors	Risk ratio	95% confidence interval	p value
Preoperative factors			
ASA class 3	3.00	1.92–4.67	<0.001
History of cirrhosis	2.15	1.19–3.86	0.011
History of previous acute cholecystitis, cholangitis, or pancreatitis	1.73	1.18–2.53	0.005
On long-term anticoagulation with warfarin	4.66	3.12–6.96	<0.001
Perioperative factors			
Type of procedure			
Low-pressure pneumoperitoneum (7 mmHg)	1.00		
Standard-pressure pneumoperitoneum (14 mmHg)	1.31	0.90–1.92	0.161
Intraoperative antiemetic drug			
Combination of dexamethasone and metoclopramide	1.00		
Ondansetron	3.04	1.00–9.30	0.051
Metoclopramide	4.33	1.31–14.30	0.016
Intraoperative cholangiogram	2.89	1.41–5.95	0.004
Operative time > 60 min	1.67	1.13–2.47	0.011
Incidental perforation of gallbladder	1.85	1.24–2.77	0.003
Use of abdominal drain	5.89	4.85–7.16	<0.001
Postoperative factors			
Postoperative nausea or vomiting	1.72	1.18–2.51	0.005
NRS pain score > 3	4.77	2.96–7.67	<0.001
Parenteral analgesia requirement > 2 doses	1.91	1.31–2.78	0.001
Oral analgesia requirement > 2 doses	5.76	3.99–8.99	<0.001
Complications	5.78	4.77–7.01	<0.001
Private ward admission	1.56	0.98–2.50	0.062

TABLE 6: Predictive factors from multivariable analysis.

Predictive factors	Adjusted risk ratio	95% confidence interval	p value
Preoperative factors			
History of cirrhosis	2.29	1.63–3.22	<0.001
History of previous acute cholecystitis, cholangitis, or pancreatitis	1.53	1.08–2.15	0.015
On long-term anticoagulation with warfarin	1.94	1.10–3.40	0.021
Perioperative factors			
Type of procedure			
Low-pressure pneumoperitoneum (7 mmHg)	1.00		
Standard-pressure pneumoperitoneum (14 mmHg)	1.48	1.03–2.14	0.034
Intraoperative antiemetic drug			
Combination of dexamethasone and metoclopramide	1.00		
Ondansetron	2.80	0.97–8.07	0.056
Metoclopramide	3.60	1.17–11.11	0.026
Postoperative factors			
NRS pain score > 3	2.38	1.48–3.82	<0.001
Oral analgesia requirement > 2 doses	3.77	2.44–5.80	<0.001
Use of abdominal drain	4.04	2.16–7.56	<0.001
Complications	3.50	1.12–10.98	0.032
Private ward admission	1.75	1.16–2.65	0.008

In our setting, there are two types of wards for patients undergoing LC, that is, general and private wards. Private wards were a popular type because there are privacy and comfort. For this reason, the patients in private wards were satisfied and wanted to stay in the postoperative period for more than one day.

However, our results also suggested that while ASA class 3, intraoperative cholangiogram, operative time of more than 60 minutes, incidental perforation of the gallbladder, parenteral analgesia requirement of more than 2 doses, and PONV were significant risk factors in the univariable analysis, they were not independent risk factors for long hospital stays in multivariable analysis. Nevertheless, these patients should be of concern as regards complications and also a potential extended hospital stay.

To avoid unnecessary longer hospital stays, intraoperative cholangiogram should be performed in only selected cases such as patients at risk for bile duct injury or patients with anomaly of bile duct. Long hospital stay was also correlated with prolonged operative time and complications in difficult cases. Thus, surgeons should be cautious about the complications in these conditions, especially the injury of the bile duct.

Although it has been found that LC in elderly patients is associated with higher complication rates and longer hospital stays [22], these findings were contradicted in our study. Our results showed that age was not associated with a longer hospital stay. In addition, our results also showed that gender, BMI [23, 24], previous upper intra-abdominal surgery history, surgeons' status, thickened gallbladder wall, and the presence of adhesions were not associated with delayed hospital stay.

In evaluating patient-related risk factors, comorbidities such as diabetes mellitus, hypertension, dyslipidemia, cardiovascular disease, chronic kidney disease, and thalassemia were also analyzed. Patients with diabetes mellitus are known to have poorer surgical outcomes and higher rates of intraoperative complications [25]. On the other hand, our results showed that more patients with diabetes mellitus and other comorbidities belonged to the short stay group. Nevertheless, careful sugar control during the perioperative course should be considered for patients with diabetes mellitus.

The limitations of this study included the bias inherent to the retrospective nature of the design. Inadequate documentation, such as underestimation of the incidence of PONV, resulted in PONV being insignificant in multivariable analysis. However, a huge patient cohort and carefully adjusted variables in the analysis method provide interesting results of influencing factors. In addition, most of our results still were concurrent with previous findings from other studies.

Our study was a retrospective review of elective LC during a 4-year period at one center. The study included all patients who underwent successful elective LC surgery without open conversion. With broad inclusion criteria, a more accurate assessment of any influencing factors for a longer hospital stay was expected. With proper patient selection and adequate preoperative preparation, more patients could benefit from a reduced postoperative hospital stay.

In terms of patient factors, patients with cirrhosis, on long-term anticoagulation medication with warfarin, or with a history of acute cholecystitis, cholangitis, or pancreatitis should be informed of the possibility of a lengthened postoperative hospital stay. In addition, the use of low-pressure pneumoperitoneum (7 mmHg) and a combination of dexamethasone and metoclopramide as intraoperative antiemetic drugs during elective LC may be helpful in reducing the length of postoperative hospital stay.

From these results, patients with ASA class 1 or 2, patients without cirrhosis, and patients with uncomplicated gallstones could be enrolled for further ambulatory LC. The proper procedure and management of PONV and postoperative pain might help to generate further ambulatory LC in our country.

References

[1] R. J. Porte and B. C. De Vries, "Laparoscopic versus open cholecystectomy: a prospective matched-cohort study," *HPB Surgery*, vol. 9, no. 2, pp. 71–75, 1996.

[2] P. A. Grace, A. Quereshi, J. Coleman et al., "Reduced postoperative hospitalization after laparoscopic cholecystectomy," *The British Journal of Surgery*, vol. 78, no. 2, pp. 160–162, 1991.

[3] M. E. Stoker, J. Vose, P. O'mara, and B. S. Maini, "Laparoscopic cholecystectomy: a clinical and financial analysis of 280 operations," *Archives of Surgery*, vol. 127, no. 5, pp. 589–595, 1992.

[4] C. P. Rubert, R. A. Higa, and F. V. B. Farias, "Comparison between open and laparoscopic elective cholecystectomy in elderly, in a teaching hospital," *Revista do Colegio Brasileiro de Cirurgioes*, vol. 43, no. 1, pp. 2–5, 2016.

[5] W. Ko-Iam, T. Sandhu, S. Paiboonworachat et al., "Metoclopramide, versus its combination with dexamethasone in the prevention of postoperative nausea and vomiting after laparoscopic cholecystectomy: A double-blind randomized controlled trial," *Journal of the Medical Association of Thailand*, vol. 98, no. 3, pp. 265–272, 2015.

[6] T. Sandhu, P. Tanvatcharaphan, and V. Cheunjongkolkul, "Ondansetron versus metoclopramide in prophylaxis of nausea and vomiting for laparoscopic cholecystectomy: a prospective double-blind randomized study," *Asian Journal of Surgery*, vol. 31, no. 2, pp. 50–54, 2008.

[7] F. Keus, J. A. de Jong, H. G. Gooszen, and C. J. van Laarhoven, "Laparoscopic versus open cholecystectomy for patients with symptomatic cholecystolithiasis," *The Cochrane Database of Systematic Reviews*, no. 4, Article ID CD006231, 2006.

[8] Y.-Y. Tsang, C.-M. Poon, K.-W. Lee, and H.-T. Leong, "Predictive factors of long hospital stay after laparoscopic cholecystectomy," *Asian Journal of Surgery*, vol. 30, no. 1, pp. 23–28, 2007.

[9] J. U. Chong, J. H. Lee, Y. C. Yoon et al., "Influencing factors on postoperative hospital stay after laparoscopic cholecystectomy," *Korean Journal of Hepato-Biliary-Pancreatic Surgery*, vol. 20, no. 1, pp. 12–16, 2016.

[10] N. O. Machado, "Laparoscopic cholecystectomy in cirrhotics," *Journal of the Society of Laparoendoscopic Surgeons*, vol. 16, no. 3, pp. 392–400, 2012.

[11] J. Strömberg, F. Hammarqvist, O. Sadr-Azodi, and G. Sandblom, "Cholecystectomy in patients with liver cirrhosis," *Gastroenterology Research and Practice*, vol. 2015, Article ID 783823, 6 pages, 2015.

[12] B. de Goede, P. J. Klitsie, S. M. Hagen et al., "Meta-analysis of laparoscopic versus open cholecystectomy for patients with liver cirrhosis and symptomatic cholecystolithiasis," *The British Journal of Surgery*, vol. 100, no. 2, pp. 209–216, 2013.

[13] S. D. Fitzgerald, P. V. Bailey, G. J. Liebscher, and C. H. Andrus, "Laparoscopic cholecystectomy in anticoagulated patients," *Surgical Endoscopy*, vol. 5, no. 4, pp. 166–169, 1991.

[14] T. Sandhu, S. Yamada, V. Ariyakachon, T. Chakrabandhu, W. Chongruksut, and W. Ko-Iam, "Low-pressure pneumoperitoneum versus standard pneumoperitoneum in laparoscopic cholecystectomy, a prospective randomized clinical trial," *Surgical Endoscopy*, vol. 23, no. 5, pp. 1044–1047, 2009.

[15] W. Ko-Iam, S. Paiboonworachat, P. Pongchairerks, S. Junrungsee, and T. Sandhu, "Combination of etoricoxib and low-pressure pneumoperitoneum versus standard treatment for the management of pain after laparoscopic cholecystectomy: a randomized controlled trial," *Surgical Endoscopy*, vol. 30, no. 11, pp. 4800–4808, 2016.

[16] T. Sandhu, S. Paiboonworachat, and W. Ko-Iam, "Effects of preemptive analgesia in laparoscopic cholecystectomy: a double-blind randomized controlled trial," *Surgical Endoscopy*, vol. 25, no. 1, pp. 23–27, 2011.

[17] J. Hua, J. Gong, L. Yao, B. Zhou, and Z. Song, "Low-pressure versus standard-pressure pneumoperitoneum for laparoscopic cholecystectomy: a systematic review and meta-analysis," *American Journal of Surgery*, vol. 208, no. 1, pp. 143–150, 2014.

[18] M. Barczyński and R. M. Herman, "A prospective randomized trial on comparison of low-pressure (LP) and standard-pressure (SP) pneumoperitoneum for laparoscopic cholecystectomy," *Surgical Endoscopy and Other Interventional Techniques*, vol. 17, no. 4, pp. 533–538, 2003.

[19] J.-J. Wang, S.-T. Ho, Y.-H. Uen et al., "Small-dose dexamethasone reduces nausea and vomiting after laparoscopic cholecystectomy: a comparison of tropisetron with saline," *Anesthesia and Analgesia*, vol. 95, no. 1, pp. 229–232, 2002.

[20] T. Bisgaard, B. Klarskov, H. Kehlet, and J. Rosenberg, "Preoperative dexamethasone improves surgical outcome after laparoscopic cholecystectomy: a randomized double-blind placebo-controlled trial," *Annals of Surgery*, vol. 238, no. 5, pp. 651–660, 2003.

[21] S.-J. Wu, X.-Z. Xiong, T.-Y. Cheng, Y.-X. Lin, and N.-S. Cheng, "Efficacy of ondansetron vs. metoclopramide in prophylaxis of postoperative nausea and vomiting after laparoscopic cholecystectomy: a systematic review and meta-analysis," *Hepato-Gastroenterology*, vol. 59, no. 119, pp. 2064–2074, 2012.

[22] S.-P. Cheng, Y.-C. Chang, C.-L. Liu et al., "Factors associated with prolonged stay after laparoscopic cholecystectomy in elderly patients," *Surgical Endoscopy*, vol. 22, no. 5, pp. 1283–1289, 2008.

[23] A. Tandon, G. Sunderland, Q. M. Nunes, N. Misra, and M. Shrotri, "Day case laparoscopic cholecystectomy in patients with high BMI: experience from a UK centre," *Annals of the Royal College of Surgeons of England*, vol. 98, no. 5, pp. 329–333, 2016.

[24] D. T. Farkas, D. Moradi, D. Moaddel, K. Nagpal, and J. M. Cosgrove, "The impact of body mass index on outcomes after laparoscopic cholecystectomy," *Surgical Endoscopy*, vol. 26, no. 4, pp. 964–969, 2012.

[25] R. Gelbard, E. Karamanos, P. G. Teixeira et al., "Effect of delaying same-admission cholecystectomy on outcomes in patients with diabetes," *The British Journal of Surgery*, vol. 101, no. 2, pp. 74–78, 2014.

25

Amelioration of Single Clove Black Garlic Aqueous Extract on Dyslipidemia and Hepatitis in Chronic Carbon Tetrachloride Intoxicated Swiss Albino Mice

Gia-Buu Tran, Sao-Mai Dam, and Nghia-Thu Tram Le

Institute of Biotechnology and Food Technology, Industrial University of Ho Chi Minh City, 12 Nguyen Van Bao Street, Ward 4, Go Vap District, Ho Chi Minh City, Vietnam

Correspondence should be addressed to Gia-Buu Tran; giabuu06cs@gmail.com

Academic Editor: Pierluigi Toniutto

Single clove garlic is the product of atypical bulbing process of garlic under specific conditions. Therefore, the number of researches on single clove garlic bioactivity is limited. Recently, the hepatoprotective effect of single clove garlic has been demonstrated. In this study, we investigated amelioration of single clove black garlic aqueous extract, a processed product from single clove garlic, on dyslipidemia and hepatitis induced by chronic administration of CCl_4. Mice were randomly divided into four groups: control, extract control, CCl_4 intoxication, and coadministrated CCl_4 and extract group. Mice were orally given a dose of 1 ml/kg body weight of CCl_4 for 28 days twice a week to establish chronic liver injury model. To evaluate the hepatoprotective effect of single clove black garlic, mice were cotreated with CCl_4 and single clove black garlic extract (200 mg/kg body weight) via gastric gauge for 30 days. Cotreatment with CCl_4 and extract could improve the changes of body weight, liver weight, and relative liver weight as compared to CCl_4 intoxicated mice. Single clove black garlic ameliorated dyslipidemia and the elevation of ALT and AST levels induced by chronic CCl_4 intoxication. Histological studies revealed that single clove black garlic could prevent mononuclear cells infiltration and hepatocyte necrosis.

1. Introduction

Liver is the vital organ in human body due to its important role in metabolism of endogenous and exogenous molecules, such as lipids, proteins and carbohydrates, and its detoxification functions. Liver is vulnerable to a variety of liver diseases including hepatic steatosis, hepatitis, fibrosis, cirrhosis, and hepatocellular carcinoma [1, 2]. It has been suggested that free radicals, reactive oxygen species, and lipid peroxidation serve a pivotal role in pathogenesis of liver diseases [3]. Therefore, antioxidant activity is considered as the key mechanism underlying the protective effect of traditional medicines which prevent and ameliorate hepatic damage in chronic liver diseases. Therefore, a large number of researches investigating identification and isolation natural hepatoprotective compounds have been documented in recent years [4].

For screening potential hepatoprotective medicines, toxic chemicals and xenobiotics such as carbon tetrachloride, thioacetamide, paracetamol, and alcohol have been used to generate pathological models [5–8]. Among these substances, carbon tetrachloride is the most common used toxicant since it provides an ideal model for studying oxidative hepatic damage due to its distinctive hepatotoxicity and its rapid metabolisms. Furthermore, carbon tetrachloride has also been used in industry such as refrigerant, fire suppression agent, and cleaning solvent; thus the risk of CCl_4 exposure has been considered. In liver, carbon tetrachloride is metabolized by hepatic cytochrome P450 leading to production of hepatotoxic metabolites such as trichloromethyl and peroxy radicals, which lead to lipid peroxidation, alteration of cell membrane permeability, and cell death [9]. It has been well documented that CCl_4 administration not only leads to fatty liver and hepatocyte necrosis, but also induces accumulation of triglycerides, decrease of reduced glutathione level, membrane damage, and loss of enzyme activity [9]. Furthermore,

Hsu and collaborators also suggested that carbon tetrachloride induced liver cirrhosis response was similar to human liver cirrhosis [10].

Garlic (*Allium sativum* L.) is a traditional herbal spice and well-known functional food in Vietnamese and Asian cuisines. It has been documented that garlic possesses many bioactive compounds, such as alliin, allicin, allylsulfides, ajoene, and 1,2-vinyldithiin, which account for many health benefits such as anticancer, antithrombotic, anti-inflammatory, antioxidant, antimicrobial, cardioprotective, and immune-modulatory activities [11]. Obioha and collaborators have indicated that garlic exerts potential hepatoprotective effect through lowering lipid peroxidation and activating antioxidant defense system [12]. Recently, garlic also is reported for its antihyperglycemic, antihyperlipidemic, and anti-inflammatory effects in type 2 diabetes mellitus associated with obesity patients [13]. However, utilization of raw garlic is strictly limited due to its peculiar flavor and its involvement in hemolytic anemia and gastrointestinal mucosa damage [14, 15].

Black garlic, the processed product which is generated by fermentation process in high temperature and high humidity, has appeared in markets for decades. Black garlic has sweet taste and eliminates unpleasant odor of raw garlic. It possesses many bioactivities including inhibition of colon and gastric cancer cells growth, antioxidant, alteration of lipid profile in diabetes, antiobesity, anti-inflammatory, and antiallergic activities [16–18]. Furthermore, black garlic extract has proven its ameliorating effect on Aβ-induced neurotoxicity and cognitive impairment [19]. Some reports also indicate that black garlic and its bioactive constituent, S-allyl-cysteine, employ hepatoprotective effects in alcohol, D-galactosamine, high fat diet, and acute carbon tetrachloride intoxicated models [20–22]. Of note, the quality and bioactive value of black garlic are diverse depended on processing method and garlic cultivars [18, 23, 24].

Due to cultivation practices and climate conditions, the bulbs of garlic sometime are not divided into cloves and generates single clove of garlic, known as single clove garlic, solo garlic, and pearl garlic. The number of researches of single clove garlic bioactivity is limited. Recently, Naji et al. (2017) suggested that single clove garlic exerted the higher hepatoprotective effect than normal garlic, which was known as "multiclove garlic" in CCl_4 intoxicated rabbit model [25]. Furthermore, the beneficial effect of multiclove black garlic on acute carbon tetrachloride intoxicated rat was proved [21]. To our knowledge, the effects of single-clove black garlic (SBE) on dyslipidemia and liver injury in hepatic pathology model have not been studied yet. In this study, we investigated the hepatoprotective effect of single clove black garlic aqueous extract on dyslipidemia and hepatitis induced by chronic administration of carbon tetrachloride in Swiss albino mice.

2. Materials and Methods

2.1. Chemicals. All reagents were provided by Sigma-Aldrich Chemical Company (St. Louis, MO, USA) unless otherwise noted. Carbon tetrachloride was obtained from Merck (1.02223.1000, Merck, Germany) and extra virgin olive oil was purchased from Sigma (W530191, Sigma, USA).

2.2. Collection and Preparation of Black Garlic Extract. Single clove garlic (*Allium sativum* L.) was cultivated from Ninh Hai District, Ninh Thuan Province, Vietnam, in March 2017. The specimen was authenticated by taxonomist at Institute of Biotechnology and Food Technology, Industrial University of Ho Chi Minh City, and voucher specimen has been deposited at local institutional herbarium for further reference.

The whole of single-clove garlic (diameter 15 ± 2 mm) was incubated in temperature and humidity controlled chamber (Shellab, USA) according to our institutional procedure. In brief, garlic was fermented at 75°C with 90% relative humidity for 20 days (Figure 1). The single clove black garlic extract was prepared by Shin et al. (2014) procedure with some modifications [21]. Single clove black garlic was peeled and mashed in 10 volumes of distilled water. Single clove black garlic cells were ruptured via assistant of pulsed microwave at 100 W for 5 minutes. The extract was prepared by refluxing in 105 ± 2°C for 1 hours, and then the extract was filtrated three times using Whatman number 1 filter paper. The filtrate was collected and concentrated in vacuum rotary evaporator to get 20°Bx. Subsequently, the aqueous extract was sterilized and divided into several 50 ml tubes and stored in −80°C until further use. Single clove black garlic extract (SBE) used in this study comprised 20.78 ± 0.21% solid materials, pH 3.64 ± 0.10.

2.3. Determination of S-Allyl-Cysteine Concentration in Aqueous Extract of Single Clove Black Garlic. For screening the presence of S-allyl cysteine, a well-known bioactive compound of black garlic in aqueous extract of single clove black garlic, we performed LC/MS analysis with the given protocol. In brief, aliquots (20 μL) of the aqueous extract were subjected to HPLC Agilent 1200 infinity liquid chromatography system (Agilent Technologies, CA, USA) coupled with MicroTOF-Q mass spectrometer (Bruker Daltonics, Germany). Separation of the analytical compounds was carried out using an ACE C18 column (4.6 × 150 mm I.D., 3.5 μm particle size, Advanced Chromatography Technologies, Aberdeen, Scotland, UK) at a flow rate of 0.3 mL/min. The solvent system consisted of two phases: mobile phase was composed of acetonitrile supplemented with 0.1% formic acid and water phase composed of 0.1% formic acid in water. The column oven temperature was maintained at 50°C. The mass spectrometer was operated with electrospray ionization source (ESI) at positive mode, and mass detection was performed in full scan mode in the range 50–3,000 m/z. The following parameters were applied to the instrument: capillary voltage 4,000 V, end plate offset −500 V, drying gas flow rate 10.0 l/min, the drying gas temperature 200°C, collision cell radio frequency 250.0 Vpp, and nebulizer 1.5 Bar. Data analysis was performed using Bruker Compass Data Analysis 4.0 software. The compounds were verified by comparison of the ESI-mass spectra and LC retention time of an authentic standard of S-allyl-cysteine where complete matching was observed.

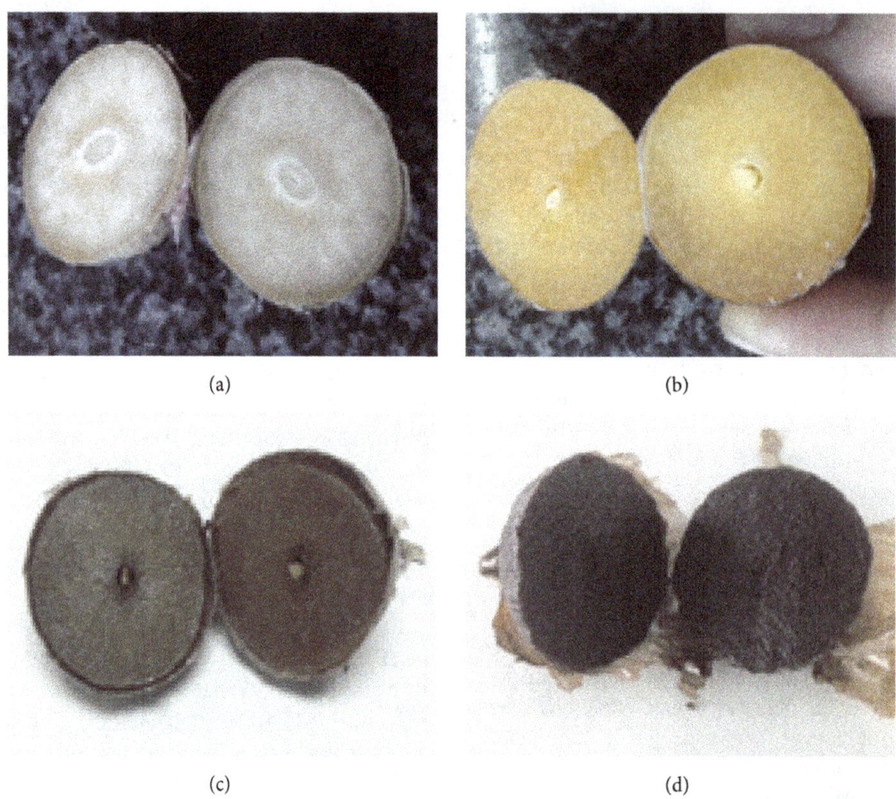

FIGURE 1: Fermentation process of single black garlic. In brief, whole bulbs of single clove garlics were fermented at 75°C in relative humidity 90% for 20 days until they obtained the particular black color. The representative samples were collected after 5 days (a), 10 days (b), 15 days (c), and 20 days (d).

2.4. Animal Experiment Design. Eight-week-old male Swiss albino mice were obtained from Pasteur Institute of Ho Chi Minh City, weighting approximately 30–32 g. The animals were randomly divided into polycarbonate cages with 5 mice for each cage. They were housed under standard husbandry conditions with 12 h light-dark cycle (8:00–20:00) for at least 1 week to acclimate with laboratory environment. They were supplied ad libitum with standard chow and distilled water. The experimental procedure was strictly compliance with Declaration of Helsinki (1964). Twenty healthy mice were randomly divided into 4 groups with 5 mice per group and treated as the protocol given below:

(1) Group 1 (control group): mice orally received equal volume of saline for 30 days. They also received olive oil at a dose 1 ml/kg body weight via gastric gavages twice per week for 28 days.

(2) Group 2 (extract control group): mice were orally received SBE (200 mg/kg body weight) for 30 days. They also received olive oil at a dose 1 ml/kg body weight via gastric gavages twice per week for 28 days.

(3) Group 3 (CCl_4 intoxicated group): hepatic injury model was induced by CCl_4 according to previous study with some modifications [26, 27]. Mice were orally given CCl_4 at the dose of 1 ml/kg body weight (in 50% in olive oil) twice per week via gastric gavages for 28 days. Then, they orally received equal volume of saline for last 2 days.

(4) Group 4 (CCl_4 and extract treated group): mice were treated with SBE (200 mg/kg body weight) daily via gastric gavages for 30 days. In addition, they were orally given CCl_4 at the dose of 1 ml/kg body weight (in 50% in olive oil) twice per week via gastric gavages for 28 days. In CCl_4 treated day, they were treated with SBE one hour before administration of mixture of CCl_4 : olive oil.

2.5. Measurement of Body Weight, Liver Weight, and Relative Liver Weight. At the end of experiment (30 days), all experimental animals were fasted overnight to reduce the difference of feeding. The body weights were directly measured using an electronic balance. Subsequently, they were anesthetized using diethyl ether. Blood was collected via cardiac puncture into heparinized tube for biochemical analysis. After that, livers were collected, washed with ice-cold saline, and weighted using an electronic balance. The relative liver weights were calculated by formula (relative liver weight (%) = liver weight/body weight × 100). Subsequently, livers were immediately fixed in 10% formalin for histological studies.

2.6. Plasma Biochemical Analysis. Blood was collected into heparinized tubes, and then the plasma was separated by centrifuge. Lipid profile including triglycerides (TG), total cholesterol (TC), high density lipoprotein cholesterol (HDL-cholesterol), low density lipoprotein cholesterol (LDL-cholesterol), and plasma levels of hepatic enzymes such as alanine aminotransferase (ALT) and aspartate transaminase (AST) were determined using commercial diagnostic kits (Diagnosticum Zrt, Hungary) according to manufacture instructions.

2.7. Histological Examination of Liver. Livers were preserved in 10% formalin and processed for histological studies with Hematoxylin and Eosin staining. The specimens were dehydrated in different grades of alcohol, cleared in xylol, embedded in paraffin wax, sectioned at 4–6 um thick, and stained with Hematoxylin and Eosin. The liver sections then were examined under microscope for estimation of extent of hepatic damage.

2.8. Statistical Analysis. Statistical analysis was performed using Statgraphics Centurion XVI software (Statpoint Technologies Inc., Warrenton, Virginia, USA). The data were presented as mean ± standard deviation. Differences between means of different groups were analyzed using ANOVA variance analysis followed with multiple range tests, and the criterion of statistical significance was set as $p < 0.05$.

3. Results and Discussions

3.1. Determination of S-Allyl-Cysteine Content in Single Clove Black Garlic Extract. There is a growing body of evidences linking black garlic with amelioration of human diseases, especially in liver disease. In previous study, Seo et al. (2009) suggested that black garlic extract could improve the lipid profile in type 2 diabetes mellitus [16]. Moreover, Jung et al. (2014) reported that consumption of black garlic extract increased HDL-cholesterol as well as ratio of LDL-cholesterol/lipoprotein B and exerted cardioprotective effect in hypercholesterolemic patients [28]. Kim et al. (2011) also proved that black garlic extract could protect liver from liver damage induced by chronic alcohol consumption [20]. Hepatoprotective effect of black garlic in carbon tetrachloride, D-galactosamine, and high fat diet treated rodents was demonstrated in previous report [21]. However, single clove black garlic aqueous extract composition and the effect of long-term administration have not been considered yet. S-Allyl-cysteine, an important sulfur-containing constituent of garlic, accumulates during manufacturing process of black garlic and exerts many biofunctions [29]. Therefore, S-allyl-cysteine content is an excellent indicator to evaluate the quality and bioactive value of black garlic. In this study, we examined S-allyl-cysteine concentration for primary evaluation of bioactive value of single clove black garlic produced by our institutional procedure. It has been found that S-allyl-cysteine existed in retention time about 7.5 min with 162.06 [M+H] and 145.03 m/z [M-H_2O+H]. The mass spectra diagram at retention time 7.5 min is presented in Figure 2. S-Allyl-cysteine concentration in extract (228.46 ± 9.61 μg/g

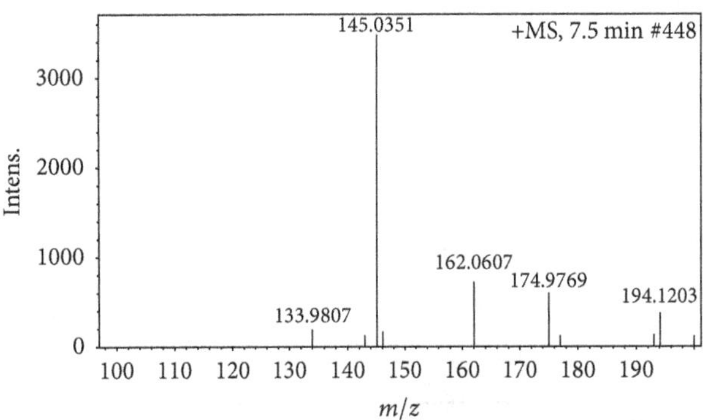

FIGURE 2: The mass spectrometry diagram of S-allyl-cysteine in single clove black garlic extract (7.5 min). The presence of bioactive compound such as S-allyl-cysteine was confirmed by LC/MS. S-Allyl-cysteine exhibited 2 peaks with m/z about 145.03 [M-H_2O+H] and 162.06 [M+H]. Thereby, we hypothesized that SBE also employed the hepatoprotective effect in liver injury induced by carbon tetrachloride administration in mice.

dry weight) is comparable with concentration of S-allyl-cysteine concentration of black garlic juice (242.3 ± 6.1 μg/g dry weight) which was produced from previous report and exhibited antidiabetic activity [30]. Furthermore, Kodai et al. (2015) have proven that S-allyl-cysteine, an important sulfur-containing constituent of black garlic, prevents liver fibrosis induced by carbon tetrachloride in rats [22]. Taken together, the data imply that single clove black garlic extract may have the beneficial effect for prevention of liver injury.

3.2. Effect of Single Clove Black Garlic Extract on Body Weight and Relative Liver Weight. In this study, we observed that there was no significant difference between body weight, liver weight, and relative liver weight of normal mice (36.26 ± 1.73 g, 1.58 ± 0.16, and 4.34 ± 0.24, resp.) and SBE administrated mice (37.24 ± 1.97, 1.68 ± 0.17, and 4.51 ± 0.29, resp., $p > 0.05$). These data implied that SBE administration did not cause the change of body weight, liver weight, and relative liver weight. On the contrary, administration of CCl_4 caused a marked reduction of body weight (33.28±2.06 g) along with a notable increase of liver weight (1.92 ± 0.22 g) as compared to normal mice ($p < 0.05$). Moreover, relative liver weight of CCl_4 treated group was significantly increased versus control group (5.76 ± 0.45% versus 4.34 ± 0.24% resp., $p < 0.05$). These results were consistent with those reported in previous studies [26, 27, 31, 32]. Of note, SBE treatment resulted in the recovery of body weight (36.04 ± 1.31 g) and reversed the change of liver weight (1.53±0.17 g) of CCl_4 intoxicated mice ($p < 0.05$). A remarkable decrease of relative liver weights (4.23 ± 0.34%) was observed in CCl_4 and SBE cotreated mice as compared to CCl_4 treated mice ($p < 0.05$). Moreover, no significant difference of body weight, liver weight, and relative liver weight between control group and coadministered CCl_4 and extract group was observed (Table 1). These results shed light on the protection effect of black garlic extract in the changes of body weight, liver weight, and relative liver weight induced by chronic CCl_4 administration.

TABLE 1: Effect of SBE on the body weight, liver weight, and relative liver weight.

	Control ($n = 5$)	SBE control ($n = 5$)	CCL_4 treated ($n = 5$)	CCl_4 + SBE treated ($n = 5$)
Body weight (g)	36.26 ± 1.73^a	37.24 ± 1.97^a	33.28 ± 2.06^b	36.04 ± 1.31^a
Liver weight (g)	1.58 ± 0.16^a	1.68 ± 0.17^{ab}	1.92 ± 0.22^b	1.53 ± 0.17^a
Relative liver weight (%)	4.34 ± 0.24^a	4.51 ± 0.29^a	5.76 ± 0.45^b	4.23 ± 0.34^a

^{a,b}Values with different letters within the row are significantly different ($p < 0.05$).

TABLE 2: Effect of SBE on lipid profile in experimental mice.

	Control ($n = 5$)	SBE control ($n = 5$)	CCL_4 treated ($n = 5$)	CCl_4 + SBE treated ($n = 5$)
Triglyceride (mg/dl)	123.55 ± 16.63^a	89.32 ± 11.83^b	195.10 ± 20.34^c	121.64 ± 15.76^a
Total cholesterol (mg/dl)	134.04 ± 8.58^a	130.24 ± 7.32^a	212.29 ± 12.47^b	151.51 ± 11.93^c
HDL-cholesterol (mg/dl)	67.66 ± 4.46^a	70.86 ± 3.80^a	49.09 ± 6.41^b	68.52 ± 2.69^a
LDL-cholesterol (mg/dl)	41.67 ± 2.97^a	41.52 ± 3.19^a	124.18 ± 6.17^b	58.66 ± 6.58^c

^{a,b,c}Values with different letters within the row are significantly different ($p < 0.05$). LDL-cholesterol: low density lipoprotein cholesterol and HDL-cholesterol: high density lipoprotein cholesterol.

In previous study, Shin et al. (2014) also reported that administration with black garlic (200 mg/kg body weight) resulted in a significant decrease in liver weight as compared to acute CCl_4 intoxicated rats [21]. The data implied that the protective effect of black garlic on liver weight was observed not only in acute CCl_4 treatment but in chronic CCl_4 treatment. Then the question has been raised that whether single clove black garlic aqueous extract could protect mice from the alteration of lipid profile of CCl_4 intoxication.

3.3. Effect of Single Clove Black Garlic Extract on Plasma Lipid Profile. A growing body of evidences from previous reports showed that CCl_4 intoxication caused alteration on plasma lipid profile [31–33]. In our study, CCl_4 treatment resulted in significant increase of TG (195.10 ± 20.34 mg/dl), TC (212.29 ± 12.47 mg/dl), and LDL-cholesterol (124.18 ± 6.17 mg/dl) levels accompanied with a remarkable decrease of HDL-cholesterol (49.09 ± 6.41 mg/dl) versus control group (123.55 ± 16.63, 134.04 ± 8.58, 41.67 ± 2.97, and 67.66 ± 4.46 mg/dl, resp., $p < 0.05$). Of note, coadministration SBE and CCl_4 to mice caused a significant decrease in plasma TG, TC, and LDL-cholesterol accompanied with a notable increase in plasma HDL-cholesterol level ($p < 0.05$) in comparison with CCl_4 group. Furthermore, SBE could improve the LDL-cholesterol level in CCl_4 treated mice ($p < 0.05$) but LDL-cholesterol level in coadministered CCl_4 and SBE group was higher than control group (58.66 ± 6.58 mg/dl versus 41.67 ± 2.97 mg/dl, resp., $p < 0.05$). We also observed a significant difference in plasma total cholesterol levels between coadministered CCl_4 and SBE mice versus normal mice (151.51 ± 11.93 mg/dl versus 134.04 ± 8.58 mg/dl, resp., $p < 0.05$). Collectively, these results suggested that black garlic extract administration could improve in lipid profile of CCl_4 intoxicated mice and decreased plasma TG level in control mice (Table 2). Furthermore, Asdaq (2015) proved that aged garlic extract and its constituent, S-allyl-cysteine, exerted antioxidative and hypolipidemic effects on high fat diet treated rats [34]. Therefore, the high concentration of S-allyl-cysteine in extract may elucidate the improvement of single clove black garlic on the alteration of blood lipid profile in SBE and CCl_4 treated. To our knowledge, the effect of single clove black garlic extract on lipid profile in CCl_4 intoxication has not been elucidated yet. Thereby, these results proved in the first time the amelioration of single clove black garlic on the change of lipid profile induced by chronic CCl_4 administration

Furthermore, there is no difference in TC, LDL-cholesterol, and HDL-cholesterol between control group and extract control group. However, chronic administration of black garlic extract reduced plasma TG level as compared to control group (89.32 ± 11.83 mg/dl and 123.55 ± 16.63 mg/dl, resp., $p < 0.05$). This finding was consolidated by the results from Ha et al. study (2015). In that report, Ha and colleagues revealed that feeding with 1.5% black garlic extract and high fat diet caused a decrease in plasma triglyceride level as compared to normal mice and high fat diet treated mice [17]. Therefore, the data implied that single clove black garlic aqueous extract has beneficial effect on lipedema not only in intoxication but also in normal physiological condition.

3.4. Effect of Black Garlic Extract on Plasma AST and ALT Levels. Hepatocellular toxicity is characterized by elevation of alanine transaminase (ALT) and alanine transaminase (AST), both enzymes involved in the transfer of amino groups of aspartate and alanine to ketoglutaric acid [35]. The concentration of ALT and AST in plasma of all experimental mice was presented in Table 3. In our study, levels of ALT and AST in normal mice (54.84±5.86 and 146.22±29.60 U/l, resp.) and SBE control mice (58.42 ± 7.13 and 141.58 ± 21.47 U/l, resp.) showed no significant difference ($p > 0.05$). These data proved that SBE administration did not cause the elevation of ALT and ALT, two markers of liver injury. On the contrary, ALT and AST levels of CCl_4 treated group (773.88 ± 126.62 and 833.44 ± 175.56 U/l, resp.) were remarkably elevated as compared to control group ($p < 0.05$). Moreover, ALT and AST levels of coadministration of SBE and CCl_4 mice (104.94 ± 14.48 U/l and 244.90 ± 40.86, resp., $p < 0.05$) were significantly lower than ALT and AST levels of CCl_4 treated mice (773.88 ± 126.62 and 833.44 ± 175.56 U/l, resp., $p < 0.05$). These results indicated that single clove black

TABLE 3: Effect of SBE on plasma ALT and AST levels in experimental mice.

	Control ($n = 5$)	SBE control ($n = 5$)	CCL_4 treated ($n = 5$)	CCl_4 + SBE treated ($n = 5$)
ALT(U/l)	54.84 ± 5.86^a	58.42 ± 7.13^a	773.88 ± 126.62^b	104.94 ± 14.48^c
AST (U/l)	146.22 ± 29.60^a	141.58 ± 21.47^a	833.44 ± 175.56^b	244.90 ± 40.86^c

[a,b,c]Values with different letters within the row are significantly different ($p < 0.05$). ALT: alanine transaminase and AST: aspartate transaminase.

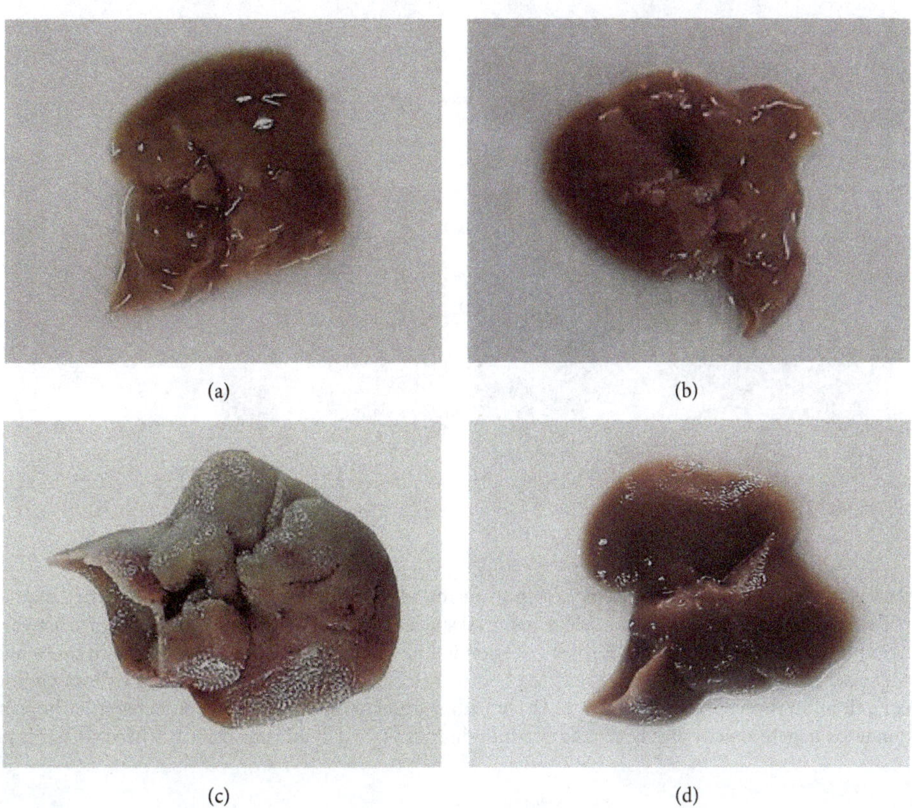

FIGURE 3: Effect of black garlic extract on gross morphology of liver from experimental mice. In gross examination, livers of normal mice showed a normal appearance with redness and soft texture, and glistering and smooth surface (a). SBE control groups showed no remarkable difference in gross morphology with livers from normal mice (b). Livers of CCl_4 intoxicated mice revealed an enlargement of livers and changed in color (pale-brown), hardness (hard texture), and coarse surface of livers as compared with livers from control group (c). Livers of coadministered CCl_4 and SBE mice improved the redness and hardness (semihard texture) but appeared slightly coarse surface comparing with CCl_4 intoxicated mice (d). Our data support the strong evidence of protective effect of black garlic extract on the change of liver morphology in CCl_4 treated mice.

garlic extract attenuated the increase of plasma ALT and AST levels induced by CCl_4 intoxication. It has been proven that black garlic treatment ameliorated the elevation of AST and ALT induced by acute CCl_4 injection [21]. Taken together, the data demonstrated that administration of single clove black garlic aqueous extract ameliorated hepatocyte toxicity induced by chronic CCl_4 treatment. Furthermore, Kodai et al. (2007) reported that S-allyl-cysteine, the main component of black garlic, could invert the elevation of ALT in CCl_4 induced acute liver injury model [36]. The lowering effects of S-allyl-cysteine and black garlic on blood ALT and AST levels were also determined in high fat diet mice [34]. As the consequence, the presence of S-allyl-cysteine in extract may account for the beneficial effect of single clove black garlic extract on ALT and AST levels in cotreated single clove black garlic extract and CCl_4 group.

3.5. Histological Analysis. The histological analysis was conducted via HE staining and gross examination for further confirmation of hepatoprotective effects of single clove black garlic extract. In gross examination, livers of normal mice showed a normal appearance with redness and soft texture, and glistering and smooth surface. There is no remarkable difference in gross morphology between livers from normal and SBE control groups. CCl_4 intoxication resulted in an enlargement of livers and changes in color (pale-brown), hardness (hard texture), and coarse surface of livers versus the livers from control group. Livers of coadministered CCl_4 and SBE mice improved the redness and hardness but showed slightly coarse surface comparing with CCl_4 intoxicated mice. The representative pictures of gross examination of livers from normal, SBE control, CCl_4 intoxicated, and coadministered CCl_4 and SBE mice are presented in Figure 3.

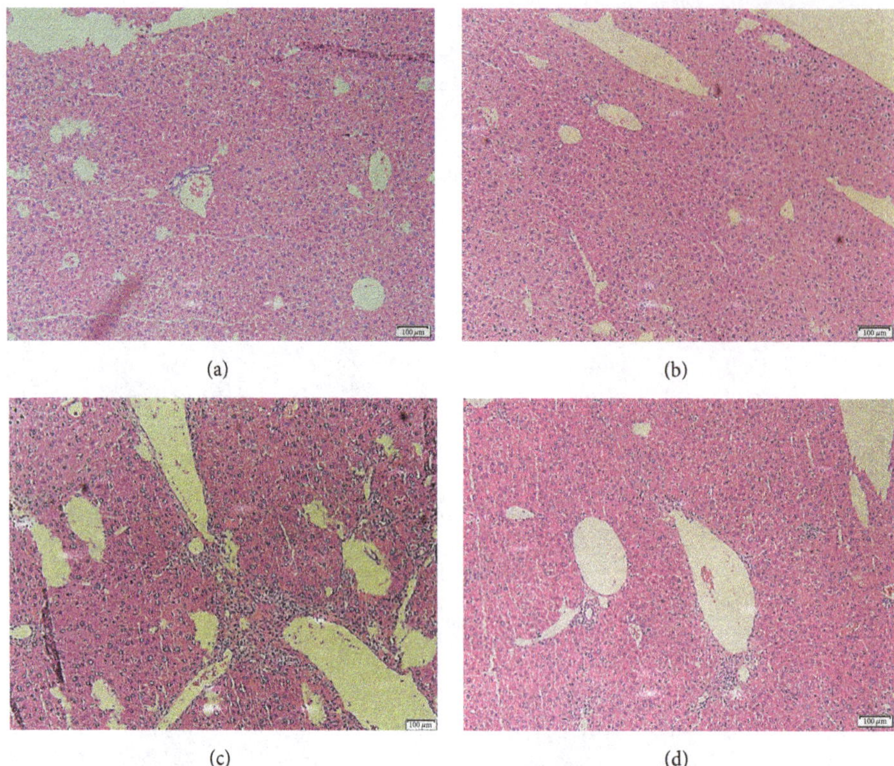

FIGURE 4: Effect of black garlic extract on liver histology from experimental mice. Liver sections from normal stained with HE revealed normal and steady architecture of hepatic parenchymal cells and portal space (a). There is no significant difference between liver sections from normal and SBE control mice stained with HE (b). CCl_4 intoxication led to severe hepatic inflammation with mononuclear cell infiltration surrounding hepatic veins accompanied by adjacent hepatocyte necrosis (c). Of note, treatment of SBE ameliorated inflammation response with mild mononuclear cell infiltration surrounding portal space with normal architecture of hepatocytes (d). The data demonstrated that black garlic extract attenuated hepatotoxicity and liver inflammation induced by CCl_4 administration. The scale bar is presented as 100 μm.

In microscope, liver sections from normal and SBE control mice stained with HE revealed normal and steady architecture of hepatocytes and portal space. CCl_4 intoxication led to severe hepatic inflammation with mononuclear cell infiltration surrounding hepatic veins accompanied by partial destruction of adjacent hepatocytes. On the contrary, treatment of SBE improved inflammation response with mild mononuclear cell infiltration surrounding portal space and normal architecture of hepatocytes and portal space (Figure 4). These data demonstrated that black garlic extract attenuated hepatotoxicity and hepatitis induced by CCl_4 administration. In previous study, Kodai et al. (2007) proved that administration of S-allyl-cysteine could attenuate hepatic cell necrosis and inflammation in acute liver injury induced by CCl_4 [36]. Furthermore, Anandasadagopan et al. (2017) reported that S-allyl-cysteine treatment could downregulate the expression of p65-NF-kB, TNF-α, and iNOS and suppressed liver inflammation in chromium- (VI-) induced hepatotoxicity model [37]. Therefore, high concentration of S-allyl-cysteine of single clove black garlic extract may elucidate the beneficial effect of single clove black garlic extract for liver histology in coadministrated CCl_4 and single clove black garlic extract group.

4. Conclusion

In conclusion, our results demonstrated that single clove black garlic aqueous extract exerted the beneficial effects on dyslipidemia and hepatitis induced by chronic carbon tetrachloride administration, a common toxin induced liver disease model, and provided more information about the bioactivity of single clove black garlic.

Abbreviations

SBE:	Single clove black garlic extract
TG:	Triglyceride
TC:	Total cholesterol
HDL-cholesterol:	High density lipoprotein cholesterol
LDL-cholesterol:	Low density lipoprotein cholesterol
AST:	Aspartate transaminase
ALT:	Alanine transaminase
HE:	Hematoxylin-Eosin.

Authors' Contributions

Gia-Buu Tran conceived and designed the study and drafted the manuscript. Gia-Buu Tran and Sao-Mai Dam performed the experiments. Nghia-Thu Tram Le handled the research data and conducted the statistical analysis of the data. Gia-Buu Tran interpreted the result, revised the manuscript, and resolved the queries of reviewers. All authors read and approved the final manuscript.

Disclosure

This research project received no specific grant from any funding agency in the public, commercial, or not-for-profit sectors.

Acknowledgments

The authors would like to express gratitude to Dr. Thi-Huyen Tran, Dr. Hong-Thien Van, and Dr. Xuan-Uyen Thuy Phan for sharing their pearls of wisdom with them during the course of this research. The authors would like to thank their colleagues from their institution for their assistance during this project.

References

[1] C. F. Lima, M. Fernandes-Ferreira, and C. Pereira-Wilson, "Drinking of Salvia officinalis tea increases CCl4-induced hepatotoxicity in mice," *Food and Chemical Toxicology*, vol. 45, no. 3, pp. 456–464, 2007.

[2] C. Loguercio and A. Federico, "Oxidative stress in viral and alcoholic hepatitis," *Free Radical Biology & Medicine*, vol. 34, no. 1, pp. 1–10, 2003.

[3] S. Li, H. Y. Tan, N. Wang et al., "The role of oxidative stress and antioxidants in liver diseases," *International Journal of Molecular Sciences*, vol. 16, no. 11, pp. 26087–26124, 2015.

[4] E. Madrigal-Santillán, E. Madrigal-Bujaidar, I. Álvarez-González et al., "Review of natural products with hepatoprotective effects," *World Journal of Gastroenterology*, vol. 20, no. 40, pp. 14787–14804, 2014.

[5] Q. Bai, H. Yan, Y. Sheng et al., "Long-term acetaminophen treatment induced liver fibrosis in mice and the involvement of Egr-1," *Toxicology*, vol. 382, pp. 47–58, 2017.

[6] L.-J. Kong, H. Li, Y.-J. Du et al., "Vatalanib, a tyrosine kinase inhibitor, decreases hepatic fbrosis and sinusoidal capillarization in CCl4-induced fbrotic mice," *Molecular Medicine Reports*, vol. 15, no. 5, pp. 2604–2610, 2017.

[7] X. Zhao, L. Wang, H. Zhang, D. Zhang, Z. Zhang, and J. Zhang, "Protective effect of artemisinin on chronic alcohol induced-liver damage in mice," *Environmental Toxicology and Pharmacology*, vol. 52, pp. 221–226, 2017.

[8] Z. Zhou, S. Park, J. W. Kim et al., "Detrimental effects of nicotine on thioacetamide-induced liver injury in mice," *Toxicology Mechanisms and Methods*, vol. 27, no. 7, pp. 501–510, 2017.

[9] R. O. Recknagel, E. A. Glende Jr., J. A. Dolak, and R. L. Waller, "Mechanisms of carbon tetrachloride toxicity," *Pharmacology & Therapeutics*, vol. 43, no. 1, pp. 139–154, 1989.

[10] Y. W. Hsu, C. F. Tsai, W. C. Chuang, W. K. Chen, Y. C. Ho, and F. J. Lu, "Protective effects of silica hydride against carbon tetrachloride-induced hepatotoxicity in mice," *Food and Chemical Toxicology*, vol. 48, no. 6, pp. 1644–1653, 2010.

[11] N. Martins, S. Petropoulos, and I. C. F. R. Ferreira, "Chemical composition and bioactive compounds of garlic (Allium sativum L.) as affected by pre- and post-harvest conditions: A review," *Food Chemistry*, vol. 211, pp. 41–50, 2016.

[12] U. E. Obioha, S. M. Suru, K. F. Ola-Mudathir, and T. Y. Faremi, "Hepatoprotective potentials of onion and garlic extracts on cadmium-induced oxidative damage in rats," *Biological Trace Element Research*, vol. 129, no. 1-3, pp. 143–156, 2009.

[13] R. Kumar, S. Chhatwal, S. Arora et al., "Antihyperglycemic, antihyperlipidemic, anti-inflammatory and adenosine deaminase-lowering effects of garlic in patients with type 2 diabetes mellitus with obesity," *Diabetes, Metabolic Syndrome and Obesity: Targets and Therapy*, vol. 6, pp. 49–56, 2013.

[14] T. Hoshino, N. Kashimoto, and S. Kasuga, "Effects of garlic preparations on the gastrointestinal mucosa," *Journal of Nutrition*, vol. 131, no. 3, pp. 11095–11135, 2001.

[15] G. Oboh, "Prevention of garlic-induced hemolytic anemia using some tropical green leafy vegetables," *Journal of Medicinal Food*, vol. 7, no. 4, pp. 498–501, 2004.

[16] Y.-J. Seo, O.-C. Gweon, J. Im, Y.-M. Lee, M.-J. Kang, and J.-I. Kim, "Effect of garlic and aged black garlic on hyperglycemia and dyslipidemia in animal model of type 2 diabetes mellitus," *Journal of Food Science and Nutrition*, vol. 14, no. 1, pp. 1–7, 2009.

[17] A. W. Ha, T. Ying, and W. K. Kim, "The effects of black garlic (Allium satvium) extracts on lipid metabolism in rats fed a high fat diet," *Nutrition Research and Practice*, vol. 9, no. 1, pp. 30–36, 2015.

[18] S. Kimura, Y.-C. Tung, M.-H. Pan, N.-W. Su, Y.-J. Lai, and K.-C. Cheng, "Black garlic: A critical review of its production, bioactivity, and application," *Journal of Food and Drug Analysis*, vol. 25, no. 1, pp. 62–70, 2017.

[19] J. H. Jeong, H. R. Jeong, Y. N. Jo, H. J. Kim, J. H. Shin, and H. J. Heo, "Ameliorating effects of aged garlic extracts against Aβ-induced neurotoxicity and cognitive impairment," *BMC Complementary and Alternative Medicine*, vol. 13, article no. 268, 2013.

[20] M. H. Kim, M. J. Kim, J. H. Lee et al., "Hepatoprotective effect of aged black garlic on chronic alcohol-induced liver injury in rats," *Journal of Medicinal Food*, vol. 14, no. 7-8, pp. 732–738, 2011.

[21] J. H. Shin, C. W. Lee, S. J. Oh et al., "Hepatoprotective effect of aged black garlic extract in rodents," *Toxicological Research*, vol. 30, no. 1, pp. 49–54, 2014.

[22] S. Kodai, S. Takemura, S. Kubo, H. Azuma, and Y. Minamiyama, "Therapeutic administration of an ingredient of agedg-arlic extracts, S-allyl cysteine resolves liver fibrosis established by carbon tetrachloride in rats," *Journal of Clinical Biochemistry and Nutrition*, vol. 56, no. 3, pp. 179–185, 2015.

[23] S. Chen, X. Shen, S. Cheng et al., "Evaluation of garlic cultivars for polyphenolic content and antioxidant properties," *PLoS ONE*, vol. 8, no. 11, Article ID e79730, 12 pages, 2013.

[24] S. E. Bae, S. Y. Cho, Y. D. Won, S. H. Lee, and H. J. Park, "Changes in S-allyl cysteine contents and physicochemical properties of black garlic during heat treatment," *LWT- Food Science and Technology*, vol. 55, no. 1, pp. 397–402, 2014.

[25] K. M. Naji, E. S. Al-Shaibani, F. A. Alhadi, S. A. Al-Soudi, and M. R. D'souza, "Hepatoprotective and antioxidant effects of single clove garlic against CCl4-induced hepatic damage in rabbits," *BMC Complementary and Alternative Medicine*, vol. 17, no. 1, article no. 411, 2017.

[26] A. J. M. Christina, G. R. Saraswathy, S. J. Heison Robert et al., "Inhibition of CCl4-induced liver fibrosis by Piper longum Linn.?" *Phytomedicine*, vol. 13, no. 3, pp. 196–198, 2006.

[27] S. R. Thaakur, G. R. Saraswathy, E. Maheswari et al., "Inhibition of CCl4-induced liver fibrosis by Trigonella foenum-graecum Linn.," *Natural Product Radiance*, vol. 6, no. 1, pp. 11–17, 2007.

[28] E.-S. Jung, S.-H. Park, E.-K. Choi et al., "Reduction of blood lipid parameters by a 12-wk supplementation of aged black garlic: A randomized controlled trial," *Nutrition Journal* , vol. 30, no. 9, pp. 1034–1039, 2014.

[29] Y. Kodera, A. Suzuki, O. Imada et al., "Physical, chemical, and biological properties of S-allylcysteine, an amino acid derived from garlic," *Journal of Agricultural and Food Chemistry*, vol. 50, no. 3, pp. 622–632, 2002.

[30] J. H. Kim, S. H. Yu, Y. J. Cho et al., "Preparation of S-Allylcysteine-enriched black garlic juice and its antidiabetic effects in streptozotocin-induced insulin-deficient mice," *Journal of Agricultural and Food Chemistry*, vol. 65, no. 2, pp. 358–363, 2017.

[31] R. Ismail, A. El-Megeid, and A. Abdel-Moemin, "Carbon Tetrachloride-Induced Liver Disease in Rats: The Potential Effect of Supplement Oils with Vitamins E and C on The Nutritional Status," *GMS German Medical Science*, vol. 7, no. 5, 2009.

[32] R. A. Khan, M. R. Khan, and S. Sahreen, "CCl_4-induced hepatotoxicity: protective effect of rutin on p53, CYP2E1 and the antioxidative status in rat," *BMC Complementary and Alternative Medicine*, vol. 12, article 178, 2012.

[33] A. E. El-Hadary and M. F. Ramadan Hassanien, "Hepatoprotective effect of cold-pressed Syzygium aromaticum oil against carbon tetrachloride (CCl4)-induced hepatotoxicity in rats," *Pharmaceutical Biology*, vol. 54, no. 8, pp. 1364–1372, 2016.

[34] S. M. B. Asdaq, "Antioxidant and hypolipidemic potential of aged garlic extract and its constituent, s-allyl cysteine, in rats," *Evidence-Based Complementary and Alternative Medicine*, vol. 2015, Article ID 328545, 2015.

[35] P. Y. Kwo, S. M. Cohen, and J. K. Lim, "ACG clinical guideline: evaluation of abnormal liver chemistries," *American Journal of Gastroenterology*, vol. 112, no. 1, pp. 18–35, 2016.

[36] S. Kodai, S. Takemura, Y. Minamiyama et al., "S-allyl cysteine prevents CC14-induced acute liver injury in rats," *Free Radical Research*, vol. 41, no. 4, pp. 489–497, 2007.

[37] S. K. Anandasadagopan, C. Sundaramoorthy, A. K. Pandurangan, V. Nagarajan, K. Srinivasan, and S. Ganapasam, "S-Allyl cysteine alleviates inflammation by modulating the expression of NF-κB during chromium (VI)-induced hepatotoxicity in rats," *Human & Experimental Toxicology*, vol. 36, no. 11, pp. 1186–1200, 2017.

26

Imaging the Abdominal Manifestations of Cystic Fibrosis

C. D. Gillespie,[1] M. K. O'Reilly,[2] G. N. Allen,[3] S. McDermott,[4] V. O. Chan,[2] and C. A. Ridge[2]

[1] *Department of Medicine, Mater Misericordiae University Hospital, Dublin, Ireland*
[2] *Department of Radiology, Mater Misericordiae University Hospital, Dublin, Ireland*
[3] *University College of Dublin School of Medicine, Dublin, Ireland*
[4] *Department of Radiology, Massachusetts General Hospital, 55 Fruit St., Boston, MA 02114, USA*

Correspondence should be addressed to C. D. Gillespie; ciaragill@gmail.com

Academic Editor: Pierluigi Toniutto

Cystic fibrosis (CF) is a multisystem disease with a range of abdominal manifestations including those involving the liver, pancreas, and kidneys. Recent advances in management of the respiratory complications of the disease has led to a greater life expectancy in patients with CF. Subsequently, there is increasing focus on the impact of abdominal disease on quality of life and survival. Liver cirrhosis is the most important extrapulmonary cause of death in CF, yet significant challenges remain in the diagnosis of CF related liver disease. The capacity to predict those patients at risk of developing cirrhosis remains a significant challenge. We review representative abdominal imaging findings in patients with CF selected from the records of two academic health centres, with a view to increasing familiarity with the abdominal manifestations of the disease. We review their presentation and expected imaging findings, with a focus on the challenges facing diagnosis of the hepatic manifestations of the disease. An increased familiarity with these abdominal manifestations will facilitate timely diagnosis and management, which is paramount to further improving outcomes for patients with cystic fibrosis.

1. Introduction

Cystic fibrosis (CF) is the most common inherited fatal disease in Caucasians. Ireland has the highest birth incidence of the disease in the world, affecting 1 in every 1600 births [1]. Its inheritance pattern is autosomal recessive but can be a result of one of over 1500 mutations of the cystic fibrosis transmembrane regulator (CFTR) gene, located on the long arm of chromosome 7 [2, 3]. The most common of these is the deletion of phenylalanine at position 508: F508del.

The CFTR gene and its product, a cyclic adenosine monophosphate (cAMP) mediated chloride channel, play a key role in hydrating bodily secretions and regulating cellular functions including sodium transport [3]. The defective gene product causes impaired chloride ion transport across exocrine gland epithelial cells [4] which leads to thickened viscous secretions affecting multiple organs including the lungs, liver, and pancreas.

With improvements in the management of the respiratory complications of CF, life expectancy in this population has increased. The abdominal manifestations of CF are common and may not present until adulthood in some cases. Many challenges remain in the diagnosis of these abdominal manifestations, particularly in the area of cystic fibrosis-related liver disease (CFLD). CFLD is an independent risk factor for mortality in CF [5] and a significant cause of morbidity and mortality in a proportion of CF patients. A reliable noninvasive method for early prediction of significant CFLD or cirrhosis is lacking. Consequently, a familiarity with the available screening tools and their limitations, the expected imaging appearances of CF abdominal disease, and the areas of research likely to impact on their diagnosis in future is paramount.

Adults comprise 45% of patients with CF in Ireland [1]. We selected the most representative abdominal imaging findings in patients with CF across all imaging modalities performed in two academic health centres. In this pictorial review, we present the typical abdominal ultrasound (US), computed tomography (CT), and magnetic resonance imaging (MRI) findings in adults with CF, with a focus on CF related liver disease.

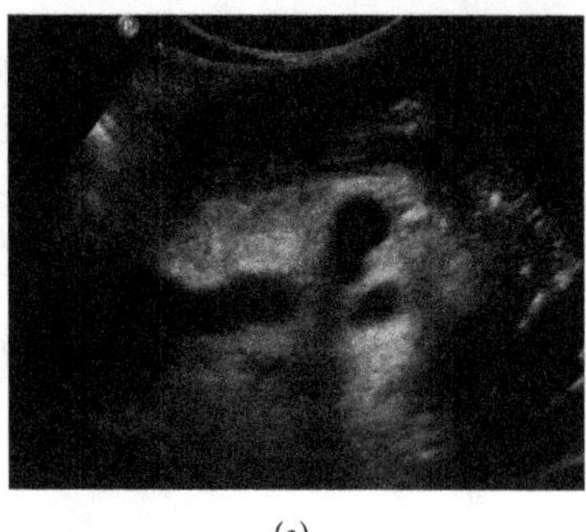

(a)

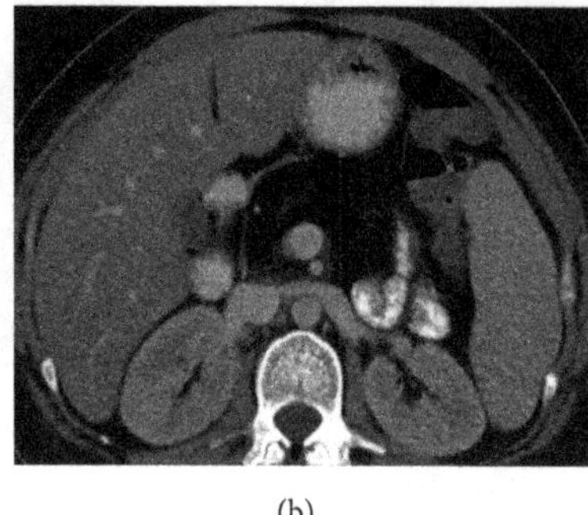

(b)

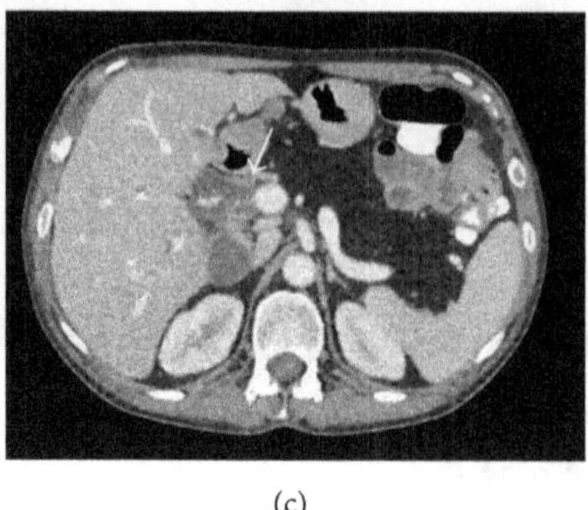

(c)

FIGURE 1: (a) Transverse abdominal ultrasound of a 34-year-old male with cystic fibrosis. Fatty infiltration of the pancreas is typically echogenic on US. (b) The pancreas is homogenously low in attenuation on CT and is often difficult to differentiate from normal retroperitoneal fat. (c) Axial portal venous phase contrast-enhanced CT performed to assess abdominal pain in a 44-year-old CF patient 2 weeks after bilateral double lung transplant demonstrates diffuse pancreatic lipomatosis which manifests as homogenous low attenuation. Note is also made of a distended common bile duct (white arrow) due to stricture.

The aim of this review is to heighten awareness of the abdominal manifestations of CF and their imaging findings, such that clinicians are better equipped to provide a timely diagnosis for what is an increasingly significant range of conditions in this population.

2. Pancreatic Manifestations

The pancreas is the most commonly affected abdominal organ in CF. The pathophysiology, clinical manifestations, and imaging findings of the typical pancreatic manifestations will be discussed.

2.1. Pathophysiology and Clinical Manifestations. Pancreatic disease is caused by inspissation of abnormally concentrated pancreatic secretions which produces proximal duct obstruction. This results in acinar atrophy, inflammation, progressive fibrosis, fatty replacement, calcification, and cyst formation.

Clinical manifestations of pancreatic dysfunction in CF include pancreatic insufficiency, pancreatitis, and an increased risk of pancreatic cancer compared to the general population [6]. Pancreatic insufficiency encompasses both exocrine and endocrine insufficiency. Exocrine occurs in 85% while endocrine occurs in 30–50% of CF patients [7]. It can lead to malabsorption and therefore malnutrition, poor health, and growth. It presents in childhood for the majority of patients, although patients who are diagnosed with CF in adulthood are less likely to have pancreatic insufficiency [7]. Pancreatitis is rare despite pathologic evidence of a chronic inflammatory process and is more common in pancreatic sufficient patients [7, 8].

2.2. Pathological and Imaging Findings

2.2.1. Pancreatic Atrophy and Steatosis. The pancreas is commonly atrophic in CF and may have a pattern of atrophy with partial fatty replacement or atrophy with complete fatty infiltration. Fatty infiltration of the pancreas is typically echogenic on US (Figure 1(a)) and homogenously low in attenuation on CT, often difficult to differentiate from normal retroperitoneal fat (Figure 1(b)). On T1 weighted MRI, there is increased signal intensity representing fatty infiltration interspersed with low signal intensity representing fibrosis. The pancreas may be enlarged and replaced with fat, known as lipomatous pseudohypertrophy [9].

The atrophic pancreas with partial fatty replacement is small in size and echogenic on US. The CT features include loss of the normal soft tissue component of the gland which may be accompanied by calcification and duct irregularity (Figures 2(a) and 2(b)).

2.2.2. Pancreatic Cystosis. Replacement of the pancreas with macroscopic cysts is rare. It is most likely a result of protein hyperconcentration, thickened secretions, and ductal ectasia (Figure 2(b)). The cysts are lined by epithelium and thus are true cysts. They replace normal pancreatic parenchyma, may displace but should not infiltrate adjacent structures, and do not exceed 5 cm in diameter as seen on US and CT (Figure 2(b)).

3. Renal Manifestations

Although renal complications in CF are infrequent, the most common manifestations include nephrolithiasis, electrolyte abnormalities, and acute kidney injury (AKI). Rarer manifestations include progression to chronic kidney disease (CKD) and parenchymal disease including amyloidosis, diabetic nephropathy, nephrocalcinosis, diffuse and nodular glomerulosclerosis, and calcineurin inhibitor toxicity in lung transplant patients [10].

Nephrolithiasis occurs in 3–6% of CF patients, three times more than age matched controls [11, 12]. It is the most common renal manifestation of CF (Figure 3). Urine is supersaturated with calcium oxalate, the main component of calculi in CF [13]. Hyperoxaluria is attributed to chronic antibiotic use, which reduces gastrointestinal colonisation by bacteria which normally degrade oxalate [12]. Oral fluids and a low oxalate diet are advised for prevention. Antegrade nephrostomy placement may be required in complicated cases.

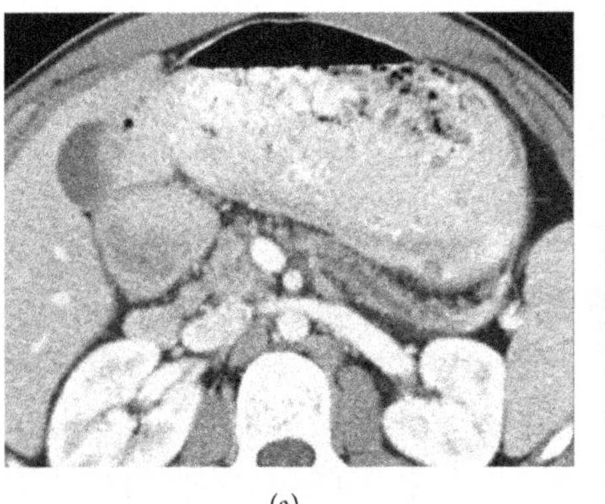

(a)

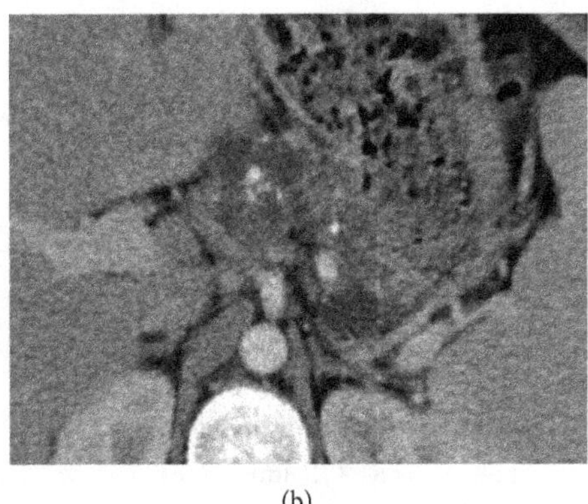

(b)

FIGURE 2: (a) Axial CT images of a 38-year-old male with cystic fibrosis. There is atrophy of the pancreas and duct irregularity. (b) Axial CT image of a 36-year-old female exhibiting pancreatic cysts, pancreatic calcification, and duct irregularity.

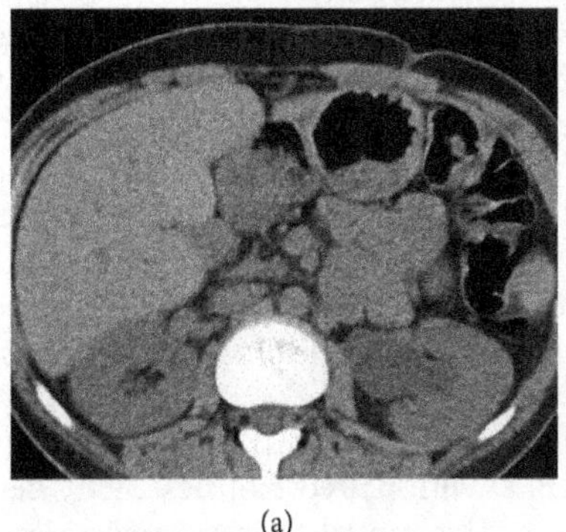

(a)

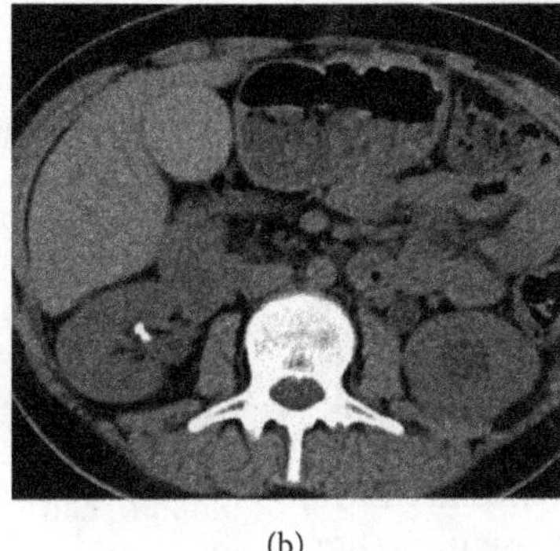

(b)

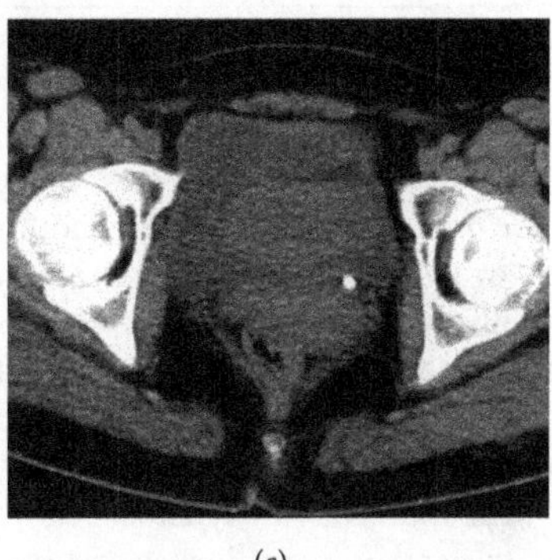

(c)

FIGURE 3: (a–c) Axial CT images of a 21-year-old female with left renal angle pain on a background of cystic fibrosis. (a) Noncontrast axial CT at the level of the renal hila demonstrates left hydronephrosis. The absence of normal pancreatic tissue and increased attenuation of the liver possibly due to haemosiderin deposition are also evident. (b) Axial CT image below the renal hila demonstrating a nonobstructing calculus in the right renal pelvis and left hydroureter. (c) Axial CT image at the level of the bladder demonstrating an obstructing left lower ureteric calculus.

CKD is rare, with an annual prevalence of 2.3% reported in one study of 12,000 CF adults. This doubled with every additional 10 years of age [14]. Recurrent episodes of AKI and aminoglycoside exposure are debated as the main contributors to CKD. Advanced CKD is rare, with a prevalence of 0.6% for stage 5 CKD and risk factors include lung transplant, CF related diabetes, and recurrent AKI [10].

4. Hepatobiliary Manifestations

CFLD encompasses a broad spectrum of hepatobiliary complications including cholestasis, elevated aminotransferases, hepatic steatosis, hepatic fibrosis, focal biliary cirrhosis, and multilobular cirrhosis with or without portal hypertension. CF is also known to be complicated by microgallbladder and hepatocellular carcinoma (HCC) has been reported in four patients in the literature [6, 15–17].

4.1. Aetiology and Classification. CFLD is due to abnormally thickened secretions within the biliary epithelium, which then accumulates within bile ducts, concentrating caustic bile components in the liver [2]. Modifier genotypes in CF may also contribute to severity of CFLD. The z-allele of the SERPINA 1 gene has a strong association (odds ratio of 5) for developing CFLD with portal hypertension [18].

The fact that CFLD lacks a consistent definition is at least in part responsible for a significant variation in reported prevalence of CFLD in the literature. Studies using broader interpretations of the term report a prevalence of 30–40%, while focal biliary cirrhosis has been reported as occurring in 20–30% of CF individuals, with multilobular cirrhosis in 5–10% [19].

Liver cirrhosis is the most important extrapulmonary cause of death in CF, accounting for 2.5% of overall mortality [20], and is therefore the most clinically significant form of CFLD. The North American CF foundation proposed a classification for CFLD based on a consensus among hepatologists convened in 2007. This separates cirrhosis and portal hypertension from other forms of hepatobiliary involvement in CF (Table 1) [19].

4.2. Biochemical Abnormalities. A diagnosis of CFLD is considered if transaminases and gamma-glutamyl transferase (GGT) are above the upper limit of normal on at least three

Table 1: Proposed classification of CFLD by North American CF Foundation (2007) adapted from Flass and Narkewicz [19].

(1) Preclinical: No evidence of liver disease on exam, imaging, or laboratory values
(2) Liver involvement without cirrhosis/portal hypertension: at least one of
Biochemical abnormalities
(a) Persistent AST, ALT, and GGT >2 times upper limit of normal
(b) Intermittent elevations of the above laboratory values
Cholangiopathy (based on US, MRI, CT, and ERCP)
Steatosis
Fibrosis
US abnormalities not consistent with cirrhosis
(3) CF related liver disease with cirrhosis/portal hypertension

AST: aspartate transaminase, ALT: alanine transaminase, and GGT: gamma-glutamyl transferase.

consecutive occasions within twelve months, with either hepatomegaly or splenomegaly on exam or ultrasound evidence of hepatobiliary abnormalities [20]. However, while basic liver function tests (LFTs) can be intermittently deranged in CF, they are largely nonspecific and are considered unreliable as a marker of severity or progression of CFLD. Meanwhile, patients with multilobular cirrhosis can have normal LFTs [20–22]. Research is ongoing to determine useful serum markers for early and reliable prediction of CFLD and its progression.

Studies have shown that different combinations of fibrogenesis markers such as collagen IV, prolyl hydroxylase, tissue inhibitor of metalloproteinase 1 levels, and monocyte chemoattractant protein 1 can distinguish patients with biopsy-proven CFLD from those with CF but no liver disease and early from late fibrosis [23, 24]. MicroRNAs also show promise, with studies showing various miRNAs can predict rapid onset of liver disease while specific combinations can distinguish fibrosis F0 from F3-4 [25]. These require further study for clinical implementation and are likely costly. Simpler biomarkers which are more readily available such as aspartate aminotransferase to platelet ratio (APRI) and Fib-4 have shown promise in one biopsy-controlled study; APRI differentiated CFLD from CF with no liver disease [sensitivity of 73%, specificity of 70%, in full agreement with histology staging 37% of the time and within one stage 73% of the time] while Fib-4 was shown to predict portal hypertension at diagnosis [25].

4.3. Biliary Manifestations. The biliary system can be involved in patients with CF but symptoms are rare. Inspissated biliary secretions cause mucosal hyperplasia in the gallbladder and bile ducts [26]. This process leads to increased sludge in the biliary tract and the development of microgallbladder, possibly through stenosis of cystic ducts and secondary atrophy of the gallbladder [6, 27].

Cholelithiasis may arise due to increased faecal bile acid secretion secondary to pancreatic insufficiency which results in lithogenic bile [28]. Cholangiopathy occurs in the form of intrahepatic bile duct dilation (Figure 1(c)), beading, or stricture formation and has been seen in children and adults with CFLD. Bile duct abnormalities have also been reported in a significant number of CF patients without clinically apparent liver disease [29]. Imaging findings include intra- and extrahepatic biliary strictures (Figures 4(a) and 4(b)), cholelithiasis, and microgallbladder (Figure 5(a)). Choledocholithiasis and cholecystitis are also reported (Figure 6).

4.4. Hepatic Steatosis. Steatosis is one of the most common hepatic manifestations in the CF population, occurring in 23–75% of CF patients [30]. Patients may present with smooth hepatomegaly but are usually asymptomatic, without signs of portal hypertension. It is represented by increased liver echogenicity on US (Figure 7), low attenuation on CT, and decreased T2 signal intensity on MRI.

Steatosis was previously accepted as a benign entity in both CF [31] and the general population [32]. However, the rising prevalence of nonalcoholic fatty liver disease (NAFLD) has brought increased focus on steatosis, and while nonalcoholic steatohepatitis (NASH) was traditionally considered the only form of NAFLD to confer considerable risk of fibrosis progression, recent studies have now drawn attention to a previously underappreciated risk of fibrosis progression in patients with steatosis [33, 34].

In a meta-analysis including 11 studies, of which 133 patients had NAFLD with paired biopsies, 39.1% developed progressive fibrosis. The annual fibrosis progression rate in NAFLD patients with stage 0 fibrosis at baseline was 0.07 stages compared with 0.14 stages for NASH patients. Pais et al. observed that 13 of 16 patients with NAFLD and mild inflammation at baseline progressed to typical NASH or bridging fibrosis, while only 1 of 5 patients with simple steatosis progressed to NASH [34]. Overall, these studies suggest that NAFLD patients can develop progressive fibrosis though at a slower rate than those with NASH and cirrhosis may develop if steatosis progresses to steatohepatitis and subsequent fibrosis. As our understanding of the natural history of steatosis in NAFLD evolves, our understanding of its significance within the CF population may also evolve.

4.5. Fibrosis: Focal Biliary Cirrhosis. Focal biliary cirrhosis (FBC), characterised by focal portal fibrosis and cholestasis, is a histopathologic lesion that is typical of CF related liver disease. It arises as a result of biliary obstruction and progressive periportal fibrosis and can progress to multilobular cirrhosis and portal hypertension, albeit very rarely [20]. It is typically clinically silent without raised transaminases.

The typical US feature is periportal echogenicity (Figures 8(a) and 8(b)). This correlates with pathologic findings of cells containing fat globules in the fibrotic portal tracts and cells in the periportal liver parenchyma which contain large fat-laden vacuoles [27]. MRI findings include high intensity signal in periportal areas on T1 weighted imaging (Figures 8(c) and 8(d)) [7].

4.6. Multilobular Cirrhosis. Although rare, multilobular cirrhosis is the most clinically significant form of CFLD and has

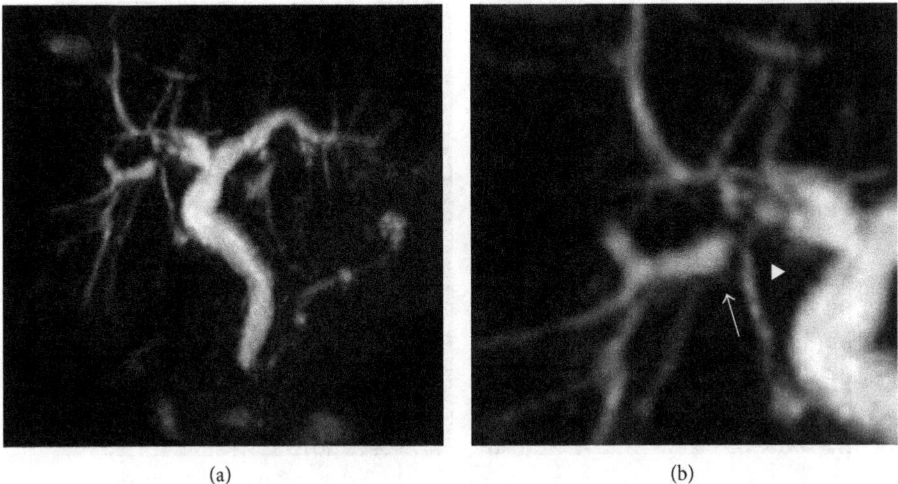

Figure 4: (a) Coronal half axis single shot turbo spin echo (HASTE) magnetic resonance cholangiopancreatography (MRCP) demonstrating intrahepatic biliary strictures in an asymptomatic 19-year-old female with CF. US performed to assess obstructive pattern abnormal liver function tests suggested biliary dilatation prompting MRCP. (b) Magnified MRCP image demonstrating focal biliary dilatation (white arrow) and biliary stricture (arrowhead).

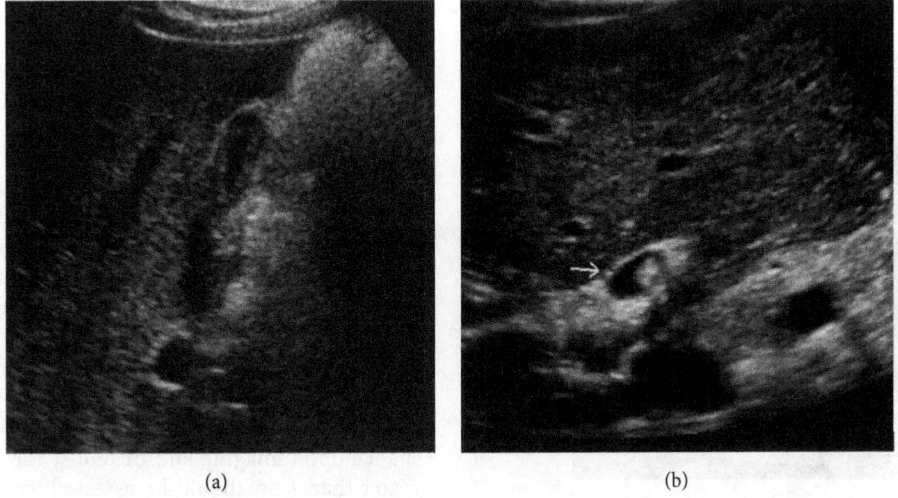

Figure 5: (a) US image of a 36-year-old female with cystic fibrosis and prior history of biliary colic demonstrating a persistently collapsed gallbladder (microgallbladder) in the longitudinal plane. (b) Gallstone in a contracted gallbladder (arrow).

an estimated average prevalence of 5.6% as per one review of 12 reports including 4446 patients [19]. A prospective study of 177 patients demonstrated a median age at diagnosis of 7 years (range; 2 months–18 years) with an incidence rate of 2.5 per 100 patient years for the first decade of life which sharply declines thereafter [35]. Multilobular cirrhosis carries with it the risk of portal hypertension and varices with a prevalence of 4.2% and 2.4%, respectively [19].

Liver disease in CF is often silent until late stages of the disease. Even with the development of multilobular cirrhosis, patients can remain asymptomatic until signs of portal hypertension develop [19]. Clinically, multilobular cirrhosis presents as a hard nodular liver with or without hepatomegaly.

Pathologically, it is characterised by diffuse cirrhosis with multiple regenerative nodules and imaging reveals a nodular liver contour with coarse heterogeneous parenchyma (Figure 8(b)) [6]. On CT and MRI, multiple regenerative nodules are seen, surrounded by bands of T2 hypointense fibrosis (Figures 8(c) and 8(d)) [27].

4.7. Complications in CF Cirrhosis

4.7.1. Portal Hypertension and Related Complications. If portal hypertension complicates the presentation of multilobular cirrhosis, patients may present with varices, ascites, or splenomegaly which can be readily identified on US and CT (Figures 8(b) and 8(c)). Siderotic nodules in the spleen,

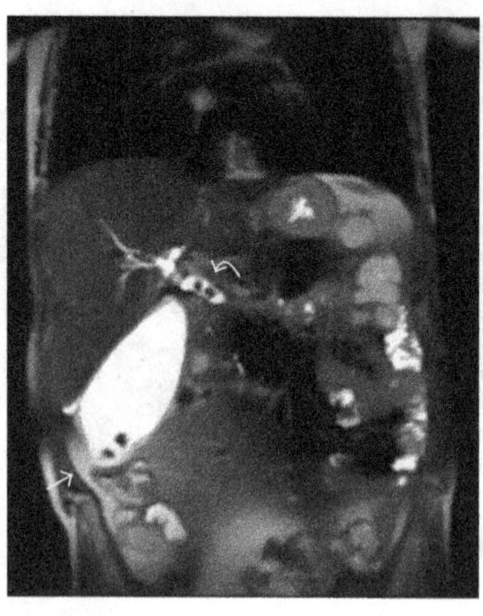

(a)

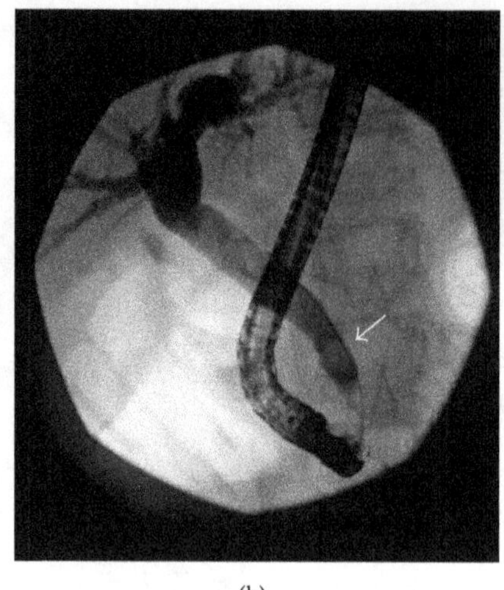

(b)

FIGURE 6: (a) Coronal T2 HASTE image of an MRCP performed to assess abdominal pain in a 44-year-old CF patient 2 weeks after bilateral double lung transplant demonstrates calculi in the distended fundus of the gallbladder. There is small volume pericholecystic fluid (arrow) and gallbladder wall thickening. Calculi are shown in the proximal common bile duct (CBD, curved arrow) consistent with choledocholithiasis. (b) Fluoroscopic image from the same patient during endoscopic retrograde cholangiopancreatogram (ERCP) and sphincterotomy. The dilated CBD is outlined by iodinated contrast with guide wire in situ. Filling defects in the distal CBD consistent with calculi (arrow).

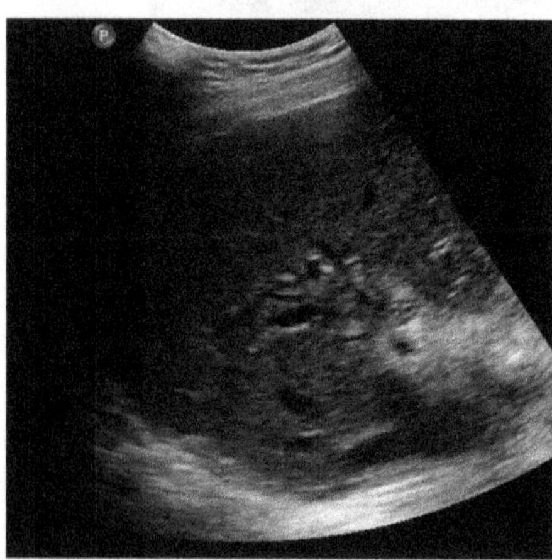

FIGURE 7: Longitudinal US of an asymptomatic 21-year-old male with cystic fibrosis performed for screening purposes. Echogenic liver parenchyma is consistent with hepatic steatosis.

also known as Gamna-Gandy bodies, are another feature of portal hypertension seen on MRI and are due to haemorrhage within the spleen (Figure 9) [27]. Of note, portal hypertension can present in noncirrhotic patients [19].

Rowland and colleagues have identified CFLD with portal hypertension as an independent risk factor for mortality, with a 10-year pair-matched cohort demonstrating an almost threefold increased risk of death compared to CF controls without liver disease [5]. However, the literature regarding this finding suggests that this is not a uniformly held opinion [35–37].

4.7.2. Hepatocellular Carcinoma. HCC can occur in patients with cirrhosis of any aetiology. With increased survival in patients with CF, there is a risk of HCC. Four such cases have been reported in the literature [6, 15–17]. Typical imaging features of this lesion in a 35-year-old male with CF and cirrhosis are depicted in Figure 9. HCC is usually characterised by a well-circumscribed lesion which is hypoechoic on US (Figure 9(a)) and low signal intensity on unenhanced T1-weighted MRI (Figure 9(b)) with avid enhancement on arterial phase MRI using gadolinium contrast (Figure 9(c)) [38]. Contrast washout on delayed phase imaging may also be seen. Similar enhancement features are seen using dynamic enhanced CT.

The American Association for the Study of Liver Disease (AASLD) guideline update in 2010 recommends biannual US for screening of HCC in any patient with cirrhosis, with reliance upon imaging and/or biopsy for diagnosis. Nodules greater than 1 cm should be assessed with 4-phase multidetector CT or dynamic contrast-enhanced MRI to assess for arterial hyperenhancement and portal venous or later phase washout. If these findings are absent, the recommendation is to proceed to further contrast-enhanced imaging or biopsy [39].

4.8. Imaging and the Challenges of Early Diagnosis of CFLD. Although CFLD is the most significant abdominal manifestation of CF from a mortality perspective, it remains the most challenging in terms of early recognition and diagnosis. We therefore dedicate this section to discussing the current challenges and future perspectives on the diagnosis of CFLD as it pertains to imaging.

Ultrasound is more sensitive than LFTs in detecting CFLD [20], with suggestions that abnormal echogenicity can precede clinical or biochemical manifestations of liver disease. However, US has been shown to have a positive predictive value of only 33% and while an abnormal US may predict the presence of moderate to severe liver disease, a normal US does not exclude significant liver fibrosis [40].

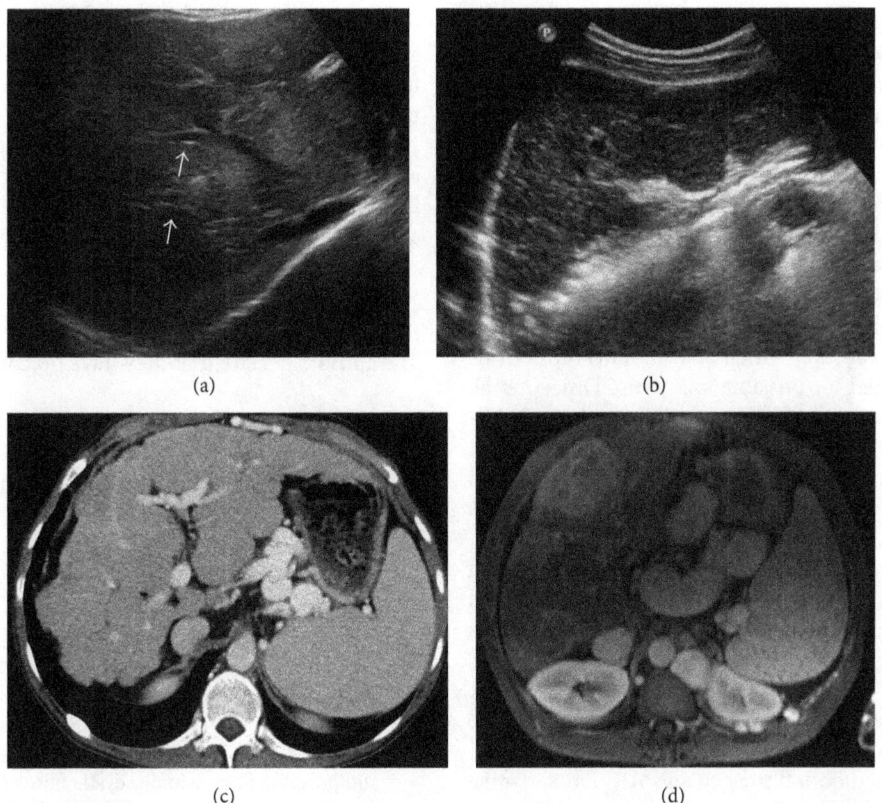

FIGURE 8: (a) Longitudinal US image of a 32-year-old male with cystic fibrosis demonstrating periportal echogenicity (arrows) consistent with periportal fibrosis. (b and c) Transverse US image and axial CT demonstrating a shrunken, nodular right lobe of liver with relative left lobe hypertrophy, varices, and splenomegaly in a CF patient with deranged LFTs at time of imaging. (d) Delayed enhanced T1-weighted axial MRI demonstrating regenerative nodules surrounded by bands of enhancing fibrotic liver parenchyma.

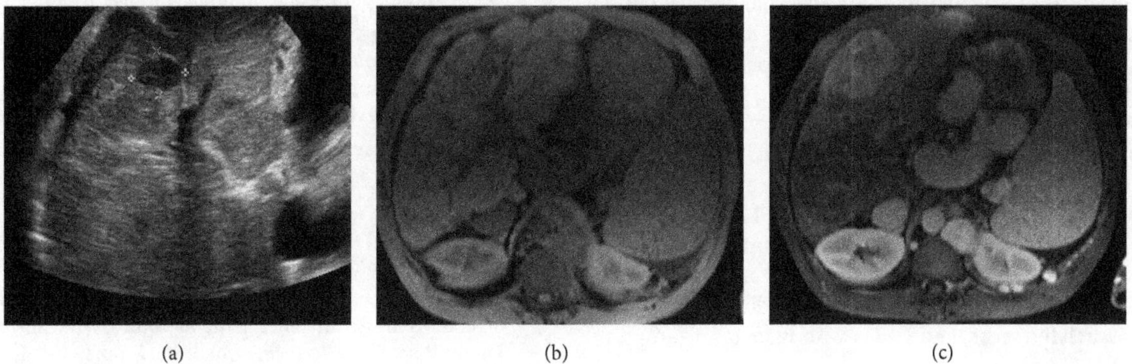

FIGURE 9: (a) Longitudinal US image of a 34-year-old male with cystic fibrosis was done as part of routine surveillance for cirrhosis in the context of stable biochemical markers. US image demonstrating a well-circumscribed hypoechoic lesion. (b and c) Noncontrast and arterial phase T1-weighted gadolinium enhanced MRI demonstrating a hyperenhancing well-circumscribed lesion in segment 4. Splenic siderotic nodules are an additional feature of portal hypertension.

Biopsy is reserved for cases of diagnostic doubt which would change management [20]. However, some studies suggest histopathological confirmation and staging of fibrosis by liver biopsy at initial diagnosis of CFLD may be warranted given its superior performance in predicting clinically significant CFLD and portal hypertension compared to noninvasive alternatives currently used in screening and follow-up [21]. In a 12-year prospective analysis of 40 children with CF, Lewindon and colleagues demonstrate that dual-pass percutaneous biopsy decreases sampling error and can predict portal hypertension while abnormal clinical exam, liver function tests (LFTs), and US failed to predict either presence of fibrosis or occurrence of portal hypertension [21].

Currently, however, best practice guidelines advise screening for CFLD using basic laboratory markers (LFTs, platelets, and INR) and abdominal US. Further imaging with CT or MRI is recommended if liver lesions or biliary tract involvement is found on US without sufficient clarity for diagnosis [20].

CT and MRI are useful in distinguishing fibrosis from steatosis, which can be difficult to determine on US, and are also useful for further investigation of focal lesions [20]. The advantage of MRI is that it is a comprehensive noninvasive investigation of the liver, biliary tract, and pancreas without ionising radiation exposure, which is an important consideration given the need for possible follow-up. Durieu et al. demonstrated the capacity of MR to detect intrahepatic biliary abnormalities in CF patients without clinically apparent liver disease, pointing to a likely underestimation by US and to MRCP as an option to identify early biliary abnormalities [29].

Transient elastography (TE) measures liver stiffness and is a mechanism for staging fibrosis which is already validated for chronic liver conditions such as hepatitis C. Early studies using TE for noninvasive assessment of liver fibrosis in CF patients showed no clear improvement over US [41]. ARFI is a novel US based elastography-method which, unlike fibroscan, can be used on both lobes of the liver [42]. Later studies proposed both fibroscan and ARFI as sensitive diagnostic tools for fibrosis [42] and provided some evidence for its use as a reliable detection tool for CF cirrhosis [43] with potential in screening for portal hypertension [44]. One prospective study using ARFI and TE supported feasibility of these tests in assessment of liver fibrosis in CF; however, further studies with longer follow-up are required [45].

A consensus on cut-off values for early diagnosis of CFLD remains elusive, and further research in this area is required, although this may in part be attributed to the absence of an accepted consensus definition of CFLD [45]. Ultimately, TE shows promise and, with further study, may improve diagnosis of liver fibrosis in CF patients if used in conjunction with current screening methods. While there are no biopsy-controlled studies for this technique in CFLD, authors cite the established evidence for TE's correlation with fibrosis in other liver diseases and have questioned the ethics of biopsy-controlled studies in paediatric populations due to its invasive nature, associated risks, and issues with respect to sampling error [41].

5. Conclusion

The abdominal manifestations of CF are of increasing importance in light of increased survival of adult populations with CF. Early recognition and diagnosis of these conditions and their complications will play an important role in improving the quality of life and further survival of patients with CF. Significant CFLD with cirrhosis or portal hypertension poses one of the biggest challenges in this respect.

Abnormal clinical examination, LFTs, and US findings are poor predictors of progression to cirrhosis or portal hypertension [21]. Investigations that reliably predict cirrhosis or portal hypertension are needed to better identify those at risk and to instigate earlier preventative measures and management of complications. A number of promising techniques may ultimately contribute to achieving this goal, but further research is awaited.

An awareness of the abdominal manifestations of CF and familiarity with their expected clinical presentation and imaging findings are paramount to the timely diagnosis and appropriate management of patients with CF.

Competing Interests

The authors declare that they have no competing interests.

References

[1] R. M. Pollock, "The treatment of cystic fibrosis in Ireland: problems and solutions," *The Cystic Fibrosis Association of Ireland*, vol. 1, pp. 1–30, 2005.

[2] T. F. Boat, "Cystic fibrosis," in *Nelson Textbook of Paediatrics*, R. E. Behrman, R. M. Kliegman, and H. B. Jenson, Eds., pp. 1437–1450, Saunders, Philadelphia, Pa, USA, 17th edition, 2004.

[3] M. R. Knowles and M. Drumm, "The influence of genetics on cystic fibrosis phenotypes," *Cold Spring Harbor Perspectives in Medicine*, vol. 2, no. 12, Article ID a009548, 2012.

[4] O. Efrati, A. Barak, D. Modan-Moses et al., "Liver cirrhosis and portal hypertension in cystic fibrosis," *European Journal of Gastroenterology and Hepatology*, vol. 15, no. 10, pp. 1073–1078, 2003.

[5] M. Rowland, C. Gallagher, C. G. Gallagher et al., "Outcome in patients with cystic fibrosis liver disease," *Journal of Cystic Fibrosis*, vol. 14, no. 1, pp. 120–126, 2015.

[6] L. P. Lavelle, S. H. McEvoy, E. Ni Mhurchu et al., "Cystic fibrosis below the diaphragm: abdominal findings in adult patients," *Radiographics*, vol. 35, no. 3, pp. 680–695, 2015.

[7] M. B. Robertson, K. A. Choe, and P. M. Joseph, "Review of the abdominal manifestations of cystic fibrosis in the adult patient," *Radiographics*, vol. 26, no. 3, pp. 679–690, 2006.

[8] C. R. Marino and F. S. Gorelick, "Scientific advances in cystic fibrosis," *Gastroenterology*, vol. 103, no. 2, pp. 681–693, 1992.

[9] M. Nakamura, N. Katada, A. Sakakibara et al., "Huge lipomatous pseudohypertrophy of the pancreas," *The American Journal of Gastroenterology*, vol. 72, no. 2, pp. 171–174, 1979.

[10] B. J. Plant, C. H. Goss, W. D. Plant, and S. C. Bell, "Management of comorbidities in older patients with cystic fibrosis," *The Lancet Respiratory Medicine*, vol. 1, no. 2, pp. 164–174, 2013.

[11] M. R. Perez-Brayfield, D. Caplan, J. M. Gatti, E. A. Smith, and A. J. Kirsch, "Metabolic risk factors for stone formation in patients with cystic fibrosis," *Journal of Urology*, vol. 167, no. 2 I, pp. 480–484, 2002.

[12] D. Nazareth and M. Walshaw, "A review of renal disease in cystic fibrosis," *Journal of Cystic Fibrosis*, vol. 12, no. 4, pp. 309–317, 2013.

[13] M. Terribile, M. Capuano, G. Cangiano et al., "Factors increasing the risk for stone formation in adult patients with cystic fibrosis," *Nephrology Dialysis Transplantation*, vol. 21, no. 7, pp. 1870–1875, 2006.

[14] B. S. Quon, N. Mayer-Hamblett, M. L. Aitken, A. R. Smyth, and C. H. Goss, "Risk factors for chronic kidney disease in adults with cystic fibrosis," *American Journal of Respiratory and Critical Care Medicine*, vol. 184, no. 10, pp. 1147–1152, 2011.

[15] D. Mckeon, A. Day, J. Parmar, G. Alexander, and D. Bilton, "Hepatocellular carcinoma in association with cirrhosis in a patient with cystic fibrosis," *Journal of Cystic Fibrosis*, vol. 3, no. 3, pp. 193–195, 2004.

[16] T. Kelleher, M. Staunton, S. O'Mahony, and P. A. McCormick, "Advanced hepatocellular carcinoma associated with cystic fibrosis," *European Journal of Gastroenterology and Hepatology*, vol. 17, no. 10, pp. 1123–1124, 2005.

[17] D. H. O'Donnell, R. Ryan, B. Hayes, D. Fennelly, and R. G. Gibney, "Hepatocellular carcinoma complicating cystic fibrosis related liver disease," *Journal of Cystic Fibrosis*, vol. 8, no. 4, pp. 288–290, 2009.

[18] J. R. Bartlett, K. J. Friedman, S. C. Ling et al., "Genetic modifiers of liver disease in cystic fibrosis," *The Journal of the American Medical Association*, vol. 302, no. 10, pp. 1076–1083, 2009.

[19] T. Flass and M. R. Narkewicz, "Cirrhosis and other liver disease in cystic fibrosis," *Journal of Cystic Fibrosis*, vol. 12, no. 2, pp. 116–124, 2013.

[20] D. Debray, D. Kelly, R. Houwen, B. Strandvik, and C. Colombo, "Best practice guidance for the diagnosis and management of cystic fibrosis-associated liver disease," *Journal of Cystic Fibrosis*, vol. 10, no. 2, pp. S29–S36, 2011.

[21] P. J. Lewindon, R. W. Shepherd, M. J. Walsh et al., "Importance of hepatic fibrosis in cystic fibrosis and the predictive value of liver biopsy," *Hepatology*, vol. 53, no. 1, pp. 193–201, 2011.

[22] C. Y. Ooi, "Letter to the Editor: ursodeoxycholic acid in cystic fibrosis-associated liver disease," *Journal of Cystic Fibrosis*, vol. 11, no. 1, pp. 72–73, 2012.

[23] T. N. Pereira, P. J. Lewindon, J. L. Smith et al., "Serum markers of hepatic fibrogenesis in cystic fibrosis liver disease," *Journal of Hepatology*, vol. 41, no. 4, pp. 576–583, 2004.

[24] G. A. Ramm, R. W. Shepherd, A. C. Hoskins et al., "Fibrogenesis in pediatric cholestatic liver disease: role of taurocholate and hepatocyte-derived monocyte chemotaxis protein-1 in hepatic stellate cell recruitment," *Hepatology*, vol. 49, no. 2, pp. 533–544, 2009.

[25] D. H. Leung, M. Khan, C. G. Minard et al., "Aspartate aminotransferase to platelet ratio and fibrosis-4 as biomarkers in biopsy-validated pediatric cystic fibrosis liver disease," *Hepatology*, vol. 62, no. 5, pp. 1576–1583, 2015.

[26] G. A. Agrons, W. R. Corse, R. I. Markowitz, E. S. Suarez, and D. R. Perry, "Gastrointestinal manifestations of cystic fibrosis: radiologic-pathologic correlation," *Radiographics*, vol. 16, no. 4, pp. 871–893, 1996.

[27] L. J. King, E. D. Scurr, N. Murugan, S. G. J. Williams, D. Westaby, and J. C. Healy, "Hepatobiliary and pancreatic manifestations of cystic fibrosis: MR imaging appearances," *Radiographics*, vol. 20, no. 3, pp. 767–777, 2000.

[28] C. C. Roy, A. M. Weber, C. L. Morin et al., "Abnormal biliary lipid composition in cystic fibrosis. Effect of pancreatic enzymes," *New England Journal of Medicine*, vol. 297, no. 24, pp. 1301–1305, 1977.

[29] I. Durieu, O. Pellet, L. Simonot et al., "Sclerosing cholangitis in adults with cystic fibrosis: a magnetic resonance cholangiographic prospective study," *Journal of Hepatology*, vol. 30, no. 6, pp. 1052–1056, 1999.

[30] U. Herrmann, G. Dockter, and F. Lammert, "Cystic fibrosis-associated liver disease," *Best Practice and Research: Clinical Gastroenterology*, vol. 24, no. 5, pp. 585–592, 2010.

[31] D. Akata and O. Akhan, "Liver manifestations of cystic fibrosis," *European Journal of Radiology*, vol. 61, no. 1, pp. 11–17, 2007.

[32] D. M. Torres, C. D. Williams, and S. A. Harrison, "Features, diagnosis and treatment of non-alcoholic fatty liver disease," *Clinical Gastroenterology and Hepatology*, vol. 10, no. 8, pp. 837–858, 2012.

[33] S. Singh, A. M. Allen, Z. Wang, L. J. Prokop, M. H. Murad, and R. Loomba, "Fibrosis progression in nonalcoholic fatty liver vs nonalcoholic steatohepatitis: a systematic review and meta-analysis of paired-biopsy studies," *Clinical Gastroenterology and Hepatology*, vol. 13, no. 4, pp. 643–654, 2015.

[34] R. Pais, F. Charlotte, L. Fedchuk et al., "A systematic review of follow-up biopsies reveals disease progression in patients with non-alcoholic fatty liver," *Journal of Hepatology*, vol. 59, no. 3, pp. 550–556, 2013.

[35] C. Colombo, P. M. Battezzati, A. Crosignani et al., "Liver disease in cystic fibrosis: a prospective study on incidence, risk factors, and outcome," *Hepatology*, vol. 36, no. 6, pp. 1374–1382, 2002.

[36] A. Chryssostalis, D. Hubert, J. Coste et al., "Liver disease in adult patients with cystic fibrosis: a frequent and independent prognostic factor associated with death or lung transplantation," *Journal of Hepatology*, vol. 55, no. 6, pp. 1377–1382, 2011.

[37] K. L. Nash, M. E. Allison, D. McKeon et al., "A single centre experience of liver disease in adults with cystic fibrosis 1995–2006," *Journal of Cystic Fibrosis*, vol. 7, no. 3, pp. 252–257, 2008.

[38] R. F. Hanna, D. A. Aguirre, N. Kased, S. C. Emery, M. R. Peterson, and C. B. Sirlin, "Cirrhosis-associated hepatocellular nodules: correlation of histopathologic and MR imaging features," *Radiographics*, vol. 28, no. 3, pp. 747–769, 2008.

[39] J. Bruix and M. Sherman, "Management of hepatocellular carcinoma: an update," *Hepatology*, vol. 53, no. 3, pp. 1020–1022, 2011.

[40] P. R. Mueller-Abt, K. J. Frawley, R. M. Greer, and P. J. Lewindon, "Comparison of ultrasound and biopsy findings in children with cystic fibrosis related liver disease," *Journal of Cystic Fibrosis*, vol. 7, no. 3, pp. 215–221, 2008.

[41] P. Witters, K. De Boeck, L. Dupont et al., "Non-invasive liver elastography (Fibroscan) for detection of cystic fibrosis-associated liver disease," *Journal of Cystic Fibrosis*, vol. 8, no. 6, pp. 392–399, 2009.

[42] M. Friedrich-Rust, N. Schlueter, C. Smaczny et al., "Non-invasive measurement of liver and pancreas fibrosis in patients with cystic fibrosis," *Journal of Cystic Fibrosis*, vol. 12, no. 5, pp. 431–439, 2013.

[43] T. Karlas, M. Neuschulz, A. Oltmanns et al., "Non-invasive evaluation of cystic fibrosis related liver disease in adults with ARFI, transient elastography and different fibrosis scores," *PLoS ONE*, vol. 7, no. 7, Article ID e42139, 2012.

[44] C. Lemaitre, S. Dominique, E. Billoud et al., "Relevance of 3D cholangiography and transient elastography to assess cystic fibrosis-associated liver disease?" *Canadian Respiratory Journal*, vol. 2016, Article ID 4592702, 8 pages, 2016.

[45] T. Karlas, M. Neuschulz, A. Oltmanns, H. Wirtz, V. Keim, and J. Wiegand, "ARFI and transient elastography for characterization of cystic fibrosis related liver disease: first longitudinal follow-up data in adult patients," *Journal of Cystic Fibrosis*, vol. 12, no. 6, pp. 826–827, 2013.

Giant Hepatic Cyst with Septal Structure: Diagnosis and Management

Toshihiro Sato,[1] Michitaka Imai,[1] Kazunao Hayashi,[1] Osamu Isokawa,[1] Tatsuya Nomura,[2] Yoshiaki Tsuchiya,[2] and Takashi Kawasaki[3]

[1] *Department of Gastroenterology, Kashiwazaki General Hospital and Medical Center, 2-11-3 Kitahanda, Kashiwazaki, Niigata 9458535, Japan*
[2] *Department of Surgery, Niigata Cancer Center Hospital, Japan*
[3] *Department of Pathology, Niigata Cancer Center Hospital, Japan*

Correspondence should be addressed to Toshihiro Sato; sato@kashiwazaki-ghmc.jp

Academic Editor: Kenya Kamimura

The hepatic cyst is a common benign liver tumor, and no surgical treatment is necessary. However, it is difficult to correctly diagnose the giant hepatic cyst containing the solid septal structures inside, from the malignant cystadenocarcinomas. The various imaging modalities such as computed tomography, magnetic resonance imaging, and ultrasonography, have been developed and are useful for the diagnosis of these liver tumors. Reviewing the other reports in this paper, the combination of more than 2 modalities will help to diagnose these tumors; however, the malignant potential is unable to be excluded if the tumor is huge. Therefore, the surgical resection should be considered for the huge hepatic cysts with septal structures if the correct diagnosis is unable to be made. For example, when the hemorrhages cause the granulation in the septa which often shows neovascularization, the imaging modalities are unable to define this situation from the malignant tissue with hypervascularity. Therefore, with the careful review of other reports, we conclude that if the imaging studies show the possible malignant potential or the sizing-up is marked, the surgical treatment should be considered with the consent from the patients.

1. Introduction

To date, cystic diseases of the liver are being encountered more frequently in the clinical setting because of advancements in various diagnostic imaging modalities. While some cases are easy to diagnose on the basis of medical history and clinical symptoms, such as metastatic hepatic tumors and hepatic abscesses, it becomes difficult to distinguish simple hepatic cysts from malignant diseases in some cases with diverse findings or intracystic hemorrhage and infection [1]. To update the information for the diagnosis of the hepatic cyst and help the therapeutic decision, we reviewed reports showing our representative hepatic cyst case mimicking the biliary cystadenocarcinoma in this paper.

2. Clinical Features of Primary Cystic Liver Tumors

2.1. Simple Cyst. Hepatic cysts are the most frequently occurring, benign, space-occupying lesions of the liver. These cysts contain fluid, and their inner walls are covered with a layer of epithelial cells [2]. It can be classified by etiology into congenital and acquired cysts. The former is divided into parenchymal and biliary cysts, and parenchymal cysts can be isolated or polycystic. Acquired cysts are broadly classified as traumatic, inflammatory (including parasitosis), and neoplastic cysts. The ultrasonography (US) shows a well-circumscribed anechoic lesion with increased through-transmission of sound and no evidence of mural nodularity. The computed tomography (CT) shows water-density lesions

TABLE 1: Comparison of simple cyst, and complicated cyst and biliary cystadenocarcinoma.

	US	CT	MRI
Simple cyst	Monolocular Anechoic lesion with increased through transmission of sound No structure	Uniformly water-density Smooth thin walls No structure No enhancement	T1WI: homogeneously hypointensity T2WI: homogeneously hyperintensity No structure No enhancement
Complicated cyst	Honeycomb pattern Increased echo levels of cystic fluid	Mural nodularity Various thickness of the walls Unclear boundary Usually no enhancement	T1WI: various intensity T2WI: hyperintense Septal and/or nodular structures Usually no enhancement
Biliary cystadenocarcinoma	Multilocular Septal and/or Nodular structures	Uneven for every locular Thick fibrous capsule Solid tumor component Increased contrast uptake	T1WI, T2WI: various intensity Septal and/or nodular structures Increased contrast uptake

T1WI: T1-weighted imaging,T2WI: T2-weighted imaging.

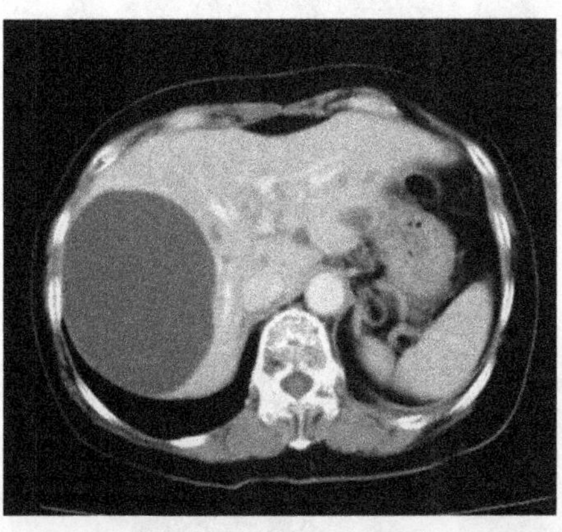

(a)

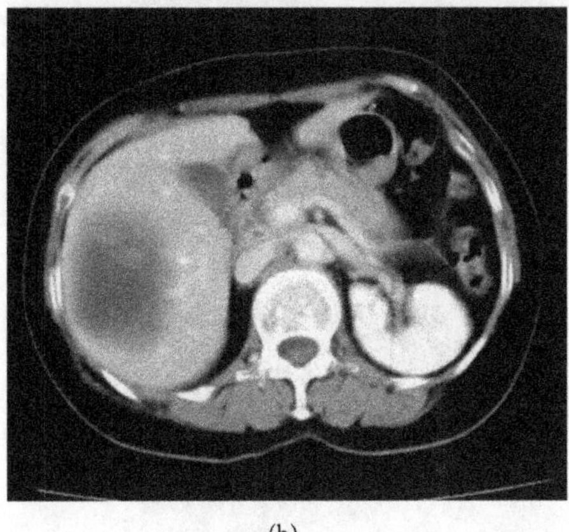

(b)

FIGURE 1: Abdominal contrast-enhanced computed tomography performed in September 2011 shows multiple cysts in both hepatic lobes. Nodular structures can be observed on the caudal side of a giant cyst.

with sharply defined margins and smooth thin walls. The magnetic resonance imaging (MRI) shows homogeneously hypointense lesion on T1-weighted imaging and homogeneously hyperintense on T2-weighted imaging (Table 1). A majority of benign hepatic cysts are frequency multiple, usually asymptomatic, and only a few centimeters in size, and usually no treatment is required. Treatment becomes necessary, however, when cysts larger than 10 cm in diameter cause pressure symptoms in the surrounding organs, when cysts are accompanied by infection and hemorrhage, or when diagnostic imaging shows evidence of malignancy [3, 4].

2.2. Complicated Cyst. Complicated cysts are rare occurring, which may be indistinguishable from cystic tumors. Intracystic hemorrhage or infection results in the development of complicated cysts. The cystic hemorrhages, internal honeycomb patterns due to coagulum adhesion to the inner surface, and fibrin deposits that form septa are observed in some simple hepatic cysts on abdominal US. The cystic fluid content can also demonstrate increased echo levels because of an increased plasma component; this hampers differentiation from malignant diseases [1]. Usually, there is no enhancement to coagulum adhesion like a mural nodularity. The same as a simple cyst, the thickening of the cyst wall of a non-bleeding part and an uninfected part is not seen, and the boundary with circumference hepatic tissue is unclear (Table 1). Most of the complicated cysts present clinically with pain and fever, so that the management may need percutaneous drainage or surgical resection [3, 4].

2.3. Biliary Cystadenocarcinoma. According to the 5th edition of the General Rules for the Clinical and Pathological Study of Primary Liver Cancer, biliary cystadenocarcinoma is defined as a malignant cystic tumor covered by mucus-producing epithelium (similar to bile duct epithelium) that exhibits papillary hyperplasia [5]. It is a rare tumor that accounts for only 0.13% of all primary hepatic cancers [6]. Multilocular lesions are most frequently accompanied by intracystic mucus secretion, and, in women, mesenchymal stromal cells may be present beneath the epithelium. Of late, this tumor has been attracting attention owing to its pathological features [7]. In the 2010 revision of the Classification of Tumors of the Digestive System by the World Health Organization, the term "biliary cystadenocarcinoma/adenoma" was eliminated and the concept of mucinous cystic neoplasm (MCN) was introduced for tumors of the hepatobiliary system. Cystic intraductal papillary neoplasm

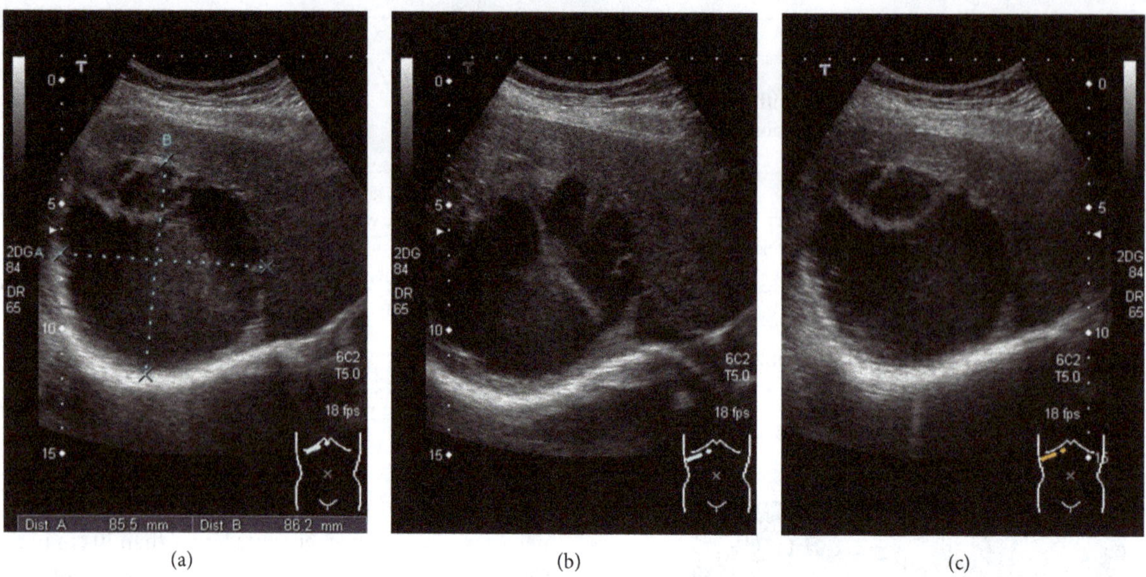

FIGURE 2: Abdominal ultrasonography performed in January 2012 reveals multiple cysts in both hepatic lobes. The cystic lesion occupying the entire right hepatic lobe shows irregular septal structures and nodules.

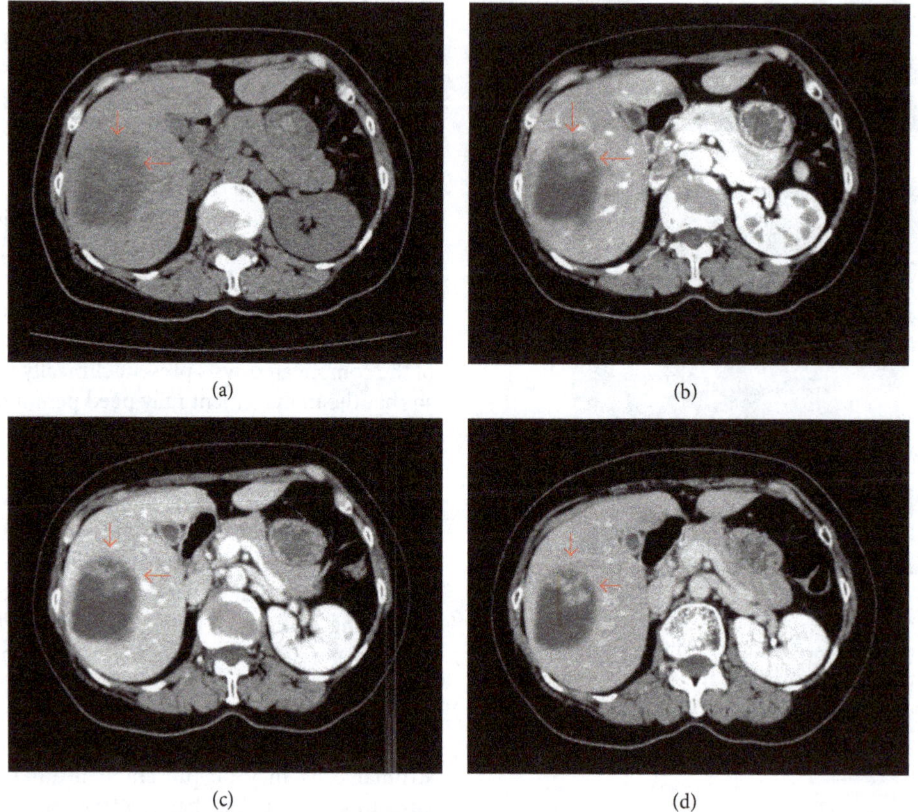

FIGURE 3: Dynamic contrast-enhanced computed tomography performed in February 2012. (a) Simple, (b) early phase, (c) portal phase, and (d) parallel phase images. The cystic mass occupying the right hepatic lobe was approximately 9.8 × 7.7 × 9.1 cm in size and had slightly increased in size since September 2011. Solid components exhibiting increased contrast uptake are observed at the base and left walls of the cyst (arrows).

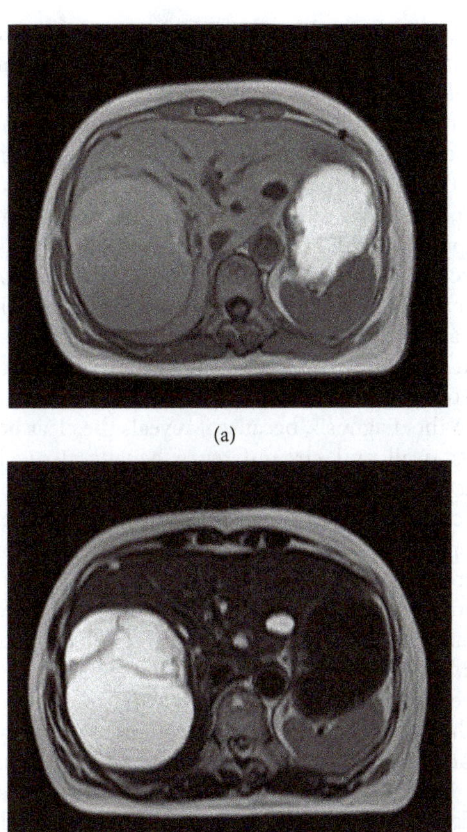

(a)

(b)

FIGURE 4: Abdominal magnetic resonance imaging and magnetic resonance cholangiopancreatography performed in February 2012. (a) T1-weighted and (b) T2WI images. The signal intensity within the cystic mass is stronger than that of simple cysts on the T1-weighted image. In addition, multilocular septal structures and nodular solid components are visible at the base. There is no clear communication with the intrahepatic bile ducts.

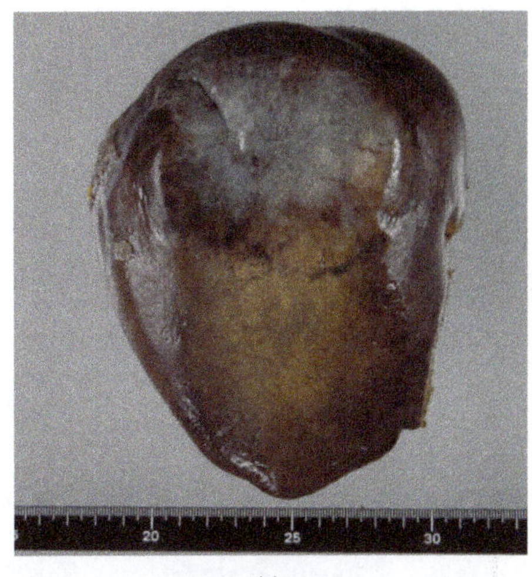

(a)

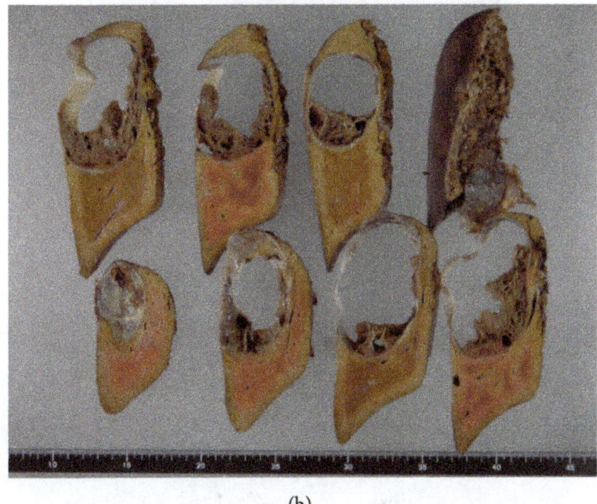

(b)

FIGURE 5: The resected specimen.

was cited as a related disease [7–10]. The characteristic appearance is a solitary complex cystic mass with well-defined thick fibrous capsule, internal septations, and mural nodularity. And solid tumor components in a cystic wall as observed on abdominal US and CT suggest a diagnosis of biliary cystadenocarcinoma, and increased contrast uptake on contrast-enhanced CT is a feature that differentiates malignant lesions from simple hepatic cysts [11, 12] (Table 1).

Biliary cystadenoma is difficult to be differentially diagnosed from cystadenocarcinoma by the imaging studies [13, 14].

Reviewing these characteristic features of cystic liver tumors, it is revealed that although the imaging studies have been developed, the careful consideration for the therapeutic decision is necessary since there are so many complicated tumors. Also as there are a few reports showing malignant potential of these tumors, the careful followup is necessary even for the tumors diagnosed as simple hepatic cyst.

3. Huge Cystic Liver Tumor with Septal Structure

The difficulty of the diagnosis of huge cystic tumor based on the imaging studies is revealed in our representative case which mimicked the cystadenocarcinoma.

Among the multiple cystic lesions in the liver detected by the CT, one of the cysts in the right hepatic lobe was approximately 10 cm in diameter, and nodular structures were seen on the caudal side of a giant hepatic cyst (Figure 1). Abdominal US revealed septal and nodular structures in the giant cyst in the right hepatic lobe (Figure 2). The dynamic CT revealed solid components that exhibited increased contrast uptake at the base and left wall of the giant cyst (Figure 3). Abdominal T1-weighted MRI showed higher signal intensity than that exhibited by simple cysts (Figure 4(a)), and T2-weighted images showed the septal structures (Figure 4(b)). These imaging studies indicate the possibility of the malignant potential of this tumor; however, the resected specimen measured showed no evidence of malignancy. A septum of fibrous connective tissue was observed on the cut surface,

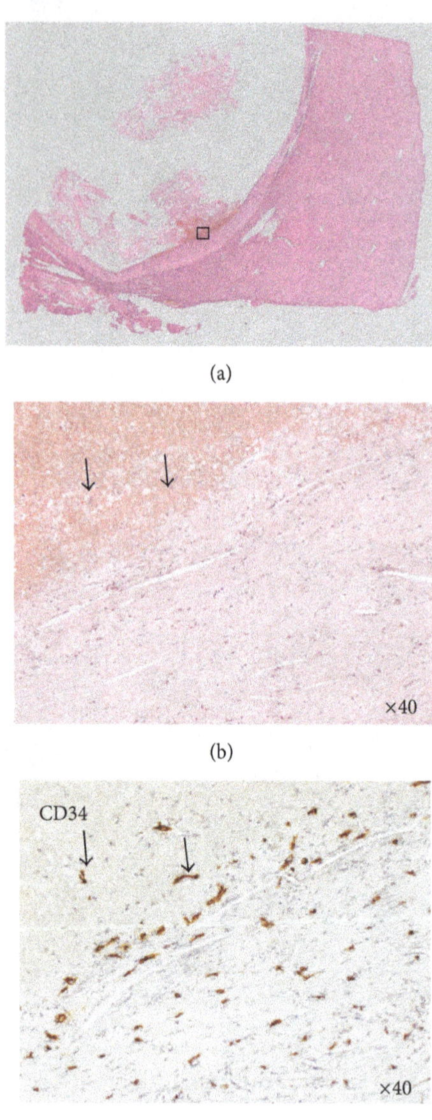

Figure 6: Histopathological images. (a) HE: magnified image, (b) HE: image ×40 magnification, (c) CD34: image ×40 magnification.

and blood serum was present in the cystic fluid (Figure 5). Histopathological examination revealed hemorrhages, fibrin, cholesterol crystals, hemosiderin-laden macrophages, foreign body-type multinucleated giant cells inside the cyst (Figures 6(a) and 6(b)), and neovascularization in the area of granulation tissue (Figure 6(c)) although there were no clear malignant components. Clarification of cells and nuclear vacuoles was observed in some of the hepatocytes in the surrounding hepatic tissue, although no other specific findings were noted. A final diagnosis of a simple hepatic cyst was made.

4. Discussion

The development of various imaging modalities helps the differential diagnosis of cystic liver tumors as summarized in Table 1. However, due to the size and septal structures, some tumors are unable to be correctly diagnosed as a benign simple cyst and the surgical resection is recommended. Since the tumor marker such as CA19-9 increases even in benign tumors [15, 16], it is difficult to make a decision by the serological findings. In these cases as shown in the figures, the puncture of cystic fluid can also be considered, however, due to the numerous of false negative, examination of cyst puncture fluid is hard to be recommended as useful. Moreover, in biliary cystadenocarcinoma, there is possibility of peritoneum sowing by puncture, and even by risking the complications, it is concluded that it is not necessary to perform cyst puncture [15–17]. In recent years, there have been reports that contrast-enhanced US with sonazoid is useful to the diagnosis, because it reveals the clear boundary of a cyst wall and circumference hepatic tissue in early vascular phase and the defect area in Kupffer's phase in biliary cystadenocarcinoma [18]. Furthermore, there have been reports on fluorodeoxyglucose (FDG) accumulation that is consistent with cystadenocarcinoma on FDG-positron emission tomography [19]. And in our case, there was a discrepancy of imaging findings between the modalities as the solid components by CT and the septal structures by MRI. Perhaps, this is a feature which suspects a simple cyst rather than biliary cystadenocarcinoma. It may be the important that the same imaging findings are acquired by two or more modalities. Studies using various diagnostic methods, including novel imaging modalities, are therefore anticipated in the future. However, there are reports on cases of biliary cystadenocarcinoma initially diagnosed as simple hepatic cyst [20] as well as cases of unresectable advanced cancer that undergo long-term followup after an initial diagnosis of cystadenoma [21]. Nevertheless, aggressive surgical resection should be considered when a definitive diagnosis of malignancy cannot be established [16, 22].

5. Conclusion

Recent reports showed that more than 2 imaging modalities help the correct diagnosis of the hepatic cystic tumors; however, due to the smaller number of the malignant cystic liver tumors and the knowledge about the images, we need to consider the surgical treatment for the cystic tumor if it shows the possible malignant potential.

References

[1] K. Shinoto, I. Oshima, S. Yoshimura et al., "A Case of A Liver Cyst with old Hemorrhage with difficulties in making the preoperative diagnosis," *Journal of Japan Surgical Association*, vol. 66, no. 10, pp. 2518–2523, 2005.

[2] F. A. Mitros, "Tumors of liver," in *Atlas of Liver Pathology: A Multimedia Textbook of Liver Pathology*, chapter 11, pp. 1–54, 1996.

[3] S. Uemoto, "Biliary cyst adenoma/adenocarcinoma of the liver," *Kan Tan Sui*, vol. 49, no. 5, pp. 624–627, 2004.

[4] B. Vachha, M. R. M. Sun, B. Siewert, and R. L. Eisenberg, "Cystic lesions of the liver," *American Journal of Roentgenology*, vol. 196, no. 4, pp. W355–W366, 2011.

[5] Liver Cancer Study Group of Japan, *The General Rules for the Clinical and Pathological Stuody of Primary Liver Cancer*, 5th edition, 2009.

[6] I. Ikai, S. Arii, M. Okazaki et al., "Report of the 17th Nationwide Follow-up Survey of Primary Liver Cancer in Japan," *Hepatology Research*, vol. 37, no. 9, pp. 676–691, 2007.

[7] S. Yamashita, N. Tanaka, S. Hata, and Y. Suzuki, "Biliary cystic tumor: report of three cases," *Japanese Journal of Gastroenterological Surgery*, vol. 43, no. 5, pp. 513–518, 2010.

[8] Y. Nakamura, "Biliary tract clinicopathology with an emphasis on biliary intraepithelial neoplasia(BilIN)," *JoJo's Bizarre Adventure*, vol. 25, pp. 31–42, 2011.

[9] W. M. S. Tsui, N. V. Adsay, J. M. Crawford et al., "Mucinous cystic neoplasm of the liver," in *WHO Classification of Tumours of the Digestive System, World Health Organization of Tumours*, F. T. Bosman, F. Carneiro, R. H. Hruban et al., Eds., pp. 246–238, International Agency for Research on Cancer, 4th edition, 2010.

[10] Y. Mano, S. Aishima, N. Fujita et al., "Cystic tumors of the liver: on the problems of diagnostic criteria," *Pathology Research and Practice*, vol. 207, no. 10, pp. 659–663, 2011.

[11] O. Hiromichi and N. Hironobu, "Diagnosis of biliary cystadenocarcinoma by ultrasonography, computed tomography and angiography," *Japanese Journal of Radiology*, vol. 43, pp. 1085–1091, 1983.

[12] J. Y. Kim, S. H. Kim, H. W. Eun et al., "Differentiation between biliary cystic neoplasms and simple cysts of the liver: accuracy of CT," *American Journal of Roentgenology*, vol. 195, no. 5, pp. 1142–1148, 2010.

[13] M. Korobkin, D. H. Stephens, J. K. T. Lee et al., "Biliary cystadenoma and cystadenocarcinoma: CT and sonographic findings," *American Journal of Roentgenology*, vol. 153, no. 3, pp. 507–511, 1989.

[14] M. Koroglu, O. Akhan, E. Akpinar, A. Oto, and B. Gumus, "Biliary cystadenoma and cystadenocarcinoma: two rare cystic liver lesions," *Journal Belge de Radiologie*, vol. 89, no. 5, pp. 261–263, 2006.

[15] H. Takeuchi, M. Suzuki, F. Kenji et al., "Clinicopathologic evaluation of 49 patients of cystic diseases of the liver," *Japanese Journal of Gastroenterological Surgery*, vol. 30, no. 3, pp. 719–723, 1997.

[16] H. Takakura, K. Tanaka, K. Takeda et al., "A hepatobiliary cystadenoma with ovarian like mesenchymal stroma, oreoperative diagnostic uncertainty," *Journal of Japan Surgical Association*, vol. 71, no. 2, pp. 489–493, 2010.

[17] M. Kobayashi, K. Araki, Y. Kohama et al., "A case of Intrahepatic bile duct cystadenoma with marked old hemorrhage," *The Japanese Journal of Gastroenterological Surgery*, vol. 27, no. 10, pp. 2248–2252, 1994.

[18] H. X. Xu, M. D. Lu, L. N. Liu et al., "Imaging features of intrahepatic biliary cystadenoma and cystadenocarcinoma on B-mode and contrast enhanced ultrasound," *Ultraschall in der Medizin*, vol. 33, no. 7, pp. 241–249, 2012.

[19] K. Suzumura, T. Hirano, Y. Iimuro et al., "A case of biliary cystadenocarcinoma with ovarian like stroma," *Japanese Journal of Gastroenterological Surgery*, vol. 44, no. 8, pp. 978–984, 2011.

[20] T. Ito, A. Noguchi, T. Saito et al., "A case of biliary cystadenocarcinoma followed up as a simple cyst of the liver," *Japanese Journal of Gastroenterological Surgery*, vol. 42, no. 6, pp. 651–656, 2009.

[21] H. Kurahara, S. Ueno, K. Nuruki et al., "Two cases of cystic tumor of the liver with impressive morphological changes duaring long-term observation," *Journal of Japan Surgical Association*, vol. 64, pp. 416–420, 2003.

[22] M. F. Hansman, J. A. Ryan Jr., J. H. Holmes IIII et al., "Management and long-term follow-up of hepatic cysts," *The American Journal of Surgery*, vol. 181, no. 5, pp. 404–410, 2001.

28

A Seven-Year Retrospective Study on the Surveillance of Hepatitis B in Laos

Phimpha Paboriboune, [1] Thomas Vial, [2] François Chassagne, [2] Philavanh Sitbounlang, [1] Sengaloun Soundala, [1] Stéphane Bertani, [2] Davone Sengmanothong, [1] Francois-Xavier Babin, [3] Nicolas Steenkeste, [3] Paul Dény, [4,5] Pascal Pineau, [6] and Eric Deharo [2]

[1] *Centre d'Infectiologie Lao-Christophe Mérieux, Vientiane, Laos*
[2] *IRD, UPS, UMR 152 PHARMADEV, Université de Toulouse, Toulouse, France*
[3] *Fondation Mérieux, Lyon, France*
[4] *Hôpitaux Universitaires Paris Seine Saint Denis, Université Paris 13, Sorbonne Paris Cité, Paris, France*
[5] *INSERM U1052, CNRS UMR 5286, Cancer Research Center of Lyon, Lyon, France*
[6] *Institut Pasteur, Organisation Nucléaire et Oncogenèse, Paris, France*

Correspondence should be addressed to Phimpha Paboriboune; phimpha@ccm-laos.org

Academic Editor: Piero Luigi Almasio

Objective. Lao PDR is one of the most highly endemic countries for hepatitis B in Asia and the second country for liver cancer incidence. Therefore, the follow-up of infected individuals through predictive serological markers is of utmost importance to monitor the progression of the pathology and take the decision on treatment. *Methods.* A retrospective-descriptive cohort study was conducted on 3,857 HBV-infected patients. Information about infection status (viral load, VL), liver function (aminotransferases), and treatments was recorded. *Results.* M/F sex ratio was 1.77 for a median age of 37. Patients under 37 displayed higher VL than older ones and men had higher VL than women. Initial VL ranged from <50 IU/mL to 2.5 10^{13} IU/mL. Median aminotransferase values were 45.5 U/L for ALAT and 44 U/L for ASAT, ranging from <8 to >2,000 U/L. Men had higher aminotransferase than women. Globally 20% of patients received treatment (mainly immunostimulant and reverse-transcriptase inhibitors); 11% had high levels of VL and liver enzymes, but only 2% of them were treated. *Conclusion.* Public health decisions should be taken urgently to rationalise vaccination and provide fair access to early diagnosis and treatment; otherwise the burden of HBV-associated diseases will be overwhelming for Laos in the near future.

1. Background

Hepatitis B (HBV) is a viral infection encountered all around the world, especially in Southeast Asia where the prevalence of persistent HBV infection is particularly high [1]. Despite efforts made to decrease the level of endemicity in the population through vaccination campaigns [2], HBV infection rates are still elevated in Laos [3]. This situation raises concerns, as chronic HBV infection leads to severe hepatic complications, such as cirrhosis and hepatocellular carcinoma (HCC). According to the Asia-Pacific HCC Trials Group, over two-thirds of people dying annually of HCC are from Asia [4]; and according to GLOBOCAN, Laos has one of the most elevated rates of liver cancer worldwide, after Mongolia which ranks first [5]. Clinically, HCC patients have a very poor prognosis with an appalling 5-year mortality rate due to HCC [6]. Consequently, early detection, serial monitoring, and appropriate treatment of HBV-infected patients are keys in order to control the burden of HCC.

With the objective of estimating the efficacy of HBV surveillance in Laos, we undertook a survey at *Centre d'Infectiologie Lao-Christophe Mérieux* (CILM) in the Lao PDR capital Vientiane. Under the auspices of the Ministry of Health, CILM is devoted to the surveillance of infectious

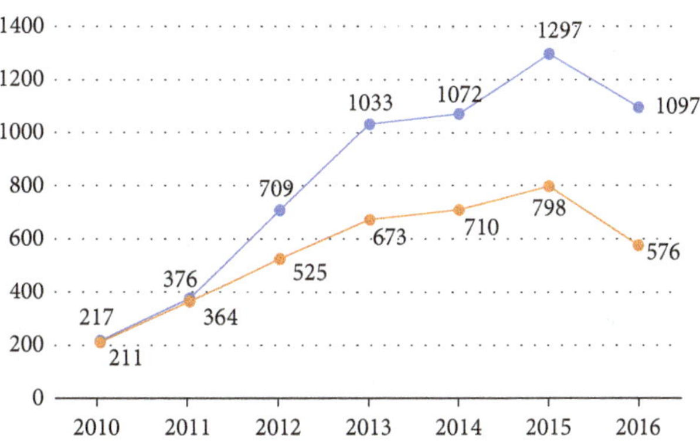

FIGURE 1: Number of patients followed (orange line) and number of samplings received and performed at CILM (blue line) from January 2010 to November 2016.

diseases among the Lao population, notably viral hepatitis, human immunodeficiency virus (HIV), and tuberculosis.

In the present study, we examined the course of HBV infection in 3,857 patients attending CILM between January 2010 and November 2016, who were previously found to be positive for the surface antigen of HBV (HBsAg). Several parameters, such as the gender, age, geographic place of living, treatment allocation, HBV DNA viral load (VL), and liver damage (as measured by aspartate (ASAT) and alanine (ALAT) aminotransferases serum levels) were analyzed.

The results presented herein are intended to help policy makers and stakeholders to apply cost-effective preventive and treatment measures against HBV and its severe health consequences in Lao PDR.

2. Methods

2.1. Data Collection. The present study was conducted retrospectively within a cohort assembled with the data of HBV-infected Lao patients attending CILM between January 2010 and November 2016.

All individuals were previously diagnosed as HBsAg-positive in local health care facilities and advised to go for HBV VL monitoring at CILM. It must be pointed out that HBeAg was not tested among these patients because this kind of test is not available in the health centres in Laos.

Sociodemographic data, health care structure location, date of HBV diagnosis, treatment history, aminotransferase (ASAT/ALAT), and viral load were registered into a database set up with Filemaker Pro Version 11. All data were exported to Microsoft Excel software version 14.4.7 to check any incongruity.

2.2. Statistics. Data were analyzed with Minitab software version 17.3.1. Comparisons between groups (numerical data) or proportions (categorical data) were performed using Student's t-test, Chi-squared test, ANOVA, or nonparametric test, as appropriate. A two-sided p value lower than 0.05 was considered to be statistically significant.

3. Results

3.1. Cohort. The laboratory received a total of 5,801 blood samples, from 3,857 patients between January 2010 and November 2016 (Figure 1). The age of patients ranged from 1 to 85 years, and median ages were 37 and 36 years for men and women, respectively (Figure 2). The cohort displayed a M/F ratio of 1.77.

About 70% of the individuals included in the survey came from public health care centres and 30% of them from the private health system. A vast majority (91%) of individuals were from Vientiane capital and only 9% of them came from provincial health care centres.

The number of follow-up blood samples varied from one to seventeen per patient, with interval between sampling ranging from one day to several months.

3.2. Laboratory Tests

3.2.1. HBV DNA Quantification. All 3,857 patients had at least one VL measurement, 23.3% (n = 898) had two measurements, 11.3% (n = 436) had three, 6% (n = 230) had four, 3.6% (n = 139) had five, and 2.3% (n = 88) had six or more assays. The mean duration to second determination of the VL was one year.

VL determination at the first follow-up sampling ranged from less than 50 to 2.5 10^{13} IU/mL. Individuals were stratified in three different classes, according to their VL at first follow-up sampling:

(i) The HBV DNA Undetectable (UD) class had 672 patients (17%) for whom the VL was <50 IU/mL. M/F ratio for this class was 1.22, and 47% of the patients were under age 37. A large majority of them, that is, 83% (n = 562), were untreated. Thirteen percent of the individuals of this class (n = 90) had a second follow-up sampling, which had a median VL value of 14,270 IU/mL.

(ii) The HBV DNA Detectable and Quantifiable (DQ) class, with a VL ranging between 50 and 10^7 IU/mL, represented the majority of the patients with 58% (n = 2,229) (Figures 3 and 4). The median value for this class was 42,234 IU/mL. M/F ratio for this class was 1.77, and 48% of the

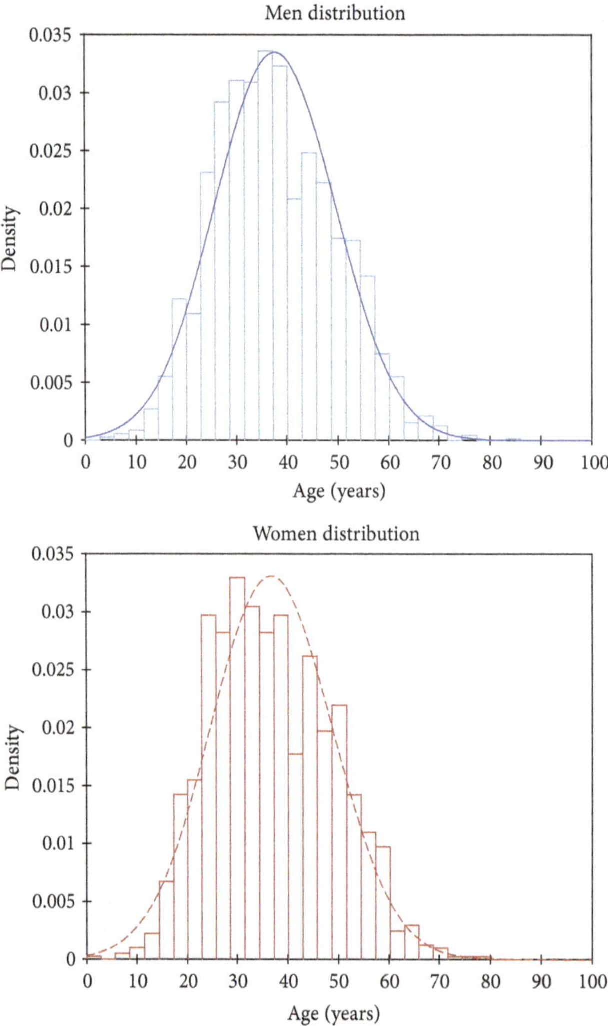

FIGURE 2: Age-based distribution of patients followed at CILM according to their gender (blue: male; red: female).

patients were under the age of 37. As observed for UD class, a very large majority of them, that is, 84% ($n = 1,872$), remained untreated. Twenty-four percent of this class ($n = 551$) had had a second follow-up sample, which had a median VL value of 40,035 IU/mL.

(iii) The HBV DNA Nonprecisely Quantifiable (NQ) class consisted of the patients for whom the VL was above 10^7. The NQ class represented 25% of the initial cohort of patients ($n = 956$). There were significantly more men than women in this class ($p < 0.0001$, 69% for men versus 39% for female). Sixty-nine percent of the NQ individuals ($n = 659$) were under age 37. Despite the extremely high VL, only 24% ($n = 228$) of them received treatment. Thirty percent ($n = 286$) had a second follow-up sample: 5.2% had an undetectable VL and 94.8% had a VL ranging from 18,000 to 40,000 IU/mL. NQ patients were significantly younger than those from UD and DQ classes ($p < 0.0001$), whereas there was no statistical difference based on age between UD and DQ individuals ($p = 0.079$).

3.2.2. Aminotransferase Levels. For aminotransferase, 40 U/L was considered as the upper limit of laboratory reference (ULN) [7]. ALAT values ranged from 5 to 3,071 U/L, with a median value of 45.5 U/L. ASAT values ranged from 8 to 2,057 U/L, with a median value of 44 U/L (Figures 4 and 5). Overall, median aminotransferase values were significantly higher in men than in women ($p < 0.0001$, ALAT for men, 812 U/L, versus ALAT for female, 457 U/L).

Patients were age-stratified in 10-year subsets, and aminotransferase levels were compared accordingly. ALAT and ASAT at first follow-up sampling were independent of age ($p > 0.05$). We then stratified aminotransferase values according to VL classes, as both VL and aminotransferases were monitored in 1,269 patients.

(i) In the UD class, 185 patients (out of 193) had a single aminotransferase determination. Both ALAT and ASAT median values were 42 IU/mL, with ranges from 7 to 1,025 U/L for ALAT and 7 to 1,855 U/L for ASAT. Eight patients had a second follow-up aminotransferase determination, with median values of 46 and 49.5 U/L for ALAT and ASAT, respectively. Both ALAT and ASAT aminotransferases had a lowest value around 30 U/L and highest one around 100 U/L.

(ii) In the DQ class, 744 patients benefited from aminotransferase determination. The median values were 42 U/L

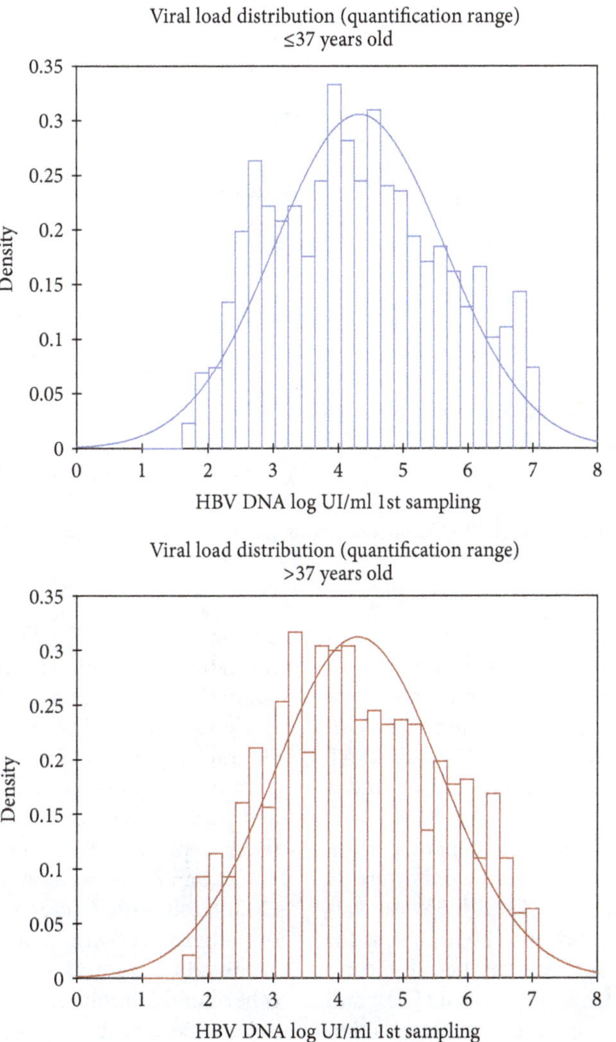

FIGURE 3: Distribution of the viral load at first sampling, according to age, in people from the "Detectable and Quantifiable" category.

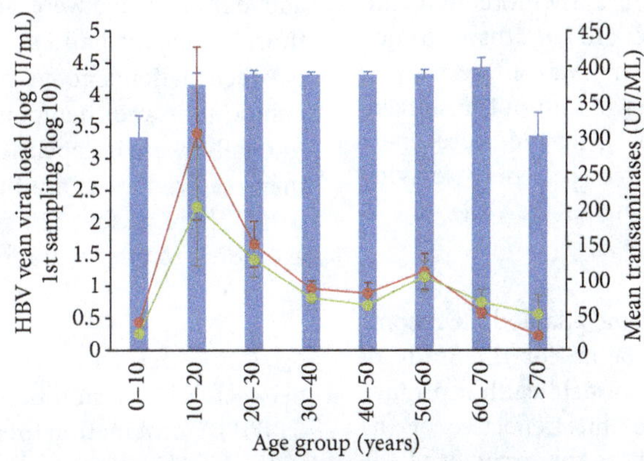

FIGURE 4: Mean viral load (blue bars) and aminotransferases (ALAT in red, ASAT in green) according to groups of age (ten years) at first sampling in the *DQ* category (only patients with VL *and* aminotransferases, excluding patients without aminotransferases).

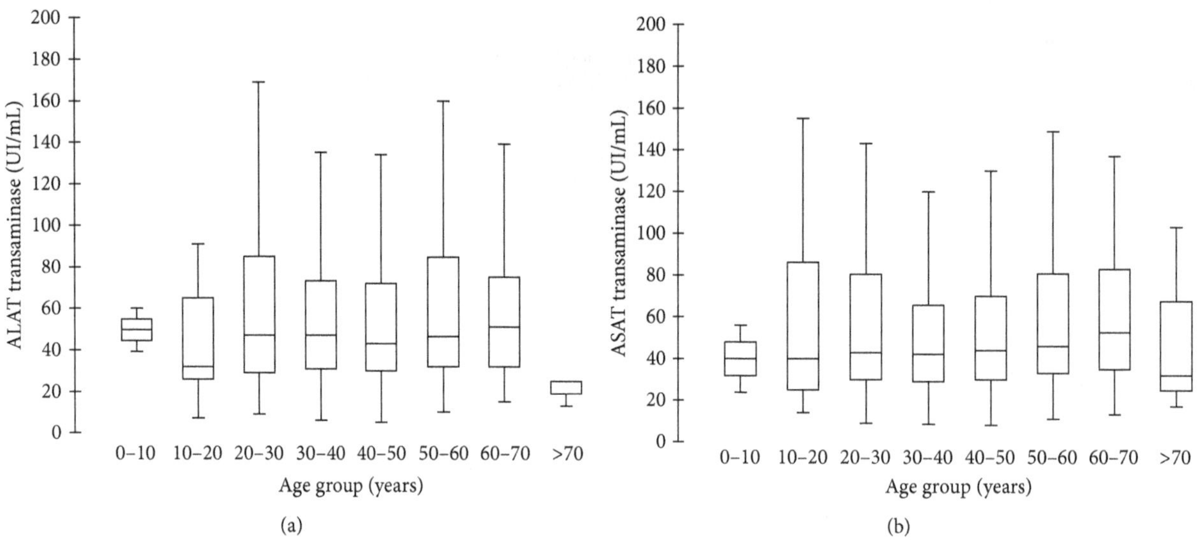

FIGURE 5: ASAT (a) and ALAT (b) concentrations according to 10-year classes of age of patients.

for ALAT and 40 U/L for ASAT, with lowest values around 7 U/L and highest ones over 2,000 U/L for both aminotransferases. 70 patients had a second follow-up aminotransferase determination, with median values of 57.7 and 51.25 U/L for ALAT and ASAT, respectively. Both ALAT and ASAT aminotransferases had a lowest value around 7 U/L and a highest one around 200 U/L.

(iii) In the NQ class, 340 NQ patients benefited from aminotransferase determination. The median values were 54 U/L for ALAT and 53.5 U/L for ASAT, with lowest values around 10 U/L and highest ones over 1,000 IU/mL for both aminotransferases. Forty-four patients had a second follow-up ALAT determination (median value: 42 U/L) and 43 patients had a second follow-up ASAT determination (median value: 38 U/L). The lowest values were around 6 U/L for both ASAT and ALAT and highest ones 296 and 170 U/L, respectively. NQ patients were younger and displayed higher ALAT and ASAT levels than UD and DQ patients ($p < 0.0001$). While considering aminotransferases levels above 40 U/L as abnormal, there were significantly more men with elevated aminotransferase level over 40 U/L than women ($p < 0.0001$). On the contrary, there were more women than men in the patient population with aminotransferases level lower than 40 U/L ($p < 0.0001$). Furthermore, there was no difference in terms of VL between patients displaying aminotransferases levels lower and higher than the 40 U/L threshold level ($p = 0.052$).

3.3. Treatments. Physicians followed and adapted the recommendations of the American Association for the Study of Liver Diseases [8]. In absence of a national health insurance system, treatments prescribed were thus reflective of the availability of drugs in Laos, as well as the capacity of the patients to pay for them.

3.3.1. Evolution of Therapeutic Schemes. The evolution of antiviral drug prescription in Laos between 2010 and 2016 is detailed in Figure 6. Overall, only 18% (693 out of 3857) of the patient population received therapy. The most prescribed compounds, regardless of therapeutic schemes, were respectively Cycloferon (33.3%), Adefovir (26.9%), and Tenofovir (14.6%) (Figure 7). Monotherapy was prescribed in 75% ($n = 520$) of the cases treated, dual therapy in 18% ($n = 127$), and triple therapy in 7% ($n = 46$). The ranking of medicines used is presented in Figure 8 for monotherapies and in Tables 1 and 2 for combination therapies. The combination of Cycloferon with Adefovir was administered to almost 44% of patients receiving dual therapy, whereas Cycloferon and Lamivudine were used in 33% of the cases, and use of the other combinations ranged from 0.8% to 7.1%. Triple therapies relied essentially on the combination of Cycloferon, Lamivudine, and Adefovir (63%).

3.3.2. Age, Gender, Origin, and Treatments. The median age of treated patients was 39 years ([IQR]: 30.6–47.8 years). Patients above median age were significantly more often treated than those under median ($p < 0.0001$). There was no difference between patients above or below the median age regarding compounds and therapeutic regimen employed. Treatments (globally) were independent of gender ($p = 0.07$), but treated men received more multitherapies than treated women ($p = 0.02$). There was no difference between therapeutic schemes according to the geographic origin of patients.

3.3.3. VL and Treatment. There was a positive correlation between VL and number of administered medications ($p = 0.0001$). Combination therapies tended to be more often used as the VL increased.

84% (583/693) of treated patients had first detectable VL whereas a small subset of patients (16% of treated patients, $n = 110/693$) was treated despite the absence of detectable VL at first quantification.

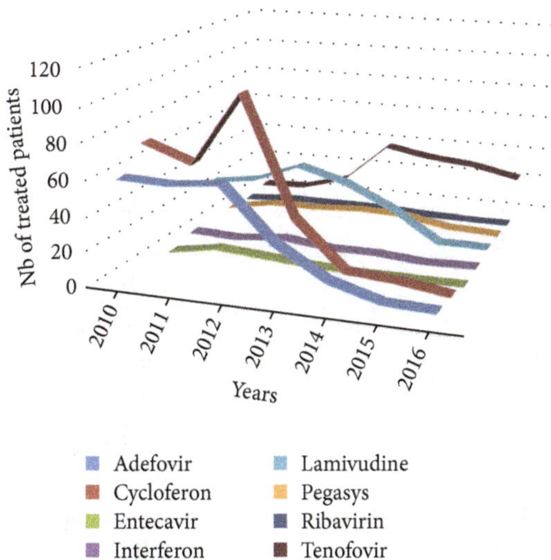

FIGURE 6: Evolution of the number of patients treated and medicines administered to patients received at CILM between January 2010 and November 2016.

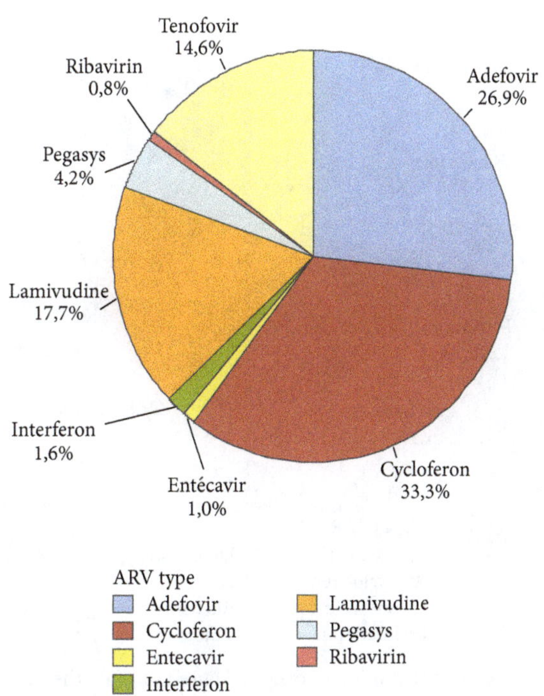

FIGURE 7: Distribution of drugs (%) used in all therapeutic schemes (single, dual, and triple).

In only 11.7% (81/693) of patients was the last VL undetectable; 65% of them were treated by monotherapy, 24% treated by dual therapy, and 11% treated by triple therapy.

3.3.4. Aminotransferases and Treatments. Among patients receiving antiviral treatments, only 12% ($n = 83/693$) were reported to have a second follow-up determination of ALAT and 10.5% (73/693) for ASAT.

In these patients, mean values for ALAT and ASAT at initial sampling were significantly higher than those observed at the last follow-up sampling (86.6 versus 46.7 U/L, $p = 0.01$; 78.8 versus 45.3 U/L, $p = 0.01$, resp.).

4. Discussion

4.1. Cohort. Between January 2010 and November 2016, nearly 4,000 patients diagnosed in Lao public or private health care facilities came to CILM for HBV diagnosis confirmation and follow-up. In this cohort, patients came mainly from the Vientiane capital public health care system. This is certainly due to the central position of CILM in the capital,

Table 1: Type of drugs, number, and % on total and dual treatments.

Dual therapies	Nb	% of total treatment (n = 693)	% of dual therapy (n = 127)
Cycloferon + Adefovir	55	7.9%	43.3%
Cycloferon + Lamivudine	42	6.1%	33.0%
Adefovir + Lamivudine	9	1.3%	7.1%
Cycloferon + Tenofovir	5	0.7%	4.0%
Tenofovir + Adefovir	4	0.6%	3.2%
Tenofovir + Lamivudine	4	0.6%	3.2%
Pegasys + Tenofovir	3	0.4%	2.4%
Pegasys + Adefovir	2	0.3%	1.6%
Entecavir + Tenofovir	1	0.1%	0.8%
Interferon + Cycloferon	1	0.1%	0.8%
Entecavir + Pegasys	1	0.1%	0.8%
Total	*126*	*18.2%*	

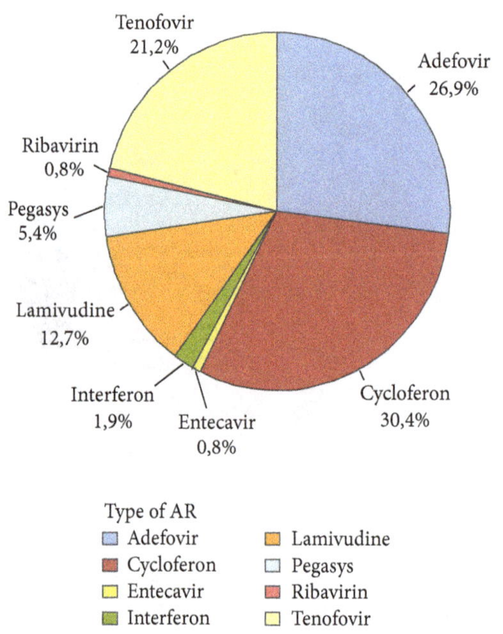

Figure 8: Distribution of drugs (%) used in monotherapy.

and also because public sector health care is less expensive than the private sector in Lao PDR. It is very unlikely that this figure reflects the prevalence of the disease, as large-scale HBV screening and treatment programs are almost nonexistent in Lao PDR. Patients come to diagnostic centres on their own discretion. The situation described in the present study is undoubtedly the tip of the iceberg: the true number of infected people in Lao PDR is probably much higher, but there is no previous study to confirm this hypothesis.

The cost of the serological diagnosis and quantification of HBV and some associated biomarkers have to be supported by people themselves, as most Lao patients do not benefit from health care insurance. This cost is around 67 US$, which represents a substantial expenditure for most people in the country. Considering that the GDP per capita in Laos was 1,500 US$ in 2016, the cost of such serological analysis constitutes almost 4% of the annual earnings for most Lao workers. Nevertheless, the number of patients attending CILM increased continually from around 200 patients in 2010 to more than 500 in 2016, with a peak of almost 800 patients in 2015 (Figure 1). This increase may reflect a dramatic increase of the number of new infections, as well as increased economic status, so people are more able to spend money

TABLE 2: Type of drugs, number, and % on total and triple treatments.

Triple therapies	Nb	% of total treatment	% of triple therapy
Cycloferon + Lamivudine + Adefovir	29	4.2%	63.0%
Cycloferon + Lamivudine + Pegasys	3	0.4%	6.5%
Adefovir + Lamivudine + Tenofovir	2	0.3%	4.3%
Adefovir + Tenofovir + Cycloferon	2	0.3%	4.3%
Lamivudine + Cycloferon + Ribavirin	2	0.3%	4.3%
Adefovir + Cycloferon + Entecavir	1	0.1%	2.2%
Adefovir + Cycloferon + Interferon	1	0.1%	2.2%
Adefovir + Cycloferon + Pegasys	1	0.1%	2.2%
Cycloferon + Interferon + Entecavir	1	0.1%	2.2%
Cycloferon + Lamivudine + Entecavir	1	0.1%	2.2%
Cycloferon + Lamivudine + Tenofovir	1	0.1%	2.2%
Interferon + Cycloferon + Lamivudine	1	0.1%	2.2%
Pegasys + Ribavirin + Tenofovir	1	0.1%	2.2%
Total	*46*	*6.6%*	

on health care. This hypothesis is supported by the fact that the GDP per capita in Laos increased by 50% from 2009 to 2016, according to Trading Economics [9]. It is also possible that increasing public awareness about the dangers of HBV makes people more willing to be tested and treated.

In the present study, there were twice more men than women attending CILM for HBV diagnosis and follow-up, whatever their geographical origin. This is similar to most studies on HBV prevalence, in which generally a higher prevalence of HBV chronic carriers is found among males than females [10]; in the majority of literature it is generally accepted that HCC affects more men than women [11, 12]. In the Asia-Pacific region, the incidence of HCC for both genders has been shown to increase over the age of 40 [13]. However, in other developing regions like Peru, the occurrence of HCC in a younger patient population has been reported [14–16]. In the present study, the patient population had rather a classical age distribution, but it was striking to observe that patients under age 37 represented almost 50% of the individuals attending CILM (Figure 2). This observation is similar to those made by a consortium of researchers from various African countries (i.e., Ghana, Ivory Coast, Malawi, Nigeria, Sudan, Tanzania, and Uganda), which have recorded that about 40% of the individuals with HBV-related HCC in Africa develop their tumour before the age of 40 [17].

4.2. Viral Load. The presence of circulating viral genomes indicates an active chronic HBV infection, presaging chronic insult to the liver. Consequently, a high HBV VL has been identified among predictive factors of liver carcinogenesis. A survey performed in a prospective cohort of chronic HBV carriers in Taiwan clearly showed the significance of the association between serum HBV DNA levels and HCC risk [18]. Other biological parameters, such as aminotransferases, have been shown to be predictive as well, when associated with VL [18]. The rigorous follow-up of these serological parameters is then of utmost importance for the stratification of patients at risk.

HBV DNA quantification represents the best marker of viral replication [19]. In our patient population, VL ranged from <50 to 2.5 10^{13} IU/mL, the group of patients showing VL of 10^7 being the most numerous.

There was no influence of the place of origin for the private/public status of health facility on the VL measured. Younger patients had a VL higher than older ones. Likewise, men displayed a higher VL than women. Almost 60% of the patient population had a VL higher than 10,000 IU/mL, the threshold value for high risk of developing HCC [20]. It is our opinion that this younger patient population should be closely monitored and treated accordingly.

Attention should also be focused on women over age 50, as a multicentre cross-sectional study in China established that the protective effect of female gender against the development of HBV-related cirrhosis gradually disappears after the age of 50 [21]. Furthermore, in the present study, 315 women of childbearing age (i.e., ≤37 years) had VL higher than 200,000 IU/mL. They should receive special attention as the use of antiviral therapies during the third trimester of pregnancy leads to a significant reduction in perinatal transmission [8].

4.3. Aminotransferases. In the present patient population, only 30% of patients attending CILM had aminotransferases records. Ideally, all patients with diagnosis of chronic HBV infection should have had aminotransferase monitoring. Unfortunately, the medical personnel transmitted incomplete laboratory-clinical charts most of the time, or patients themselves admitted their records had been lost.

In a survey conducted on 4,000 people in China, the upper cut-off values for ALAT and ASAT were, respectively, 22.15 IU/L and 25.35 IU/L in healthy men and 22.40 IU/L and 24.25 IU/L for healthy women [22]. In our study, median aminotransferase values at the first follow-up sampling were around 65 U/L for both enzymes. Mean ALAT and ASAT values in the most numerous median age groups (30–40 years) were almost three times higher than the normal level reported in the Chinese study. There was a significant difference between people under 37 and people above 37 for both biomarkers; younger people had higher levels of aminotransferase (30% higher for ALAT, 20% higher for ASAT).

According to Marcellin et al. [23], the risk of developing HCC in patients with compensated cirrhosis with normal ALAT levels is not low, and the long-term treatment is associated with reduced HCC risk, indicating that prompt treatment is necessary, even for those with normal aminotransferase levels.

When both serum HBV DNA and aminotransferase levels are elevated, treatment is recommended for patients with chronic hepatitis; however, for patients with compensated cirrhosis, treatment is recommended when serum HBV DNA levels are elevated, irrespective of serum aminotransferase levels [7]. In our cohort, 10.6% of patients had both a high level of HBV DNA (over 10,000 IU/mL) and aminotransferases, but among them only 2.4% received treatments. This should be seriously taken into account as it has been clearly demonstrated that HBV treatments, which suppress viral replication, can reverse liver fibrosis and cirrhosis and subsequently reduce the incidence of HCC [24, 25].

4.4. Treatments. Merely 18% of the patients reported receiving antiviral treatments and the number of people receiving treatment has been decreasing since 2012. Patients coming from Vientiane or the provinces received the same therapeutic attention. The more elevated the VL, the greater the number of drugs administered.

According to our data, eight different medicines were used by clinicians, irrespective of gender. Three therapeutic schemes were used: monotherapies, dual therapies, and triple therapies. The drug classes included nucleosides analogues including adenosine analogues (Adefovir and Tenofovir), guanosine analogues (Entecavir and Ribavirin), cytidine analogue (Lamivudine), immunostimulant (Cycloferon), and Interferon-like analogues (Interferon, Pegylated Interferon alpha-2a).

Monotherapy was reported for 75% of the treated group, dual therapy in 18%, and triple therapy in 7% of treated people; that is, less than 15%, 4%, and 2% of the whole population received monotherapy, dual therapy, or triple therapy, respectively.

Three drugs were predominantly prescribed: Cycloferon, Adefovir, and Tenofovir. Cycloferon and Adefovir were clearly decreasing since 2012, in favour of Tenofovir. Lamivudine and Pegasys had had a small increase in use between 2013 and 2014. Tenofovir was the only drug that persisted at a stable and high level from 2013 to 2016. Monotherapy was the primary treatment scheme of choice in Laos over the last 7 years.

Among the monotherapies, nucleosides analogues were preferred as they represented 62.3% of the treatments.

Adefovir and Tenofovir which are both acyclic nucleoside phosphonate analogues, reverse-transcriptase inhibitors (a crucial HBV enzyme [26]), were used for almost 27% and 21% of treated patients, respectively. Adefovir is almost three times less expensive than Tenofovir (see below).

Entecavir and Tenofovir monotherapy has been shown to achieve inhibition of HBV replication in almost all adherent patients [27]. These drugs are known to improve liver fibrosis and reverse cirrhosis in a majority of patients. In Laos, Tenofovir (21%) was preferred over Entecavir, which was anecdotally used (i.e., 0.8% of monotherapies).

Although Ribavirin is part of the World Health Organization's list of essential medicines, the most important medication needed in a basic health system [28], it was rarely used (0.8% of monotherapies).

Finally, Lamivudine was mentioned in only 12.7% of monotherapies, although it is the least expensive. It was probably little used because of its tendency to cause resistance in most patients over a five-year period [29].

Interferon-like drugs and immunostimulants were used in 37.7% of monotherapies. Pegylated Interferon-α (around 5.4%) and Interferon (1.9%) are cytokines that are claimed to have a limited duration of therapy in HBV therapeutic schemes (if pursued for at least 48 weeks), the absence of drug resistance, and an opportunity to obtain a durable posttreatment response [27]. Cycloferon is an early inductor of types 1 and 2 Interferon, administered orally or through the parenteral route. This is an association between acridone acetic acid and meglumine. Imported from Russia into Laos, it is particularly cheap and was used extensively when Russian doctors were present in the public health system. Cycloferon was used in 30.4% of treated people in our survey mostly alone and sometimes in combination. According to these doctors (some are now working in private clinics in Vientiane), Cycloferon is particularly effective but should be administered in combination with other antiviral drugs. Nevertheless, only 25% of treated patients received multitherapies. Interestingly, more than 90% of the combinations associate nucleoside analogues and Interferon-like molecules, especially Cycloferon.

Unfortunately, medical staff did not indicate which criteria were used to select a therapeutic scheme preferentially.

Strikingly, 11% of patients had both a high level of VL (≥10,000 IU/mL) and high liver enzymes (>40 U/L) but among them only 2% received treatments. Moreover, among all treated patients, only 12% had undetectable VL after treatment. Nevertheless, results on the impact of therapies on VL and aminotransferases should be cautiously interpreted, as we cannot be confident that the patients strictly respected their treatment protocols.

To reduce the length and the associated cost of the therapy, some authors [30] suggested discontinuing long-term nucleoside therapy, if close follow-up can be ensured in patients without advanced liver disease. Therefore, precise valuation of disease status and appropriate beginning of antiviral therapy should be clearly redesigned for the cost-effective management of patients in Lao PDR.

4.5. Other Parameters. Additional systematic biological parameters should be introduced to improve HBV infection follow-up in Laos. As mentioned above, determination of HBeAg and anti-HBe should be implemented to differentiate patients in the immune clearance phase from those in the reactivation phase that usually heralds severe complications such as HCC. Platelet and aminotransferase levels should also be taken into account to estimate an index to detect subjects with severe fibrosis when >3.25 [31].

AFP reinforced by transabdominal ultrasonography has also been shown to be extremely valuable parameter giving key information on the ongoing tumour process and should be then added in the clinical-biological monitoring of patients [30].

Finally, other variables known to be associated with HCC risk (e.g., socioeconomic status, alcohol intake, smoking, excess weight, infection with *Opisthorchis*, and drug treatment) should be collected in the near future to delineate the degree of HCC risk in Laos more accurately.

5. Conclusion

The picture drawn from the results obtained from this survey is alarming. More than 60% of the patients included had a very high HBV VL; they were mostly young people with aggravating factors such as high aminotransferases. It is also evident from our survey that the level of treatment is critically low. It is obvious that all of the factors are already in place for an increase in HCC cases in the near future.

In Lao PDR, tools and skills are present to rewrite the scenario of this predictable health catastrophe. Only an immediate political decision could slow this fatal trend by firstly improving large-scale national vaccination campaigns, which have been shown to be very effective in Asia [21], secondly, supporting a very precise and vigorous serial biological and medical imaging follow-up of patients, and, finally, putting a system in place for management of at-risk infected patients.

This strategy could be successful only if supplemented by efficient prevention campaigns, better coordination between medical staff and the laboratory, improvement of up-to-date online surveillance networks, and, last but not least, affordability of diagnosis and treatments.

Authors' Contributions

Phimpha Paboriboune, Thomas Vial, François Chassagne, Philavanh Sitbounlang, and Eric Deharo made substantial contributions to conception and design, acquisition of data, and analysis and interpretation of data; Sengaloun Soundala, Stéphane Bertani, Davone Sengmanothong, Francois-Xavier Babin, Nicolas Steenkeste, Paul Dény, and Pascal Pineau were involved in drafting the manuscript and revising it critically for important intellectual content.

Acknowledgments

The authors would like to express their sincere thanks to the Fondation Mérieux for providing financial support and to medical staff and patients. Phimpha Paboriboune was supported by CILM, IRD, Campus France, and Fondation Mérieux. François Chassagne was supported by Fondation pour la Recherche Médicale (FDM20140731352), Paul Sabatier University of Toulouse, and the Third Cancer Plan of the French National Alliance for Life Sciences and Health (ENV201408). The authors are grateful to Elizabeth Elliott and Brian Gadd for editing assistance.

References

[1] R. Zampino, A. Boemio, C. Sagnelli et al., "Hepatitis B virus burden in developing countries," *World Journal of Gastroenterology*, vol. 21, no. 42, pp. 11941–11953, 2015.

[2] Centers for Disease Control and Prevention (CDC), "Hepatitis B vaccine birthdose practices in a country where hepatitis B is endemic - Laos," *Morbidity and Mortality Weekly Report (MMWR)*, vol. 62, pp. 587–590, 2013.

[3] A. P. Black, P. Nouanthong, N. Nanthavong et al., "Hepatitis B virus in the Lao People's Democratic Republic: a cross sectional serosurvey in different cohorts," *BMC Infectious Diseases*, vol. 14, article 457, 2014.

[4] N. H. Y. Kong and P. K. H. Chow, "Conducting randomised controlled trials across countries with disparate levels of socio-economic development: The experience of the Asia-Pacific Hepatocellular Carcinoma Trials Group," *Contemporary Clinical Trials*, vol. 36, no. 2, pp. 682–686, 2013.

[5] Globocan 2012 - Home. Available from: http://globocan.iarc.fr/Default.aspx.

[6] J. M. Llovet, A. Villanueva, A. Lachenmayer, and R. S. Finn, "Advances in targeted therapies for hepatocellular carcinoma in the genomic era," *Nature Reviews Clinical Oncology*, vol. 12, no. 7, pp. 408–424, 2015.

[7] S. K. Sarin, M. Kumar, G. K. Lau et al., "Asian-Pacific clinical practice guidelines on the management of hepatitis B: a 2015 update," *Hepatology International*, vol. 10, no. 1, pp. 1–98, 2015.

[8] N. A. Terrault, N. H. Bzowej, K.-M. Chang, J. P. Hwang, M. M. Jonas, and M. H. Murad, "AASLD guidelines for treatment of chronic hepatitis B," *Hepatology*, vol. 63, no. 1, pp. 261–283, 2016.

[9] Laos GDP per capita — 1984-2016 — Data — Chart — Calendar — Forecast — News. Available from: http://www.tradingeconomics.com/laos/gdp-per-capita.

[10] B. S. Blumberg, "Sex differences in response to hepatitis b virus," *Arthritis & Rheumatism*, vol. 22, no. 11, pp. 1261–1266, 1979.

[11] J. Ferlay, I. Soerjomataram, R. Dikshit et al., "Cancer incidence and mortality worldwide: sources, methods and major patterns in GLOBOCAN 2012," *International Journal of Cancer*, 2014.

[12] J. W. Park, M. Chen, M. Colombo et al., "Global patterns of hepatocellular carcinoma management from diagnosis to death:

the BRIDGE Study," *Liver International*, vol. 35, no. 9, pp. 2155–2166, 2015.

[13] R. X. Zhu, W.-K. Seto, C.-L. Lai, and M.-F. Yuen, "Epidemiology of hepatocellular carcinoma in the Asia-Pacific region," *Gut and Liver*, vol. 10, no. 3, pp. 332–339, 2016.

[14] S. Bertani, P. Pineau, S. Loli et al., "An Atypical Age-Specific Pattern of Hepatocellular Carcinoma in Peru: A Threat for Andean Populations," *PLoS ONE*, vol. 8, no. 6, Article ID e67756, 2013.

[15] A. Marchio, S. Bertani, T. Rojas Rojas et al., "A peculiar mutation spectrum emerging from young peruvian patients with hepatocellular carcinoma," *PLoS ONE*, vol. 9, no. 12, Article ID e114912, 2014.

[16] E. Ruiz, T. Rojas Rojas, F. Berrospi et al., "Hepatocellular carcinoma surgery outcomes in the developing world: A 20-year retrospective cohort study at the National Cancer Institute of Peru," *Heliyon*, vol. 2, no. 1, Article ID e00052, 2016.

[17] J. D. Yang, A. Gyedu, M. Y. Afihene et al., "Hepatocellular carcinoma occurs at an earlier age in Africans, particularly in association with chronic Hepatitis B," *American Journal of Gastroenterology*, vol. 110, no. 11, pp. 1629–1631, 2015.

[18] X. Chen, F. Wu, Y. Liu et al., "The contribution of serum hepatitis B virus load in the carcinogenesis and prognosis of hepatocellular carcinoma: Evidence from two meta-analyses," *Oncotarget*, vol. 7, no. 31, pp. 49299–49309, 2016.

[19] J.-M. Pawlotsky, G. Dusheiko, A. Hatzakis et al., "Virologic Monitoring of Hepatitis B Virus Therapy in Clinical Trials and Practice: Recommendations for a Standardized Approach," *Gastroenterology*, vol. 134, no. 2, pp. 405–415, 2008.

[20] C.-J. Chen, H.-I. Yang, and U. H. Iloeje, "Hepatitis B virus DNA levels and outcomes in chronic hepatitis B," *Hepatology*, vol. 49, no. 5, pp. S72–S84, 2009.

[21] H. You, Y. Kong, J. Hou et al., "Female gender lost protective effect against disease progression in elderly patients with chronic hepatitis B," *Scientific Reports*, vol. 6, Article ID 37498, 2016.

[22] P. Zhang, C.-Y. Wang, Y.-X. Li, Y. Pan, J.-Q. Niu, and S.-M. He, "Determination of the upper cut-off values of serum alanine aminotransferase and aspartate aminotransferase in Chinese," *World Journal of Gastroenterology*, vol. 21, no. 8, pp. 2419–2424, 2015.

[23] P. Marcellin, T.-T. Chang, S. G. Lim et al., "Adefovir dipivoxil for the treatment of hepatitis B e antigen-positive chronic hepatitis B," *The New England Journal of Medicine*, vol. 348, no. 9, pp. 808–816, 2003.

[24] P. Marcellin, E. Gane, M. Buti et al., "Regression of cirrhosis during treatment with tenofovir disoproxil fumarate for chronic hepatitis B: a 5-year open-label follow-up study," *The Lancet*, vol. 381, no. 9865, pp. 468–475, 2013.

[25] C.-Y. Wu, J.-T. Lin, H. J. Ho et al., "Association of nucleos(T)ide analogue therapy with reduced risk of hepatocellular carcinoma in patients with chronic hepatitis B - A nationwide cohort study," *Gastroenterology*, vol. 147, no. 1, pp. 143–e5, 2014.

[26] E. De Clercq and G. Li, "Approved antiviral drugs over the past 50 years," *Clinical Microbiology Reviews*, vol. 29, no. 3, pp. 695–747, 2016.

[27] WHO — WHO Model Lists of Essential Medicines. Available from: http://www.who.int/medicines/publications/essentialmedicines/).

[28] F. Suzuki, Y. Suzuki, A. Tsubota et al., "Mutations of polymerase, precore and core promoter gene in hepatitis B virus during 5-year lamivudine therapy," *Journal of Hepatology*, vol. 37, no. 6, pp. 824–830, 2002.

[29] G. Papatheodoridis, I. Vlachogiannakos, E. Cholongitas et al., "Discontinuation of oral antivirals in chronic hepatitis B: A systematic review," *Hepatology*, vol. 63, no. 5, pp. 1481–1492, 2016.

[30] F. Izzo, M. Piccirillo, V. Albino et al., "Prospective screening increases the detection of potentially curable hepatocellular carcinoma: Results in 8900 high-risk patients," *HPB*, vol. 15, no. 12, pp. 985–990, 2013.

[31] M. Fusco, P. Piselli, S. Virdone et al., "Infection with hepatitis viruses, FIB-4 index and risk of hepatocellular carcinoma in southern Italy: a population-based cohort study," *Infectious Agents and Cancer*, vol. 11, no. 1, pp. 1–8, 2016.

29

Hepatotoxicity of Nonsteroidal Anti-Inflammatory Drugs: A Systematic Review of Randomized Controlled Trials

Pajaree Sriuttha, Buntitabhon Sirichanchuen, and Unchalee Permsuwan

Faculty of Pharmacy, Chiang Mai University, Chiang Mai, Thailand

Correspondence should be addressed to Pajaree Sriuttha; mookpj@gmail.com

Academic Editor: Maria Buti

Background. Nonsteroidal anti-inflammatory drugs (NSAIDs) are the most widely used medication in several countries, including Thailand. NSAIDs have been associated with hepatic side effects; however, the frequency of these side effects is uncertain. *Aim of the Review.* To systematically review published literature on randomized, controlled trials that assessed the risk of clinically significant hepatotoxicity associated with NSAIDs. *Methods.* Searches of bibliographic databases EMBASE, PubMed, and the Cochrane Library were conducted up to July 30, 2016, to identify randomized controlled trials of ibuprofen, naproxen, diclofenac, piroxicam, meloxicam, mefenamic acid, indomethacin, celecoxib, and etoricoxib in adults with any disease that provide information on hepatotoxicity outcomes. *Results.* Among the 698 studies, 18 studies met the selection criteria. However, only 8 studies regarding three NSAIDs (celecoxib, etoricoxib, and diclofenac) demonstrated clinically significant hepatotoxic evidence based on hepatotoxicity justification criteria. Of all the hepatotoxicity events found from the above-mentioned three NSAIDs, diclofenac had the highest proportion, which ranged from 0.015 to 4.3 ($\times 10^{-2}$), followed by celecoxib, which ranged from 0.13 to 0.38 ($\times 10^{-2}$), and etoricoxib, which ranged from 0.005 to 0.930 ($\times 10^{-2}$). *Conclusion.* Diclofenac had higher rates of hepatotoxic evidence compared to other NSAIDs. Hepatotoxic evidence is mostly demonstrated as aminotransferase elevation, while liver-related hospitalization or discontinuation was very low.

1. Introduction

Nonsteroidal anti-inflammatory drugs (NSAIDs) are the most widely used medication in several countries, including Thailand, for treatment of symptoms of pain and inflammation, such as osteoarthritis (OA) and rheumatoid arthritis (RA) [1, 2]. It has been reported that 12.1% of the US population took NSAIDs at least three times per week for more than 3 months [3]. In Thailand, NSAIDs are both widely prescribed by physicians and available for purchase over-the-counter without a physician's prescription in drug stores.

Based on the data of Thai Food and Drug Administration (Thai FDA) during 1984–2016, medications used for musculoskeletal system disorders were the second-most common cause of adverse drug events (ADE), resulting in 14% of all reported ADEs. Ibuprofen and diclofenac were listed among the top 15 drugs to cause ADE [4]. While the major adverse effects of NSAIDs such as gastrointestinal mucosa injury are well known, NSAIDs have also been associated with hepatic side effects ranging from asymptomatic elevations in serum aminotransferase levels and hepatitis with jaundice to fulminant liver failure and death [5]. In 2008, lumiracoxib was withdrawn from the market in several countries, mostly due to its potential to cause severe hepatic failure [6], which is classified as one type of hepatotoxicity.

Drug-induced hepatotoxicity leads to abnormalities in liver tests or liver dysfunction. An elevation of ALT, ALP or conjugated bilirubin was confirmed as "$> 2 \times$ ULN" according to CIOMS criteria [7, 8]. At present, the thresholds and the cutoffs for ALT have been modified; the $5 \times$ ULN has been suggested in a recent state-of-the art paper written by international experts [9].

Hepatotoxicity is more frequently discovered during postmarketing studies or, even, much later. This is due to the slightly low incidence rate of NSAIDs associated with hepatotoxicity [5, 10, 11]. The sample size of the premarketing studies designed to assess the efficacy or safety of NSAIDs might not be sufficient to provide the true incidence rate of hepatotoxicity. Although clinically apparent liver injury from NSAIDs is rare (~1–10 cases per 100,000 prescriptions) [5], NSAIDs are consumed in massive amounts worldwide; hence, despite the overall low incidence rate of NSAID-induced hepatotoxicity, their widespread use makes them an important cause of drug-induced liver injury.

In 2005, Rostom et al. [12] conducted a systematic review of randomized controlled trials (RCT) of diclofenac, naproxen, ibuprofen, celecoxib, rofecoxib, valdecoxib, and meloxicam in arthritis patients. The authors defined hepatic toxicity as aminotransferase elevations > 3 × ULN, liver-related drug discontinuation, serious hepatic adverse events, liver-related hospitalizations, and liver-related deaths. They concluded that diclofenac and rofecoxib had higher rates of aminotransferases, three times greater than ULN when compared with either placebo or other NSAIDs. However, none of these studies found high rates of serious hepatic adverse events, hospitalization, or death. These results are in concordance with the findings reported by Rubenstein and Laine [11] who evaluated the incidence and risk of serious liver-related NSAID toxicity using published literature for population-based observational studies (case-control, controlled cohort, and single cohort population-based studies). They found that the incidence rate of hepatotoxicity associated with hospital admission was in the range of 3.1–23.4/100000 patient-years. The incidence rate of hepatotoxicity associated with NSAIDs, also obtained from a retrospective study, was found to be in the range of 1.4–9/100000 patient-years [13–15].

Therefore, randomized, controlled trials that assessed the risk of clinically significant hepatotoxicity associated with NSAIDs that are commonly used in Thailand were systematically reviewed. Those NSAIDs included ibuprofen, naproxen, diclofenac, piroxicam, meloxicam, mefenamic acid, indomethacin, celecoxib, and etoricoxib.

2. Methods

2.1. Search Methods for Identification of Studies. The relevant articles were identified by searching the following databases for data up to July 30, 2016: the Cochrane Library, EMBASE, and PubMed. A comprehensive search was systematically performed, and the search was limited to the English language. The electronic search terms are summarized in supplement 1. Manual searching for relevant publications from extracted articles was also performed.

2.2. Study Selection. A total of 9 NSAIDs that are commonly used in Thailand were chosen. There were ibuprofen, naproxen, diclofenac, piroxicam, meloxicam, mefenamic acid, indomethacin, celecoxib, and etoricoxib. In contrast to a previous study [12] which included randomized controlled trials of at least 4 weeks, this study did not limit the study duration of the randomized controlled trial. This is because the apparent mechanism by which almost all NSAIDs cause hepatic injury is idiosyncrasy rather than intrinsic toxicity (except acetaminophen and aspirin). As a result, the time to onset of liver injury varies from within a week to several months after starting any drugs [34]. The criteria considered for drug-induced hepatic injury in this study were elevation of transaminases (alanine aminotransferase or aspartate aminotransferase) to >3 × ULN or ALP to >2 × ULN threshold as a significant elevation because it is the most commonly used initial screen for hepatic injury [35]. Therefore, randomized controlled trials of adults (age ≥18 years) with any diseases were included for data extraction if (1) the studies described at least one of the following NSAIDs: ibuprofen, naproxen, diclofenac, piroxicam, meloxicam, mefenamic acid, indomethacin, celecoxib, and etoricoxib and (2) hepatotoxicity outcomes were reported as the number of events related to at least one of the following outcomes: elevation of aspartate aminotransferase (AST) > 3 × ULN, elevation of ALT > 3 × ULN, elevation of ALT, AST or both > 3 × ULN, elevation of ALP > 2 × ULN, Hy's case (ALT > 3 × ULN and total bilirubin > 1.5 × ULN), liver-related treatment discontinuations, and liver-related hospitalization.

Eligibility assessment was performed independently in an unblinded standardized manner by two reviewers (PS and BS) to identify potential relevant articles. Disagreement between reviewers was resolved by consensus. All duplicated studies and nonrelevant articles were excluded. Data extraction and quality assessment were then performed for all included studies (Figure 1).

2.3. Data Extraction and Quality Assessment. The included full text articles were reviewed, and data related to study characteristics and safety outcome were extracted. Then, all the extracted data were entered into a standardized prepared table.

The data were extracted from each of the included studies according to the following criteria: (1) characteristics of the trial participants (including gender, age, comorbidity, alcohol use, and indication of NSAIDs); (2) type of intervention (including type, dose, duration, and frequency of the NSAID); versus placebo, or versus another NSAID; and (3) type of safety outcomes that were measured, such as elevation of AST or ALT < 3 × ULN, elevation of AST or ALT > 3 × ULN, elevated total bilirubin > 2 × ULN, elevation of ALP > 2 × ULN, serum ALT elevation > 3 × ULN accompanied by a serum bilirubin elevation > 2 × ULN (Hy's case), liver-related treatment discontinuation, hospitalization due to hepatic cause and acute liver failure, transplant, or death.

To ascertain the validity of the eligible RCTs, the methodological quality of the included studies was assessed independently by two reviewers (Pajaree Sriuttha and Buntitabhon Sirichanchuen) using the Jadad score [36]. The Jadad score is composed of the following issues: (1) adequacy of randomization and concealment of allocation; (2) blinding of patients, health care providers, data collectors, and outcome assessors; and (3) extent of loss to follow-up (i.e., proportion of patients in whom the investigators were not able to ascertain outcomes). Conflicts were resolved by consensus.

2.4. Analysis. The characteristics of the included studies are described in detail. The hepatotoxic outcomes were identified based on the "above" criterion of this study. The percentage of hepatotoxic events was calculated and classified in terms of the study and the individual drug. The estimate of the

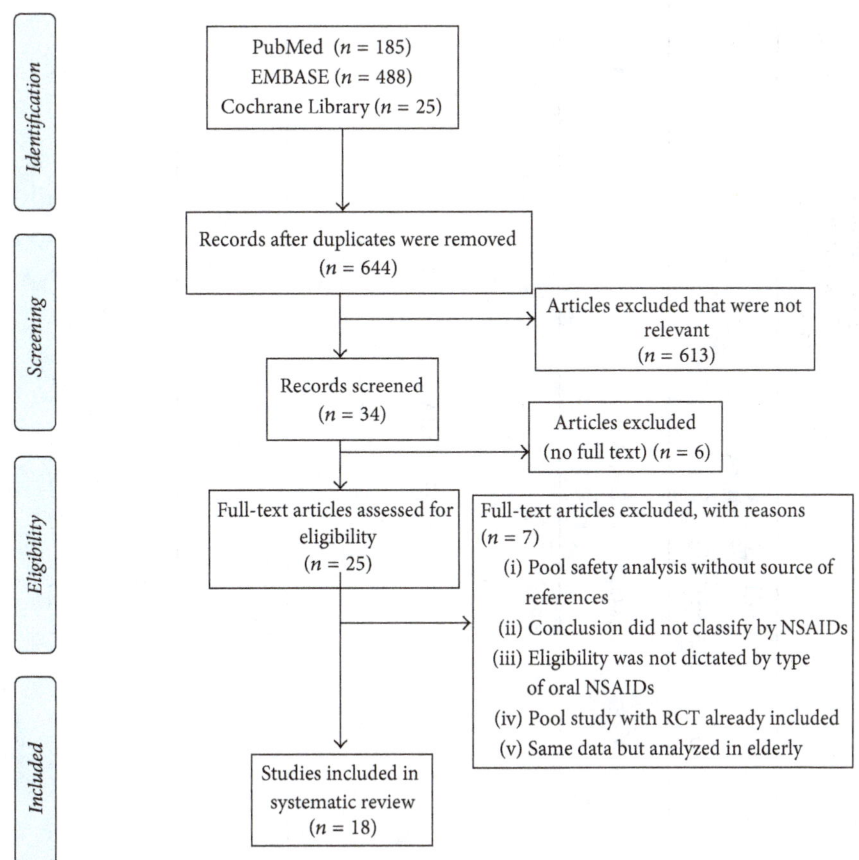

FIGURE 1: The flowchart of the selected studies in this systematic review.

hepatotoxic events was also pooled and displayed as a graph.

3. Results

Of the total of 698 studies from Medline, EMBASE, and Cochrane Library, there were 644 left after deleting duplicate studies. Of these 644 articles, 613 were discarded due to their not satisfying the study inclusion criteria, and 6 studies were deleted due to unavailability of full text.

The full text of the remaining 25 citations was retrieved and examined in more detail. It was found that 7 studies failed to satisfy the study inclusion criteria as described. Therefore, 18 studies were finally included for data analysis, as shown in Figure 1.

3.1. Characteristics of Included Studies. Table 1 presents the characteristics of all the included studies. Of the 18 included studies, 2 studies were presented as pooled analyses from other studies, and the remaining 16 studies were individual RCT. Four studies were placebo control trials [21, 23, 24, 29], and the remaining 14 studies were active control trials. Diclofenac was reported as having been found by 11 studies [19–25, 27, 28, 32, 33]; naproxen by 5 studies [17–19, 26, 30]; celecoxib by 4 studies [23, 28, 29, 31]; ibuprofen, piroxicam, and indomethacin by only 1 study [16, 19, 24]; and etoricoxib by 1 study [27]. In all listed NSAIDs in this study, no study of mefenamic acid was found. Two trials were presented in the form of pooled analyses from multiple studies [18, 27]. The total number of samples in the 18 studies was 45,705. The NSAID use in most of the studies were indicated in osteoarthritis (13 studies) or rheumatoid arthritis (2 studies), or both (2 studies), except for one trial with low back pain [30]. It was found that 14 trials reported a higher number of female patients than male patients, while the rest of the trials did not report the gender [18, 19, 30, 31]. The patients' ages were in the range of 18–90. A majority of the patients treated had age >50 years. All the studies provided data of use of more than 1 NSAID. The duration of intervention was 4 weeks or less for 4 studies (22.2%), 6 weeks for 1 study (5.6%), 12 weeks for 6 studies (33.3%), and 16 weeks or longer for 7 studies (38.9%). The Jadad methodological quality assessment scores ranged from 2 to 5. Two studies (11.1%) had a score of 2, and 7 studies (38.8%) had a score of 5.

3.2. Outcomes. All the 18 studies reported safety assessment as both clinical laboratory test results and clinical symptoms of adverse events at different time points. The biomarkers most commonly used to report were AST and ALT with 88.9% and 83.3%, respectively. Alkaline phosphatase was reported in 9 studies (50.0%) and total bilirubin was reported in 7 studies (38.9%). Two studies (11.1%) reported liver

Table 1: Characteristics of studies included in systematic review.

Number	Study	Study design	Intervention (dose/day)	Number of samples	Characteristics of patients Female (%)	Age (mean ± SD) (years)	Indication	Duration (weeks)	Jadad score
1	Buxton et al. 1978 [16]	A crossover, double-blind, two cycles of four-week treatment study	Indomethacin 75 mg	20	70.0	64	OA	2 wk fenbufen 2 wk placebo 2 wk indomethacin	3
			Fenbufen 600 mg	20					
2	Verbruggen et al. 1982 [17]	A crossover, double-blind study	Naproxen 500 mg	11	90.0	66 (median)	OA	2	3
			Nabumetone 1000 mg	10	64.0	62.5 (median)			
3	Turner 1988 [18]	Two randomized, double-blind studies	Naproxen 750 mg	286	N/A	52.3 (all)	RA	24	3
			Naproxen 1500 mg	300					
4	Eversmeyer et al. 1993 [19]	A randomized, open-label, multicenter study	Diclofenac 100–200 mg	296	N/A	N/A Age > 18	OA and RA	12	2
			Nabumetone 1500–2000 mg	3315					
			Naproxen 500–1500 mg	279					
			Ibuprofen 1200–3200	296					
			Piroxicam 10–20 mg	286					
5	Kennedy et al. 1994 [20]	A randomized, double-blind, parallel, multicenter study	Diclofenac 150 mg	121	70.0	64.6 ± 9.7	OA	16	5
			Ketoprofen ER 200 mg	118	70.0	63.3 ± 10.8			
6	Schmitt et al. 1999 [21]	A randomized, double-blind, multicenter study	Diclofenac, enteric coated 150 mg	112	98.9	60 ± 9	OA	12	5
			Diclofenac dual release capsule 150 mg	111	82.9	61 ± 9			
			Diclofenac capsule 75 mg	114	85.1	61 ± 10			
			Placebo	56	82.1	62 ± 9			
7	Morgan et al. 2001 [22]	A randomized, double-blind, parallel, multicenter study	Diclofenac 100–150 mg	168	70.0	72 ± 6	OA	12 wk	3
			Nabumetone 1000–2000 mg	167	71.0	72 ± 6			

Table 1: Continued.

Number	Study	Study design	Intervention (dose/day)	Number of samples	Characteristics of patients: Female (%)	Characteristics of patients: Age (mean ± SD) (years)	Indication	Duration (weeks)	Jadad score
8	McKenna et al. 2001 [23]	A placebo-controlled, randomized, double-blind comparison study	Celecoxib 200 mg	201	68.0	61.9	OA	6 wk	4
			Diclofenac 150 mg	199	62.0	62.7			
			Placebo	200	66.0	60.4			
9	Furst et al. 2002 [24]	A randomized, double-blind, double-dummy, parallel study	Diclofenac 150 mg	181	77.9	54.7 ± 12.8	RA	12 wk	4
			Meloxicam 7.5 mg	175	78.9	56.3 ± 11.5			
			Meloxicam 15 mg	184	75.5	55.6 ± 12.1			
			Meloxicam 22.5 mg	177	73.4	56.7 ± 11.8			
			Placebo	177	75.1	56.0 ± 12.1			
10	Tugwell et al. 2004 [25]	A randomized, double-blind, double-dummy, equivalence study	Diclofenac 150 mg	311	57.0	63 ± 10	OA	12 wk	5
			Topical diclofenac 1.5% w/w 1.55 ml	311	57.0	64 ± 10			
11	Temper et al. 2006 [26]	A randomized, double-blind, single-dummy, control parallel, multicenter study	Naproxen 750 mg	Group 1, 239; and group 2, 52	71.8	59.5	OA	group 1, 52 wk; and group 2, 42 wk	5
			Acetaminophen 4 g	Group 1, 237; and group 2, 53	66.6	59.1			
12	Laine et al. 2009 [27]	Three randomized, double-blind studies: the MEDAL study, EDGE study, and EDGE II study	Diclofenac 150 mg	17,289	74.2	63.2 ± 8.5	OA and RA	72	3
			Etoricoxib 60 or 90 mg	17,412	74.2	63.2 ± 8.5			
13	Dahlberg et al. 2009 [28]	A randomized, double-blind, parallel, multicenter study	Celecoxib 200 mg	463	68.0	71	OA	52	5
			Diclofenac 100 mg	462	69.0	71			
14	Sampalis and Brownell 2012 [29]	A randomized, double-blind, placebo, and active comparator controlled pilot study	Celecoxib 200 mg	15	67.0	57.6 ± 12.6	OA	12	4
			UP446 250 mg	15	67.0	62.8 ± 10.8			
			UP446 500 mg	15	60.0	54.6 ± 14.8			
			Placebo	15	67.0	55.3 ± 14.3			

Table 1: Continued.

Number	Study	Study design	Intervention (dose/day)	Number of samples	Characteristics of patients: Female (%)	Age (mean ± SD) (years)	Indication	Duration (weeks)	Jadad score
15	Shell et al. 2012 [30]	A randomized, double-blind, controlled study	Naproxen 250 mg Medical food alone Both medical food and naproxen	42 43 44		18–75	pain Low back	4	3
16	Chopra et al. 2013 [31]	A randomized, double-blind, parallel, multicenter study	Celecoxib 200 mg SGCG & SCG Glucosamine 2 g	110 220 110	NA	56.6 55.5 55.3	OA	24	5
17	Altman et al. 2015 [32]	An open-label, multicenter study	Low dose SoluMatrix diclofenac 75–105 mg	601	59.7	61.9	OA	52	2
18	Pinsornsak et al. 2015 [33]	A randomized, double-blind, controlled study	Diclofenac 75 mg Sahastara (SHT) 3000 mg	33 33	90.3 90.0	58.2 60.4	OA	4	5

TABLE 2: Reported biochemistry markers and evidence of hepatotoxicity.

Laboratory test for screening hepatotoxicity	Number of studies (n = 18)	%
Individual laboratory test		
AST	16	88.9
ALT	15	83.3
ALP	9	50.0
Total bilirubin	7	38.9
Reported as liver function tests	2	11.1
Combined laboratory test		
AST or ALT	6	33.3
AST and ALP and total bilirubin	1	5.5
AST or ALT and ALP	3	16.7
AST or ALT and total bilirubin	1	5.5
AST or ALT and ALP and total bilirubin	5	27.8
Evidence of hepatotoxicity		
No evidence, or not clinically significant	10	55.6
Evidence reported, with clinical significance	8	44.4

function tests without specifying whether any biochemistry markers were used. A combination of laboratory tests was used to confirm drug-induced liver injury (hepatocellular, cholestatic, or mixed type) in 9 studies (50.0%), while either AST or ALT was used to confirm the same in 6 studies (33.3%), as shown in Table 2 (see supplement 2 and Table 1 for details).

The time points for monitoring liver tests of 18 studies were mostly done at different time points from the pretreatment phases to the end of the study. In five studies, the duration of study was ranged from 2 to 12 weeks and the monitoring was done at the pretreatment phases and the end of the study [17, 23, 25, 29, 30].

It was found that a variety of criteria was used for hepatotoxicity assessment in the various included studies. Eight studies did not mention the criteria in their methodology, 2 studies indicated the criteria as "marked change from baseline," and 5 studies used 2-3 × ULN of aminotransferase as cut points. Only 3 studies used the combination of aminotransferase elevation > 2-3 × ULN with either ALP > 1.5–2 × ULN or total bilirubin > 2 × ULN as cut points to justify and assess the abnormality of liver function.

3.3. Evidence of Hepatotoxicity. Clinically significant evidence of hepatotoxicity was found in 8 studies [16, 20, 23, 25, 27, 28, 31, 32], which accounted for 44.4%. It was found that almost all studies reported AST or ALT, which indicates hepatotoxicity. According to the criteria adopted in this study for hepatotoxicity, 7 of 8 studies (87.5%) demonstrated the elevation of either AST or ALT, or both enzymes, >3 × ULN during the study period [16, 20, 23, 25, 27, 31, 32] (Table 3 and supplement 3; Table 2 for full information). One study did not report the magnitude of elevated AST or ALT enzymes but reported liver-related discontinuation [28].

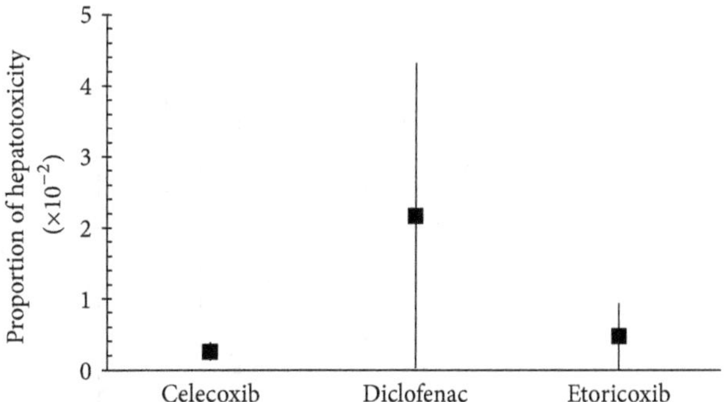

FIGURE 2: Proportion of hepatotoxicity induced by NSAIDs.

One study assessed liver injury using both AST and ALP elevations [16]. Diclofenac and etoricoxib showed >5 × ULN of aminotransferase elevations. In addition, 2 diclofenac studies reported Hy's cases [27, 32]. It was found that most studies used high doses of diclofenac, around 100–150 mg, except for 1 study that used a lower dose, in SoluMatrix dosage form [32]. In 3 studies, it was found that diclofenac users discontinued the drug due to liver-related injury [27, 28, 32].

In 8 studies with clinically significant hepatotoxicity (Table 3), the drug that caused hepatotoxicity in 1 study did not in our interest which was fenbufen [16]. For the remaining 7 studies, the drugs that caused hepatotoxicity were diclofenac (6 studies), celecoxib (2 studies), and etoricoxib (1 study).

Of the total of 789 patients who received celecoxib, from 4 studies [23, 28, 29, 31], only 2 patients (0.002%) had ALT > 3 × ULN and 1 patient (0.0013%) had liver-related discontinuation. Hence, the hepatotoxicity events ranged from 0.13 to 0.38 ($\times 10^{-2}$). Only 1 study reported hepatotoxicity events from etoricoxib, which were in the range of 0.005–0.930 ($\times 10^{-2}$). Of those 17,412 total samples, 162 patients (0.009%) had aminotransferase elevation > 3 × ULN, 1 patient (0.00005%) had Hy's case, and 57 patients (0.0032%) had liver-related discontinuation. Compared with 2 drugs mentioned above, diclofenac had the highest proportion of hepatotoxic events which ranged from 0.015 to 4.3 ($\times 10^{-2}$). Patients with AST elevation > 3 × ULN were found in 395/19998 (0.02%), ALT elevation > 3 × ULN in 864/19998 (0.04%), AST/ALT elevation > 3 × ULN in 19/19998 (0.001%), and Hy's case in 3/19998 (0.0002%), in addition to liver-related discontinuation and hospitalization in 492/19998 (0.024%) and 4/19998 (0.0002%), respectively (Table 4 and Figure 2).

4. Discussion

Since the clinical apparent liver injury from NSAIDs is rare and hardly found during the premarketing studies, this study was conducted to systematically review the RCTs of NSAIDs, which assessed the risk of significant hepatotoxicity. Three electronic databases (PubMed, EMBASE, and Cochrane Library) were searched from inception to July 30, 2016.

Overall 698 studies were found (185 from PubMed, 488 from EMBASE, and 25 from Cochrane Library). Only 18

Table 3: Outcome of studies indicating hepatotoxicity in this systematic review.

Number	Study	Intervention (dose/day)	Number of patients included	Hepatotoxic outcome Number of events (percentage of events)						
				AST > 3 ULN	ALT > 3 ULN	ALT, AST, or both > 3 ULN	ALP > 2 ULN	Hy's cases[a]	Liver-related discontinuation	Liver-related hospitalization
1	Buxton et al. 1978 [16]	Fenbufen 600 mg	20	2 (10.0)[c]			3 (15.0)			
5	Kennedy et al. 1994 [20]	Diclofenac 150 mg	121			14 (12.0) 5 (4.1)[d]				
8	McKenna et al. 2001 [23]	Diclofenac 150 mg	199	2 (1.0)	5 (2.5)					
10	Tugwell et al. 2004 [25]	Diclofenac 150 mg	311	4 (1.4)	13 (4.7)					
		Topical diclofenac 1.5% w/w 1.55 ml	311	1 (0.4)	3 (1.1)					
12	Laine et al. 2009 [27]	Diclofenac 150 mg	17289	246 (1.4) 104 (0.6)[c] 31 (0.2)[e]	511 (3.0) 228 (1.3)[c] 83 (0.5)[e]			2 (0.012)	461 (2.7)	4 (0.023)
		Etoricoxib 60 mg or 90 mg	17412			116 (0.7) 38 (0.2)[c] 8 (0.05)[e]		1 (0.006)	57 (0.3)	
13	Dahlberg et al. 2009 [28]	Diclofenac 100 mg	462						8 (1.7)	
		Celecoxib 200 mg	463						1 (0.2)	
16	Chopra et al. 2013 [31]	Celecoxib 200 mg	110		2 (1.9)					
		SGCG & SCG	220		10 (4.5)[b]				7 (3.2)	
17	Altman et al. 2015 [32]	Low dose SoluMatrix diclofenac 75–105 mg	601	8 (1.4)	24 (4.1)		16 (2.7)[f]	1 (0.2)	23 (3.8)	

Remark. [a]Hy's cases: ALT > 3 ULN, and bilirubin ≥ 2 ULN; [b]more than 3–6 ULN; [c]more than 5 ULN; [d]more than 8 ULN; [e]more than 10 ULN; [f]more than 1.5 ULN.

Table 4: Safety outcomes of NSAIDs included in this study.

Drug	Number of trials included	Total number of patients included	Number of events							Range of hepatotoxic events[b]	Range of proportion ($\times 10^{-2}$)
			AST > 3 ULN	ALT > 3 ULN	ALT, AST, or both > 3 ULN	ALP > 2 ULN	Hy's Law[a]	Liver-related discontinuation	Liver-related hospitalization		
Celecoxib	4	789	—	2	—	—	—	—	1	1-2	0.13–0.38
Diclofenac	11	19998	395	864	19	—	3	492	4	3–864	0.015–4.3
Etoricoxib	1	17412	—	—	162	0	1	57	—	1–162	0.005–0.930

Remark. [a]Hy's Law: ALT > 3 ULN, and bilirubin ≥ 2 ULN; [b]calculated from the minimal event and the maximal event due to the possibility of overlapping of patients.

studies met the selection criteria. There were several issues in those 18 included studies needed to be discussed.

The first one is the indication of NSAIDs use. Of those 18 studies, 13 studies were dispensed for the indication of osteoarthritis (OA), while 5 studies were used for rheumatoid arthritis (RA). The underlying diseases of RA and OA are different in their pathology. The inflammation of OA is distinct from that in RA. OA is chronic, comparatively low-grade, and mediated primarily by the innate immune system [37]. Therefore, the dose of NSAIDs used in OA is less than RA. As a consequence, the NSAID use in OA is less likely to influence the development of liver toxicity.

The second one is the treatment duration. We found that most studies had long-term use of NSAIDs (>12 weeks). Duration of NSAID use is not drug-related risk factor for idiosyncratic drug-induced liver injury (DILI) because this mechanism can cause DILI at any time. In relation to the occurrence of DILI, high lipophilicity and high daily dose are associated with DILI [38]. The importance is that patients should be periodically monitored appropriately.

The third one is related to the hepatotoxicity events. We found that all the hepatotoxicity events are likely to be of the hepatocellular type according to the pattern of classification of liver injuries (hepatocellular, cholestatic, and mixed hepatocellular-cholestatic) which has been defined based upon the pattern of enzyme elevations [7, 39]. This might be due to several reasons. Firstly, the number of biomarker uses considered is not sufficient. For example, the study reported only either AST or ALT; it did not report ALP. Therefore, the pattern of hepatotoxicity injury is likely to be of the hepatocellular type. However, these two biomarkers (ALT and AST) might be appropriate for evaluating diclofenac which is the most reported type of pattern of injury in the hepatocellular type. However, only two biomarkers being above (ALT and AST) is not sufficient to confirm the other two patterns of hepatotoxicity injury (cholestatic and mixed hepatocellular-cholestatic) that occur from celecoxib [40–42] or other NSAIDs such as naproxen and piroxicam [39, 43]. Assessment of liver safety data needs to take into account not only classic safety biomarkers such as the standard liver tests of ALT, AST, ALP, and total bilirubin but also patient demographics, medical history, adverse events, and concomitant medication [44]. Next, the biomarker used is not specific enough to define liver injuries. For example, the AST biomarker was used without ALT. Serum ALT is more liver-specific than AST [39]. AST can be used instead of ALT only when the latter is unavailable and when there is no known muscle pathology driving the rise in AST. In addition, time points for monitoring liver tests should be periodical since the latency of drug-induced liver injury varies. For example, the time to onset of diclofenac varies from within a week to over a year after starting the drug [39, 43, 45]. In addition, timing of the blood test is critical in defining the pattern of the enzyme elevation accurately. In some instances, an enzyme pattern that is initially hepatocellular can evolve into a mixed or even cholestatic pattern. Blood samples that are taken very early in the course of injury are more likely to show a hepatocellular pattern of injury, while samples taken late in the course of icteric cases of drug-induced liver injury are more likely to show a cholestatic pattern [39]. It was found that almost all the included 18 studies had several monitoring time points from the pretreatment phases to the end of the study.

The fourth one is related to the criteria to justify the significant hepatotoxicity events. The hepatotoxicity criteria of this study were quite rigid (elevation of ALT/AST > 3 × ULN or elevated total bilirubin > 2 × ULN, and ALP > 2 times threshold as a significant elevation; the hepatotoxic events were also defined as Hy's Law cases, liver-related treatment discontinuation, hospitalization due to hepatic cause and acute liver failure, transplant, or death). However, there was a variety of criteria used in the included studies, and these criteria might not have been rigid enough compared with this study's criteria. As a result, those studies might identify the hepatotoxicity events, but, at the same time, might not meet this study's criteria. At present, the consensus on criteria for DILI increases the cut-off level of ALT elevation to 5 × ULN. Therefore, it is more likely to exclude clinically unimportant and self-limited drug-related events as well as nonalcoholic steatohepatitis not related to DILI [9]. If these updated criteria were chosen, it would be that only two of the studies reported ALT elevation > 5 × ULN [20, 27].

The fifth one is the daily dose used for NSAIDs. The mechanism of liver injury from NSAIDs is not well understood, and it has been proposed that acidic moiety of NSAIDs or reactive adducts of NSAID metabolites may bind to host proteins and cause cellular injury in susceptible individuals [45]. Aithal and Day [46] proposed a multistep theory for diclofenac-induced liver injury; the liver injury was dose-dependent and seen mostly at the dose of 150 mg or higher. Additionally, Rostom et al. [12] found that increased doses did appear to increase the risk of elevated levels of aminotransferases with diclofenac. The results of this study support this content because a daily dose of 150 mg was reported in 8 of 11 diclofenac studies.

The findings of our study indicate that, from 18 studies, only 8 studies with 3 NSAIDs (celecoxib, etoricoxib, and diclofenac) reported clinically significant hepatotoxicity based on the hepatotoxicity justification criteria [16, 20, 23, 25, 27, 28, 31, 32]. Of all the hepatotoxicity events found from those 3 NSAIDs, diclofenac had the highest proportion which was in the range of 0.015–4.3 ($\times 10^{-2}$), followed by celecoxib which was in the range of 0.13–0.38 ($\times 10^{-2}$), and etoricoxib which was in the range of 0.005–0.930 ($\times 10^{-2}$). On the other hand, no study was found to have reported hepatotoxicity from mefenamic acid. This might be due to infrequent use of mefenamic acid in chronic diseases.

Our findings were not in line with the systematic review conducted by Rubenstein and Laine [11] which indicated no hepatotoxicity from diclofenac. This might be due to differences in the research design (RCTs versus observational studies) and more outcome measurement in this study (elevation of aminotransferase, total bilirubin, ALP, Hy's Law cases, liver-related treatment discontinuation, hospitalization due to hepatic cause and acute liver failure, transplant, or death) than in Rubenstein's study (hospitalizations and deaths). Another systematic review of RCTs conducted by Rostom et al. [12] reported hepatotoxicity from diclofenac justified by elevation of aminotransferases (ALT/AST), which agreed with the findings of this study. However, Rostom et al. [12] did not find any hospitalization from diclofenac, which was in contrast to this study's findings.

Celecoxib and etoricoxib seem to be associated with lesser risk of liver damage even though the quality of the available data is inadequate to define accuracy of incidence [47]. Soni et al. [48] confirmed low incidence of hepatotoxicity by pooling the results of 41 RCTs. In addition, in a study conducted by Silverstein et al. [49], the RCT of celecoxib, compared with other NSAIDs, showed an increase in transaminase enzyme in 0.6% of samples, of which 0.02% had elevated ALT > 3 × ULN. These pieces of evidence were in line with the findings of this study which indicated very low proportions of clinically significant hepatotoxic events (0.0013–0.003).

As for etoricoxib, which has not been approved in the USA, 1 study reported hepatotoxicity in this systematic review. Up until present, no case of etoricoxib-induced severe hepatotoxicity has been published in PubMed. This apparent low rate of liver injury induced by etoricoxib was due to the fact that most studies analyzing this drug were underpowered to detect clinical events [47]. However, warning about potential hepatotoxicity is written in the product summary.

In summary, to report liver safety assessment from randomized controlled trials, the requirements for the studies should be uniform; for example, necessary criteria such as precise definitions and report outcome should be clearly specified. We found that, among 9 NSAIDs, diclofenac has the greatest proportion of hepatotoxic events, with low liver-related hospitalization. To minimize potential risk of hepatotoxicity from NSAIDs, especially diclofenac, the lowest effective dose is recommended and avoid dispensing those NSAIDs as the first-line drug if other safer NSAIDs are available.

References

[1] L. M. Ornbjerg, H. B. Andersen, P. Kryger, and B. Cleal, "What do patients in rheumatologic care know about the risks of NSAIDs?" *J Clin Rheumatol: practical reports on rheumatic & musculoskeletal diseases*, vol. 14, no. 2, pp. 69–73, 2008.

[2] S. Shah and V. Mehta, "Controversies and advances in non-steroidal anti-inflammatory drug (NSAID) analgesia in chronic pain management," *Postgraduate Medical Journal*, vol. 88, no. 1036, pp. 73–78, 2012.

[3] Y. Zhou, D. M. Boudreau, and A. N. Freedman, "Trends in the use of aspirin and nonsteroidal anti-inflammatory drugs in the general U.S. population," *Pharmacoepidemiology and Drug Safety*, vol. 23, no. 1, pp. 43–50, 2014.

[4] Health Product Vigilance Center, Food and Drug Administration, Adverse Events data from 1984, 2016, http://thaihpvc.fda.moph.go.ththaihvcpublic/News/uploads/hpvc_5_13_0_100591.pdf.

[5] P. Sarges, J. M. Steinberg, and J. H. Lewis, "Drug-induced liver injury: highlights from a review of the 2015 literature," *Drug Safety*, vol. 39, no. 9, pp. 801–821, 2016.

[6] A. Techman, "Novartis Withdraws Lumiracoxib (Prexigeń) in Australia in Response to Decision From Therapeutic Goods Administration to Cancel Registration," *CIAOMed*, 2007.

[7] G. Danan and C. Benichou, "Causality assessment of adverse reactions to drugs—I: a novel method based on the conclusions of international consensus meetings: application to drug-induced liver injuries," *Journal of Clinical Epidemiology*, vol. 46, no. 11, pp. 1323–1330, 1993.

[8] C. Benichou, G. Danan, and A. Flahault, "Causality assessment of adverse reactions to drugs—II: an original model for validation of drug causality assessment methods: case reports with positive rechallenge," *Journal of Clinical Epidemiology*, vol. 46, no. 11, pp. 1331–1336, 1993.

[9] G. P. Aithal, P. B. Watkins, R. J. Andrade et al., "Case definition and phenotype standardization in drug-induced liver injury," *Clinical Pharmacology & Therapeutics*, vol. 89, no. 6, pp. 806–815, 2011.

[10] H. Kromann-Andersen and A. Pedersen, "Reported adverse reactions to and consumption of nonsteroidal antiinflammatory drugs in Denmark over a 17 year period," *Dan Med Bull*, vol. 35, no. 2, pp. 187–192, 1988.

[11] J. H. Rubenstein and L. Laine, "Systematic review: The hepatotoxicity of non-steroidal anti-inflammatory drugs," *Alimentary Pharmacology & Therapeutics*, vol. 20, no. 4, pp. 373–380, 2004.

[12] A. Rostom, L. Goldkind, and L. Laine, "Nonsteroidal anti-inflammatory drugs and hepatic toxicity: A systematic review of randomized controlled trials in arthritis patients," *Clinical Gastroenterology and Hepatology*, vol. 3, no. 5, pp. 489–498, 2005.

[13] LA. Garcia Rodriguez, S. Perez Gutthann, A. M. Walker, and L. Lueck, "The role of non-steroidal anti-inflammatory drugs in acute liver injury," *BMJ*, vol. 305, no. 6858, pp. 865–898, 1992.

[14] F. J. De Abajo, D. Montero, M. Madurga, and L. A. García Rodríguez, "Acute and clinically relevant drug-induced liver injury: A population case-control study," *British Journal of Clinical Pharmacology*, vol. 58, no. 1, pp. 71–80, 2004.

[15] G. Traversa, C. Bianchi, R. Da Cas, I. Abraha, F. Menniti-Ippolito, and M. Venegoni, "Cohort study of hepatotoxicity associated with nimesulide and other non-steroidal anti-inflammatory drugs," *BMJ*, vol. 327, no. 7405, pp. 18–22, 2003.

[16] R. Buxton, D. M. Grennan, and D. G. Palmer, "Fenbufen compared with indomethacin in osteoarthrosis," *Current Medical Research and Opinion*, vol. 5, no. 9, pp. 682–687, 1978.

[17] L. A. Verbruggen, E. Cytryn, and H. Pintens, "Double-Blind Crossover Study of Nabumetone versus Naproxen in the Treatment of Osteoarthritis," *Journal of International Medical Research*, vol. 10, no. 4, pp. 214–218, 1982.

[18] R. Turner, "Hepatic and renal tolerability of long-term naproxen treatment in patients with rheumatoid arthritis," *Seminars in Arthritis and Rheumatism*, vol. 17, no. 3, pp. 29–35, 1988.

[19] W. Eversmeyer, M. Poland, R. E. DeLapp, and C. P. Jensen, "Safety experience with nabumetone versus diclofenac, naproxen, ibuprofen, and piroxicam in osteoarthritis and rheumatoid arthritis," *American Journal of Medicine*, vol. 95, no. 2, pp. 2A10S–2A8S, 1993.

[20] A. C. Kennedy, B. J. Mullen, S. H. Roth et al., "A double-blind comparison of the efficacy and safety of ketoprofen extended-release (200 mg once daily) and diclofenac (75 mg twice daily) for treatment of osteoarthritis," *Current Therapeutic Research*, vol. 55, no. 2, pp. 119–132, 1994.

[21] W. Schmitt, K. Walter, and H. J. Kurth, "Clinical trial on the efficacy and safety of different diclofenac formulations: Multiple-unit formulations compared to enteric coated tablets in patients with activated osteoarthritis," *Inflammopharmacology*, vol. 7, no. 4, pp. 363–375, 1999.

[22] G. J. Morgan Jr., J. Kaine, R. DeLapp, and R. Palmer, "Treatment of elderly patients with nabumetone or diclofenac: Gastrointestinal safety profile," *Journal of Clinical Gastroenterology*, vol. 32, no. 4, pp. 310-314, 2001.

[23] F. McKenna, D. Borenstein, H. Wendt, C. Wallemark, J. B. Lefkowith, and G. S. Geis, "Celecoxib versus diclofenac in the management of osteoarthritis of the knee: A placebo-controlled, randomised, double-blind comparison," *Scandinavian Journal of Rheumatology*, vol. 30, no. 1, pp. 11-18, 2001.

[24] D. E. Furst, K. S. Kolba, R. Fleischmann et al., "Dose response and safety study of meloxicam up to 22.5 mg daily in rheumatoid arthritis: a 12 week multicenter, double blind, dose response study versus placebo and diclofenac," *The Journal of Rheumatology*, vol. 29, no. 3, pp. 436-446, 2002.

[25] P. S. Tugwell, G. A. Wells, and J. Z. Shainhouse, "Equivalence study of a topical diclofenac solution (pennsaid)compared with oral diclofenac in symptomatic treatment of osteoarthritis of the knee:a randomized controlled trial," *Journal of Rheumatology*, vol. 31, no. 10, pp. 2002–2012, 2004.

[26] A. R. Temple, G. D. Benson, J. R. Zinsenheim, and J. E. Schweinle, "Multicenter, randomized, double-blind, active-controlled, parallel-group trial of the long-term (6-12 months) safety of acetaminophen in adult patients with osteoarthritis," *Clinical Therapeutics*, vol. 28, no. 2, pp. 222–235, 2006.

[27] L. Laine, L. Goldkind, S. P. Curtis, L. G. Connors, Z. Yanqiong, and C. P. Cannon, "How common is diclofenac-associated liver injury? Analysis of 17,289 arthritis patients in a long-term prospective clinical trial," *American Journal of Gastroenterology*, vol. 104, no. 2, pp. 356–362, 2009.

[28] L. E. Dahlberg, I. Holme, K. Høye, and B. Ringertz, "A randomized, multicentre, double-blind, parallel-group study to assess the adverse event-related discontinuation rate with celecoxib and diclofenac in elderly patients with osteoarthritis," *Scandinavian Journal of Rheumatology*, vol. 38, no. 2, pp. 133–143, 2009.

[29] J. S. Sampalis and L. A. Brownell, "A randomized, double blind, placebo and active comparator controlled pilot study of UP446, a novel dual pathway inhibitor anti-inflammatory agent of botanical origin," *Nutrition Journal*, vol. 11, no. 1, article 21, 2012.

[30] W. E. Shell, E. H. Charuvastra, M. A. Dewood, L. A. May, D. H. Bullias, and D. S. Silver, "A double-blind controlled trial of a single dose naproxen and an amino acid medical food theramine for the treatment of low back pain," *American Journal of Therapeutics*, vol. 19, no. 2, pp. 108–114, 2012.

[31] A. Chopra, M. Saluja, G. Tillu et al., "Ayurvedic medicine offers a good alternative to glucosamine and celecoxib in the treatment of symptomatic knee osteoarthritis: a randomized, double-blind, controlled equivalence drug trial," *Rheumatology*, vol. 52, no. 8, Article ID ket414, pp. 1408-1417, 2013.

[32] R. D. Altman, V. Strand, M. C. Hochberg et al., "Low-dose solumatrix diclofenac in the treatment of osteoarthritis: A 1-year, open-label, phase III safety study," *Postgraduate Medical Journal*, vol. 127, no. 5, pp. 517–528, 2015.

[33] P. Pinsornsak, P. Kanokkangsadal, and A. Itharat, "The clinical efficacy and safety of the sahastara remedy versus diclofenac in the treatment of osteoarthritis of the knee: A double-blind, randomized, and controlled trial," *Evidence-Based Complementary and Alternative Medicine*, vol. 2015, Article ID 103046, 2015.

[34] N. P. Chalasani, P. H. Hayashi, H. L. Bonkovsky, V. J. Navarro, W. M. Lee, and R. J. Fontana, "ACG clinical guideline: the diagnosis and management of idiosyncratic drug-induced liver injury," *American Journal of Gastroenterology*, vol. 109, no. 7, pp. 950–966, 2014.

[35] N. Kaplowitz, "Rules and laws of drug hepatotoxicity," *Pharmacoepidemiology and Drug Safety*, vol. 15, no. 4, pp. 231–233, 2006.

[36] A. R. Jadad, R. A. Moore, D. Carroll et al., "Assessing the quality of reports of randomized clinical trials: Is blinding necessary?" *Controlled Clinical Trials*, vol. 17, no. 1, pp. 1-12, 1996.

[37] W. H. Robinson, C. M. Lepus, Q. Wang et al., "Low-grade inflammation as a key mediator of the pathogenesis of osteoarthritis," *Nature Reviews Rheumatology*, vol. 12, no. 10, pp. 580–592, 2016.

[38] M. Chen, A. Suzuki, J. Borlak, R. J. Andrade, and M. I. Lucena, "Drug-induced liver injury: Interactions between drug properties and host factors," *Journal of Hepatology*, vol. 63, no. 2, pp. 503–514, 2015.

[39] United States Library of Medicine, "Liver Tox Clinical and Research Information on Drug Induced Liver Injury," 2016, http://livertox.nih.gov.

[40] A. Grieco, L. Miele, A. Giorgi, I. M. Civello, and G. Gasbarrini, "Acute cholestatic hepatitis associated with celecoxib," *Annals of Pharmacotherapy*, vol. 36, no. 12, pp. 1887–1889, 2002.

[41] M. V. Galan, S. C. Gordon, and A. L. Silverman, "Celecoxib-induced cholestatic hepatitis [4]," *Annals of Internal Medicine*, vol. 134, no. 3, p. 254, 2001.

[42] S. Nachimuthu, L. Volfinzon, and L. Gopal, "Acute hepatocellular and cholestatic injury in a patient taking celecoxib," *Postgraduate Medical Journal*, vol. 77, no. 910, pp. 548–550, 2001.

[43] F. Bessone, "Non-steroidal anti-inflammatory drugs: What is the actual risk of liver damage?" *World Journal of Gastroenterology*, vol. 16, no. 45, pp. 5651–5661, 2010.

[44] M. Merz, K. R. Lee, G. A. Kullak-Ublick, A. Brueckner, and P. B. Watkins, "Methodology to Assess Clinical Liver Safety Data," *Drug Safety*, vol. 37, no. 1, pp. 33–45, 2014.

[45] P. A. Schmeltzer, A. S. Kosinski, D. E. Kleiner et al., "Liver injury from nonsteroidal anti-inflammatory drugs in the United States," *Liver International*, vol. 36, no. 4, pp. 603–609, 2016.

[46] G. P. Aithal and C. P. Day, "Nonsteroidal anti-inflammatory drug-induced hepatotoxicity," *Clinics in Liver Disease*, vol. 11, no. 3, pp. 563–575, 2007.

[47] F. Bessone, N. Hernandez, M. G. Roma et al., "Hepatotoxicity induced by coxibs: how concerned should we be?" *Expert Opinion on Drug Safety*, vol. 15, no. 11, pp. 1463–1475, 2016.

[48] P. Soni, B. Shell, G. Cawkwell, C. Li, and H. Ma, "The hepatic safety and tolerability of the cyclooxygenase-2 selective NSAID celecoxib: Pooled analysis of 41 randomized controlled trials," *Current Medical Research and Opinion*, vol. 25, no. 8, pp. 1841–1851, 2009.

[49] F. E. Silverstein, G. Faich, J. L. Goldstein, L. S. Simon, T. Pincus, A. Whelton et al., "Gastrointestinal toxicity with celecoxib vs nonsteroidal anti-inflammatory drugs for osteoarthritis and rheumatoid arthritis: the CLASS study: a randomized controlled trial. Celecoxib Long-term Arthritis Safety Study," *Journal of the American Medical Association*, vol. 284, no. 10, pp. 1247–1255, 2000.

30

Prognostication of Learning Curve on Surgical Management of Vasculobiliary Injuries after Cholecystectomy

Abu Bakar Hafeez Bhatti,[1] Faisal Saud Dar,[1] Haseeb Zia,[1] Muhammad Salman Rafique,[2] Nusrat Yar Khan,[1] Mohammad Salih,[3] and Najmul Hassan Shah[3]

[1] *Department of HPB and Liver Transplantation, Shifa International Hospital, Islamabad 44000, Pakistan*
[2] *Department of Radiology, Shifa International Hospital, Islamabad 44000, Pakistan*
[3] *Department of Hepatology, Shifa International Hospital, Islamabad 44000, Pakistan*

Correspondence should be addressed to Abu Bakar Hafeez Bhatti; abubakar.hafeez@yahoo.com

Academic Editor: Daisuke Morioka

Background. Concomitant vascular injury might adversely impact outcomes after iatrogenic bile duct injury (IBDI). Whether a new HPB center should embark upon repair of complex biliary injuries with associated vascular injuries during learning curve is unknown. The objective of this study was to determine outcome of surgical management of IBDI with and without vascular injuries in a new HPB center during its learning curve. *Methods.* We retrospectively reviewed patients who underwent surgical management of IBDI at our center. A total of 39 patients were included. Patients without (Group 1) and with vascular injuries (Group 2) were compared. Outcome was defined as 90-day morbidity and mortality. *Results.* Median age was 39 (20–80) years. There were 10 (25.6%) vascular injuries. E2 injuries were associated significantly with high frequency of vascular injuries (66% versus 15.1%) ($P = 0.01$). Right hepatectomy was performed in three patients. Out of these, two had a right hepatic duct stricture and one patient had combined right arterial and portal venous injury. The number of patients who developed postoperative complications was not significantly different between the two groups (11.1% versus 23.4%) ($P = 0.6$). *Conclusion.* Learning curve is not a negative prognostic variable in the surgical management of iatrogenic vasculobiliary injuries after cholecystectomy.

1. Introduction

Around 750000 cholecystectomies are performed in the United States annually [1]. Laparoscopic cholecystectomy offers several advantages including less wound pain, better cosmesis, and early return to normal activity. Main disadvantage is a slightly higher risk of biliary injury than open cholecystectomy, that is, 0.5% versus 0.2% [2–4]. Variations in biliary anatomy, failure in identifying these variations, and a rising trend of performing cholecystectomy in the acute phase of inflammation may lead to more frequent occurrence of biliary injuries [1, 5]. In addition, use of laparoscopic approach not only provides environment more conducive to occurrence of iatrogenic bile duct injury (IBDI) but also increases the risk that these injuries would not be identified intraoperatively [1].

Once a biliary injury has occurred, surgical repair by experienced hepatobiliary surgeon is the most critical factor determinant of outcome [6]. It has been shown that outcomes of surgery for biliary injuries even in specialized centers have a learning curve. What constitutes a learning curve is unclear but 10–15 repairs a year have generally been referred to as "learning curve periods" by experienced centers [7, 8]. It has been shown that quality of life in patients who suffer an IBDI is compromised even after 10 years of successful intervention, costs up to 182,000 (hospital and society) pounds, and is frequently associated with malpractice litigation [9, 10]. As many as 9 different techniques have been developed to identify biliary anatomy preoperatively and intraoperatively and prevent IBDI, critical view of safety (CVS) being the one best validated [10]. With such impact of IBDI on patient lives, there are certain questions regarding associated vascular injuries in IBDI that remain unanswered. We remain unaware of the exact incidence of vascular injuries associated with biliary injuries, their impact on operative morbidity and long term biliary complications, and role of hepatectomy [11]. This raises the question that whether new HPB centers in their learning curve should embark upon IBDI associated with vascular injuries.

The objective of the current study was to demonstrate results of IBDI repair in a new HPB center during its learning phase and determine impact of concomitant vascular injuries on outcome.

2. Methods

We retrospectively reviewed patients who underwent surgery for iatrogenic biliary injuries at Department of HPB and Liver Transplantation, Shifa International Hospital, Islamabad, between August 2011 and December 2014. All patients were referred from other centers and no IBDI was experienced in our department. A minimum follow-up of 3 months was assured to correctly document 90-day morbidity and mortality.

All patients were seen at HPB out-patient clinic or emergency. A thorough history and physical exam were followed by relevant lab tests. We performed MRCP/ERCP for preoperative assessment of biliary tree depending upon patient's presentation and previous investigations. In addition dynamic CT scan liver was performed in all patients to assess vascular injuries and liver. These patients were discussed in a multidisciplinary team before a treatment plan was formulized. This team comprised of gastroenterologists, radiologists, and surgeons. Patients who had a failed ERCP or were not candidates for ERCP underwent surgical exploration. For classification of biliary injuries, we utilized Strasberg's classification [12]. Various biliary injuries (bile duct injuries) based on Strasberg's classification have been described as follows.

A: leak from cystic duct or an accessory duct.

B: occlusion of an accessory duct with no continuity with common bile duct.

C: leak from bile duct with no continuity with common bile duct.

D: lateral and partial injuries to main bile ducts without complete loss of continuity.

E1: complete section of common bile duct; CHD stump > 2 cm.

E2: complete section of common bile duct; CHD stump < 2 cm.

E3: no CHD available, but right and left hepatic duct confluence intact.

E4: loss of confluence with no communication between right and left hepatic ducts.

E5: aberrant right sectoral duct involved alone or in combination with CHD stricture.

For grading of complications Clavien-Dindo grading system was used [13].

We generally used right subcostal incision but, in case a patient was operated on before, scar of previous surgery was used. Roux-en-Y hepaticojejunostomy was performed in all patients and a single drain was placed near anastomosis. After operation, patients were kept in surgical step down for one day before being shifted to the ward. Broad spectrum antibiotics were administered in the postoperative period given the previous history of biliary peritonitis or obstructive jaundice.

For the purpose of this study, patients were divided into two groups, that is, Group 1 IBDI and Group 2 IBDI with vascular injury. The two groups were compared for variables including demographics, predominant symptoms, past history of surgeries, and endoscopic intervention. Operative variables including type of biliary injury, associated vascular injuries, and type of repair were also compared. Outcome was assessed on basis of 90-day morbidity and mortality. Categorical variables were assessed using chi square and Fischer's test while t-test was used for interval variables. SPPS version 20 was used for statistical analysis. The study was performed in accordance with declaration of Helsinki. It was a noninterventional study and no potential identifiers were present. Hospital ethics committee granted exemption from formal review of this study (IRB number 582-030-2016).

3. Results

A total of 39 patients underwent surgical management of IBDI. Median age of our cohort was 39 (20–80) years. Male-to-female ratio was 1:5.5. Median time to cholecystectomy and presentation was 72 (3–920) days in patients with associated vascular injury and 312 (5–5436) days in patients without vascular injury and was not significantly different (P = 0.5). There were 9 (23%) patients with concomitant vascular injuries. No difference was observed between Groups 1 and 2 with respect to gender, presenting symptom, surgical access, and radiological interventions as shown in Table 1.

3.1. Operative Details. Table 2 demonstrates types of vascular and biliary injuries in our patients. Based on Strasberg's classification of biliary injuries, 27 (69.2%) patients had E3 and E4 injuries. All patients underwent Roux-en-Y hepaticojejunostomy. There were 9 (23%) patients with 10 (25.6%) vascular injuries. All patients except 1 had injury to right vascular structures. In this patient left portal vein was also injured and thrombosed along with right hepatic artery. She was managed with hepaticojejunostomy and PTFE graft from main portal vein to left portal vein. Only one patient underwent right hepatectomy due to combined arterial and portal venous injury. Other patients with vascular injuries were managed with HJ alone. A right hepatectomy was performed in three patients. Out of these, two had a right hepatic duct stricture associated with right lobe atrophy and one patient had combined right arterial and portal venous injury with resultant liver infarction.

3.2. Outcome. Mean follow up time was 8 ± 8.3 months and ranged between 3 to 34 months. Mean hospital stay was

Table 1: Patient characteristics.

		IBDI with vascular injury $N = 9$		IBDI $N = 30$		P value
		Number	Percent	Number	Percent	
Gender	Male	1	11.1	5	16.6	1.0
	Female	8	88.9	25	83.4	
Presenting symptom	Abdominal pain	5	55.5	14	46.6	0.4
	Bile in drain	1	11.1	1	3.4	
	Jaundice	3	33.4	15	50	
Cholecystectomy	Laparoscopic	2	22.2	9	30	1.0
	Open	7	77.8	21	70	
Radiological intervention	ERCP	6	66.7	23	76.6	0.2
	PTC	1	11.1	0	0	

Table 2: Biliary and vascular injuries.

		Number	Percent
Type of injury	C	2	5.2
	D	3	7.7
	E1	1	2.5
	E2	6	15.4
	E3	20	51.3
	E4	7	17.9
Type of vascular injury	Right PV ligated	1	2.6
	Left portal vein thrombosis	1	2.6
	Right PV thrombosis	1	2.6
	Right hepatic artery clipped	3	7.8
	Right hepatic artery ligated	4	10.2

Table 3: Outcome based on 90-day morbidity.

			Number	Percent
Morbidity	Grade II	Wound infection	7	17.9
	Grade III A	Pleural effusion	2	5.2
	Grade IV	Sepsis	1	2.6

6.1 ± 2.1 days. Overall 90 day morbidity was 10 (25.7%) and there were only 3 (7.6%) grade III and above complications as shown in Table 3. There was no mortality.

3.3. Comparison of Surgical Details. Out of 39 patients, who suffered an IBDI, 11 (28.2%) had previous history of laparoscopic cholecystectomy. In only 4 (10.2%) patients, a biliary injury was recognized intraoperatively. Around half of all patients (51.3%) were explored at least once for surgical repair of biliary injury before they were referred to us. Out of these 11 patients underwent a hepaticojejunostomy, that is, 9 at the first surgery and 2 in the second exploration. Table 4 represents various surgical variables compared between the two groups. E2 injuries were associated with a high frequency of vascular injuries (66% versus 15.1%) ($P = 0.01$). The number of patients who developed postoperative complications was not significantly different between the two groups. All patients who underwent hepatectomy had an underlying vascular injury ($P = 0.009$).

4. Discussion

Vascular injuries are frequently associated with biliary injuries after cholecystectomy. Although majority of them can be managed expectantly, some require major surgical intervention. Roux-en-Y hepaticojejunostomy represents an excellent surgical technique even in patients with previous failed attempts at bile duct repair. Limitations of the current study include its retrospective design, potentially missed preoperative and postoperative variables, and relatively short follow-up. In addition a multivariate analysis of independent prognostic factors could not be performed due to low numbers of observed complications.

We classified biliary injuries based on Strasberg's classification which is a well renowned classification system [12]. A number of other classifications exist in the literature [14–16]. Complex anatomy of portal region, frequent variations in anatomy, multitude of injury mechanisms, and diagnostic and treatment modalities available have produced a spectrum of biliary injuries that cannot be fully explained by any single classification.

Certain variations in biliary anatomy predispose to iatrogenic injuries after cholecystectomy. Anatomical variations in biliary anatomy might be seen in as high as 20% patients undergoing cholecystectomy [17, 18]. Cystic artery and duct anomalies are the most frequent and might be seen in up to 15% patients. Cystic duct opens at variable levels on bile duct. A short cystic duct makes its identification difficult and also predisposes to clip slippage whereas a long cystic duct might be confused with CBD. A short cystic artery risks damage to right hepatic artery. Among variations in hepatic arterial anatomy, Moynihan's hump is one of the most significant and predisposes to uncontrollable bleeding, misidentification with clipping, and stricture formation. Development of CVS is very important to minimize risk of IBDI. This involves dissection of Calot's triangle from all fatty tissue, mobilization of lowest part of gall bladder, and unambiguous identification of cystic duct and artery entering gall bladder [10].

TABLE 4: Comparison between patients IBDI with and without vascular injury.

		IBDI with vascular injury $N = 9$		IBDI $N = 30$		P value
		Number	Percent	Number	Percent	
Previous surgical attempts	Yes	3	33.4	18	60	0.2
	No	6	66.6	12	40	
IBDI recognized intraoperatively	Yes	1	11.1	4	13.4	1.0
	No	8	88.9	26	86.6	
Type of previous surgery	Drain placement	1	11.1	10	33.3	0.5
	Hepaticojejunostomy	2	22.2	7	23.4	
Number of surgical attempts	1	2	22.2	8	26.8	0.5
	2	1	11.1	10	33.3	
Vasculobiliary injury association	E2	4	44.5	2	6.7	0.01
	Others	5	55.5	28	93.3	
Final surgery	Hepaticojejunostomy	7	77.7	21	70	0.6
	Redo HJ	2	22.3	9	30	
Hepatectomy	Yes	3	33.3	0	0	0.009
	No	6	66.7	30	100	
Complications	No	8	88.9	23	76.6	0.6
	Yes	1	11.1	7	23.4	

The true incidence of concomitant vascular injuries with IBDI is not well known but can range between 12 and 61% [3, 19, 20]. This variation primarily is representative of differences in patient groups included in these studies. There were 9 (23%) patients with 10 (25.6%) vascular injuries in the current study. Although majority of patients were managed expectantly in terms of their vascular injury, two patients required an additional surgical procedure including hepatectomy and PTFE graft reconstruction. We advocate routine use of dynamic liver CT to properly identify vascular injuries and assess liver status before a surgical attempt is finalized. We found a statistically significant association between vascular injury and E2 injuries. It has been shown that majority of vascular injuries that occur alongside biliary injury are E1/E2. That is because the RHA usually skirts around the common hepatic duct at this level. However, at the time of final intervention many injuries have progressed to E3/E4 levels depending upon exact level of biliary ischemia [21, 22]. That probably is why E3/E4 injuries were more frequent in the current study. Impact of vascular injury on outcome is also a matter of debate with studies reporting conflicting results [23–29]. With this ambiguity it is difficult for a new HPB center in its learning curve to ascertain whether to embark upon bile duct repairs with vascular injuries or refer these cases to more experienced centers. In the current study, there was no difference in postoperative complication rate between patients with and without concomitant vascular injuries. A postop complication rate between 20 and 26% and hospital mortality of 3% have been shown with IBDI repairs [7, 8, 30–32]. We had a comparable complication rate, no anastomotic leak/stricture was observed, and the hospital mortality was zero. Several factors might have played a pivotal role in achieving these acceptable results. It has been shown that skills acquired in living donor liver transplant setting could facilitate and ease out complex biliary surgeries [33, 34]. It is possible that, as >20 transplants/year, we had achieved effective technical skills in dealing with biliary injuries due to our living donor liver transplant experience. Use of fine sutures like 7/0 and 8/0 prolene and PDS, preservation of microcirculation of bile duct, and making anastomosis under loupe magnification in LDLT allow better understanding of portal anatomy and refinement in surgical technique. A multidisciplinary approach with thorough discussion with interventional gastroenterologists and radiologists allowed better understanding of extent of biliary injury, exact level of injury, and whether vascular structures were involved or not. A dynamic CT scan accurately identified liver status, integrity of hepatic arteries and portal vein, and possibilities of reconstruction in the event where there was a vascular injury. It also helped us in identifying patients who would need a liver resection. Surgeon's experience was a crucial factor as the primary surgeon had more than 10-year experience in dealing with various types of hepatobiliary cases and construction of biliary anastomosis. Follow-up in the current study is relatively short and our results do not reflect upon long term outcomes. An element of follow-up loss in our patients cannot be excluded as they were referred from remote regions of the country and once they resumed their normal life, they did not seek follow-up. Strasberg et al. suggested that patients with an underlying vascular injury who undergo biliary repair within days are more likely to develop anastomotic strictures than patients who are operated on later [11, 35]. Out of 9 patients in Group 2, two had a repair at day 3 and day 4 while the rest were operated on at least after 4 or more weeks.

Combined vasculobiliary injury may lead to slow atrophy of right lobe of liver [36, 37]. Atrophy is more likely to occur with E4 injuries since they disrupt hilar collaterals from the left hepatic artery in case of right hepatic arterial injury [9, 37]. Three patients required right hepatectomy in our series. All had E4 injuries. Underlying arterial injury was present in all of them while one patient had a combined hepatic arterial and portal venous injury.

5. Conclusion

The current study demonstrates acceptable surgical outcomes from a new HPB center in management of complex biliary injuries. Concomitant vascular injuries can be effectively managed during learning curve and an active liver transplant program may help in achieving improved outcomes. Dynamic CT scan should be performed in all patients to correctly assess vascular status. A multidisciplinary approach should be taken and long term follow-up of patients with vasculobiliary injury should be performed to identify late complications and assess quality of life.

Competing Interests

None of the authors have any competing interests.

References

[1] L. Stewart, "Iatrogenic biliary injuries: identification, classification, and management," *Surgical Clinics of North America*, vol. 94, no. 2, pp. 297–310, 2014.

[2] A. Waage and M. Nilsson, "Iatrogenic bile duct injury: a population-based study of 152 776 cholecystectomies in the Swedish Inpatient Registry," *Archives of Surgery*, vol. 141, no. 12, pp. 1207–1213, 2006.

[3] D. J. Deziel, K. W. Millikan, S. G. Economou, A. Doolas, S.-T. Ko, and M. C. Airan, "Complications of laparoscopic cholecystectomy: a national survey of 4,292 hospitals and an analysis of 77,604 cases," *The American Journal of Surgery*, vol. 165, no. 1, pp. 9–14, 1993.

[4] R. Vecchio, B. V. MacFadyen, and S. Latteri, "Laparoscopic cholecystectomy: an analysis on 114,005 cases of United States series," *International Surgery*, vol. 83, no. 3, pp. 215–219, 1998.

[5] K. S. Gurusamy, C. Davidson, C. Gluud, and B. R. Davidson, "Early versus delayed laparoscopic cholecystectomy for people with acute cholecystitis," *The Cochrane Database of Systematic Reviews*, vol. 6, Article ID CD005440, 2013.

[6] J. Pekolj, F. A. Alvarez, M. Palavecino, R. Sánchez Clariá, O. Mazza, and E. de Santibañes, "Intraoperative management and repair of bile duct injuries sustained during 10,123 laparoscopic cholecystectomies in a high-volume referral center," *Journal of the American College of Surgeons*, vol. 216, no. 5, pp. 894–901, 2013.

[7] M. Á. Mercado, B. Franssen, I. Dominguez et al., "Transition from a low- to a high-volume centre for bile duct repair: changes in technique and improved outcome," *HPB*, vol. 13, no. 11, pp. 767–773, 2011.

[8] M. A. Mercado and I. Domínguez, "Classification and management of bile duct injuries," *World Journal of Gastrointestinal Surgery*, vol. 3, no. 4, pp. 43–48, 2011.

[9] P. R. de Reuver, M. A. G. Sprangers, E. A. J. Rauws et al., "Impact of bile duct injury after laparoscopic cholecystectomy on quality of life: a longitudinal study after multidisciplinary treatment," *Endoscopy*, vol. 40, no. 8, pp. 637–643, 2008.

[10] K. T. Buddingh, V. B. Nieuwenhuijs, L. van Buuren, J. B. F. Hulscher, J. S. De Jong, and G. M. Van Dam, "Intraoperative assessment of biliary anatomy for prevention of bile duct injury: a review of current and future patient safety interventions," *Surgical Endoscopy*, vol. 25, no. 8, pp. 2449–2461, 2011.

[11] S. M. Strasberg and W. S. Helton, "An analytical review of vasculobiliary injury in laparoscopic and open cholecystectomy," *HPB*, vol. 13, no. 1, pp. 1–14, 2011.

[12] S. M. Strasberg, M. Hertl, and N. J. Soper, "An analysis of the problem of biliary injury during laparoscopic cholecystectomy," *Journal of the American College of Surgeons*, vol. 180, no. 1, pp. 101–125, 1995.

[13] D. Dindo, N. Demartines, and P.-A. Clavien, "Classification of surgical complications: a new proposal with evaluation in a cohort of 6336 patients and results of a survey," *Annals of Surgery*, vol. 240, no. 2, pp. 205–213, 2004.

[14] H. Bismuth, "Postoperative strictures of the bile ducts," in *The Biliary Tract V*, L. H. Blumgart, Ed., pp. 209–218, Churchill-Livingstone, New York, NY, USA, 1982.

[15] J. E. Healey and P. C. Schroy, "Anatomy of the biliary ducts within the human liver: analysis of the prevailing pattern of branchings and the major variations of the biliary ducts," *Archives of Surgery*, vol. 66, no. 5, pp. 599–616, 1953.

[16] D. Castaing, "Surgical anatomy of the biliary tract," *HPB*, vol. 10, no. 2, pp. 72–76, 2008.

[17] K. A. H. Talpur, A. A. Laghari, S. A. Yousfani, A. M. Malik, A. I. Memon, and S. A. Khan, "Anatomical variations and congenital anomalies of extra hepatic biliary system encountered during laparoscopic cholecystectomy," *Journal of the Pakistan Medical Association*, vol. 60, no. 2, pp. 89–93, 2010.

[18] M. M. Hasan, E. Reza, M. R. Khan, S. Z. Laila, F. Rahman, and M. H. Mamun, "Anatomical and congenital anomalies of extra hepatic biliary system encountered during cholecystectomy," *Mymensingh Medical Journal*, vol. 22, no. 1, pp. 20–26, 2013.

[19] H. Bektas, H. Schrem, M. Winny, and J. Klempnauer, "Surgical treatment and outcome of iatrogenic bile duct lesions after cholecystectomy and the impact of different clinical classification systems," *British Journal of Surgery*, vol. 94, no. 9, pp. 1119–1127, 2007.

[20] A. Alves, O. Farges, J. Nicolet, T. Watrin, A. Sauvanet, and J. Belghiti, "Incidence and consequence of an hepatic artery injury in patients with postcholecystectomy bile duct strictures," *Annals of Surgery*, vol. 238, no. 1, pp. 93–96, 2003.

[21] A. Koffron, M. Ferrario, W. Parsons, A. Nemcek, M. Saker, and M. Abecassis, "Failed primary management of iatrogenic biliary injury: incidence and significance of concomitant hepatic arterial disruption," *Surgery*, vol. 130, no. 4, pp. 722–731, 2001.

[22] A. M. Davidoff, T. N. Pappas, E. A. Murray et al., "Mechanisms of major biliary injury during laparoscopic cholecystectomy," *Annals of Surgery*, vol. 215, no. 3, pp. 196–202, 1992.

[23] L. Stewart, T. N. Robinson, C. M. Lee, K. Liu, K. Whang, and L. W. Way, "Right hepatic artery injury associated with laparoscopic bile duct injury: incidence, mechanism, and consequences," *Journal of Gastrointestinal Surgery*, vol. 8, no. 5, pp. 523–531, 2004.

[24] R. S. Brittain, T. L. Marchioro, G. Hermann, W. R. Waddell, and T. E. Starzl, "Accidental hepatic artery ligation in humans," *The American Journal of Surgery*, vol. 107, no. 6, pp. 822–832, 1964.

[25] J. R. Madariaga, S. F. Dodson, R. Selby, S. Todo, S. Iwatsuki, and T. E. Starzl, "Corrective treatment and anatomic considerations for laparoscopic cholecystectomy injuries," *Journal of the American College of Surgeons*, vol. 179, no. 3, pp. 321–325, 1994.

[26] S. C. Schmidt, J. M. Langrehr, R. E. Hintze, and P. Neuhaus, "Long-term results and risk factors influencing outcome of major bile duct injuries following cholecystectomy," *British Journal of Surgery*, vol. 92, no. 1, pp. 76–82, 2005.

[27] M. A. Silva, C. Coldham, A. D. Mayer, S. R. Bramhall, J. A. C. Buckels, and D. F. Mirza, "Specialist outreach service for on-table repair of iatrogenic bile duct injuries—a new kind of 'travelling surgeon'," *Annals of the Royal College of Surgeons of England*, vol. 90, no. 3, pp. 243–246, 2008.

[28] Ø. Mathisen, O. Søreide, and A. Bergan, "Laparoscopic cholecystectomy: bile duct and vascular injuries: management and outcome," *Scandinavian Journal of Gastroenterology*, vol. 37, no. 4, pp. 476–481, 2002.

[29] G. Tzovaras and C. Dervenis, "Vascular injuries in laparoscopic cholecystectomy: an underestimated problem," *Digestive Surgery*, vol. 23, no. 5-6, pp. 370–374, 2006.

[30] S. C. Schmidt, J. M. Langrehr, U. Settmacher, and P. Neuhaus, "Surgical treatment of bile duct injuries following laparoscopic cholecystectomy. Does the concomitant hepatic arterial injury influence the long-term outcome?" *Zentralblatt fur Chirurgie*, vol. 129, no. 6, pp. 487–492, 2004.

[31] J. Karvonen, R. Gullichsen, S. Laine, P. Salminen, and J. M. Grönroos, "Bile duct injuries during laparoscopic cholecystectomy: primary and long-term results from a single institution," *Surgical Endoscopy and Other Interventional Techniques*, vol. 21, no. 7, pp. 1069–1073, 2007.

[32] S. C. Chan, C. M. Lo, and S. T. Fan, "Simplifying living donor liver transplantation," *Hepatobiliary and Pancreatic Diseases International*, vol. 9, no. 1, pp. 9–14, 2010.

[33] T. T. Cheung, R. T. P. Poon, K. S. H. Chok et al., "Pancreaticoduodenectomy with vascular reconstruction for adenocarcinoma of the pancreas with borderline resectability," *World Journal of Gastroenterology*, vol. 20, no. 46, pp. 17448–17455, 2014.

[34] E. R. Winslow, E. A. Fialkowski, D. C. Linehan, W. G. Hawkins, D. D. Picus, and S. M. Strasberg, "'Sideways': results of repair of biliary injuries using a policy of side-to-side hepaticojejunostomy," *Annals of Surgery*, vol. 249, no. 3, pp. 426–434, 2009.

[35] A. Laurent, A. Sauvanet, O. Farges, T. Watrin, E. Rivkine, and J. Belghiti, "Major hepatectomy for the treatment of complex bile duct injury," *Annals of Surgery*, vol. 248, no. 1, pp. 77–83, 2008.

[36] J.-Q. Yan, C.-H. Peng, J.-Z. Ding et al., "Surgical management in biliary restricture after Roux-en-Y hepaticojejunostomy for bile duct injury," *World Journal of Gastroenterology*, vol. 13, no. 48, pp. 6598–6602, 2007.

[37] E. de Santibañes, M. Palavecino, V. Ardiles, and J. Pekolj, "Bile duct injuries: management of late complications," *Surgical Endoscopy*, vol. 20, no. 11, pp. 1648–1653, 2006.

31

Comparative Protective Effects of N-Acetylcysteine, N-Acetyl Methionine, and N-Acetyl Glucosamine against Paracetamol and Phenacetin Therapeutic Doses–Induced Hepatotoxicity in Rats

Tahia H. Saleem,[1] Nagwa Abo El-Maali,[2] Mohammed H. Hassan,[3] Nahed A. Mohamed,[1] Nashwa A. M. Mostafa,[4] Emaad Abdel-Kahaar,[5,6] and Azza S. Tammam[2]

[1]*Department of Medical Biochemistry, Faculty of Medicine, Assiut University, Assiut, Egypt*
[2]*Department of Chemistry, Faculty of Science, Assiut University, Assiut, Egypt*
[3]*Department of Medical Biochemistry, Faculty of Medicine, South Valley University, Qena, Egypt*
[4]*Department of Histology, Faculty of Medicine, Assiut University, Assiut, Egypt*
[5]*Department of Medical Pharmacology, Faculty of Medicine, South Valley University, Qena, Egypt*
[6]*Institute of Pharmacology of Natural Products & Clinical Pharmacology, Ulm University, Ulm, 89081, Germany*

Correspondence should be addressed to Mohammed H. Hassan; mohammedhosnyhassaan@yahoo.com

Academic Editor: Dirk Uhlmann

Background and Aims. Both paracetamol (PA) and phenacetin (PH) are analgesic and antipyretic agents. Part of phenacetin therapeutic activity is attributed to its metabolism into paracetamol. Paracetamol causes direct hepatic oxidative stress damage. The present study aimed to investigate the possible damaging effects of both PA and PH, when used in therapeutic doses, on rat liver and to compare the antioxidant and hepatoprotective effects of N-acetylcysteine (NAC), N-acetyl-methionine (NAM), and N-acetylglucosamine (NAG) against PA- or PH-induced hepatic damage. *Methods.* 90 male Wistar albino rats (120-140 gm) were undertaken, categorized randomly into 9 groups of 10 rats each, and administered by gavage for 2 weeks with DMSO 1% (controls), PA, PA+NAC, PA+NAM, PA+NAG, PH, PH+NAC, PH+NAM, and PH+NAG. Biochemical assays of malondialdehyde (MDA), nitric oxide (NO), reduced glutathione (GSH), total thiols, and alpha-fetoprotein (AFP) in liver homogenates and serum assays of ALT, AST, 8-hydroxy guanine (8-OH-Gua), and AFP were done. Also histopathological examinations of liver tissues in various groups were done. *Results.* PA and PH cause significant increase in hepatic levels of MDA, NO, and AFP and serum ALT, AST, and 8-OH-Gua levels, with significant decrease in hepatic GSH and total thiols. NAG and NAC significantly improve the PA- and PH-induced hepatic and blood, biochemical, and histopathological disturbances, respectively. *Conclusions.* Both PA and PH induce oxidative stress in rat liver within their therapeutic doses. NAG and NAC in pharmacological doses can antagonize the oxidative damaging effect of both PA and PH.

1. Introduction

Liver is frequently exposed to metabolic insults due to its major role in metabolism and detoxification of endogenous and exogenous compounds including drugs and xenobiotics [1]. Both phenacetin (mostly due to its conversion to paracetamol) and paracetamol are hepatotoxic in animals [2].

Phenacetin was extensively used as an analgesic and fever-reducing agent for many years; however, its use was prohibited in the late 1970s due to its potential to cause renal nephropathy [3]. Phenacetin was replaced by the metabolite paracetamol (acetaminophen) which is nowadays one of the most commonly used antipyretic and analgesic drugs [4], and one of the well-known experimental models of hepatotoxicity [5]. Part of phenacetin therapeutic activity is attributed to its metabolism into paracetamol [6]. Acetaminophen is converted N-acetyl-p-benzoquinone imine (NAPQI) as an intermediate toxic metabolic product via cytochrome P450, which is nullified in the liver via binding to nonprotein sulfhydryl reduced glutathione (GSH) resulting in direct

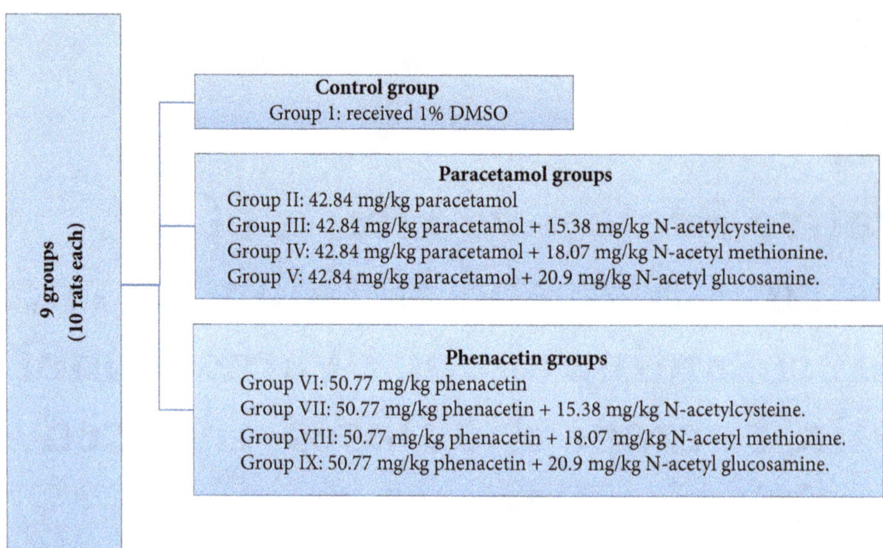

FIGURE 1: Study design: rats were divided randomly into 9 groups of 10 rats each.

hepatic oxidative stress damage due to depletion of the antioxidant capacity (glutathione peroxidase) of the liver [7, 8]. Many studies prove the antioxidant properties of N-acetyl cysteine, N-acetyl methionine, and N-acetyl glucosamine [9–11].

N-acetylcysteine (NAC) is a precursor of the amino acid L-cysteine which is a component of the biologic antioxidant glutathione (GSH). In addition to its indirect antioxidant effect (through incorporation in GSH formation), NAC exhibits also direct antioxidant properties through the interaction of its free thiol group with the electrophilic groups of ROS [12].

N-acetyl-L-methionine (NAM) is capable of replacing the dietary requirements for methionine. Methionine is an essential methyl donor in mammals and acts as an efficient scavenger of several oxidizing molecules. Methionine is also required for synthesis of cysteine which is the limiting amino acid for GSH synthesis [13].

N-acetylglucosamine, an amide of glucosamine and acetic acid, has a beneficial effect in the treatment of joint disorders, e.g., osteoarthritis and rheumatoid arthritis [14]. Previously, it was also reported that NAG has the ability to inhibit the release of superoxide anion from human polymorphonuclear leukocytes. The mechanism of this effect is not fully understood [15].

Several studies have investigated the damaging effects of paracetamol, when used in toxic doses, on the liver or the efficacy of various antioxidants to neutralize such effect, but studies regarding phenacetin could seldom be found. This is the first study aiming to carry out biochemical and histopathological assessments of possible hepatic-oxidative stress induced by paracetamol and phenacetin, when used in therapeutic doses, in male albino rats and also to compare and detect which of the three antioxidants (N-acetylcysteine, N-acetylmethionine, and N-acetylglucosamine) has the best antioxidant and hepatoprotective efficacy against the drug-induced liver injury, if any.

2. Materials and Methods

2.1. Experimental Animals. In this study, 90 male Wister albino rats, obtained from the Animal House of the Faculty of Medicine, Assiut University, Assiut, Egypt, were used. Their body weights ranged from 120 to 140 gm. Rats were housed in cages, kept at room temperature with normal 12h light/12h dark cycle, and treated according to the guidelines of the Animal House of Assiut University, where standard commercial pellets for feeding, water *ad libitum*, and other animal health conditions during the course of the experiment were performed.

2.2. Design of the Experiment. The included rats were divided randomly into 9 groups of 10 rats each. All chemicals were dissolved in 1% dimethyl sulfoxide (DMSO) and rats were treated daily for 15 days. The different groups of the rats and their treatment regimens were illustrated in Figure 1.

(i) All used chemicals were purchased from Sigma Aldrich Chemical Co. (UK). All used reagents were of analytical grade and highest purity. The CAS numbers for PA, PH, NAC, NAM, and NAG were 103-90-2, 62-44-2, 616-91-1, 65-82-7, and 7512-17-6, respectively.

(ii) Calculations of NAC, NAM, and NAG doses were based on theoretical chemistry from previously published work [16]. We calculated the doses of these chemicals according to their molecular weight ratio (1:1), starting with the average of therapeutic dose of paracetamol 3gm/ 24h (in adults) with its maximum dose (4g/ 24h) [4].

2.3. Blood Samples Collection. Rats of the different groups were anesthetized using diethyl ether inhalation and killed by cervical dislocation 24 hours after the last dose. At time of scarifying, the blood samples were collected from the retroorbital veins into plain tubes and were centrifuged at

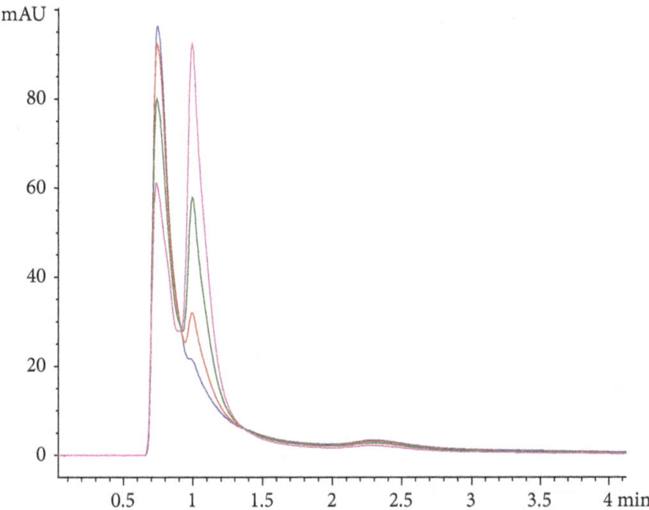

Figure 2: Calibration curves for HPLC assay of 8-OH-Gua at concentrations 1, 5, 15, and 25 mg/L.

4,000 r.p.m for 10 min, and the separated sera were used for alanine transaminase (ALT), aspartate transaminase (AST), alfa fetoprotein (AFP), and 8-hydroxy-guanine (8-OH-Gua) measurements.

2.4. Preparation of Liver Samples. Rats' livers were quickly removed and washed with isotonic saline solution 0.9%, and each one was divided into two parts.

The first part was fixed immediately in 10% neutral buffered formalin for 48 hours at room temperature and then processed to prepare the paraffin sections. Serial sections of 7 μm thickness were cut and subjected to haematoxylin and eosin staining (H&E) to examine the general histological changes of the liver. All these histological techniques were done in Histology Department, Faculty of Medicine, Assiut University, according to Bancroft and Gamble [17].

The second part was frozen in ice bath during scarifying and then washed, and 300 mg of the liver tissue was homogenized in 3 ml (0.1M) phosphate buffer (pH 7.4) to prepare 10% W/V homogenates, using homogenizer (Glas-Col, USA). The homogenates were centrifuged at 6,000 r.p.m for 1 hour at 4°C (MIKRO 220R Germany) and the isolated supernatants were preserved at -20°C for the subsequent biochemical measurements in the form of malondialdehyde (MDA), nitric oxide (NO), reduced GSH, total thiols, and AFP.

2.5. Biochemical Assays. (1) Serum AST and ALT measurements were done, by colorimetric method (UNICO 1200), using commercially available assay kits supplied by Egyptian Company for Biotechnology (S.A.E) with catalog no. 292002 and 291002, respectively.

(2) AFP assays in serum and hepatic tissue homogenates assays were done, using commercially available ELISA assay kits supplied by CHECK, INC (USA) with catalog no. 40-052-115007.

(3) Serum 8-OH-Gua determination was done, using high performance liquid chromatography (HPLC; Agilent Technologies 1200 Series, G1315D DAD): a 20 μl serum was centrifuged at 13,000 rpm for 5 min. After centrifugation, the sample was automatically injected into the HPLC column (Zorbax Extend C18 Analytical 4.6 × 150 mm 5-um). The detector Diode Array Detector (DAD) was at 254 nm. The conditions for the HPLC were as follows: mobile phase: 100.0% (NaOAc 50 mM); pH: 4.6; flow rate: 1.5 ml/min.; column temperature: 35°C. The concentration of 8-OHG was calculated from the obtained standard curve (Figure 2).

(4) MDA, NO, reduced GSH, total thiols, and total proteins measurements in hepatic tissue homogenates were done using chemical methods (SpectraMax Plus, Molecular Devices, USA) according to Wills [18], Paya et al. [19], Beutler [20], Ellman [21], and Lowry et al. [22], respectively.

2.6. Statistical Analysis. Statistical Package for Social Science (SPSS) for Windows, version 5.0 (Graph Pad software, Inc., San Diego, CA, USA) was used. Experimental data were expressed as mean ± standard deviation (SD). The results were analyzed using one way analysis of variance (ANOVA) followed by Newman-Keuls multiple comparison test as a posttest to determine significant differences between means. The level of significance was considered when $p<0.05$.

3. Results

3.1. Biochemical Analysis Results. The mean ± SD values of serum alanine aminotransferase (ALT), aspartate aminotransferase (AST) levels, AFP, and 8-OH-Gua among the studied groups were presented in (Table 1). Phenacetin causes significant increase in the serum levels of ALT and 8-OH-Gua (127.1 U/l ± 24 and 4.643 mg/l ± 1.033, $p<0.001$) more than paracetamol (124.9 U/l ± 38.25 and 3.643± 1.011mg/l, $p<0.01$), when compared with the control group (81.45 U/l ± 37.8 and 2.240 mg/l ± 1.072), respectively. Both PA and PH cause significant increase in the AST serum levels (150.5 U/l ± 50.77 and 150.7 U/l ± 57.52, $p<0.01$) in comparison with the control group (100.2 U/l ± 27.84), with nonsignificant changes

Table 1: Mean ± SD of serum alanine aminotransferase (ALT), aspartate aminotransferase (AST) levels, AFP, and 8-OH-Gua among the studied groups.

Animal groups	N	ALT (U/L)	AST (U/L)	AFP(ng/ml)	8-OH-Gua(mg/l)
Controls	10	81.45 ± 37.8	100.2 ± 27.84	12.23 ± 0.4265	2.240 ± 1.072
Paracetamol groups					
PA	10	124.9 ± 38.25a**	150.5 ± 50.77a**	12.58 ± 0.6175a ns	3.643 ± 1.011a**
PA+NAC	10	73.11 ± 17.08b***	66.93 ± 32.64b***	12.45 ± 0.2716b ns	0.8158 ± 0.3600a*b***
PA+NAM	10	63.34 ± 10.03b***	53.34 ± 14.24b***	12.43 ± 0.4281b ns	1.981 ± 0.3059b**
PA+NAG	10	60.58 ± 12.23b***	55.38 ± 15.22b***	12.50 ± 0.2986b ns	1.097 ± 0.2448b***
Phenacetin groups					
PH	10	127.1 ± 24a***	150.7 ± 57.52a**	12.74 ± 0.6226a ns	4.643 ± 1.033a***
PH+NAC	10	55.46 ± 17.76b***	76.82 ± 26.64b***	12.22 ± 0.3991bns	1.535 ± 0.1212b***
PH+NAM	10	52.85 ± 13.29b***	60.57 ± 7.75b***	12.03 ± 0.6099bns	1.892 ± 0.7727b***
PH+NAG	10	54.46 ± 14.37b***	59.00 ± 14.23b***	12.28 ± 0.2771bns	1.026 ± 0.4326b***

*p<0.05, **p<0.01, ***p<0.001; ns: nonsignificant (p>0.05); a: comparison with control group, b: comparison with the drug only (PA or PH) group. PA: paracetamol; PH: phenacetin; NAC: N-acetyl cysteine; NAM: N-acetyl methionine; NAG: N-acetyl glucosamine; AFP: alpha fetoprotein; 8-OH-Gua: 8-hydroxyguanine.

Table 2: Mean ± SD of liver homogenate levels of oxidants (MDA and NO), antioxidants (GSH and total thiols), and AFP among the studied groups.

Animal groups	N	MDA (nmol/mg tissue protein)	NO (nmol/mg tissue protein)	GSH (nmol/mg tissue protein)	Total thiols (nmol/mg tissue protein)	AFP (nmol/mg tissue protein)
Controls	10	55.78 ± 16.08	549.0 ± 101.1	493.9 ± 98.85	2062 ± 667.5	312.2 ± 38.44
Paracetamol groups						
PA	10	76.20 ± 10.55a**	621.7 ± 51.87a*	354.0 ± 61.68a**	1299 ± 173.9a**	375.9 ± 33.65a*
PA+NAC	10	63.56 ± 9.84b*	566.0 ± 94.18b*	494.4 ± 94.35b**	1542 ± 376.0b ns	282.9 ± 26.32b**
PA+NAM	10	54.13 ± 13.9b**	520.0 ± 124.6b*	449.3 ± 111.9b*	1640 ± 465.4b ns	258.1 ± 65.42b**
PA+NAG	10	55.50 ± 14.48b**	449.4 ± 68.64b**	508.8 ± 87.9b**	1536 ± 369.6b ns	223.9 ± 65.42b***
Phenacetin groups						
PH	10	80.25 ± 10.5a*	776.5 ± 154.3a**	331.3 ± 60.81a*	1215 ± 209.1a**	433.2 ± 20.03a**
PH+NAC	10	58.11 ± 20.13b*	630.1 ± 154.5b*	531.3 ± 179.5b**	1401 ± 167.4b**	300.1 ± 66.74b**
PH+NAM	10	66.33 ± 21.16bns	581.5 ± 161.3b*	450.0 ± 101.8bns	1615 ± 361.3b ns	277.4 ± 75.51b**
PH+NAG	10	53.63 ± 14.98b*	495.4 ± 111.2b**	507.5 ± 77.97b*	1504 ± 428.5b ns	234.7 ± 55.39b***

*p<0.05, **p<0.01, ***p<0.001; ns: nonsignificant (p>0.05); a: comparison with control group, b: comparison with the drug only (PA or PH) group. PA: paracetamol; PH: phenacetin; NAC: N-acetyl cysteine; NAM: N-acetyl methionine; NAG: N-acetyl glucosamine; MDA: malondialdehyde; NO: nitric oxide; GSH: reduced glutathione; AFP: alpha fetoprotein.

in serum levels of AFP (12.58 ng/ml ± 0.6175 and 12.74 ng/ml ±0.6226), when compared with the controls (12.23 ng/ml ± 0.4265, p>0.05), respectively.

Cotreatment of the rats with NAC, NAM, or NAG was associated with a significant decrease in serum levels of ALT, AST, and 8-OH-Gua in the paracetamol (73.11 U/l ± 17.08, 63.34 U/l ± 10.03, and 60.58 U/l ± 12.23; 66.93 U/l ± 32.64, 53.34 U/l ± 14.24, and 55.38 U/l ± 15.22; 0.8158 mg/l ± 0.3600, 1.981 mg/l ± 0.3059, and 1.097 mg/l ± 0.2448) and phenacetin groups (55.46 ± 17.76 U/l, 52.85 U/l ± 13.29, and 54.46 U/l ± 14.37; 76.82 U/l ± 26.64, 60.57 U/l ± 7.75, and 59.00 U/l ± 14.23; 1.535 mg/l ± 0.1212, 1.892 mg/l ± 0.7727, and 1.026 mg/l ± 0.4326), respectively, when compared with drug-only groups. The levels of significance were similar (p<0.001) among paracetamol and phenacetin groups treated with either NAC or NAG but phenacetin-NAM group showed higher significant decrease in the serum 8-OH-Gua levels (p<0.001) than in paracetamol-NAM group (p<0.01).

The mean ± SD values of hepatic homogenate levels of oxidants (MDA and NO), antioxidants (GSH and total thiols), and AFP among the studied groups are shown in (Table 2). Both paracetamol and phenacetin significantly increase the liver homogenate levels of MDA, nmol/mg tissue protein (76.20 ± 10.55 and 80.25 ± 10.5); NO, nmol/mg tissue protein (621.7 ± 51.87 and 776.5 ± 154.3); and AFP, nmol/mg tissue protein (375.9 ± 33.65, and 433.2 ± 20.03) with significant decrease in GSH, nmol/mg tissue protein (354.0 ± 61.68 and 331.3 ± 60.81), and total thiols, nmol/mg tissue protein (1299 ± 173.9 and 1215 ± 209.1), in comparison with the controls (55.78 ± 16.08, 549.0 ± 101.1, 312.2 ± 38.44, 493.9 ± 98.85, and 2062 ± 667.5, respectively).

Regarding the cotreated NAC, NAM, and NAG-paracetamol groups, there was significant reduction in the MDA (63.56 ± 9.84, 54.13 ± 13.9, and 55.50 ± 14.48), NO (566.0 ± 94.18, 520.0 ± 124.6, and 449.4 ± 68.64), and AFP (282.9 ± 26.32, 258.1 ± 65.42, and 223.9 ± 65.42), with significant increase in GSH levels (494.4 ± 94.35, 449.3 ± 111.9, and 508.8 ± 87.90), respectively, when compared with the PA-only group, except for total thiols which showed nonsignificant changes ($p>0.05$). These antioxidant effects were more obvious in NAG-treated group ($p<0.01$ for MDA, NO, and GSH; $p<0.001$ for AFP) than in NAC-PA and NAM-PA groups.

Regarding the cotreated phenacetin groups, the least antioxidant effect was for those received NAM as there were nonsignificant effects on homogenate levels of MDA (66.33 ± 21.16), GSH (450.0 ± 101.8), or total thiols (1615 ± 361.3), but there was significant decrease in both NO (581.5 ± 161.3, $p<0.05$) and AFP (277.4 ± 75.51, $p<0.01$), in comparison to the PH-only group. The best antioxidant effects were for those receiving NAC which cause significant decrease in MDA (58.11 ± 20.13) and NO (630.1 ± 154.5) with $p<0.05$ for both, AFP (300.1 ± 66.74, $p<0.01$), with significant increase in GSH (531.3 ± 179.5) and total thiols (1401 ± 167.4) with $p<0.01$ for both, when compared with the PH-only group. Those treated with NAG revealed significant decrease in MDA (53.63 ± 14.98, $p<0.05$), NO (495.4 ± 111.2, $p<0.01$), and AFP (234.7 ± 55.39, $p<0.001$), with significant increase in GSH (507.5 ± 77.97, $p<0.05$), but nonsignificant effect has been noticed on the total thiols, in comparison to the PH-only group.

3.2. Histopathological Examination Results of the Liver Sections. Histopathological changes in the liver architecture of various study groups have been described in Figures 3 and 4. The overall results showed that both paracetamol and phenacetin cause disturbances in the liver architecture in the form of dilated congested central vein, deeply stained hepatocytic nuclei with vacuolated cytoplasm (more in paracetamol treated group), and cellular infiltrations (more in phenacetin treated group), with improvement of these changes approaching the control architecture in variable degrees among groups receiving antioxidants with the best notable improvement for PA-NAG group as regards paracetamol groups and for PH-NAC group as regards phenacetin groups, which were in line with the biochemical analysis results.

4. Discussion

Drug-induced hepatotoxicity is a frequent event, which is difficult to determine, due to underreporting, incomplete observation of exposure, and difficulties in diagnosis or detection [23]. We choose in our study a rat model because PA-induced hepatic damage in rats resembles human liver damage, at both biochemical and histological levels [24].

Although serum AFP is primarily used as a marker for hepatocellular carcinoma, it can be also regularly elevated in a range of nonneoplastic liver diseases such as acute liver injury with extensive necrosis [25]. AFP was found to be increased in severe acetaminophen-induced liver injury and this increase was associated with a favorable outcome [26]. In the present study, there was nonsignificant change in serum AFP in PA-only group or PH-only group when compared with the controls. This indicates that the drug doses were used within the therapeutic range and did not reach the toxic doses that cause hepatic necrosis with subsequent rise in the AFP serum levels. There was a significant rise in the serum ALT and AST levels in PA-only group and PH-only group versus the control, which confirms that both PA and PH, even when used within the therapeutic doses, still induce acute liver damage and inflammation. On the other hand, the level of AFP in liver homogenate was found to be significantly increased among PA- and PH-only-treated groups with subsequent decrease among other groups cotreated with antioxidants, which indicates the occurrence of PA and PH-induced hepatic inflammation which also was confirmed with the histopathological findings of the liver sections, which was in line with Patil et al. [27] and Abd-Elfatah et al. [28], who both reported increased AFP levels in hepatic inflammation. The hepatoprotective effects of the used drugs (NAC, NAM, and NAG) have been indicated via the associated significant decrease in the serum levels of ALT and AST and the hepatic levels of AFP, which were of more or less equal effects among the cotreated PA and PH groups.

In our experiment, the PA- and PH-induced hepatic oxidative damage was evidenced by the liver histopathological findings and the significant increased hepatic levels of MDA and NO and serum levels of 8-OH-Gua, with significant decreased hepatic GSH and total thiols among PA-only and PH-only treated groups when compared with the controls. These findings were in agreement with many studies [29–33].

Although there is considerable evidence for the safety and efficacy of NAC in management of PA-induced liver injury [34], no previous studies could be traced in literature as regards the comparison between hepatoprotective and antioxidant activity of NAC, NAM, and NAG against PA- and PH-induced liver damage when used in the therapeutic doses, as most if not all researches investigate the role of many herbal products in protecting against PA overdose or toxic doses. The present study revealed that, among the three studied antioxidants, N-acetyl glucosamine has the best hepatoprotective (based on histopathological findings) and antioxidant effect (based on biochemical analysis), in preserving the liver against PA hazardous effect, even better than the well-known NAC. While, for PH-induced liver damage, NAC showed the best antagonizing effects on biochemical and histopathological levels.

In conclusions, the present original study confirms that both PA and PH can induce mild degree of hepatic inflammation and oxidative stress, when used within their therapeutic doses, which was not previously investigated. NAG showed better effect than the well-known NAC, in neutralizing the hepatic oxidative stress induced by PA. PA and PH can be used safely after mixing with the pharmacological dose of NAG and NAC, respectively, and could be trialed as

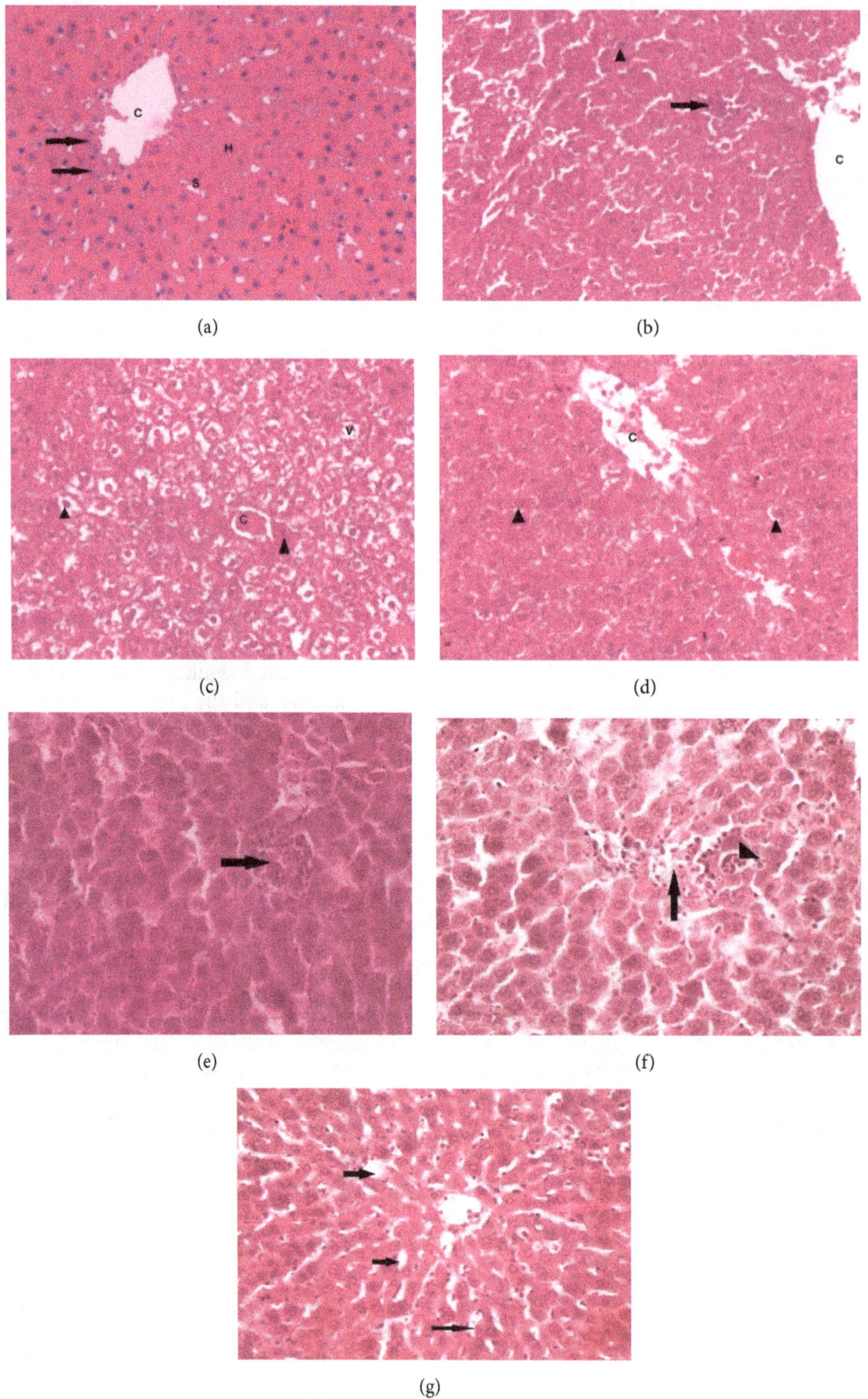

FIGURE 3: **Histological changes in the rats' liver of various paracetamol groups.** (a) Photomicrograph of a section in the liver of ***group I*** showing a normal hepatic structure. The hepatocytes are arranged in the form of plates radiating from the central vein (C). They are polyhedral with acidophilic granular cytoplasm (H). Binucleated cells are common arrows. Hepatic sinusoids appear as narrow spaces between the hepatic plates (S). (b) ***Group II*** showing dilated central vein (C) with areas of cellular infiltration in between the hepatocytes (arrow). Notice the hepatocytes with deeply stained nuclei (arrowhead). (c) ***Group II*** showing congested central vein (C). Notice many hepatocytes with vacuolated cytoplasm (V). (d) ***Group III*** showing decrease in hepatocytes vacuolation but still there are deeply stained nuclei (arrowhead) and dilated congested central veins (C) with exfoliated cells. (e) ***Group IV*** showing minimal cellular vacuolation but there is moderate cellular infiltration (Arrow). (f) ***Group V*** showing moderate cellular infiltration in between hepatocytes (arrow head) and in liver sinusoids (arrow). (g) ***Group V*** showing slight dilatation of blood sinusoids (arrow). H&E x400.

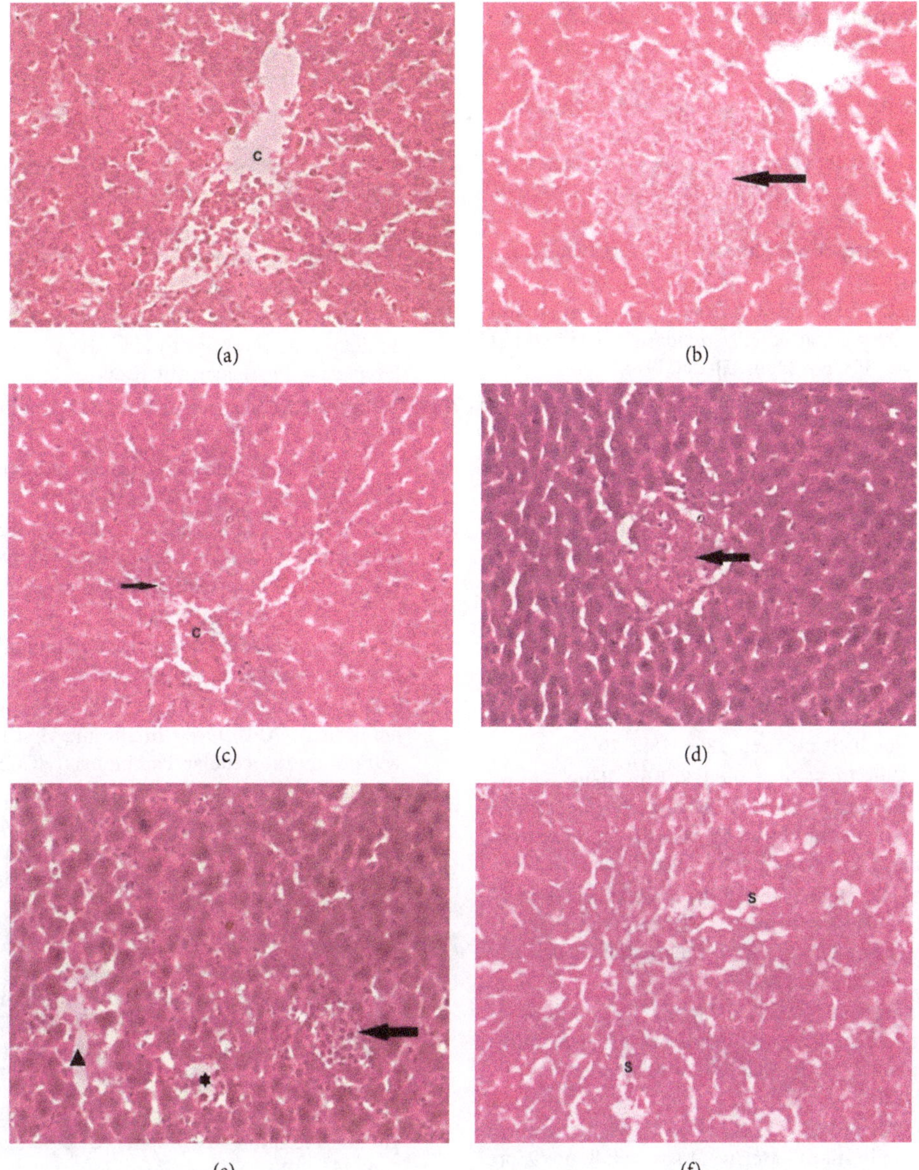

(a) (b) (c) (d) (e) (f)

FIGURE 4: **Histological changes in the rats' liver of various phenacetin groups.** (a) Photomicrograph of a section in the liver of ***group VI*** showing dilated central vein with many cells in the lumen (C). (b) ***Group VI*** showing large irregular area of disturbed liver architecture (arrow). (c) ***Group VII*** showing minimal cellular infiltration (arrow) with dilated congested central veins (C). (d) ***Group VIII*** showing a localized area of disturbed architecture that contains many cells with vacuolated cytoplasm (arrow). (e) ***Group IX*** showing area of cellular infiltration (arrow) and the other area showing degenerated hepatocytes with many spaces (arrow head). Notice the dilated blood sinusoids with some cells in the lumen(∗). (f) ***Group IX*** showing dilated blood sinusoids (S). H&E x400.

targeted therapeutic potential in PA or PH overdose induced hepatotoxicity.

Authors' Contributions

All authors contributed equally to this work and approved the final version of the manuscript.

References

[1] M. Nitin, K. Prasad, D. Shah, and B. Limbani, "Hepatoprotective activity of aqueous extract of Butea monosperma leaf extract in paracetamol induced hepatotoxicity in rats," *Journal of Pharmacy Research*, vol. 5, pp. 1914-1915, 2012.

[2] L. Prescott, "Hepatotoxicity of mild analgesics.," *British Journal of Clinical Pharmacology*, vol. 10, no. S2, pp. 373S–379S, 1980.

[3] F. V. Abbott and M. I. Fraser, "Use and abuse of over-the-counter analgesic agents," *Journal of Psychiatry & Neuroscience*, vol. 23, no. 1, pp. 13–34, 1998.

[4] R. Tittarelli, M. Pellegrini, M. G. Scarpellini, E. Marinelli, and

V. Bruti, "Hepatotoxicity of paracetamol and related fatalities," *European Review for Medical and Pharmacological Sciences*, vol. 21, pp. 95–101, 2017.

[5] M. J. Tuñón, M. Alvarez, J. M. Culebras, and J. González-Gallego, "An overview of animal models for investigating the pathogenesis and therapeutic strategies in acute hepatic failure," *World Journal of Gastroenterology*, vol. 15, no. 25, pp. 3086–3098, 2009.

[6] S. P. Clissold, "Paracetamol and Phenacetin," *Drugs*, vol. 32, no. 4, pp. 46–59, 1986.

[7] W. Nakamura, S. Hosoda, and K. Hayashi, "Purification and properties of rat liver glutathione peroxidase," *Biochimica et Biophysica Acta*, vol. 358, no. 2, pp. 251–261, 1974.

[8] G. B. Concorn, J. R. Mitchell, and Y. N. Vaishnav, "Evidence that acetaminophen and N-hydroxy acetaminophen form a common arylation intermediate, N-acetyl-P-benzoquinone," *Mol Pharmacol*, vol. 18, pp. 536–538, 1980.

[9] Y. Samuni, S. Goldstein, O. M. Dean, and M. Berk, "The chemistry and biological activities of N-acetylcysteine," *Biochimica et Biophysica Acta (BBA) - General Subjects*, vol. 1830, no. 8, pp. 4117–4129, 2013.

[10] Y. Kouno, M. Anraku, K. Yamasaki et al., "N-acetyl-l-methionine is a superior protectant of human serum albumin against photo-oxidation and reactive oxygen species compared to N-acetyl-l-tryptophan," *Biochimica et Biophysica Acta (BBA) - General Subjects*, vol. 1840, no. 9, pp. 2806–2812, 2014.

[11] M. S. Azam, E. J. Kim, H.-S. Yang, and J. K. Kim, "High antioxidant and DNA protection activities of N-acetylglucosamine (GlcNAc) and chitobiose produced by exolytic chitinase from Bacillus cereus EW5," *Springer Plus*, vol. 3, no. 1, pp. 1–11, 2014.

[12] C. Kerksick and D. Willoughby, "The antioxidant role of glutathione and N-acetyl-cysteine supplements and exercise-induced oxidative stress," *Journal of the International Society of Sports Nutrition*, vol. 2, no. 2, pp. 38–44, 2005.

[13] T. Smith, M. S. Ghandour, and P. L. Wood, "Detection of *N*-acetyl methionine in human and murine brain and neuronal and glial derived cell lines," *Journal of Neurochemistry*, vol. 118, no. 2, pp. 187–194, 2011.

[14] J.-K. Chen, C.-R. Shen, and C.-L. Liu, "N-acetylglucosamine: Production and applications," *Marine Drugs*, vol. 8, no. 9, pp. 2493–2516, 2010.

[15] M. Kamel and M. Alnahdi, "Inhibition of superoxide anion release from human polymorphonuclear leukocytes by N-acetyl-galactosamine and N-acetyl-glucosamine," *Clinical Rheumatology*, vol. 11, no. 2, pp. 254–260, 1992.

[16] A. El-Shahawy, N. Abo El-Maali, and H. El-Hawary, "Averting cancer effect of paracetamol and phenacetin by n-acetylcysteine and its analogues," *International Journal of Pharmaceutical Sciences and Research (IJPSR)*, vol. 5, pp. 4159–4169, 2014.

[17] J. D. Bancroft and M. Gamble, *Theory and Practice Histological Techniques*, Elsevier, China: Churchill Livingstone, 2008.

[18] E. D. Wills, "Lipid peroxide formation in microsomes. Relationship of hydroxylation to lipid peroxide formation.," *Biochemical Journal*, vol. 113, no. 2, pp. 333–341, 1969.

[19] D. Paya, V. Maupoil, C. Schott, L. Rochette, and J.-C. Stoclet, "Temporal relationships between levels of circulating NO derivatives, vascular NO production and hyporeactivity to noradrenaline induced by endotoxin in rats," *Cardiovascular Research*, vol. 30, no. 6, pp. 952–959, 1995.

[20] E. Beutler, "Improved method for the determination of blood glutathione," *Journal of Laboratory and Clinical Medicine*, vol. 61, pp. 882–888, 1963.

[21] G. L. Ellman, "Tissue sulfhydryl groups," *Archives of Biochemistry and Biophysics*, vol. 82, no. 1, pp. 70–77, 1959.

[22] O. H. Lowry, N. J. Rosebrough, A. L. Farr, and R. J. Randall, "Protein measurement with the Folin phenol reagent," *The Journal of Biological Chemistry*, vol. 193, no. 1, pp. 265–275, 1951.

[23] D. Singh, W. C. Cho, and G. Upadhyay, "Drug-Induced Liver Toxicity and Prevention by Herbal Antioxidants: An Overview," *Frontiers in Physiology*, vol. 6, 2016.

[24] L. F. Prescott, "New perspectives on acetaminophen," *Drugs*, vol. 63, pp. 51–55, 2003.

[25] K. Taketa, "α-fetoprotein: revaluation in hepatology," *Hepatology*, vol. 12, no. 6, pp. 1420–1432, 1990.

[26] L. E. Schmidt and K. Dalhoff, "Alpha-fetoprotein is a predictor of outcome in acetaminophen-induced liver injury," *Hepatology*, vol. 41, no. 1, pp. 26–31, 2005.

[27] M. Patil, K. A. Sheth, and C. K. Adarsh, "Elevated Alpha Fetoprotein, No Hepatocellular Carcinoma," *Journal of Clinical and Experimental Hepatology*, vol. 3, no. 2, pp. 162–164, 2013.

[28] S. Abd-Elfatah and F. Khalil, "Evaluation of the role of alpha-fetoprotein (AFP) levels in chronic viral hepatitis c patients, without hepatocellular carcinoma (HCC)," *Al-Azhar Assiut Medical Journal (AAMJ)*, vol. 12, pp. 131–154, 2014.

[29] G. G. Kostopanagiotou, A. D. Grypioti, P. Matsota et al., "Acetaminophen-induced liver injury and oxidative stress: Protective effect of propofol," *European Journal of Anaesthesiology*, vol. 26, no. 7, pp. 548–553, 2009.

[30] Y. Cigremis, H. Turel, K. Adiguzel et al., "The effects of acute acetaminophen toxicity on hepatic mRNA expression of SOD, CAT, GSH-Px, and levels of peroxynitrite, nitric oxide, reduced glutathione, and malondialdehyde in rabbit," *Molecular and Cellular Biochemistry*, vol. 323, pp. 31–38, 2009.

[31] C. Saito, C. Zwingmann, and H. Jaeschke, "Novel mechanisms of protection against acetaminophen hepatotoxicity in mice by glutathione and *N*-acetylcysteine," *Hepatology*, vol. 51, no. 1, pp. 246–254, 2010.

[32] E. I. Kandil, W. E. Zahran, A. S. Helmy, and N. H. Ahmed, "Attenuation of Hepatorenal Toxicity Induced By Paracetamol and Gama Irradiation with Coenzyme Q10 Co-Supplementation in Male Albino Rats," *Egy. J. Pure Appl. Sci*, vol. 53, pp. 35–43, 2015.

[33] F.-C. Liu, H.-C. Lee, C.-C. Liao, A. H. Li, and H.-P. Yu, "Tropisetron Protects Against Acetaminophen-Induced Liver Injury via Suppressing Hepatic Oxidative Stress and Modulating the Activation of JNK/ERK MAPK Pathways," *BioMed Research International*, vol. 2016, Article ID 1952947, 9 pages, 2016.

[34] M. F. Chughlay, N. Kramer, M. Werfalli, W. Spearman, M. E. Engel, and K. Cohen, "N-acetylcysteine for non-paracetamol drug-induced liver injury: a systematic review protocol," *Systematic Reviews*, vol. 4, no. 1, 2015.

Permissions

 Every chapter published in this book has been scrutinized by our experts. Their significance has been extensively debated. The topics covered herein carry significant findings which will fuel the growth of the discipline. They may even be implemented as practical applications or may be referred to as a beginning point for another development.

The contributors of this book come from diverse backgrounds, making this book a truly international effort. This book will bring forth new frontiers with its revolutionizing research information and detailed analysis of the nascent developments around the world.

We would like to thank all the contributing authors for lending their expertise to make the book truly unique. They have played a crucial role in the development of this book. Without their invaluable contributions this book wouldn't have been possible. They have made vital efforts to compile up to date information on the varied aspects of this subject to make this book a valuable addition to the collection of many professionals and students.

This book was conceptualized with the vision of imparting up-to-date information and advanced data in this field. To ensure the same, a matchless editorial board was set up. Every individual on the board went through rigorous rounds of assessment to prove their worth. After which they invested a large part of their time researching and compiling the most relevant data for our readers.

The editorial board has been involved in producing this book since its inception. They have spent rigorous hours researching and exploring the diverse topics which have resulted in the successful publishing of this book. They have passed on their knowledge of decades through this book. To expedite this challenging task, the publisher supported the team at every step. A small team of assistant editors was also appointed to further simplify the editing procedure and attain best results for the readers.

Apart from the editorial board, the designing team has also invested a significant amount of their time in understanding the subject and creating the most relevant covers. They scrutinized every image to scout for the most suitable representation of the subject and create an appropriate cover for the book.

The publishing team has been an ardent support to the editorial, designing and production team. Their endless efforts to recruit the best for this project, has resulted in the accomplishment of this book. They are a veteran in the field of academics and their pool of knowledge is as vast as their experience in printing. Their expertise and guidance has proved useful at every step. Their uncompromising quality standards have made this book an exceptional effort. Their encouragement from time to time has been an inspiration for everyone.

The publisher and the editorial board hope that this book will prove to be a valuable piece of knowledge for researchers, students, practitioners and scholars across the globe.

Contributors

Chris R. Kenyon
Sexually Transmitted Infections, HIV/STI Unit, Institute of Tropical Medicine, Nationalestraat 155, 2000 Antwerpen, Belgium

Robert Colebunders
Infectious Diseases, University of Antwerp (UA), HIV/STD Unit, Institute of Tropical Medicine, Nationalestraat 155, 2000 Antwerpen, Belgium

Y. Maor
Department of Gastroenterology and Hepatology, Sheba Medical Center, 52621 Tel-Hashomer, Israel

S.Malnick
Department of Internal Medicine C, Kaplan Medical Center,The Hebrew University of Jerusalem, 76100 Rehovot, Israel

Ran Jin, Andrew Willment, Astrid Kosters
Department of Pediatrics, School of Medicine, Emory University, 2015 Uppergate Drive NE, Atlanta, GA 30322, USA
Children's Healthcare of Atlanta, Atlanta, GA 30329, USA

Miriam B. Vos
Department of Pediatrics, School of Medicine, Emory University, 2015 Uppergate Drive NE, Atlanta, GA 30322, USA

Shivani S. Patel
Medical University of South Carolina, Charleston, SC 29425, USA

Xiaoyan Sun
Department of Statistics, Emory University, Atlanta, GA 30322, USA

Ming Song and Yanci O.Mannery
School of Medicine, University of Louisville, Louisville, KY 40202, USA

Craig McClain
School of Medicine, University of Louisville, Louisville, KY 40202, USA
Robley Rex Louisville VAMC, Louisville, KY 40206, USA

N. Chaudhary, S.Mehrotra, M. Srivastava and S. Nundy
Department of Surgical Gastroenterology and Liver Transplantation, Sir Ganga Ram Hospital, Rajinder Nagar, Room No. 2222, SSR Block, New Delhi 110060, India

Kenichi Harada
Department of Human Pathology, Kanazawa University School of Medicine, Kanazawa 920-8640, Japan

Yasuni Nakanuma
Department of Human Pathology, Kanazawa University School of Medicine, Kanazawa 920-8640, Japan
Department of Pathology, Shizuoka Cancer Center, Shizuoka 411-8777, Japan

Paulette Bioulac-Sage and Brigitte Le Bail
Service d'Anatomie Pathologique, Hôpital Pellegrin, CHU Bordeaux, 33076 Bordeaux, France
U1053 Université Bordeaux 2, 33076 Bordeaux, France

Charles Balabaud
U1053 Université Bordeaux 2, 33076 Bordeaux, France

Jean Frédéric Blanc
U1053 Université Bordeaux 2, 33076 Bordeaux, France
Service d'Hépatologie, Gastro-enterologie, Hôpital St André CHU Bordeaux, 33000 Bordeaux, France

Christine Sempoux
Service d'Anatomie Pathologique, Cliniques Universitaires Saint Luc, Université Catholique de Louvain, 1200 Brussels, Belgium

Laurent Possenti
Service d'Hépatologie, Gastroentero-logie, Hôpital St André CHU Bordeaux, 33000 Bordeaux, France

Nora Frulio, Hervé Laumonier and Hervé Trillaud
Service de Radiologie, Hôpital St André CHU Bordeaux, 33000 Bordeaux, France

Christophe Laurent and Jean Saric
Service de Chirurgie Digestive, Hôpital St André CHU Bordeaux, 33000 Bordeaux, France

Laurence Chiche
Service Hépatobiliare et Pancréatique, Hôpital Haut Lévêque CHU Bordeaux, 33604 Pessac, France

Aftab Ahmed and Ijlal Akbar Ali
Department of Internal Medicine, Oklahoma University Health Sciences Center,Williams Pavilion 1130, Oklahoma City, OK 73104, USA

Hira Ghazal
Dow Medical College, Mission Road, Karachi 74200, Pakistan

Javid Fazili and Salman Nusrat
Section of Digestive Diseases and Nutrition, Oklahoma University Health Sciences Center, Williams Pavilion 1345, 920 SL Young Boule-vard,Oklahoma City, OK 73104, USA

M. Del Ben, L. Polimeni, F. Baratta, S. Bartimoccia, R. Carnevale, L. Loffredo, P. Pignatelli and F. Violi
Department of Internal Medicine and Medical Specialities, Sapienza University, Rome, Italy

F. Angelico
Department of Internal Medicine and Medical Specialities, Sapienza University, Rome, Italy
Department of Public Health and Infectious Disease, Sapienza University, Rome, Italy

Alireza Abdollahi and Elham Zare
Department of Pathology, Imam Hospital Complex, Tehran University of Medical Sciences (TUMS), Tehran, Iran

Sara Sheikhbahaei and Nima Hafezi-Nejad
Department of Pathology, Imam Hospital Complex, Tehran University of Medical Sciences (TUMS), Tehran, Iran
Students' Scienti ic Research Center (SSRC), Tehran University of Medical Sciences (TUMS), Tehran, Iran

Mohamed Ahmed Khedr, Ahmad Mohamed Sira and Magdy Anwar Saber
Department of Pediatric Hepatology, National Liver Institute, Menofiya University, Shebin El-koom, Menofiya 32511, Egypt

Gamal Yousef Raia
Department of Clinical Pathology, National Liver Institute, Menofiya University, Shebin El-koom, Menofiya 32511, Egypt

John P.McGahan, John Webb, Ramit Lamba and Michael T. Corwin
Davis Medical Center, Department of Radiology, University of California, 4860 Y Street, Suite 3100, Sacramento, CA 95817, USA

John Bishop and Lydia Howell
Davis Medical Center, Department of Pathology, University of California, 4400 V Street, Path Building, Sacramento, CA 95817, USA

Natalie Torok
Davis Medical Center, Department of Internal Medicine, University of California, 4150 V Street, Suite 3500, Sacramento, CA 95817, USA

Zahra Hesami and Akbar Vahdati
Department of Biology, Science and Research Branch, Islamic Azad University, Fars, Iran

Akram Jamshidzadeh
Pharmaceutical Sciences Research Center, Shiraz University of Medical Sciences, Shiraz, Iran

Maryam Ayatollahi and Bita Geramizadeh
Transplant Research Center, Shiraz University of Medical Sciences, Shiraz, Iran

Omid Farshad
International Branch, Shiraz University of Medical Sciences, Shiraz, Iran

Yasunori Sato, Kenichi Harada and Motoko Sasaki
Department of Human Pathology, Kanazawa University Graduate School of Medicine, 13-1 Takara-machi, Kanazawa 920-8640, Japan

Yasuni Nakanuma
Department of Human Pathology, Kanazawa University Graduate School of Medicine, 13-1 Takara-machi, Kanazawa 920-8640, Japan
Department of Pathology, Shizuoka Cancer Center, 1007 Shimonagakubo, Nagaizumi-cho, Sunto-gun, Shizuoka 411-8777, Japan

Masayuki Ohtsuka, Hiroaki Shimizu, Hideyuki Yoshitomi, Katsunori Furukawa and Masaru Miyazaki
Department of General Surgery, Graduate School of Medicine, Chiba University, 1-8-1 Inohana, Chuoh-ku, Chiba 260-8670, Japan

Toshio Tsuyuguchi, Yuji Sakai and Osamu Yokosuka
Department of Medicine and Clinical Oncology, Graduate School of Medicine, Chiba University, Chiba 260-8670, Japan

Atsushi Kato, Akemi Tsutsui, Xiang Shan Ren, Kenichi Harada, Yasunori Sato and Motoko Sasaki
Department of Human Pathology, Kanazawa University Graduate School of Medicine, Kanazawa 920-8640, Japan

Yasuni Nakanuma
Department of Human Pathology, Kanazawa University Graduate School of Medicine, Kanazawa 920-8640, Japan
Department of Pathology, Shizuoka Cancer Center, Shizuoka 411-8777, Japan

Cheng Ji
USC Research Center for Liver Disease, Department of Medicine, Keck School of Medicine of USC, University of Southern California, 2011 Zonal Avenue, HMR-101, Los Angeles, CA 90089, USA

Lewis W. Teperman
Division of Transplant Director, Mary Lea Johnson Richards Organ Transplantation Center, New York University Langone Medical Center, Rivergate 3, 403 E 34th Street, New York, NY 10016, USA

Janet M. Wojcicki and Philip Rosenthal
Department of Pediatrics, University of California, San Francisco, CA, USA

David Rehkopf
Department of Medicine, Stanford University, Stanford, CA, USA

Elissa Epel
Department of Psychiatry, University of California, San Francisco, CA, USA

Allison M. Bell, Jamie L.Wagner and Katie E. Barber
Department of Pharmacy Practice, University of Mississippi School of Pharmacy, Jackson, MS 39216, USA

Kayla R. Stover
Department of Pharmacy Practice, University of Mississippi School of Pharmacy, Jackson, MS 39216, USA

Department of Medicine-Infectious Diseases, University of Mississippi Medical Center, Jackson, MS 39216, USA

Yunxia Tang, Qiongshu Li, FanweiMeng, Xingyu Huang, Chan Li, Xin Zhou, Xiaoping Zeng, Yixin He, Jia Liu, Xiang Hu and Tao Li
Shenzhen Beike Cell Engineering Research Institute, Yuanxing Science and Technology Building, Nanshan, Shenzhen 518057, China

Ji-Fan Hu
Stem Cell and Cancer Center, First Hospital, Jilin University, Changchun 130012, China
Stanford University Medical School, Palo Alto Veterans Institute for Research, Palo Alto, CA 94304, USA

Abidullah Khan, Maimoona Ayub and Wazir Mohammad Khan
KTH Peshawar, Peshawar, Pakistan

Subrata Deb
Department of Pharmaceutical Sciences, College of Pharmacy, Larkin University, Miami, FL 33169, USA

Prasanth Puthanveetil and Prashant Sakharkar
Roosevelt University College of Pharmacy, Schaumburg, IL 60173, USA

Antje Bruckbauer, Jheelam Banerjee and Michael B. Zemel
NuSirt Biopharma Inc., 11020 Solway School Rd, Knoxville, TN 37931, USA

Lizhi Fu, Fenfen Li, Qiang Cao, Xin Cui, RuiWu, Hang Shi and Bingzhong Xue
Center for Obesity Reversal, Department of Biology, Georgia State University, 33 Gilmer Street SE, Atlanta, GA 30302, USA

Wasana Ko-iam
Clinical Epidemiology, Faculty of Medicine, Chiang Mai University, Chiang Mai,Thailand
Department of Surgery, Faculty of Medicine, Chiang Mai University, Chiang Mai,Thailand

Trichak Sandhu, Anon Chotirosniramit, Narain Chotirosniramit, Kamtone Chandacham, Tidarat Jirapongcharoenlap and Sunhawit Junrungsee
Department of Surgery, Faculty of Medicine, Chiang Mai University, Chiang Mai,Thailand

Sahattaya Paiboonworachat
Department of Anesthesiology, Faculty of Medicine, Chiang Mai University, Chiang Mai,Thailand

Paisal Pongchairerks
Department of Surgery, Bumrungrad International Hospital, Bangkok, Thailand

Gia-Buu Tran, Sao-Mai Dam and Nghia-Thu Tram Le
Institute of Biotechnology and Food Technology, Industrial University of Ho Chi Minh City, 12 Nguyen Van Bao Street,Ward 4, Go Vap District, Ho Chi Minh City, Vietnam

C. D. Gillespie
Department of Medicine, Mater Misericordiae University Hospital, Dublin, Ireland

M. K. O'Reilly, V. O. Chan and C. A. Ridge
Department of Radiology, Mater Misericordiae University Hospital, Dublin, Ireland

G. N. Allen
University College of Dublin School of Medicine,Dublin, Ireland

S. McDermott
Department of Radiology, Massachusetts General Hospital, 55 Fruit St., Boston, MA 02114, USA

Toshihiro Sato, Michitaka Imai, Kazunao Hayashi and Osamu Isokawa
Department of Gastroenterology, Kashiwazaki General Hospital and Medical Center, 2-11-3 Kitahanda, Kashiwazaki, Niigata 9458535, Japan

Tatsuya Nomura and Yoshiaki Tsuchiya
Department of Surgery, Niigata Cancer Center Hospital, Japan

Takashi Kawasaki
Department of Pathology, Niigata Cancer Center Hospital, Japan

Phimpha Paboriboune, Philavanh Sitbounlang, Sengaloun Soundala and Davone Sengmanothong
Centre d'Infectiologie Lao-Christophe Mérieux, Vientiane, Laos

Thomas Vial, François Chassagne, Stéphane Bertani and Eric Deharo
IRD, UPS, UMR 152 PHARMADEV, Université de Toulouse, Toulouse, France

Francois-Xavier Babin and Nicolas Steenkeste
Fondation Mérieux, Lyon, France

Paul Dény
Hôpitaux Universitaires Paris Seine Saint Denis, Université Paris 13, Sorbonne Paris Cité, Paris, France
INSERM U1052, CNRS UMR 5286, Cancer Research Center of Lyon, Lyon, France

Pascal Pineau
Institut Pasteur, Organisation Nucléaire et Oncogenèse, Paris, France

Pajaree Sriuttha, Buntitabhon Sirichanchuen and Unchalee Permsuwan
Faculty of Pharmacy, Chiang Mai University, Chiang Mai,Thailand

Abu Bakar Hafeez Bhatti, Faisal Saud Dar, Haseeb Zia and Nusrat Yar Khan
Department of HPB and Liver Transplantation, Shifa International Hospital, Islamabad 44000, Pakistan

Muhammad Salman Rafique
Department of Radiology, Shifa International Hospital, Islamabad 44000, Pakistan

Mohammad Salih and Najmul Hassan Shah
Department of Hepatology, Shifa International Hospital, Islamabad 44000, Pakistan

Tahia H. Saleem and Nagwa Nahed A.Mohamed
Department of Medical Biochemistry, Faculty of Medicine, Assiut University, Assiut, Egypt

Abo El-Maali and Azza S. Tammam
Department of Chemistry, Faculty of Science, Assiut University, Assiut, Egypt

Mohammed H. Hassan
Department of Medical Biochemistry, Faculty of Medicine, South Valley University, Qena, Egypt

Nashwa A. M. Mostafa
Department of Histology, Faculty of Medicine, Assiut University, Assiut, Egypt

Emaad Abdel-Kahaar
Department of Medical Pharmacology, Faculty of Medicine, South Valley University, Qena, Egypt
Institute of Pharmacology of Natural Products and Clinical Pharmacology, Ulm University, Ulm, 89081, Germany

Index

www.ingramcontent.com/pod-product-compliance
Lightning Source LLC
Chambersburg PA
CBHW080455200326
41458CB00012B/3973
* 9 7 8 1 6 3 2 4 1 6 3 6 0 *